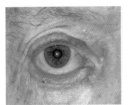

ECTROPION

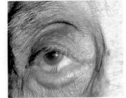

ENTROPION

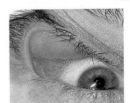

FLOPPY LID SYNDROME

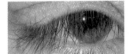

TRICHIASIS

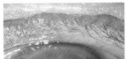

ANTERIOR SEBORRHEIC
BLEPHARITIS

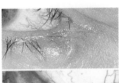

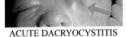

ACUTE DACRYOCYSTITIS

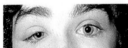

POSTERIOR BLEPHARITIS

BASAL CELL CARCINOMAS

PRESEPTAL CELLULITIS

THYROID EXOPHTHALMOS

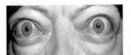

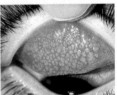

ORBITAL CELLULITIS

OCULAR ALLERGY or
VIRAL CONJUNCTIVITIS.

CONJUNCTIVAL PAPILLARY
HYPERTROPHY

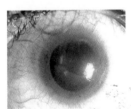

LIMBAL VERNAL
ALLERGY

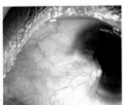

PTERYGIUM

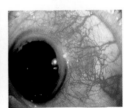

EPISCLERITIS

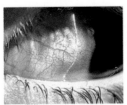

NODULAR SCLERITIS

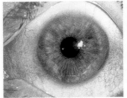

DRY EYES - ROSE BENGAL

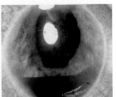

HYPHEMA

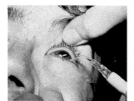

IRRIGATION TECHNIQUE

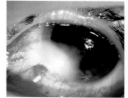

MODERATE CHEMICAL BURN

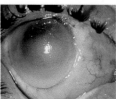

SEVERE CHEMICAL BURN

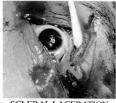

SCLERAL LACERATION

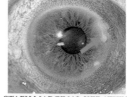

STAPH MARGINAL KERATITIS

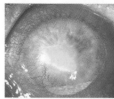

BACT. HYPOPYON ULCER

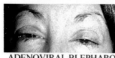

ADENOVIRAL BLEPHARO-
CONJUNCITIVITS

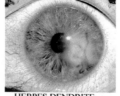

HERPES DENDRITE
& DISCIFORM EDEMA

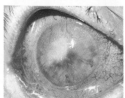

VIRAL INTERSTITIAL
KERATITIS

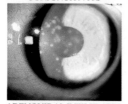

ADENOVIRAL INFILTRATES

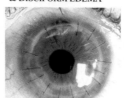

CORNEAL TRANSPLANT

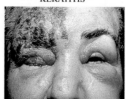

ACUTE ZOSTER

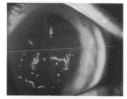

ZOSTER DENDRITES

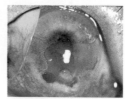

TROPHIC ULCER & T-SCL

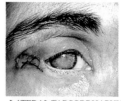

LATERAL TARSORRHAPHY

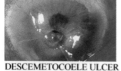

DESCEMETOCOELE ULCER

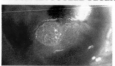

GLUED ULCER

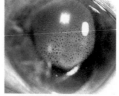

IRITIS - KERATIC
PRECIPITATES

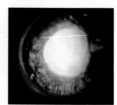

IRIS ATROPHY -
TRANSILLUMINATION

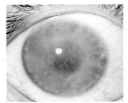
MACULAR DYSTROPY

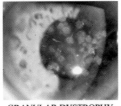
GRANULAR DYSTROPHY

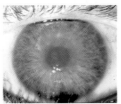
FUCH'S DYSTROPHY - EDEMA

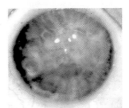
BULLOUS KERATOPATHY

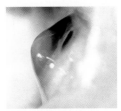
KERATOCONUS

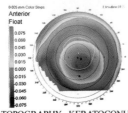
TOPOGRAPHY - KERATOCONUS

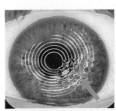
KERATOSCOPY: FOCAL
IRREGULAR ASTIGMATISM

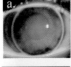
HCL FIT: a. GOOD. b. TOO FLAT.
c. TOO ASTIGMATIC. d. TOO STEEP.

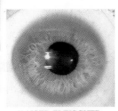
KAISER-FLEISCHER
COPPER RING

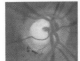
ASYMMETRIC CUPPING

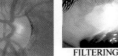
FILTERING BLEB

ANTERIOR CHAMBER:
a. SHALLOW. b. DEEP

GONIOSCOPY: OPEN ANGLE

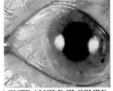
ACUTE ANGLE CLOSURE
GLAUCOMA

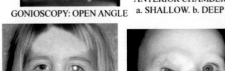
WHITE PUPIL SIGN

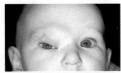
HEMANGIOMA UPPER LID

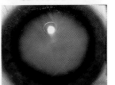
NUCLEAR CATARACT

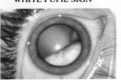
RETINOBLASTOMA

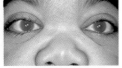
HURLER'S SYNDROME

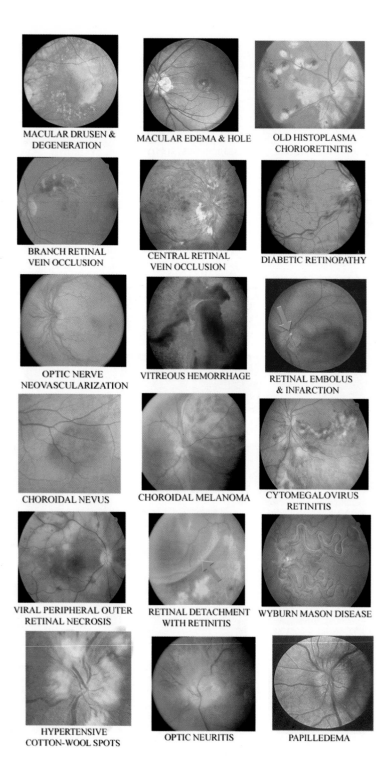

MACULAR DRUSEN &
DEGENERATION

MACULAR EDEMA & HOLE

OLD HISTOPLASMA
CHORIORETINITIS

BRANCH RETINAL
VEIN OCCLUSION

CENTRAL RETINAL
VEIN OCCLUSION

DIABETIC RETINOPATHY

OPTIC NERVE
NEOVASCULARIZATION

VITREOUS HEMORRHAGE

RETINAL EMBOLUS
& INFARCTION

CHOROIDAL NEVUS

CHOROIDAL MELANOMA

CYTOMEGALOVIRUS
RETINITIS

VIRAL PERIPHERAL OUTER
RETINAL NECROSIS

RETINAL DETACHMENT
WITH RETINITIS

WYBURN MASON DISEASE

HYPERTENSIVE
COTTON-WOOL SPOTS

OPTIC NEURITIS

PAPILLEDEMA

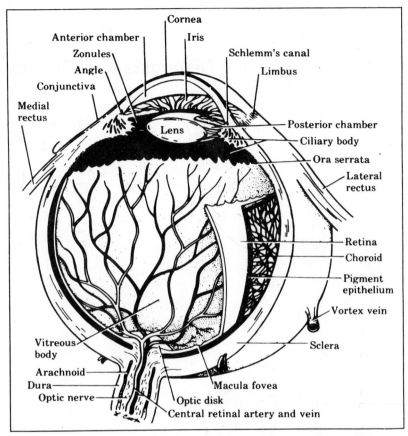

The internal structures of the human eye. (Adapted from the original drawing by Paul Peck. *Anatomy of the Eye*. Courtesy of Lederle Laboratories, Pearl River, N.Y.)

Manual of Ocular Diagnosis and Therapy

Fifth Edition

Manual of Ocular Diagnosis and Therapy

Fifth Edition

Editor

Deborah Pavan-Langston, M.D., FACS

Associate Professor of Ophthalmology
Harvard Medical School
Surgeon, Director of Clinical Virology
Massachusetts Eye and Ear Infirmary
Clinical Research Consultant
Schepens Eye Research Institute
Boston, Massachusetts

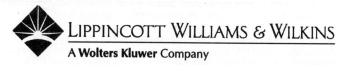

LIPPINCOTT WILLIAMS & WILKINS
A **Wolters Kluwer** Company
Philadelphia • Baltimore • New York • London
Buenos Aires • Hong Kong • Sydney • Tokyo

Acquisitions Editor: *Jonathan Pine*
Developmental Editor: *Kerry Barrett*
Production Editor: *Thomas Boyce*
Manufacturing Manager: *Benjamin Rivera*
Cover Designer: *Deborah Pavan-Langston*
Compositor: *TechBooks*
Printer: *Vicks Lithograph*

© 2002 by LIPPINCOTT WILLIAMS & WILKINS
530 Walnut Street
Philadelphia, PA 19106 USA
LWW.com

Printed in the USA
Previous editions: 1995, 1991, 1985, 1980

Library of Congress Cataloging-in-Publication Data

ISBN 0-7817-3298-0

Care has been taken to confirm the accuracy of the information presented and to
describe generally accepted practices. However, the authors, editor, and publisher
are not responsible for errors or omissions or for any consequences from application
of the information in this book and make no warranty, expressed or implied, with
respect to the currency, completeness, or accuracy of the contents of the publication.
Application of this information in a particular situation remains the professional
responsibility of the practitioner.

The authors, editor, and publisher have exerted every effort to ensure that drug
selection and dosage set forth in this text are in accordance with current
recommendations and practice at the time of publication. However, in view of
ongoing research, changes in government regulations, and the constant flow of
information relating to drug therapy and drug reactions, the reader is urged to check
the package insert for each drug for any change in indications and dosage and for
added warnings and precautions. This is particularly important when the
recommended agent is a new or infrequently employed drug.

Some drugs and medical devices presented in this publication have Food and Drug
Administration (FDA) clearance for limited use in restricted research settings. It is
the responsibility of the health care provider to ascertain the FDA status of each
drug or device planned for use in their clinical practice.

10 9 8 7 6 5 4 3 2 1

CONTENTS

CONTRIBUTING AUTHORS

Dimitri T. Azar, M.D.
*Associate Professor of Ophthalmology,
Harvard Medical School;
Associate Surgeon, Director, Cornea
and Refractive Surgery, Massachusetts
Eye and Ear Infirmary, Boston,
Massachusetts*

Nathalie Azar, M.D.
*Instructor in Ophthalmology,
Harvard Medical School; Director,
Pediatric Ophthalmology and
Strabismus Service, Assistant in
Ophthalmology, Massachusetts Eye
and Ear Infirmary, Boston,
Massachusetts*

William P. Boger III, M.D.
*Associate in Ophthalmology,
Children's Hospital; Instructor in
Ophthalmology, Harvard Medical
School, Boston, Massachusetts*

Cynthia L. Grosskreutz, M.D., Ph.D.
*Assistant Professor of Ophthalmology,
Co-Director, Glaucoma Service,
Associate Surgeon, Massachusetts Eye
and Ear Infirmary, Boston,
Massachusetts*

Sheri Morneault-Sparks, O.D., Ph.D.
*Instructor in Ophthalmology,
Harvard Medical School;
Adjunct Professor of Optometry,
The New England College of
Optometry; Director, Contact Lens
Service, Massachusetts Eye and Ear
Infirmary, Boston, Massachusetts*

Peter Reed Pavan, M.D.
*Professor and Chairman,
Department of Ophthalmology,
University of South Florida
College of Medicine, Tampa, Florida*

Deborah Pavan-Langston, M.D., FACS
*Associate Professor of Ophthalmology,
Harvard Medical School; Surgeon,
Director of Clinical Virology,
Massachusetts Eye and Ear Infirmary;
Clinical Research Consultant,
Schepens Eye Research Institute,
Boston, Massachusetts*

Victor L. Perez, M.D.
*Cornea and Uveitis Clinical Fellow,
Massachusetts Eye and Ear Infirmary,
Harvard Medical School, Boston,
Massachusetts; Associate Staff,
Cole Eye Institute Cleveland Clinic
Foundation, Cleveland, Ohio*

Robert A. Petersen, M.D.
*Assistant Professor of Ophthalmology,
Harvard Medical School; Senior
Associate in Ophthalmology, Children's
Hospital; Consultant Staff,
Massachusetts Eye and Ear Infirmary,
Boston, Massachusetts*

Peter A.D. Rubin, M.D.
*Associate Professor of Ophthalmology,
Harvard Medical School; Associate
Surgeon, Director, Eye Plastics and
Orbital Surgery, Massachusetts Eye
and Ear Infirmary, Boston,
Massachusetts*

Shirley H. Wray, M.D., Ph.D.
*Professor of Neurology,
Harvard Medical School; Director,
Neurovisual Sciences, Massachusetts
General Hospital, Boston,
Massachusetts*

PREFACE

This fifth edition of the Manual has, in many areas, undergone extensive revision from previous editions—revision promoted by the gratifying advances made in clinical and laboratory diagnosis, high technology, and new approaches in drug development. The object of the original exercise, however, remains unchanged: to publish a highly practical and specific book on ocular diagnosis and therapy that will be of use to the doctor on the "front lines," the one sitting face to face with a patient. This updated book is written for the widest possible audience: practicing eye care specialists, family practitioners, emergency room physicians, internists, neurologists, and pediatricians; that is, seasoned practitioners and house officers in virtually any discipline, as well as medical students first learning about ocular disease. It is for anyone involved in decisions concerning either care of the eyes or what the eyes can tell us about other care needed by the patient.

Each chapter covers the clinical findings of a multitude of ocular problems, diagnostic tests, differential diagnoses, and detailed treatments. The subject matter varies widely and includes the latest information on topics from the simple removal of corneal foreign bodies to new diagnostic techniques, management of hyphema, chemical burns, infections (bacterial, viral, fungal, parasitic), the great variety of glaucomas, cataract extraction and intraocular lenses, pediatric problems, extraocular muscle imbalance, neuroophthalmic disease, and the use of antiinfectives, corticosteroids, immunosuppressives, antiglaucoma drugs, and numerous other therapeutic agents. The updated indications and techniques of refractive surgery, laser therapy for the front and back of the eye, and expanded chapters on retinal and uveal disease are presented in the light of today's knowledge. The ocular findings in systemic disease and an extensive listing of the ocular toxicities of systemic drugs are thoroughly tabulated by disease and drug for easy reference. The straightforward outline form of the text, and the index, drug formulary, drawings, and tables are all designed so that information can be rapidly located and a pertinent review brought quickly to hand.

The contributing authors were selected primarily for their skills as practicing physicians or surgeons with widely acknowledged expertise in the area covered. Eight are currently the directors of their specialized clinical divisions. All are knowledgeable in clinical and laboratory research as well and are, therefore, up to date on new developments in the field. I am indebted to these fine physicians for their contributions to this book.

For the first time in the history of this manual, color plates have been included. Eighty-one full-color clinical photographs were contributed from the private collections of the authors. These labeled figures progress anatomically from the external ocular tissues to the anterior ocular segment and on to the back of the eye.

Kerry Barrett, Jonathan Pine, and Thomas Boyce of Lippincott Williams & Wilkins have been very encouraging and extremely helpful. For countless hours of copyediting, typing, and retyping with enthusiasm when exasperation was the easier reaction, I thank my long-time assistant, Mary Lou Moar. I also acknowledge the excellent drawings of Laurel Cook and Peter Mallen, and I am most indebted to Mrs. Georgiana Stevens for her generous support, and to my daughter, Wyndy, for her thoughtful advice. Without the help of all these people and countless others too numerous to mention by name, this book would not exist.

Deborah Pavan-Langston, M.D., FACS

ACKNOWLEDGMENT

Clinical photographs for the color plates were generously contributed from the collections of the following authors: Deborah Pavan-Langston, M.D., Peter Reed Pavan, M.D., Peter Rubin, M.D., Sheri Morneault-Sparks, O.D., Ph.D., William P. Boger, M.D., Shirley H. Wray, M.D., Ph.D., and Claes Dohlman, M.D., Ph.D.

1. OCULAR EXAMINATION TECHNIQUES AND DIAGNOSTIC TESTS

Deborah Pavan-Langston

I. **General principles**
  A. **Physical examination and evaluation of the ocular system** are greatly facilitated by a number of techniques that may be performed in the office, using equipment readily available through any optical or medical supply house. Some of the more complicated techniques, however, must be performed by a specialist in a hospital setting. These techniques are discussed with a view to (a) their indications, (b) how they are performed, so that the referring examiner can explain to a patient what might be expected, and (c) the necessary information to aid the examiner in management of the patient.
  B. **Order of examination.** Examination of the eye and its surrounding tissues with and without special aids may yield valuable information for the diagnosis and treatment of primary ocular disease or disease secondary to systemic problems. So that nothing is overlooked, a systematic routine should be adopted and particular attention given to those factors that brought the patient to testing in the first place. With time and increased experience, an examination that initially may take a somewhat prolonged period of time can be shortened significantly with no loss of accuracy and frequently with increased accuracy of perception. Individual chapters should be referred to for related detail.
  C. **The general order for nonemergency examination** is as follows:
    1. **History.** Present complaints, previous eye disorders, family eye problems, present and past general illnesses, medications, and allergies.
    2. **Visual acuity.** Distant and near without and with glasses, if used, and with pinhole if less than 20/30 is obtained.
    3. **Extraocular muscle function.** Range of action in all fields of gaze, stereopsis testing, and screening for strabismus and diplopia.
    4. **Color vision testing.**
    5. **Anterior segment examination** under some magnification if possible (loupe or slitlamp), with and without fluorescein or rose bengal dyes.
    6. **Intraocular pressures (IOPs).**
    7. **Ophthalmoscopy** of the fundi.
    8. **Visual field testing.**
    9. **Other tests** as indicated by history and prior examination:
      a. Tear film adequacy and drainage.
      b. Corneal sensation.
      c. Transillumination.
      d. Exophthalmometry.
      e. Keratoscopy.
      f. Keratometry.
      g. Gonioscopy.
      h. Corneal topography.
      i. Corneal pachymetry.
      j. Specular microscopy.
      k. Confocal slit-scanning microscopy.
      l. Fluorescein and indocyanine green angiography.
      m. Electroretinography (ERG) and electrooculography (EOG).
      n. Ultrasonography.
      o. Radiology, tomography, magnetic imaging.
      p. Keratocentesis.
      q. Scanning laser retinal nerve fiber analysis.

Procedures **e.** through **o.** are done by specialists in eye care, and referral should be made if such testing is indicated.

II. Routine office examination techniques

A. Visual acuity. Determination of visual acuity is a test of macular function and should be part of any eye examination, regardless of symptomatology or lack thereof.

1. **Distant visual acuity.** Visual acuity is examined one eye at a time, the other eye being occluded. Pressure on the occluded eye should be avoided so that there will be no distortion of the image when that eye is tested subsequently. If the patient normally wears glasses, the test should be made both with and without corrected lenses and recorded as "uncorrected" and "corrected" (sc or cc).

   a. **The chart** most commonly used for distance vision with literate patients is the Snellen chart, which is situated 20 ft (approximately 6 m) away from the patient and diffusely illuminated without glare. At this distance the rays of light from the object in view are almost parallel, and no effort of accommodation (focusing) is necessary for the normal eye to see the subject clearly. The Snellen chart is made up of letters of graduated sizes; the distance at which each size subtends an angle of 5 minutes is indicated along the side of the chart. The farther one is from an object, the smaller the retinal image. By combining the two factors of size and distance, it is possible to determine the minimum visual angle, i.e., the smallest retinal image that can be seen by a given eye. A normal visual system can identify an entire letter subtending an angle of 5 minutes of arc and any components of the letter subtending 1 minute of arc at a distance of 20 ft. Some patients, however, may resolve letters subtending even smaller visual angles. The vision of a normal eye is recorded as 20/20, or 6/6 in metric measurement. If the patient is able to read down only to the 20/30 line, the vision is recorded as 20/30. If the patient is unable to read even the large E at the top, which subtends an arc of 400 degrees, he or she may be moved closer so that the distance measurement is changed. The visual acuity may then be recorded as 10/400, for instance, if the patient is able to read this letter at 10 ft from the chart.

   b. **Pinhole vision** is tested if the patient is unable to read the 20/30 line. A pinhole aperture is placed in front of the eye to ascertain any improvement in acuity. The use of a pinhole will correct for any uncorrected refractive error such as nearsightedness, farsightedness, and astigmatism (regular or irregular from corneal surface abnormalities) without the need for lenses. Through the pinhole a patient with a refractive error should read close to 20/20. If the pinhole fails to improve the patient's visual acuity score, the examiner must suspect another cause for the reduced vision, such macular or optic nerve disease.

   c. **Preschool children** or **patients who are unable to read** should be shown the Illiterate E chart, which is made up entirely of the letter E facing in different directions. Patients are instructed to point their finger in the direction of the bars of the E. Children as young as 3 years of age may be able to cooperate in this testing. Another form of testing is with Allen cards, which are small cards with test pictures printed on each one; at a distance of 20 ft, a visual acuity of 20/30 may be tested. If the patient is unable to identify the pictures at that distance, the distance at which the picture is identified is recorded, e.g., 10/30, 5/30, and so on.

   d. **If a patient is unable to identify any letter** on the chart at any distance, visual acuity is recorded as counting fingers (CF) at whatever distance the patient is able to perform this function, e.g., CF 3. Vision less than CF is recorded as hand motion or light perception (LP). If an eye is unable to perceive light, the examiner should record no light perception rather than the misleading term *blind*.

e. Tests of light projection may demonstrate normal retinal function when vision is extremely poor and the **examiner is unable to see the retina,** as in the presence of mature cataract or severe corneal scarring.

This test is done by covering the other eye completely and holding a light source in four different quadrants in front of the eye in question. The patient is asked to identify the direction from which the light is approaching the eye. A red lens is then held in front of the light and the patient is asked to differentiate the red from the white light. If all answers are correct, the examiner may be reasonably certain that retinal function is normal. It is important to note that normal retinal and macular function may be present despite abnormal LP due to unusually dense anterior segment disease, which prevents light sufficient to give the retina proper stimulation from reaching it.

f. The potential acuity meter (PAM) is a reasonably accurate device for differentiating between visual loss from anterior segment (corneal scarring, cataract) and macular disease. It allows a preoperative prediction for what the potential postoperative vision might be. For example, if the vision is 20/400 by routine testing but 20/40 with PAM, one can, in most cases, assume good macular function and good correction of vision once the anterior segment defect has been corrected. Conversely, if the vision is 20/400 both by regular and PAM testing, one can assume that almost all of the visual loss is due to macular disease and that anterior segment surgery or medical therapy will be to no avail. The PAM attaches easily to a standard slitlamp and projects a Snellen acuity chart into the eye using a 1.5-mm-diameter pinhole aperture. In cases in which the cornea is clear but cataract obstructs vision, the patient is tested at different points on the cornea in an attempt to project through clearer areas in the lens and allow the best possible reading.

g. Macular photostress test. Very early macular dysfunction, whether from spontaneous or toxic degeneration, may be detected by the macular photostress test. The patient looks at a flashlight held 2 cm from the eye for 10 seconds. The time it takes for visual recovery to one line less than the visual acuity determined prior to this test is measured. Normal time is about 55 seconds. Recovery taking longer than this (90 to 180 seconds) indicates macular dysfunction, even though the area may appear anatomically normal.

h. Macular function may be tested in the presence of **opaque media** by gently massaging the globe through closed lids with the lighted end of a small flashlight. If the macula is functioning normally, the patient will usually see a red central area surrounded by retinal blood vessels. If macular function is abnormal, the central area will be dark rather than red and no blood vessels will be seen.

i. Legal blindness. Visual acuity correctable by glasses or contact lenses to 20/200 or less in both eyes, or visual fields in both eyes of less than 10 degrees centrally, constitutes legal blindness in the United States. Its presence requires that the patient be reported to the Commission for the Blind in the patient's home state. Report forms are short and readily available from the Commission.

2. Close visual acuity is usually measured using a multipurpose reading card such as the Rosenbaum Pocket Vision Screener or the Lebensohn chart. The patient holds the chart approximately 35 cm from the eye and, reading separately with each eye with and without glasses, reads the smallest print he or she is able to identify. This may then be recorded directly from the chart as 20/30, 20/25, or as Jaeger equivalents J-1, J-2. In patients older than the late 30s, the examiner should suspect uncorrected presbyopia if the patient is unable to read a normal visual acuity at 35 cm, but is able to read it completely or at least better if the card is held farther away. Abnormally low close vision in an elderly patient without reading glasses is meaningless per se, except for comparative purposes in serial examinations of the severely ill.

B. Extraocular muscle function. The movement of the eyes in all fields of gaze should be examined (see Chapter 12, secs. **I.** and **XI.**).

   1. In the primary position of gaze (i.e., straight ahead) the straightness, or orthophoria, of the eyes may be ascertained by observing the reflection of light on the central corneas. The patient is asked to look directly at a flashlight held 30 cm in front of the eye. Normally, the light reflection is symmetric and central in both corneas. The asymmetric positioning of a light reflex in one eye indicates deviation of that eye. Location of the reflex on the nasal side of the central cornea indicates that the eye is aimed outward, or exotropic; location of the reflex temporal to the central cornea indicates that the eye is deviated inward, or esotropic. Each millimeter of deviation is equivalent to 7 degrees or 15 diopters (D) of turn. A paretic or paralyzed extraocular muscle is the cause of such ocular deviation. Vertical deviation may be determined by noting the location of a light reflex above or below the central cornea. In some patients, the light reflex will be slightly inside or outside the central cornea due to a normal difference between the visual axis and the anatomic axis between the central cornea and the fovea. This angle is referred to as the **angle kappa** and is positive if the eye appears to be deviating outward, and negative if the eye appears to be deviating inward. No ocular movement will occur on cover–uncover testing if the apparent deviation is due to angle kappa alone (see Chapter 12, sec. **III.B.**).

   2. Cardinal positions of gaze. The patient is asked to look in the six cardinal positions of gaze, i.e., left, right, up and right, up and left, down and right, and down and left. **Congruity** (parallelism) of gaze between the two eyes should be noted as well as the extent of the excursion. The examiner should check for restriction of gaze in any direction or for double vision in any field of gaze due to restriction of one eye. Occasionally, involuntary movement may occur in normal patients at the extremes of gaze; this movement is referred to as *end-gaze* or *physiologic nystagmus*. **Nystagmus** is a short-excursion, back and forward movement of the eye that may be fine or coarse, slow or rapid. Occasionally, fine rotational nystagmus may also be observed. Except in end-gaze nystagmus, this rotational nystagmus may bear further investigation (see Chapter 12, secs. **XI.** and **XIII.**).

   3. The near point of conversion (NPC) is the point closest to the patient at which both eyes converge on an object as it is brought toward the eyes. This point is normally 50 to 70 mm in front of the eye. The moment one eye begins to deviate outward, the limit of conversion has been reached. An NPC greater than 10 cm is considered abnormal and may result in excessive tiring of the eyes on close work such as reading or sewing.

   4. Stereopsis is tested grossly by having the patient touch the end of one finger to the tip of the examiner's finger coming in horizontally end to end. Past pointing may indicate lack of depth perception in the absence of central nervous system (CNS) disease. More refined testing is done using the Wirt test fly, circle, and animal figures with three-dimensional (3-D) glasses. Stereopsis may be graded from the equivalent of 20/400 (large fly) to 20/20 (nine circle depth perception) using this commercially available test. Simultaneous perception of four red and green lights while wearing glasses with a red lens over one eye (eye sees only red) and a green lens over the other (eye sees only green) indicates a more gross but significant form of fusion. This test is the Worth four-dot test and is also available commercially.

C. Color vision testing

   1. Purpose. Demonstration of adequate color vision is mandatory for certain jobs in a number of states and for obtaining a driver's license. Jobs affected are armed services trainees, transportation workers, and others whose occupations require accurate color perception. Color vision, particularly red perception, may be disturbed in early macular disease, whether toxic or idiopathic degenerative, and in optic nerve, chiasmal, or bilateral occipital lobe disease. Some of the earliest and reversible drug toxicities, such as that from chloroquine and avitaminosis A are detected by repeated color vision testing; regression and progression may also be documented. These tests are designed for:

    a. **Screening defective color vision from normal.**

    b. **Qualitative classification** as to type of defect. Protans and deutans are red-green deficient and are found in 4.0% of all males and 0.4% of all females; tritans and tetartans are very rare and are thus blue-yellow deficient.

    c. **Quantitative analysis** of degree of deficiency: mild, medium, or marked.

  2. Technique. The progressively more subtle and difficult polychromatic plates of Ishihara, Stilling, or Hardy-Rand-Ritter are made up of dots of primary colors printed on a background of similar dots in a confusion of colors or grays. These dots are set in patterns, shapes, numbers, or letters that would be recognized by a normal individual but not perceived by those with color perception defects. Patients are shown a series of plates, the number of correct answers is totaled in various color test areas, and the type and severity of any deficiency are thus defined. The anomaloscopic 100 hue test detects earlier, more subtle changes.

D. Anterior segment examination (see frontispiece)

  1. Magnifying loupes. The external examination of the eye itself is greatly facilitated by the use of a bright light source, such as a flashlight or transilluminator, and a magnifying loupe. Many different kinds of loupes are available, but basically they may be divided into two categories. One form is worn as a spectacle loupe and has magnification ranging from 2× to 5×, with working distances ranging between 20 and 35 cm. These magnifying spectacles may be mounted on the normal prescription glasses if these are worn by the examining physician. The second form of loupe is a headband loupe, which can range in power from 1.75× to 5.25× with working distances ranging between 20 and 50 cm. Loupes are of great help in evaluating not only local tissue changes and location of corneal abrasions and staining, but also in minor surgical procedures and the removal of corneal foreign bodies. Handheld magnifiers do not leave both hands free for other purposes.

  2. Slitlamp biomicroscopy of anterior segment and fundus. Biomicroscopy involves examination of the external ocular structures and the front of the eye to a depth of the anterior vitreous using a specially designed microscope and light source. Slitlamps are most commonly stand-mounted, but for bedside exam, handheld lamps are available. Use of a slitlamp is indicated in any condition in which examination is facilitated and made more accurate by a well-illuminated and highly magnified view of the anterior segment of the eye, e.g., corneal ulcerations, iris tumors, cataract evaluation. Patient and examiner are seated on either side of the slitlamp, the patient placing the chin on a chin rest and the *forehead against a frame* while the examiner views the eye through the microscope. By moving the microscope in and out with a hand control, the examiner can adjust the depth of focus so that the object of interest is brought clearly into view. The general order of examination is to start with the lids and then progress to the conjunctiva, cornea, anterior chamber, iris and pupil, lens, and anterior vitreous. The fundi are seen by use of double ashperic 60, 78, or 90 D lenses handheld before the eye. The examiner shines the slit beam straight through the (usually) dilated pupil to focus on the retina, thus obtaining a stereoscopic but inverted view. This is useful for evaluating macular edema, optic nerve lesions, or other posterior pole lesions. It is less useful for the peripheral retina beyond the equator. Other techniques for views of the deeper vitreous, retina, and optic nerve are described below.

a. **Special dyes** such as fluorescein to detect ulcerations or rose bengal to detect dead and dying cells on the ocular surface may be used. With fluorescein, a cobalt filter is swung into place to delineate clearly the areas of epithelial absence. A white or green light is used for rose bengal staining.
b. **The slitlamp beam** may be widened to a full circle to illuminate the entire front of the eye or narrowed to a tiny slit that will assist the examiner in determining the thickness of various anterior segment structures. The tissue illuminated by the narrow beam is referred to as an *optical section* and represents an optical cut through the various depths of tissue. The cornea and lens under magnification and illuminated by the intense narrow beam of focal light passing from the slitlamp may be seen to be made up of multiple layers of different optical densities. Layers seen in a normal cornea are epithelium, stroma, and endothelium; those in a normal lens are cortex and nucleus. Opacities and other local pathologic processes can be located with great accuracy in the anterior segment using the slitlamp.
c. **The slitlamp beam may also be narrowed to a single fine point of light** that can be focused through the front of the eye to reveal changes in the density of the **aqueous fluid** in the anterior chamber. Such changes are particularly significant in the presence of intraocular inflammation or trauma. Cells or increased protein in the aqueous or cells in the vitreous, invisible with ordinary illumination and magnification, may be seen using the narrow beam of the slitlamp (the Tyndall phenomenon). In a normal person the aqueous humor is clear or optically empty, but with increased protein content, as in intraocular inflammation, the beam is visible and referred to as aqueous flare. Its intensity may be measured by a subjective rating used by the observer, ranging from 0 to 4+ (see Chapter 9, sec. **III.**).
E. **Anterior ocular structures**
   1. **Eyelids and palpebral fissures.** Under good lighting conditions the lashes and eyebrows should be inspected for the presence of inflammation, scaling, or dandruff, and the lashes also for orientation, i.e., being turned in or out, misdirected, missing, or present as more than one row. Focal changes in pigmentation are also important to note. The observer should inspect the general appearance of the lid margins as to color, texture, swelling, position, and motility. Note should be made of signs of inflammation, pouting of the meibomian gland openings, rash, unusual vascularity, or old scars. The normal lid margins should overlie the corneal limbus by 1 to 2 mm above and below with no exposure of sclera. Voluntary lid closure should be complete with no inferior exposure. Involuntary blinking should occur every 3 to 6 seconds with complete closure of the lids. Both upper lids should elevate well on upward gaze and drop on downward gaze. The space between the upper and lower lid margin ranges normally between 9 and 13 mm. This measurement is not so critical as is a disparity in the size of this measurement between the two eyes in a given patient. The lid margins should follow the globe synchronously on downward and upward gaze without evidence of lid lag. The borders should have good anatomic apposition to the globe with the tear puncta (upper and lower punctal openings are located 2 to 4 mm temporal to the medial canthus in contact with the tear film that they drain).
   2. **Lid eversion.** The upper lid may easily be everted for inspection of the palpebral conjunctiva by having the patient look down while the examiner grasps the lashes with one hand, pulling out and down, pressing on the lid with a cotton-tipped applicator stick 1 cm above the edge of the lid margin, i.e., at the superior border of the tarsal plate, and flipping the lid over the stick (Fig. 1.1). In the presence of pain, a topical anesthetic may assist in this part of the examination. To restore the everted upper lid, the examiner simply asks the patient to look up and simultaneously pulls the lashes down gently. The lower palpebral conjunctiva is easily seen by

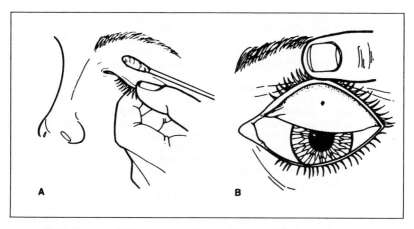

FIG. 1.1. A: Technique of lid eversion. **B:** Foreign body is easily located with the everted lid held against upper orbital rim. An internal cartilaginous tarsal plate holds the lid firm.

pressing down over the bony maxilla to pull the lid down with a finger and asking the patient to look up.

3. **The main lacrimal gland** is situated at the superotemporal quadrant of the orbit. It may be seen as a globulated pink mass under the upper eyelid when the patient is asked to look down and nasally, and traction is placed on the upper outer eyelid. Tears are carried from this gland as well as from the accessory lacrimal glands in the conjunctiva from the superotemporal quadrant of the eye down toward the infranasal area, where tears pass through the lacrimal canaliculi via the puncta and down into the lacrimal sac. From there they enter the nasolacrimal duct opening under the inferior turbinate of the nose. Tears flow down the back of the throat, occasionally giving patients the taste of medication instilled into the conjunctival culde-sac.

4. **The bulbar (eyeball) conjunctiva** is examined by gently separating the lids and asking the patient to look in all directions of gaze—up, down, right, and left. The normal conjunctiva is a thin membrane almost entirely transparent and appearing white, although a few patients may normally have hyperemic (red) eyes due to dilation of the many fine conjunctival vessels running throughout the membrane. In general, the examiner should be able to observe the white sclera through the transparent bulbar conjunctiva without difficulty, although occasionally deposits of pigment may be seen. On either side of the limbus a slightly raised yellow area (pinguecula) may normally be seen and may with age turn slightly yellow, due to benign degeneration of elastic tissue. Benign pigmented nevi may be present; these are flat and often translucent under magnification.

5. **The palpebral conjunctiva** is seen by lid eversion and varies in appearance with age. Above and below the tarsal plate it has many shallow folds; frequently, small bumps that represent follicles or lymphoid tissue formation are present. Follicles are normally absent in infants, prominent in children, and less notable in adults. Over the tarsal plate the conjunctiva is firmly bound to the fibrous plate and normally shows no follicles. The examiner may see faint yellow lines of the meibomian gland running vertically in the tarsal plate through the translucent overlying tissue. **Conjunctival lacerations or abrasions** are easily detected with a drop of sterile fluorescein solution or the application of a sterile fluorescein paper strip to the

tear film. A white light will show the injured area as yellow-green. A cobalt blue light will show the area as bright green.

6. **Deep to the conjunctiva are the episcleral vessels,** which run in a *radial* direction from the cornea. Inflammation in these vessels is indicative of deeper disease than inflammation involving just the conjunctival tissues.

7. **The normal corneal surface** is so smooth that it is analogous to a convex reflecting surface. Any minor disruption in this surface will be readily apparent, particularly under magnification, as a break in a normally perfect light reflex. The size of each cornea should be noted and normally measures 13 mm horizontally and 12 mm vertically in an adult. A flashlight and loupe are extremely useful for examination in the absence of a slitlamp.

   a. **Scars, old and active vessels, and deposits** in the stroma and on the back of the cornea are difficult to see with the unaided eye. **Small foreign bodies** may be missed without illumination and magnification. The application of a sterile **fluorescein or rose bengal dye strip** (wet with sterile saline) to the tear film is extremely important in detecting the presence of abrasions or foreign bodies on the corneal surface. Under white light, an abrasion will stain yellow-green and under cobalt blue light, bright green. Rose bengal stain will stain and outline the defect in red and is easily seen with a white light. A drop of local anesthetic will greatly aid the examination of a patient suffering lid spasm secondary to a corneal lesion.

   b. **Corneal sensitivity (esthesiometry)** should be ascertained prior to the instillation of topical anesthetics, particularly if the examiner is suspicious of herpetic viral disease. To determine corneal sensitivity, the cornea is lightly touched with a **wisp of cotton** drawn out to a few threads while the lids are held apart. The approach should be from the side so that the patient does not see the cotton tip coming toward him or her and reflexively close the eye. One eye should be compared with the other on a 0 to 10 scale and note made of reduced sensitivity. A more accurate measurement of corneal sensitivity may be made with the **Cochet-Bonnet anesthesiometer.** By adjusting the length of a retractable nylon thread, the examiner can measure in units the length at which the thread is first detected by each cornea and compare the readings.

8. **Anterior chamber** (see frontispiece). Detailed examination of the anterior chamber is difficult without the use of a slitlamp biomicroscope, but a good light and the use of the naked eye or a magnifying loupe will allow the examiner to detect chamber depth, clearness or cloudiness of the aqueous fluid, and the presence of blood, either diffuse or settled out in hyphema layering. Hypopyon (the accumulation of pus in the anterior chamber) may also be detected in the inferior anterior chamber.

9. **Iris.** The color of each iris should be noted and differences in color, texture, and pattern recorded. Under magnification the examiner may detect the presence of nevi, abnormal areas of very dark pigmentation, new vessels, atrophy, tears, or surgical openings. Transillumination is useful here, because abnormalities will show up against the red pupillary–iris reflex (see sec. **L.2.,** below).

10. **The pupils** should be inspected for size, shape, and reaction to direct and consensual (in the opposite pupil) light as well as the accommodation reflex. All of these reflexes involve decrease in pupil size on exposure to light or on attempted near focus.

    a. **Normal pupils** are equal in size, although in blue-eyed patients there may be a 0.5-mm difference under normal conditions. The range of normal pupils is 3 to 5 mm in room light. Pupils smaller than 3 mm in diameter are miotic; pupils larger than 7 mm are mydriatic. Pupils may be miotic if the patient is taking certain drugs for glaucoma or is taking heroin. They may be abnormally large in cases of ocular contusion, systemic poisoning, and neurologic disease of the midbrain (see Chapter 13, sec. **III.**).

b. **The pupil is normally** round in shape. In the absence of surgical manipulation, irregularity is almost always pathologic. The shape may be affected by congenital abnormality, scarring down from iritis, syphilis, trauma, or the presence of surgically placed intraocular lenses (IOLs).

c. **The direct light reflex** is tested in a semidark room with a light brought in from the side. The pupil should contract to direct light as well as when light is shined in the pupil of the opposite side; this latter response is the **consensual** reaction to light. Reaction to accommodation is tested by holding a finger approximately 10 cm away from the eye being tested. The patient is asked to look at the finger and then at the far wall directly beyond it. The pupil normally constricts when looking at the near object and dilates when looking at the far object. Under normal conditions, if the pupil reacts to light, it will react to accommodation as well. The Argyll Robertson pupil is a condition due to CNS lues and occasionally to herpes zoster in which there is a failure of direct and consensual light response, but a normal reaction to accommodation. Adie tonic pupil responds to either stimulation, but does so abnormally slowly (see Chapter 13).

11. **The lens** may be observed under magnification for opacity using either a loupe or the plus lenses of an ophthalmoscope. This procedure is more easily done with the pupil dilated so that as much of the lens as possible can be seen. The examiner should also note the central location of the lens and its stability in position (partially dislocated lenses are tremulous) as well as its translucency. Difficulty in viewing the fundus through the lens is indicative of a significant cataract or vitreous opacity. The hazier the view into the eye, the hazier the view out of it for the patient.

F. **IOP measurements for glaucoma or hypotony**

1. **Finger tension.** A rough estimate of IOP may be made by palpation of the eyeball through closed lids. The patient is asked to look down (but not close the eyes) and the examiner places two forefingers on the upper lid over the globe, exerting pressure alternately with each forefinger while the other rests on the globe. Pressure just sufficient to indent the globe slightly should be applied. In the absence of inflammation this is a painless procedure, but it should be avoided if rupture of the globe is suspected. After experience with palpating a number of normal eyeballs, the examiner will learn what normal resistance is and by comparison may determine whether an eyeball is either "too hard or too soft."

2. **Tonometry.** Accurate IOP may be determined by use of tonometers. If the IOP is between 22 and 25 mm Hg or more, ocular hypertension or glaucoma must be considered. Visual field and ophthalmoscopic study of the nerve head should be performed. Tonometry readings may be repeated at different hours of the day to determine diurnal curve (see sec. **II.F.3.**). Pressures greater than 25 mm Hg are generally accepted as representative of ocular hypertension. In the presence of a visual field defect or asymmetric or marked cupping of the optic nerve head, the diagnosis of glaucoma can be definitely established.

a. **Technique of Schiötz tonometry.** After the instillation of local anesthesia, such as one drop of proparacaine or tetracaine, the patient is placed in a supine position and asked to look directly upward, fixing on some object such as his or her extended hand. The physician separates the lids to keep them from contacting the eyeball, taking care not to exert pressure on the globe **(Fig. 1.2A).** The instrument is placed gently in a vertical position directly over the cornea, and the plunger is allowed to exert its full weight. With the instrument held steady the pointer will stay fixed at a single scale, with slight oscillations 0.5 mm in either direction because of alterations in the internal pressure caused by the arterial pulse in the eye. If the reading with the 5.5-g weight is between

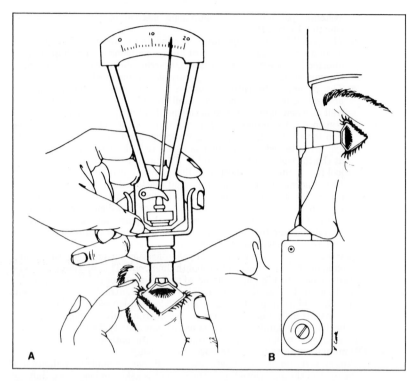

FIG. 1.2. A: Technique of Schiötz tonometry. Digital pressure on the globe is avoided. **B:** Applanation tonometry. The applanation tonometer may be handheld or mounted on a slitlamp biomicroscope. (Adapted from Paton D, Craig J. *Glaucomas: diagnosis and management.* Clinical Symposia. Summit, NJ: Ciba Pharmaceutical Co., 1976.)

3 and 6 on the scale, this reading may be used. Readings below 3 are inaccurate with this instrument, and a 7.5-g weight should be added and the reading taken again. If the reading is still below 3, the 10-g weight should be used. If the patient squeezes his or her lids, this will raise the IOP; note should be made of this, because a falsely high pressure may be recorded. Schiötz tonometry tends to be less accurate in myopic patients or patients with thyroid ocular disease. Applanation tonometry is more accurate in these patients.

    b. **Applanation tonometry.** This very accurate method for measuring IOP may be performed with an applanation tonometer mounted on a routine slitlamp biomicroscope or with a handheld applanation tonometer (Fig. 1.2B). After local anesthesia is induced as with Schiötz tonometry, fluorescein paper strips are inserted into the lower cul-de-sac to place dye in the tear film. The tonometer scale is set at 0 and the head is then brought gently against the anterior corneal surface with the patient looking straight ahead. On contact and with the cobalt blue light in place, two fluorescein semicircles are seen through the microscope, one higher than the other; the top with the outer curve up and the bottom with the outer curve down. The semicircles should be equal in size and in the middle of the field of view. Their steady pulsation indicates that the instrument is in the correct position. Pressure on the eye is increased by turning the calibrated dial of the tonometer until the inner border of each semicircle just touches and overlaps with each pulsation. The pressure reading (in millimeters Hg) is determined directly by reading from the measuring drum. This machine is more accurate than Schiötz tonometry in patients with altered scleral rigidity (myopia, thyroid disease), but appears to be less accurate than the pneumotonometer or tonopen in post-laser-assisted in situ keratomileusis (LASIK) patients. The flow of volumetric displacement of 9.56 nm increases the IOPs by only 2.5%, as compared with the much greater volumetric displacement encountered with Schiötz tonometry.

    c. **The pneumotonometer** is an electronic tonometer that has its greatest use in patients with corneal scarring or altered corneal shape such that conventional Schiötz or applanation tonometers cannot be employed with any accuracy. The soft tip of a blunt pencil-like device connected by wire to an electronic recorder is momentarily touched to the anesthetized cornea. Pressure is calculated by the jump in scale readings from baseline noncontact curve to that of the momentary touch flattening the cornea or indicated directly on a digital screen. The **tonopen** is portable, battery operated, and similar in use to the pneumotonometer.

    d. **The air puff noncontact tonometer** is a reasonably accurate electronic tonometer that has the advantage of use without topical anesthetic. The patient sits with the head in a slitlamp-like device, and a 3-millisecond puff of air (a blink takes 10 milliseconds) is blown against the cornea. The indentation pattern is detected by the tonometer eye. The pressure is calculated by the amount of corneal flattening by the fixed air puff pressure and displayed on digital readout. This machine can be used in mass glaucoma-screening programs.

3. **Tonography** is an electronic Schiötz measurement over 4 minutes to determine the rate of aqueous outflow from the anterior chamber. It is currently used infrequently. A coefficient of outflow factor less than 0 is suspicious of glaucoma.

G. Direct ophthalmoscopy

    1. **Examination of the posterior segment of the eye** (vitreous, optic nerve head or disk, vessels, retina, choroid) is performed with the aid of an ophthalmoscope. A satisfactory examination of the posterior pole can usually be made through an undilated pupil, provided that the media (aqueous, lens, vitreous) are clear. However, a greater extent of the peripheral posterior segment can be examined through a dilated pupil. Ophthalmoscopy is best done in a darkened room.

    2. **For optimum dilated fundus examination,** mydriatic agents in common use are cyclopentolate 0.5% or tropicamide 1%/phenylephrine 2.5%; the latter should be used with caution in any patient with a history of significant cardiovascular disease. No mydriatic agent should be instilled in an eye in which a shallow anterior chamber is suspected. An estimate of the anterior chamber depth can be made by illuminating it from the side with a penlight. **If the iris seems abnormally close to the cornea, dilation is contraindicated because of the risk of inducing acute angle-closure glaucoma** (see Chapter 10, sec. III.). A slitlamp beam depth of less than 3 to 4 corneal thicknesses centrally is also indicative of a possible shallow chamber and is a relative contraindication to dilation.

    3. **Ophthalmoscopes.** There are many forms of ophthalmoscopes, the most commonly used being handheld **direct** ophthalmoscopes designed to provide a direct magnified (14×) view. The source of illumination is projected by means of a mirror or prism coinciding with the observer's line of vision through the aperture.

    4. **Technique of ophthalmoscopy.** The ophthalmoscope is held close to the observer's eye and approximately 15 cm from the patient's eye in the observer's right hand to examine the patient's right eye and in the observer's left hand to examine the patient's left eye. The observer uses his or her right eye for the patient's right eye and his or her left eye for the patient's left eye. The patient should have no glasses on, have chin straight, and be fixating on a distant target with the eye as steady as possible. From time to time the patient may have to be reminded to refixate on a distant target to avoid accommodation from interfering with the observer's level of focus within the eye. The physician may have to adjust the ophthalmoscope power setting to accommodate for the patient's or his or her own refractive error—red-numbered minus lenses are used for nearsighted errors, black-numbered plus lenses are used for farsighted errors. Eyes that have undergone cataract removal but no lens implantation (aphakia) should be examined with a +8 to +12 lens to obtain a view of the fundus. If both patient and examiner have normal eyes and the lens is set at 0, a red reflex will be seen and is considered normal. Moving the ophthalmoscope as close to the patient's eye as possible, the observer uses black or positive lenses. Lens settings of +4 to +8 will focus the ophthalmoscope on the anterior segment to reveal corneal opacities or changes in the iris and lens. The retina in a normal eye will focus at 0, provided that no refractive error is present. By decreasing the power of the lens from positive toward negative, the depth of focus will become greater so that the examiner may move from the anterior segment progressively through structures until the vitreous and retina are reached.

5. **Vitreous opacities** such as hemorrhages and floaters should be localized and noted, and changes in the posterior segment structures focused and studied.

6. **The optic nerve head** should be brought into focus and examined. This structure is generally circular to oval with vertical orientation and pink in color. The temporal side is usually lighter pink than the nasal side. The center of the disk may have some depression, which is referred to as the *physiologic cup*, the bottom of which may be fibrous in appearance and represents the fibers of the lamina cribrosa of the sclera. Normal cupping is round and may vary from absence to 80% involvement of the nerve head. In the presence of extensive, vertically elongated, or asymmetric cupping, glaucoma should be suspected. In optic atrophy the entire nerve head will be pale; in papilledema or papillitis it will be swollen and congested. The size of the normal nerve head may vary with the refractive error of the patient, being small in farsighted patients and large in myopic patients. The border of the nerve head is usually discretely demarcated from the retina, but may merge gradually into the surrounding tissue without any clear-cut edge. A white border representing a scleral ring or crescent is often present and formed by exposure of sclera between the choroidal vasculature and the opening for the optic nerve. There may be excessive choroidal pigment in this area.

7. **Fundus lesions** should be measured using the disk diameter (dd) as a reference size. For example, a retinal scar may be described as being 3 dd in size and located 5 dd nasal to the nerve head at 1 o'clock. Elevation of this lesion may also be measured by noting the difference between lens powers that clearly focus the top of the lesion and an adjacent normal area of the fundus. Elevation of 3 D lens change would be equivalent to approximately 1 mm in actual elevation. Multiples of this may be made according to the size and height of the lesion.

8. **Retinal arteries and veins (AV).** The arteries are red and smaller than the veins in about a 4:5 ratio. Because of a thicker wall, the arteries have a shiny central reflex stripe. The column of blood traversing these vessels may be seen through the transparent walls. Branching is variable. The examiner should evaluate the transparency of the vessels, the presence of pressure effects such as AV compression (nicking) where vessels cross each other, and presence of focal narrowing of arterioles, as well as increased tortuosity and widening of venules, hemorrhages, and exudates around the vessels. Round hemorrhages may occur in patients with diabetes mellitus and are

generally located between the posterior vitreous face and the retina. Flame-shaped hemorrhages are usually intraretinal and are commonly found in patients with high blood pressure and blood dyscrasias.

9. **The macular area** located about 2 dd temporal to the optic nerve head is darker than the surrounding retina and in a young person will have a lustrous central yellow point called the fovea centralis (see frontispiece). This appears as a small area of dark red with a tiny yellow light reflex at the center of the fovea. The foveal reflex dulls with age or certain drug-induced retinal toxicities.

10. **The periphery of the fundus** can be examined by the movement of the ophthalmoscope in various directions as well as by having the patient move the eye in various quadrants horizontally and vertically. Through a dilated pupil, the periphery can be seen directly with a direct ophthalmoscope up to 1.5 mm from the peripheral retinal attachment (ora serrata).

11. **Normal variations of the fundus.** With increased experience, the observer will become acquainted with a wide range of normal variations. Vasculature is particularly variable. Vessels may appear from the temporal half of the nerve head and run to the macular area. These cilioretinal vessels originate from the vascular circle of Zinn behind the nerve head in the sclera and are formed by branches from the short posterior ciliary arteries. They represent anastomosis between the choroidal (ciliary) and retinal circulation. Occasionally, a tuft of connective tissue arises from the nerve head on its nasal side and projects forward into the vitreous. This embryonic remnant of the hyaloid artery is located in the surrounding canal of Cloquet. If located near the edge of the nerve head, the disk margin may appear blurred or even elevated. Such persistent hyaloid remnants do not interfere with vision unless associated with other ocular defects.

Myelinated nerve fibers are another normal variation and may be seen as striking projections of white feathery tissue originating from the optic disk and extending for variable distances into the peripheral retina. Visual field defects may be present in the area of myelination of the nerve fibers running in this area. Drusen, small round hyaline excrescences formed on Bruch membrane, may create variations in elevation of the nerve head or scalloping of its border, or they may more commonly occur as scattered small yellow lesions in the peripheral fundus. They may occasionally produce pseudopapilledema of the nerve head, but no visual field defect will be present except for enlargement of the blind spot. **Macular drusen** may precede subretinal neovascularization. Fluorescein angiography may be indicated.

H. **Indirect ophthalmoscopy** is a technique generally used by specialists and involves the use of a head-mounted, prism-directed light source coupled with use of double aspheric (+14, +20, or +28) diopter condensing lenses to see the retinal image.

1. **Optics.** Several designs of indirect ophthalmoscopes are available, but all produce a stereoscopic image that is inverted, real, and capable of being seen on a semitransparent film held at the focal plane of the lens. Although most indirect ophthalmoscopes are designed for use through dilated pupils, some may be used through a miotic or undilated pupil; this is a great advantage in patients who cannot be dilated either because they do not respond to topical drugs, are at risk of angle-closure glaucoma, or have pupil scarred to the lens.

2. **The image** covers approximately ten times the area usually seen in the field of the direct ophthalmoscope, but is smaller than a direct ophthalmoscope (3×), although the larger field of view gives great perspective to the entire fundus and is helpful in locating multiple lesions or in evaluating retinal detachment. Another advantage is stronger illumination, which allows light to pass through opacities of the vitreous obstructive to a direct ophthalmoscope. See sec. **D.,** above, for the use of lenses to obtain a magnified stereoscopic view of the posterior pole.

I. **Visual field testing** (see Chapter 13, sec. **I.**).

  1. **The purpose** of visual field testing is to determine both the outer limits of visual perception by the peripheral retina and the varying qualities of vision within that area. Visual field interpretation is important for diagnosing disease, localizing it in the visual pathway between the retina and the occipital cortex in the brain, and noting its progress, stability, or remission. As a result, repeated tests of the visual field are important both diagnostically and in ascertaining the effects of therapy. Each eye is tested separately. With one eye fixing on a given distant test object, the sensitivity of various areas of the visual field may be tested with varying size and color of test objects moved throughout that field. The greatest sensitivity, of course, is at the fovea and represents the highest visual acuity of central fixation. This visual acuity decreases rapidly as the test objects are moved away from central fixation. Colored objects offer less stimulus to the retina than white objects of similar size. Therefore, an object may be too small to be detected by peripheral retinal receptors, but quite effective in mapping out central visual field within 10 to 15 degrees of foveal fixation.

  2. **Techniques.** Visual fields are examined most frequently by four methods: Amsler grid, confrontation, perimetry, and tangent screen.

    a. **Amsler charts** for qualitative vision evaluation make it possible to analyze the earliest maculopathies and their progression, as well as to detect any scotomatous defects encroaching on the central 10 degrees of vision.

      (1) **Technique.** The small book of six charts contains diffusely dotted or lined square grids 10 cm on the side, the latter with smaller 5-mm squares within. With the chart held at 30 cm from the patient's eye, the linear measurements correspond to visual angles of 20 degrees and 1 degree, respectively. The patient stares at the center of the squares one eye at a time. Alterations in perception of the regular patterns indicate various field defects.

      (2) **Purpose.** The examiner may find central scotomas (focal area of decreased or lost retinal sensitivity) as in macular scarring, cecocentral scotomas as in toxic amblyopias, paracentral scotomas as in chorioretinitis, and metamorphopsia (distortion of vision) as in very early maculopathies. The edge of a glaucomatous Bjerrum scotoma, a peripheral field defect secondary to CNS or peripheral retinal disease encroaching on the central 10 degrees of vision, will also be detected.

    b. **Confrontation.** No special instruments are required for this form of visual field testing, which provides a rough estimate of the patient's visual field by comparing it with the examiner's visual field. It is assumed that the examiner's visual field is normal.

      (1) **Technique.** The patient and examiner face each other at a distance of 1 m. With the left eye covered, the patient is instructed to look with the right eye at the left eye of the examiner, whose own right eye is covered. A small object such as a pencil or a larger one such as a wiggling finger may be used as a target. The examiner places his or her hand midway between the patient and him- or herself and initially beyond the limits of field of vision of either in a given meridian, e.g., far temporal to both patient and examiner. As the test object is moved slowly toward the line of vision between patient and examiner, the patient is asked to respond as soon as he or she is able to see the target. The physician compares this to the time when he or she is able to perceive the target. This is repeated at eight to ten equally spaced meridians at approximately 360 degrees. The visual field is considered normal if the patient sees the target 90 degrees temporally, 50 degrees nasally, 50 degrees upward, and 65 degrees downward. The test is then repeated on the other eye. With careful testing the blind spot and focal scotomas can be detected.

(2) **Purpose.** This test may also detect gross alterations in field defects due to ocular disease, such as chorioretinitis or advanced glaucoma, or to intracranial disease such as brain tumor or hemorrhage (see also Chapter 10, sec. **II.E.**, Fig. 10.2 [glaucoma]; and Chapter 13, Figs. 13.3–13.5 [neuroophthalmic fields]).

c. **Perimetry** is done to obtain accurate examination of the peripheral extent of the visual field. Perimetry may be done as manual *kinetic* (moving target from nonseeing to seeing areas of vision) or *static* (nonmoving target flashed at different locations in visual field) using a **Goldmann** type bowl perimeter, or by *automated static perimetry* using a bowl perimeter such as the **Humphrey** visual field analyzer or the **Octopus.** In addition to varying target size, perimeters vary target brightness as well, presenting them at threshold (the dimmest spot detected during testing) or suprathreshold levels. Size I is 0.25 mm^2 and size V is 64 mm^2 with gradations in between. Luminance varies from 32 to 1,000 apostilbs with ten gradations in between. Most automated perimeters provide normal values and compare the patient to normal in the printout of the results. The Humphrey analyzer will also give a probability that any test location is not normal dependent on patient age and location in the visual field. The standard glaucoma field is 30-2, with follow-up fields either 30-2 or 24-2. In addition to automated static perimetry, there is now **short-wavelength automated perimetry (SWAP)** which appears to detect visual field defects earlier than automated static perimetry, and **frequency doubling perimetry,** which is a 1-minute screening test that is very good in detecting moderate to advanced glaucoma.

The Octopus detects threshold sensitivity to a light stimulus at 72 points in the visual field. The intensity of the stimulus is carried to below threshold and worked up to suprathreshold. Its advantages are that the Octopus picks up the earliest, most subtle field defects, the results are reproducible, and progression of subtle or gross defects can easily be documented. The disadvantages of all automated perimeters are subjective patient fatigue, the expense of the machines, and the need for trained personnel to run them.

Visual field examination is indicated when the physician detects or suspects a disorder that has constricted the side, paracentral, or central vision. In uncooperative patients, the results of this test are unreliable.

(1) **Technique.** The patient is seated at the perimeter with one eye covered and the chin on the chin rest. The patient must fix his or her vision on the central target of the perimeter and a test target, static or kinetic as just described, is presented at some location in the field. The patient is asked to signal immediately when he or she sees the target, indicate when it disappears, and indicate again when it reappears. By the end of the test, the entire 360 degrees of field have been mapped.

(2) **Purpose.** The examiner may accurately map defects in the peripheral vision all the way from the far extent of the field into central or foveal fixation. The smaller the test target used, the greater the possibility of discovering scotomas in the field.

d. **Tangent screen.** Up to 90% of all visual field defects in the central 30 degrees may be picked up using this method of kinetic perimetry (a suprathreshold stimulus moving from nonseeing to seeing areas of vision). It is not as sensitive in picking up early defects as the Goldmann and automated perimeters.

(1) **Technique.** The patient is seated 1 m from a 2-m^2 black screen with a direct line of fixation on the central object in the tangent screen. One eye is tested at a time. A 3- to 50-mm white test object is brought in from the periphery, exploring 8 to 10 meridians from periphery to central fixation, as in perimetry. The patient indicates immediately when the object appears and disappears so that the examiner can

map areas of decreased or absent vision. The blind spot should be outlined carefully and early in the examination to show the patient the nature of scotoma mapping. The findings, including the size and color of the test object and the distance from the screen, are charted. *Color fields* with red and blue test objects are most useful in the central 10 to 15 degrees of vision and may be the test that picks up early toxic retinopathy soonest.

J. **Tear film adequacy: clinical tests.** The testing of tear film adequacy can be divided into three separate areas: (a) tear quantity, (b) tear quality, and (c) tear film stability. Each is of importance in determining the role of the tear film in the symptomatology and pathologic changes noted in dry eye syndromes.

1. **Tear quantity test.** Tear secretion may be divided into basal and reflex secretion. Basal secretion is maintained by the accessory conjunctival lacrimal glands of Krause and Wolfring. Reflex secretion is a product of the main lacrimal gland. Accurate interpretation of tests requires assessment of the role that reflex tearing played during the test. The average basal tear volume is from 5 to 9 μL with a flow rate of 0.5 to 2.2 μL per minute. Unlike reflex tearing, this parameter is not age dependent, and basal volume or flow rate does not normally decrease in elderly persons. The majority of clinical complications of tear volume, however, result from hyposecretion. The epithelium, cornea, and conjunctiva are extremely sensitive to decreased tear volume, especially in the exposed interpalpebral area. The early effects of dryness are degeneration and death of epithelial cells, which may progress in severe cases to keratinization of the cornea and conjunctiva.

a. **Schirmer test.** The purpose of this test is the measurement of the **total (reflex and basal) tear secretion.** To minimize reflex tearing, the eyes should not be manipulated before starting this test. There is no contraindication to this test. The materials used are commercially available Whatman no. 41 filter paper strips 5 mm wide × 30 mm in length, known as Schirmer tear test filter strips. The patient is seated in a dimly lit room, and the filter paper strips are folded 5 mm from the end. The folded end is placed gently over the lower palpebral conjunctiva at its lateral one-third. The patient keeps the eyes open and looks upward. Blinking is permissible. After 5 minutes the strips are removed and the amount of wetting is measured from the folded end. If the strips are completely wetted before 5 minutes, they may be removed prematurely. A normal patient will wet from 10 to 30 mm in 5 minutes; this is age dependent and decreases after the age of 60 years, but is rarely less than 10 mm in 5 minutes. Measurements greater than 30 mm at 5 minutes indicate that reflex tearing is intact but not controlled and, therefore, are of little diagnostic value. Between 10 and 30 mm of tear secretion may be normal, or basal secretion may be low but compensated for by reflex secretion. Values less than 5 mm on repeated testing indicate hyposecretion of basic tearing. There is a 15% chance of diagnostic error in this test.

b. **Basic secretion test.** The purpose of this most commonly used test is to measure the basal secretion by eliminating reflex tearing. Topical anesthetic is instilled into the conjunctiva and a few minutes allowed to pass until reactive hyperemia has subsided. The room is darkened and the procedure is the same as in the Schirmer test I. Interpretation of the results is also similar. The difference between the results of this test and those of the Schirmer test I is a measurement of reflex secretion contraindications and any contraindication to the local anesthetic. Materials used are the Schirmer strip and proparacaine 0.5%.

c. **Tear film breakup time (TFBUT).** The TFBUT is the time between a complete blink and appearance of the first random corneal dry spot, and indicates relative tear film stability. It should be performed *before any drops* are instilled. Saline-wetted fluorescein strip is touched to the lower tear meniscus to enhance visibility of dry spots. A shortened TF-BUT of 1 to 2 seconds suggests mucin deficiency or other ocular surface abnormalities. Normal TFBUT is 10 to 15 seconds.

d. **Rose bengal staining.** The purpose of this test is to ascertain indirectly the presence of reduced tear volume through *detection of damaged epithelial cells.* The eye is anesthetized topically with proparacaine 0.5%. Tetracaine or cocaine may give false-positive tests because of their softening effect on corneal epithelium. One drop of 1% rose bengal solution or a drop from a *saline-wetted* rose bengal strip is instilled in each conjunctival sac. Rose bengal is a vital stain taken up by dead and degenerating cells that have been damaged by the reduced tear volume, particularly in the exposed interpalpebral area. This test is particularly useful in early stages of conjunctivitis sicca and keratoconjunctivitis sicca syndrome. A positive test will show triangular stipple staining of the nasal and temporal bulbar conjunctiva in the interpalpebral area and possible punctate staining of the cornea, especially in the lower two-thirds. False-positive staining may occur in conditions such as chronic conjunctivitis, acute chemical conjunctivitis secondary to hair spray use and drugs such as tetracaine and cocaine, exposure keratitis, superficial punctate keratitis secondary to toxic or idiopathic phenomena, and foreign bodies in the conjunctiva. The stain will also color mucus and epithelial debris, which may mask the results. Certain patients who are normal will show some positive staining to rose bengal on the cornea. Because of this, conjunctival as well as corneal staining should be present before the diagnosis of keratoconjunctivitis sicca is made.

2. **Tear quality test** involves tests for the presence of mucus, protein, and tear film stability. Mucin lowers the surface tension of the tears and converts the hydrophobic corneal epithelial surface to a wettable hydrophilic surface. Mucin is produced by conjunctival goblet cells and spread by the action of the lids over the corneal epithelium. Mucin-deficient diseases such as Stevens-Johnson syndrome and pemphigus result in corneal desiccation despite normal tear volume, due to the lack of mucus as a wetting agent.

a. **A conjunctival biopsy** may be done to ascertain the presence or absence of mucin-producing goblet cells. Four percent cocaine solution on a cotton-tipped swab is applied directly to the lower nasal fornix, an area containing the highest population of goblet cells. After 60 seconds, a Vannas scissors and a jeweler's forceps are used to excise a conjunctival sample 5 mm long × 2 mm deep. The tissue is spread gently on a 2 × 2 cm cardboard, epithelial side up until it is flat. The cardboard is placed in 95% alcohol and sent to the pathology laboratory with a request for periodic acid–Schiff (PAS) stain. Histologically, the normal lower nasal fornix contains from 10 to 14 goblet cells per field at 200×. In a mucin-deficient state, this population is markedly diminished or absent. This procedure is extremely simple and painless. The conjunctiva heals rapidly over a 24- to 48-hour period. Local antibiotic ointment such as erythromycin or bacitracin should be instilled.

b. **A qualitative mucous assay** may be performed to determine the presence of mucus. Cotton strips 3 × 10 mm are placed in the inferior cul-de-sac of the unanesthetized eye for 5 minutes. Each strip is then placed on a glass slide and stained with PAS reagent. Color change is noted 1 minute later and compared with a sample from a known normal subject. If adequate mucus is present the strip will show a positive PAS reaction, turning dark purple. In the absence of mucus the reaction is negative. This test may be meaningful only in those eyes containing at least some tear film.

K. **Tear secretion tests.** Tests of tear secretion are important in ascertaining the **etiology of chronic tearing (epiphora).** The causes of epiphora can be divided into (a) partial or complete obstruction of the excretory canal, (b) increased lacrimal secretion (see sec. **II.J.1.,** above), and (c) decreased basal lacrimal secretion with secondary reflex tearing (see sec. **II.J.1.**, above). Tear excretion involves the pumping action of the lids and good anatomic apposition of the patent punctal openings against the globe. Any lid abnormality such as entropion, ectropion, or punctal occlusion may be associated with chronic tearing. Examination of the eyelids prior to the test may reveal an anatomic etiology for chronic tearing, rather than a deficiency of the deeper nasolacrimal canal drainage system.

1. **Regurgitation test** is the test of the excretory patency medial to the lacrimal sac (canalicular canals running in the lid margin). The examiner gently compresses the skin over and around the medial canthal ligament while observing the punctum under magnification. Obstruction medial to the lacrimal sac, i.e., in the canal, results in regurgitation of fluid, often mucoid or purulent, through the punctum when pressure is applied over the lacrimal sac. This obstruction is almost always complete and is usually associated with inflammation in the sac (dacryocystitis).

2. **The primary dye test** is used to test the patency of the entire excretory system (the nasolacrimal drainage system into the back of the nose). Fluorescein is instilled into the lower cul-de-sac. A small wisp of cotton on the end of a wire cotton applicator or a sterile cotton tip is placed 3.8 cm into the nose under the inferior meatus. (This is along the floor of the nasal canal.) After 2 minutes the cotton is removed and examined. If the cotton is fluorescein-stained, the test is positive and the system is patent and functioning. If there is no dye on the cotton, either the cotton was misplaced or the excretory mechanism is obstructed. There is no localizing value regarding the site of obstruction within the nasolacrimal canal.

3. **The secondary dye test** (lacrimal irrigation test) is another test of the excretory patency and is used if the primary dye test is negative. A 2-mL syringe is filled with saline and a lacrimal cannula attached to it. This cannula is placed in the lower canaliculus, entering through the lower punctum, and the saline is injected. The patient leans forward and the naris on the ipsilateral side is observed. If the patient tastes the saline in his or her throat or if fluorescein fluid comes from the naris, the test is positive. If the primary dye test is negative and the secondary dye test positive, the system is partially blocked. If both tests are negative, the excretory system is totally blocked. There is no localizing value to this test for lesions within the nasolacrimal system. Because the pressure of the injection may open a partially obstructed system, lacrimal irrigation without performing the primary dye test may be misleading.

4. **Canaliculus testing** is a test for the patency of the canaliculi or canals running in the lid margin. Clear saline is injected through the punctum of one canaliculus using a 2-mL syringe and lacrimal cannula. The opposite punctum on the same eye is observed. If saline returns through the other canaliculus, both are patent and the obstruction is in or beyond the common canaliculus beyond the medial canthus. If no fluid comes from the opposite punctum, at least one of the canaliculi is obstructed. This test is contraindicated in the presence of acute inflammation of the lacrimal sac.

5. **Dacryocystography** for localization of obstruction site is discussed under radiographic techniques (see sec. **III.I.8.**, below).

L. **Corneal sensation** is tested prior to topical anesthetics by gently touching the cornea with a wisp of cotton (drawn out from the end of a cotton-tip applicator) and comparing each eye against the other on a 0 to 10 scale of increasing sensitivity. A more precise reading may be achieved using the Cochet-Bonnet anesthesiometer, which gives a scale reading relative to the length of a retractable nylon filament extended from the end of the handle.

M. **Transillumination**

1. **Intraocular tumors** may often be detected by transillumination of the globe. Intense light, such as that from a small handheld flashlight, placed on the sclera in successive quadrants behind the ciliary body will be transmitted inside the eye, where it produces a red reflex in the pupil. Intraocular

masses, such as malignant melanoma containing pigment, will block the light when it is placed over the tumor, thus diminishing or preventing the red reflex. The presence of tumor under a retinal detachment (detachments are commonly caused by intraocular tumors) may be detected in this manner; the test is also useful for distinguishing a retinal detachment resulting from causes other than tumor. Normally, retinal detachment will not interfere with the normal red reflex so produced.

    2. **Atrophy of the iris pigment layer** or ciliary body may also be revealed by transillumination. Such atrophy is frequently seen in patients with chronic intraocular inflammation. This test should be performed in a completely darkened room, with the examiner dark adapted and the instrument placed 8 mm posterior to the limbus to avoid the ciliary body, which would normally cut off light entering the eye.

N. **Exophthalmometry.** The exophthalmometer (**Hertel**) is used to determine the degree of anterior projection or prominence of the eyes. This instrument is helpful in diagnosing and in following the course of exophthalmos.

    1. **Technique.** The patient holds the head straight and looks directly at the examiner's eyes. Two small concave attachments of the exophthalmometer are placed against the lateral orbital margins, and the distance between these two points is recorded from the central bar. This distance must be constant for all successive examinations in order to judge accurately the status of ocular protrusion. The examiner views the cornea of the patient's right eye in the mirror while the patient fixes the right eye on the examiner's left eye. Simultaneously, the cornea is lined up in the mirror with the scale, which reads directly in millimeters. A similar reading is then taken from the left eye with the patient fixing on the examiner's right eye. The bar reading and the degree of exophthalmos are then recorded in millimeters; e.g., a bar reading of 100 might have right eye 17 mm, left eye 18 mm.

    2. **Interpretation.** The normal range of exophthalmometry readings is 12 to 20 mm. The readings are normally within 2 mm of each other and indicate the anterior distances from the corneas to the lateral orbital margins. Exophthalmos is present if the reading is greater than 20 mm in one eye and may indicate a search for an underlying cause such as thyroid ocular disease or orbital tumor. A disparity of 3 mm or greater between readings taken from each eye during a test is also an indication for further investigation, even though both readings may fall within the normal range.

O. **Placido disk and Klein keratoscope.** These simple instruments are useful in the qualitative diagnosis of corneal reflex regularity and irregular astigmatism. The presence of a pathologic state, such as subtle or gross scarring or early keratoconus, will cause the normally regular concentric circles viewed through the keratoscope or disk to be asymmetric or frankly distorted and irregular. The examiner holds the disk or keratoscope to his or her eye and observes the illuminated cornea of the patient through the aperture. Distortion or roughening of the rings may account for a marked decrease in vision through a cornea that may appear normal on initial examination. A focally indented area in the rings indicates a shortening of that meridian such as from a tight suture that may need to be cut to relieve astigmatism.

P. **Keratometry.** The keratometer is an instrument generally used for measuring corneal astigmatism in two main meridians. It is particularly useful in the fitting of corneal contact lenses, but may also be used to detect irregular astigmatism and early pathologic states such as keratoconus. Successive readings several months apart will indicate progression or stability of corneal disease. The device is similar to a slitlamp in use. The corneal reflex is evaluated for regularity and measured at 90-degree axes in the two meridians of greatest difference, i.e., the flattest and steepest planes.

Q. **Gonioscopy.** The visually inaccessible **anterior chamber angle** may be viewed directly with gonioscopic techniques that involve the use of a contact lens, focal illumination, and magnification. The contact lens eliminates the corneal curve and allows light to be reflected from the angle so that its structures may be seen in detail.

1. **Technique.** This procedure may be performed with topical anesthetic drops at the slitlamp and such lenses as the Alan-Thorpe, Goldmann, or Zeiss lenses, all of which have periscopic mirrors by which the angle is examined with reflected light. The patient may also undergo gonioscopy without the slitlamp while in the supine position when the Koeppe contact lens is used. The angle is viewed through a handheld microscope with the Barkan light held in the other hand giving bright focal illumination. Greater magnification is achieved with the Koeppe lens than with lenses on the slitlamp, thereby allowing greater magnification of details of the angle, but this technique is used less frequently because of relative inconvenience compared to lenses applied with the patient at the slitlamp.

2. **Purpose.** This technique is most useful in determining various *forms of glaucoma,* such as open-angle, narrow-angle, angle-closure, and secondary angle-closure glaucoma, by allowing evaluation of the angle width (distance of the iris root from the trabecular meshwork) and study of the tissues in the angle of the glaucomatous eyes at various stages (see Chapter 10). Gonioscopy is also of great use in examining *other problems* within the anterior chambers, such as retained intraocular foreign bodies hidden in the recess of the angle. It is useful in the study of iris tumors and cysts as well as in the evaluation of trauma to the tissues in the area of the angle. With wide pupillary dilation the area behind the iris (posterior chamber), including ciliary processes, zonules, lens, and equator, may be seen in many patients.

III. **Hospital or highly specialized office techniques**
   A. **Corneal topography** is done with computerized machines which use video capture of concentric circle Placido disk images to produce videokeratographs in the form of color-coded dioptric contour maps which show even subtle variations in power distribution plots, and can calculate the power and location of the steepest and flattest meridians, similar to values given by a keratometer. Cool colors are lower in power than warm colors, e.g., blue = flat, red = steep, green = normal. The corneal modeling system uses 32 rings with 256 points analyzed on each ring with a power change resolution of 0.25 d. The EyeSys uses 16 rings with a fast-imaging processing time. Corneal *diagnosis and changes* may be monitored by sequential topography and include disorders such as keratoconus, contact lens warping of the cornea, postoperative healing patterns (keratoplasty, cataract, tight sutures, radial keratotomy, excimer laser photorefractive keratectomy), marginal degenerations, and keratoglobus.
   B. **Corneal pachymetry.** Pachymeters measure corneal thickness (normal 0.50 to 0.65 mm, thicker peripherally) and are good indicators of endothelial function as well as being useful in calculating blade set for radial keratotomy. Optical pachymeters attach to the slitlamp and are quite reliable, but are subject to reader variation. Ultrasonic pachymeters can record readings at multiple corneal sites with a vertical applanating tip, thus minimizing errors caused by tilting, but also making peripheral readings more difficult.
   C. **Specular photomicroscopy.** This camera-mounted, slitlamp-like instrument allows visualization and photography of the corneal endothelial mosaic. Wide-field microscopy encompasses 200 cells per frame and can be done at multiple corneal sites. Normal endothelial density averages 2,400 cells per mm^2 (1,500 to 3,500 range) and decreases with age. Cell shape is normally hexagonal. Microscopy will detect pleomorphism (cells deviating from normal shape), cell dropout as in Fuchs dystrophy, and polymegetheism (abnormal cell size variation). All may contribute to endothelial dysfunction and corneal edema and may be seen in diabetes; following anterior segment surgery; in inflammation, glaucoma, and contact lens wear; and following intracameral drug administration.

D. **Confocal scanning slit microscopy** allows a direct, highly magnified, high-resolution viewing of corneal cells, structures, and organisms in patients. The instrument focuses on a single plane in the cornea while eliminating light from all other planes. The field of view is expanded via the scanning system and has a magnification of 200× and resolution of 9 μm. Confocal microscopy is used to follow healing after laser or traditional surgery and to help identify infectious organisms such as fungi and bacteria.

E. **Fluorescein and indocyanine green (ICG) angiography of the fundus**
   1. **Purpose. Fluorescein** angiography (FA) has proved to be a valuable tool in the diagnosis and management of a large number of retinal disorders that affect either the retinal vascular system or the choriocapillaris, Bruch membrane, or the pigment epithelial layers. Disease states particularly amenable to evaluation by angiography include diabetic retinopathy, ocular histoplasmosis, macular edema, idiopathic preretinal macular fibrosis, retrolental fibroplasia, vascular occlusive disease, flecked retina syndrome, sickle cell retinopathy, viral retinopathy, retinal telangiectasis, von Hippel-Lindau disease, Eales disease, choroidal tumor, both primary melanoma and metastatic carcinoma, and benign hemangioma. **ICG** methodology is similar to FA. Compared to FA, ICG produces better choroidal vessel resolution but lesser resolution of retinal vessels. ICG is mainly used to detect occult choroidal neovascular membranes or their recurrence posttreatment, and for suspected retinal epithelial detachment. The fundic FA may provide three kinds of information:
      a. **Documentation of the fine anatomic detail** of the fundus.
      b. **Physiologic information** pertinent to the index of flow of blood to the eye and flow through the retinal circulation.
      c. **Documentation of fundic pathology** when dye is seen passing vascular barriers that are ordinarily impermeable.
   2. **Technique.** After the patient's pupils have been dilated, he or she is seated at a slitlamp mounted with a fundus camera and equipped with both exciter and barrier interference filters. These filters will allow only green light from the fluorescent dye passing through the vessels to be recorded on the film, thus exclusively outlining the vascular pattern and pathologic structures contained therein. Five milliliters of sodium fluorescein 10%, a harmless and painless dye, is injected into the antecubital vein. Photographs of one eye are taken at 5 seconds and then every second thereafter for 15 more seconds. Photographs will then be taken for up to 1 minute at 3- to 5-second intervals and then repeated at 20 minutes in both eyes. Occasionally, in patients with sensory epithelial detachments or diffuse retinal edema, photographs will be taken at 1 hour or more.
   3. **Side effects.** Normally, the patient will have some afterimage effect and a yellowish discoloration of the skin, both of which will disappear within a matter of a few hours. The urine will also be discolored for approximately 1 day. Transient episodes of nausea may occur, and rarely there may be transient vomiting. Fainting is uncommon but may be seen, particularly in young male patients. Such patients should be held in the office for 1 hour to ascertain that there is no more severe reaction following. Severe allergic reactions such as anaphylaxis or cardiorespiratory problems are extremely rare and should be handled by a competent medical team.
   4. **Stages of the normal angiogram.** Dye is visible in the choroidal circulation approximately 1 second before its appearance in the retinal arterioles (arterial phase). It lasts until the retinal arteries are completely filled. The AV phase of the transit involves complete filling of both retinal arteries and capillaries and the early stages of laminar flow in the veins. The venous phase of the dye transit includes initial laminar flow along the walls of the veins and then complete venous filling. The transit time in the macula is the most rapid, and the retinal capillary bed is best resolved in the macula because of increased pigmentation in the retinal pigment epithelium (RPE), which will block out underlying choroidal fluorescence.

5. **In interpreting the angiogram** the examiner may refer to a few terms that need definition.

   a. **Pseudofluorescence** results from fluorescein leakage into the vitreous and is a reflected illumination from this body.

   b. **Autofluorescence** pertains to true fluorescence of structures in the retinal area, such as drusen of the optic nerve head.

   c. **A window defect** is a localized deficiency of pigment granules in the RPE through which choroidal fluorescence is seen.

   d. **Pooling** is an accumulation of dye in a tissue space such as that between the RPE and Bruch membrane.

   e. **Staining** is an increased accumulation of dye within tissue substance, such as the sensory retinal capillary bed.

   f. **Blocked fluorescence** is interference with visualization of the normal underlying choroidal fluorescence, as in increased RPE thickness, increased choroidal pigmentation as in a nevus, or the presence of retinal hemorrhages or exudates in the sensory retina beneath the pigment epithelium.

   g. **A filling defect** is an area of decreased fluorescence where circulation is occluded. It occurs in either the choroidal or retinal vascular bed. The rate of filling, emptying, and configuration assists the examiner in diagnosis and evaluation of various disease states of the fundus such as ischemic diabetic retinopathy.

F. **FA of the iris** is performed to document abnormal vascular patterns, tumors, ischemia, and inflammatory patterns. Unfortunately, the iris pigment often absorbs emitted fluorescein enough to make this test worthwhile only in light- to medium-(hazel) pigmented eyes. It may be performed on the fundus fluorescein camera by dialing a plus lens into the optical system, pulling the camera farther back, and focusing on the iris. Photography is delayed a few seconds longer than in retinal angiography because of the longer arm-to-iris circulation time for the injected fluorescein.

G. **ERG**

   1. **Purpose.** The ERG is an important instrument in the detection and evaluation of hereditary and constitutional disorders of the retina. These disorders include: partial and total color blindness, night blindness, retinal degeneration such as retinitis pigmentosa, chorioretinal degenerations or inflammations including choroideremia, Spielmeyer-Vogt disease, leutic chorioretinitis, Leber congenital amaurosis, retinal ischemia secondary to arteriosclerosis, giant-cell arteritis, central retinal artery or vein occlusion, and carotid artery insufficiency. Toxicity secondary to administration of drugs such as hydroxychloroquine, chloroquine, and quinine may be detected and quantitated by the ERG. Siderosis, whether from local iron deposit or systemic disease, will also produce abnormal changes in the recording. Frequently, the ERG will not distinguish among these, but will indicate the presence of diffuse abnormalities. Retinal detachment will reduce the recording levels of the ERG, although ultrasonography is probably a better way to detect such detachment in the presence of an opacity of the ocular media. Systemic diseases associated with low-voltage ERG include hypovitaminosis A, mucopolysaccharidosis, hypothyroidism, and anemia. The ERG may also be used to rule out the retina as the level of blindness in certain conditions such as cortical blindness, dyslexia, and hysteria.

   2. **ERG** is a **technique** of placing an ocular fitted contact lens electrode on the patient's eye so that recordings of electrical responses from various parts of the retina to external stimulation by light of varying intensity may be made. The A and B waves originate in the outer retinal layers, the A wave being produced by the photoreceptor cells and the B wave by the interconnecting Müller cells.

   3. **Disadvantages.** The ganglion cells do not contribute to the ERG because their electrical signals are in the former spike, which cannot be recorded

externally. Therefore, a normal ERG may be recorded in the absence of ganglion cells and in the presence of total optic nerve atrophy or advanced retinal diseases, such as Tay-Sachs disease, in which the metabolic defect is located in the ganglion cells. In addition, because the ERG is a mass response from the retina, diseases of the macula that represent only a small part of the retina will not be recorded on the ERG.

H. EOG is an electrical recording based on the standing potential of the eye.

    1. Use in retinal disease. The EOG is useful in situations in which the ERG is not sufficiently sensitive to detect macular degeneration. This includes Best's disease (vitelliform macular degeneration), in which the ERG is abnormal even in carriers, and early toxic retinopathies such as those caused by chloroquine or other antimalarial drugs. Supranormal EOGs have been found in albinism and aniridia, in which chronic excessive light exposure appears to have resulted in attendant peripheral retinal damage. The EOG records metabolic changes in RPE as well as in the neuroretina. Therefore, it serves as a test that is supplemental and complementary to the ERG and, in certain disease states, more sensitive than the ERG.

    2. Use in eye movements. By placing the skin electrodes around the eye and using the cornea as the positive electrode with respect to the retina, eye movements of both eyes can be recorded either separately or together, using bitemporal electrodes. This technique is most useful in recording various forms of nystagmus, and is particularly useful for clinicians who desire objective recordings of spontaneous and caloric-induced nystagmus. The technique is highly specialized, and the information produced therefrom is of use to only a fairly small number of clinicians.

I. Ultrasonography (echography). Diagnostic ocular ultrasonography has made possible the detection of intraocular abnormalities not visualized clinically because of opacification of the cornea, anterior chamber, lens, or vitreous, as well as pathologic processes involving the periorbital tissues. It provides much the same information as a computed tomography (CT) scan. Ultrasonography is analogous in many ways to soft tissue x-ray and consists of the propagation of high-frequency sound waves through soft tissue, with the differential reflection of these waves from objects in the beam pathway. The reflected waves create echoes that are displayed on an oscilloscope screen as in sonar or radar systems, producing a picture that is amenable to clinical interpretation. This technique has an advantage over x-rays or CT scans because it is a dynamic examination allowing innumerable views including studies of the moving globe. The main disadvantage is the need for direct contact with the globe or lid. Because of the highly sophisticated and expensive equipment involved and the necessity of dynamic interpretation of data, this technique is performed only by specialists within the field.

    1. Forms of ultrasonic testing commonly used are A-mode, B-mode, high-frequency ultrasound; optical coherence tomography (OCT); and confocal scanning laser ophthalmoscopy.

        a. A-mode is a one-dimensional time-amplitude representation of echoes received along the beam path. The distance between the echo spikes recorded on the oscilloscope screen provides an indirect measurement of tissue such as globe length or lens thickness. The height of the spike is indicative of the strength of the tissue sending back the echo; e.g., cornea, lens, retina, or sclera produce very high amplitude spikes, and vitreous membranes or hemorrhage produces lower spikes. In B-mode ultrasound the same echoes produced in A-mode may be presented as dots instead of spikes. By the use of a scanning technique, these dots can be integrated to produce an echo representation of a two-dimensional (2-D) section of the eye rather than the one dimension seen with A-mode. The location, size, and configuration of structures are rapidly apparent with this technique. The combination of both A-mode and B-mode techniques simultaneously produces the most successful results in ultrasonic testing.

   b. **Routine B-scan ultrasound** is performed using 10 MHz or less and is useful in detecting retinal detachments, swollen cataracts, hyphemas, and ciliary body detachment in hypotonous eyes.
   c. **High-frequency ultrasound** is a newer, more sensitive technique using up to 50 to 60 MHz and detecting anterior segment pathology in great detail. It requires a water bath because depth of penetration is less than the 10 MHz ultrasound, reaching to 4 to 5 mm behind the cornea to iris, lens, and ciliary body. It detects ciliary body detachment, plateau iris, anterior chamber angle outline, adhesions, trabecular membranes, and small foreign bodies in the angle. **Tridimensional high-frequency scanning** also is being used to image the posterior segment and localize lesions and detachments in a 3-D image. Very high frequency scans are being developed, up to 150 MHz, particularly for corneal evaluation, e.g., for use with excimer laser surgery.
   d. **OCT** complements all of the ultrasound techniques described in this section in posterior segment evaluation. It is a noncontact, noninvasive cross-sectional imaging technique that does not require immersion of the eye and can detect and measure changes in tissue thickness with micron-scale sensitivity to produce high-resolution measurements and images of the eye. Imaging of the anatomic layers within the retina and quantitation of the *optic nerve fiber layer* is quite accurate and correlates well with *glaucoma status*. The **confocal scanning laser ophthalmoscope** is a further complement to ultrasound in creating 3-D images of the optic nerve head using a series of tomographic optical sections of the structure being imaged. Such parameters as cup area and volume, cup/disk ratio, rim volume, and peripapillary nerve fiber layer (NFL) thickness may be calculated in the computer data system.
2. **Technique.** Both A and B types of ultrasound may be performed by either contact or immersion methods, both with the patient lying on a table.
   a. **In the contact method,** a transducer probe shaped like a pencil is held in direct contact with the eye or closed lid, using a topical anesthetic with a viscous coupling agent. In A-mode ultrasound, the examiner moves the probe around the eyes systematically until abnormal areas are found. These abnormal echoes are then tested with electronic variables to characterize them in terms of location, density, thickness, and shape. Because this equipment is portable, the examination may be done at the patient's bedside or in the operating room. In uncooperative young children the contact method may be the only practicable method. The major drawback is obscuration of the first few millimeters of the anterior segment and ciliary body.

   B-scan contact techniques are similar to those employed with A-mode instruments. Without immersion, echo characterization is limited to determining tissue configuration and density, and resolution suffers somewhat due to the continuous rapid display on the oscilloscope. The anterior segment and adjacent areas are obscured by electronic artifact, as with the A-mode. B-scan using the contact method is satisfactory for detecting most kinds of intraocular pathologies, but is of limited value in the orbit.
   b. **Immersion.** The most successful use of ultrasound is with immersion methods, where the eye is in direct contact with a water bath, with the transducer tip held just beneath the water surface but not against the eye. Anterior segment examination as well as examination of the deeper ocular and orbital structures is very successful under these conditions. Although untoward experience is unlikely, immersion techniques are not used on recently traumatized or postoperative eyes unless the information derived will influence treatment.
3. **Interpretation.** Ultrasonic techniques may be used to ascertain the size, shape, and integrity of the wall of the globe and are frequently useful in detecting hidden anterior as well as posterior penetrating wounds. Collapse

of the globe would be obvious on ultrasound, as is phthisis bulbi (end-stage shrinkage of the globe).

a. **Anterior segment examination** reveals chamber depth and configuration as well as debris. Cataractous changes and subluxation of the lens may be identified most easily by B-scan techniques. Iris abnormalities such as iris bombé, recession of the root, cysts, and tumors may be shown if they are sufficiently large. Ultrasonography does not determine the functional status of the angle relative to outflow of aqueous in glaucoma, only its physical status.

b. **Examination of the posterior segment** by either A- or B-scan ultrasound may pick up subtle vitreous changes such as asteroid hyalosis or synchysis scintillans. Membrane opacities such as retinal detachment, choroidal detachment, vitreous membranes, diffuse debris, and organized tissue are also easily detected. In cases of penetrating injury, the path followed by a foreign body may be detected on ultrasound as a track of moderate-amplitude echoes from hemorrhage or debris. An echo track may indicate the location of a foreign body exiting from the eye posteriorly. Intraocular tumors may be located, and configuration and degree of choroidal excavation may be helpful clues to differentiating melanomas from metastatic tumors and benign hemangiomas; however, these criteria are not highly reliable with present techniques. Other masses such as subretinal hemorrhage and diskiform chorioretinopathy may simulate the tumor pattern. Vitreous membranes, retinal detachments, and choroidal detachments all produce distinctive pictures that may differentiate one from the other.

c. **The localization of foreign bodies** is most accurately detected and located by a combination of A- and B-scan ultrasound. Radiographic techniques, however, have long been in use and also provide very accurate information about the localization and nature of most intraocular foreign bodies. Radiologically there is no way to differentiate among iron, copper, stone, or leaded glass fragments. Foreign bodies such as vegetable matter, nonleaded glass, or plastic, however, may not be sufficiently radiopaque to show up on film, whereas they would show up on ultrasound. Not only may the foreign body be located within the globe, but the amount and density of tissue damage or tissue reactions surrounding it may also be determined. Ultrasound is superior to CT scan if the foreign body is localized near the ocular wall, because a foreign body CT artifact may obscure whether the object is inside or outside of the eye. The magnetic character of a foreign body may be ascertained by pulsing a weak magnet over the eye and observing the behavior of the foreign body echo on the oscilloscope. Orbital foreign bodies, unlike intraocular ones, are much more difficult to locate with ultrasound because of the high reflection from the surrounding fat, muscle, and associated bony structures. Although in theory there is no limit to the size of foreign bodies that may be detected, practically speaking, small foreign bodies may be missed because the examiner may search randomly with the probe, not passing the beam through the exact area of the foreign body. Consequently, a negative report does not exclude foreign body in the eye, whereas the positive finding of foreign body is usually quite definite and highly localizing.

d. **Orbital ultrasonography** is most useful in evaluation of soft tissue lesions causing exophthalmos. Pseudoproptosis due to a large globe or a shallow orbit may be detected, and cystic, solid, angiomatous, and infiltrative mass lesions may be differentiated from each other. Inflammatory disease such as pseudotumor oculi, Graves' disease, neuritis, and cellulitis are also amenable to localization and differentiation, as is retrobulbar hemorrhage. Fractures of orbital walls are not amenable to ultrasonic evaluation; radiographic study should be used in such situations.

e. **Surgical implications.** Ultrasonography has been an invaluable technique for determining the potential functional status of an eye in which the ocular media has made impossible ordinary clinical examination. ERG is frequently unreliable in the presence of opaque media; under such circumstances ultrasound may be the sole means of determining the integrity of intraocular contents. Ascertaining of normal posterior segment will allow a surgeon to proceed with keratoplasty or cataract extraction with greater confidence of good results than when forced to operate on an eye with no knowledge of the status of the posterior segment. This technique is a noninvasive, well-tolerated, safe procedure with no known toxicity.

f. **Intraocular lenses (IOLs).** A very frequent use of ultrasonography is the determination of certain ocular measurements such as anterior chamber depth and global length. This, coupled with keratometry readings, will allow a surgeon to determine which implant power will make a cataract patient emmetropic, hyperopic, or myopic postoperatively (see Chapter 7, sec. **VII.B.**).

J. Scanning laser polarimetry (SLP) evaluation of retinal nerve fiber layer (NFL). The NFL is composed of the axons of the 1 to 2×10^6 retinal ganglion cells. The nerve fiber analyzer and the GDx combine polarimetry with the scanning laser ophthalmoscope. With the aid of digital enhancement, scanning laser ophthalmoscopes can show the NFL with high lateral resolution and contrast even through a small pupil and unclear media. SLP is done using a scanning laser ophthalmoscope coupled with a polarization modulator, which detects the birefringent properties of the retinal NFL resulting from its microtubule substructure. Data obtained are *relative*, not absolute, NFL thickness. The focal NFL defects are more sensitive indicators of **glaucomatous optic atrophy** than changes in cup size. Abnormally shaped disks, e.g., tilted or myopic, can also be evaluated more accurately for neurological loss.

K. Radiologic studies of the eye and orbit. Radiologic examination of the eye and orbit is useful in evaluating trauma, foreign bodies, and tumors.

1. **Anatomy.** Each orbit is a four-sided pyramidal cavity with the apex aimed posteromedially and the base opening onto the face. It is made up of seven bones and divided into the roof, lateral wall, medial wall, and the floor. Detailed anatomy is described in Chapter 4.

2. **Routine radiologic views,** in many cases, will reveal as much information as a CT scan and are indispensable in cases in which a patient cannot cooperate for the longer scanning procedure. They are of little use in soft tissue injuries of the eye. X-ray studies of the orbits are more difficult than x-rays of other sites of the body because of the superimposition of other bones of the skull. The patient is placed on the radiographic table, usually in the prone position. The head may be adequately adjusted and immobilized by a clamp device, headband, or sandbags. Several variations of position may be used as well as tomographic techniques to localize at a particular depth.

a. **Caldwell view** is a posterior–anterior (PA) projection of the orbit. The patient is in prone position with the forehead and nose resting on the table. This position offers the following **advantages:** (a) the petrous ridges are projected downward and there is a clear visualization of the **orbital rim and roof,** (b) the **greater wing of the sphenoid** is easily detected as it forms the large part of the lateral wall, (c) the **orbital section of the lesser wing of the sphenoid** is projected close to the medial wall, (d) the **superior orbital fissure** is clearly seen between the greater and lesser wings of the sphenoid, and (e) the **foramen rotundum** is projected under the inferior rim of the orbit.

b. **Waters view.** This PA film allows additional visualization of the orbital and periorbital structures. The patient is again prone with the head extended so that the chin lies on the table and the tip of the nose is approximately 4 cm above the table. The Waters view allows a clear **view of** the **maxillary antrum** separate from the superimposed petrous bones; the petrous ridges are projected downward, whereas the antral contours are complete and not deformed. Visualization of the maxillary antrum is of use in revealing orbital pathology. The **inferior orbital rim, the lateral wall, the zygomatic arch, and frontal and ethmoidal sinuses** are all demonstrated in this view.

  c. **The oblique view** is used for visualization of the outer wall of the orbit and should be taken from both sides. The patient rests with cheek, nose, and brow of the side of interest resting on the table. The x-rays are projected through the occiput and exit through the center of the orbit. This technique obtains better visualization of the **outer rim of the orbit** and is of particular interest if orbital rim fracture is suspected.

  d. **The Rhese position** is useful for demonstration of the **optic canal.** The patient is prone with head adjusted so that the zygoma, nose, and chin rest on the table. The structures that are visualized are the optic canal (appearing in the lateral quadrant of the orbit), the ethmoid cells, the lesser wing of the sphenoid, and the superior orbital fissure. If the patient is unable to lie prone, this film may be taken in the supine position as well.

  e. **The lateral view** is useful for localization of **foreign bodies.** The patient lies on the side, and the outer canthus of the orbit of interest is placed against the film. The x-rays are directed vertically through the canthus.

3. **Orbital tomography.** Body section radiography (**polytomography**) is a method whereby the examiner may blur the superimposed surrounding structures and clearly visualize a given spot at a given depth. During exposure the x-ray tube is moved in one direction above the object and the film is moved in the opposite direction with the tube adjusted so that the fulcrum point is at the level of anatomic interest. This plane will then be shot focused against the blurred anatomic structures around it. Tomography is of use particularly in **localizing small fractures** as well as in determining the **extent of linear fractures** and the presence of **orbital tumors.** In conjunction with specialized routine views, polytomograms are believed by most radiologists to be as informative as a CT scan.

4. **CT scan.** The CT scan's ability to delineate tissues of varying density make it an invaluable diagnostic tool. Routine CT scans are usually multiple axial or transverse "cuts," 8, 2, or even 1 mm apart, depending on the lesions being evaluated, starting at the skull vertex and going to the skull base. As such, the orbital walls, eye, and extraocular muscles are sectioned longitudinally in the horizontal plane. Orbital and extraocular examinations are enhanced by coronal and sagittal sections. Radiopaque medium may be injected during the scan to demonstrate vascular abnormalities. The CT is the study of choice in soft tissue inquiries. Spatial resolution of better than $1 \times 1 \times 1.5$ mm^3 provides fine detail. Cuts 1 to 2 mm should be used especially for injuries such as potential optic nerve damage or localization of ocular or orbital foreign bodies of varying composition and density. Blowout fractures with muscle incarceration are best seen with coronal sections through the orbital floor and maxillary antrum. Incarceration of muscle may be distinguished from that of fat. Other diagnoses possible with CT scanning include tumors or hematomas of the lids, extraocular muscles, orbit, or optic sheath, transected muscle or optic nerve, incarcerated muscle, ruptured globe, dislocated lens, vitreous hemorrhage, choroidal or retinal detachment, fractures of the optic canal, fracture of any wall, and secondary sinus involvement. The main disadvantages of CT scanning are poor contrast between some different soft tissues, possible radiation hazards (orbital CT scan = 2 to 3 rad, similar to an orbital series of skull x-rays), beam-hardening artifacts created by metallic objects or cortical bone, and lack of direct scanning in the sagittal plane. Indicated uses of CT versus magnetic resonance imaging (MRI) are discussed in sec. **III.K.5.,** below. CT

is not sensitive enough to be the sole diagnostic factor for open globe injury, but must only complement other clinical findings.

5. **MRI** is the procedure of choice for soft tissue anatomy and pathology and vascularized lesions of global, orbital, and neuroophthalmic structures from the orbit through the brain.

   a. **Advantages and disadvantages.** The patient is in a magnetic field and not exposed to ionizing radiation. Application of a radiofrequency pulse to various tissue protons causes a change in the intrinsic spin and magnetic vector in many nuclei. The superior soft-tissue contrast is a result of differing T1 (longitudinal or spin–lattice relaxation time) and T2 (transverse or spin–spin relaxation time). Simply said, long T1 values yield a dark (hypointense) signal and long T2 values yield a bright (hyperintense) signal. The technique is therefore extremely safe as long as the area examined is *free of foreign magnetic metal* and the patient has *no cardiac pacemaker,* which may be turned off or on by the MRI.

   Other advantages of MRI are that the technique is not hampered by bone, which, because of low molecular mobility, is relatively invisible on the images. Soft tissues are thus seen in an unobstructed fashion; anatomic delineation of normal and abnormal structures as well as a metabolic profile of those structures is obtained. Better resolution is obtained with 3-D isotropic images where thinner slices (2 mm) are taken, and better contrast is obtained on 2-D images with thicker slices (3 to 5 mm), which give greater signal to noise ratios. Lesions smaller than 2 mm are best seen on 3-D images, because they do not blend into their surrounding tissues, whereas larger lesions can be demonstrated on either 2-D or 3-D imaging. MRI is capable of differentiating hemorrhages, ischemia, multiple sclerosis, and tumors of the brain as well as virtually all ocular and orbital structures.

   b. **Ocular indications** for use of MRI (usually 3-D) and/or CT include ocular trauma, tumors within opaque media when ultrasound is equivocal, and suspected intraocular foreign bodies. *MRI should not be used* if the intraocular foreign body is thought to be ferromagnetic (e.g., BBs, iron, unknown composition), however, and CT and ultrasound should be used for such evaluations. IOL haptics of titanium or platinum are not a contraindication to MRI. MRI can distinguish retinoblastoma (low-intensity mass) from hemorrhage or exudate, which appears brighter, and from Coats's disease or toxocariasis because of the latter two having bright T2-based signals. MRI will distinguish choroidal melanotic melanomas from nonpigmented tumors and effusions, but not from fat.

   c. **Orbital indications** for CT and/or MRI are proptosis, papilledema, and orbital inflammatory, infectious, or neoplastic disease. Two-dimensional imaging is commonly used. Excellent contrast is provided between fine cortical bone, orbital fat, extraocular muscles, optic nerve, the globe, and the numerous disease processes that may involve these structures. Dye-contrasted CT and MRI resolve vascular lesions with excellent delineation, e.g., hemangiomas, carotid–cavernous sinus fistulas, and thrombosed ophthalmic veins.

   d. **Neuroophthalmic indications** for CT and/or MRI include the above orbital disorders, if unexplained after orbital evaluation, plus unexplained optic and cranial neuropathies, eye movement disorders, visual field defects, or any other signs or symptoms of intracranial disease. MRI images are generally superior to CT in delineating vascular or solid lesions in the sella turcica, cavernous sinus, optic chiasm, posterior fossa, and brain stem. MRI also shows multiple sclerosis plaques and hemorrhages better than CT, but CT is superior if a calcified lesion is under evaluation. The election of CT, MRI, or both must be based on clinical suspicion of the nature of the disease, but with faster scan time, finer resolution use of paramagnetic contrast agents, increased availability, lack of radiation exposure, and decreasing cost taken into consideration. MRI may progressively become the procedure of first choice over CT scanning.

6. **Magnetic resonance angiography** is a noninvasive method for imaging the carotid arteries and major cerebral blood vessels. The technique is based on phase shift in the velocity of blood flow through the vasculature and can detect atherosclerotic plaques, aneurysms, and dissections. Intraarterial angiography is still superior for detecting aneurysms.

7. **Other noninvasive tests for carotid disease** include oculoplethysmography and pneumoplethysmography, transcranial or external Doppler, and carotid ultrasonography with duplex scanning.

8. **Dacryocystography** is the radiographic evaluation of the excretory system in an attempt to localize the precise **site of obstruction.** The procedure will vary with the radiologist. Water-soluble contrast medium such as cyanographin or salpix is used. The lacrimal irrigation test (secondary dye test) with the patient at an x-ray machine is performed and 1 mL of contrast solution is injected through the lower canaliculus. AP Waters and lateral projections are taken of the excretory system. If both sides are injected simultaneously, a back view should be taken in case the lateral views overlap. The results of radiographic examination will reveal the site of obstruction. This is of particular value in partial or intermittent obstruction, obstruction secondary to trauma, or obstruction associated with diverticulum or fistula. **Contraindications** to the test are radiologic contraindications as determined by the radiologist, acute dacryocystitis, and allergy to iodide.

L. **Anterior chamber aspiration (keratocentesis)**

1. **Indications.** Diagnostic aspiration of aqueous from the anterior chamber is indicated for (a) specific identification of intraocular microbes, (b) identification of inflammatory cell types indicative of disease type, and (c) determination of specific antibodies in the aqueous and comparison of these to serum antibodies against the same antigen in an attempt to localize antigens to the eye.

2. **Technique.** Keratocentesis may be carried out on an outpatient basis in the minor surgery room. A lid speculum is applied and, after a single proparacaine drop is instilled, a cotton-tipped applicator moistened with cocaine 4% is applied for approximately 15 seconds to an area of conjunctiva near the inferior limbus. This area is thereby anesthetized so that it may be grasped firmly with a toothed forceps. A 30-gauge disposable needle attached to a disposable tuberculin syringe is then inserted into the cornea near the forceps with minimum pressure while the examiner slowly turns the syringe barrel back and forth in his or her finger. As the bevel of the needle enters the anterior chamber, the examiner's assistant withdraws the plunger, thereby aspirating 0.1 to 0.2 mL of aqueous. The needle tip is kept over the iris at all times to avoid hitting deeper ocular structures. If the chamber shallows so that the anterior surface of the iris approaches the site of needle penetration, the bevel should be withdrawn and the procedure halted regardless of the amount of fluid withdrawn. At the end of the procedure, antibiotic ointment and cycloplegic drops should be applied, and a light patch put over the eye for a few hours. Keratocentesis is basically painless, although hyphema may develop in patients with neovascularization of the iris; it is, therefore, not recommended in such a clinical situation. There may be a transient increase in IOP for 12 hours after paracentesis, particularly in patients with Behçet syndrome. The etiology of this pressure increase is unknown.

3. **Diagnostic tests.** The aqueous fluid so withdrawn is very limited in quantity; consequently, the clinician should have a clear idea of which tests are desired at the time of the tap so that no fluid is wasted. Tests include bacterial cultures, parasitic or cytologic examination using conventional stains, or fluorescent antibody stains for viruses and dark-field examination for treponemas. Aqueous can be concentrated on a filter disk (Millipore,

Bedford, MA) for electron microscopic examination or prepared by wet fixation for Papanicolaou testing for malignancy. Serologic examination of the aqueous humor is of value if specific antibody is present in the aqueous in higher concentration than in the circulating serum. This finding is indicative of the presence of antigen within the eye; such antigen is most likely the cause of a given disease state, e.g., toxoplasma. Serologic examination must be done in a hospital university research laboratory or by the state laboratory. In case of **endophthalmitis,** aqueous cultures and smears are of **limited use.** Vitrectomy is the diagnostic procedure of choice (see Chapter 9).

2. BURNS AND TRAUMA

Deborah Pavan-Langston

I. **Anterior segment burns** may be chemical, thermal, radiation, or electrical.
   A. **Chemical burns** are the most urgent and are caused usually by **alkali** or **acid. Other forms of anterior segment burns** that should be managed as chemical burns are those due to **tear gas** and **mace.** These are generally thought not to cause permanent ocular damage; however, there have been reports of eyes lost after such burns. Ocular injury from **sparklers** and **flares** containing magnesium hydroxide should also be managed as chemical rather than as thermal burns.
   B. **Pathology of chemical burns.** The most serious chemical burns are produced by alkali material such as lye (NaOH); caustic potash (KOH); fresh lime [$Ca(OH)_2$], i.e., plaster, cement, mortar, whitewash; and ammonia (NH_4), which is present in household cleaner, fertilizers, magnesium OH (sparklers), and refrigerant.
      1. **Alkali burns** are more severe than acid burns because of their rapid penetration, often less than 1 minute, through the cornea and anterior chamber, combining with cell membrane lipids, thereby resulting in disruption of the cells and stromal mucopolysaccharide with concomitant tissue softening. Damage from alkali burns is related more to the degree of alkalinity (pH) than to the actual cation. Permanent injury is determined by the nature and concentration of the chemical as well as by the time lapsed before irrigation.
      2. **Acid burns,** such as those caused by battery acid, industrial cleaner (H_2SO_4), laboratory glacial acetic acid or HCl, fruit and vegetable preservatives, bleach, refrigerant (H_2SO_3), industrial solvents, mineral refining agents, gas alkylation agents, silicone production agents, and glass etching agents (HFl), cause their maximum damage within the first few minutes to hours and are less progressive and less penetrating than alkaline agents. Acids precipitate tissue proteins that rapidly set up barriers against deep penetration by the chemical. Damage is therefore localized to the area of contact, with the exception of burns from hydrofluoric acid or from acids containing heavy metals, both of which tend to penetrate the cornea and anterior chamber, ultimately giving rise to intraocular scarring and membrane formation.
      3. **Mace** (chloroacetophenone) and other **tear gas** compounds are variable in their toxic contents and clinical effects. If sprayed, as recommended, from more than 6 feet away, not directed at the eyes, and at a conscious individual, only minor chemical conjunctivitis occurs. More direct and concentrated spray toward the eyes in a person whose defensive reflexes are compromised will result in severe injury clinically similar to an alkali burn. Mace and other lacrimator ocular burns should be managed in the same manner as alkali burns.
   C. **Classification and prognosis** of the chemically burned eye is most useful for alkali burns, but also extends to acid and toxic chemical injuries of the eye.
      1. Thoft classification includes the following groups. **I.** Epithelial damage, no ischemia, good prognosis. **II.** Cornea hazy, iris detail seen, less than one-third limbal ischemia, good prognosis. **III.** 100% epithelial loss and stromal haze blurs iris, one-third to one-half limbal ischemia, guarded prognosis. **IV.** Opaque cornea, greater than one-half limbal ischemia, poor prognosis.
      2. A **mild** alkali burn will exhibit sluggish reepithelialization and mild corneal haze with ultimate minimum visual handicap regardless of treatment. **Moderately severe** burns take variable courses, depending

31

on the extent of the injury. There may be moderate stromal opacification with increased corneal thickness and heavy proteinaceous aqueous exudation in a markedly hyperemic eye. Superficial neovascularization of the cornea may follow the advancing edge of regenerating epithelium, and there may be persistent epithelial defects that ultimately lead to stromal thinning and perforation. A scarred and vascularized cornea will result in permanent visual impairment. In the most **severe** burns, the corneal stromal integrity may be undisturbed for the first 2 weeks, although anterior iritis may be severe and go undetected. As epithelium begins to heal back across the stroma, ulceration begins and perforation may ensue secondary to the release of collagenases, elastases, and other enzymes from epithelium, polymorphonuclear neutrophil leukocytes, and keratocytes, and decreased collagen synthesis due to severe ascorbate deficiency in alkali-burned eyes.

D. Therapy is classified by time postinjury.

1. **Immediate treatment** for chemical burns is copious irrigation using the most readily available source of water (shower, faucet, drinking fountain, hose, or bathtub). The greater the time is between injury and decontamination, the worse the prognosis. The victim should not wait for sterile physiologic or chemical neutralizing solutions. The lids should be held apart and water irrigated continuously over the injured globe(s). The initial lavage at the site of the injury should continue for several minutes, so that both eyes receive copious irrigation. Orbicularis spasm may make this difficult. Use of a cloth material on the lids will help the irrigator to hold otherwise slippery spastic lids. Skin irrigation may be started simultaneously by pouring water over the affected area, but is unquestionably secondary to ocular lavage.

2. **After the initial lavage,** the patient should be taken immediately to an emergency room with a phone call made ahead so that treatment is waiting by the time the patient arrives. In the emergency room **topical anesthetic is** instilled immediately and q20 minutes to relieve some of the considerable pain, and immediate lavage is begun with at least 2,000 mL of normal saline 0.9% over a minimum period of 1 hour. Lid retractors should be used if necessary. The conjunctival fornices and palpebral conjunctiva should be swept with sterile cotton-tipped applicators to remove any foreign matter that may have been retained at the time of injury. Cotton-tipped applicators moistened with 0.05 mol/L of 10% ethylenediaminetetraacetic acid (EDTA) make sticky CaOH easier to remove. If eversion of upper or lower lids reveals chemical still embedded in the tissue, 0.01 to 0.05 mol EDTA solution should be used as irrigant or the fornices further swabbed with cotton-tipped applicators soaked in EDTA. Careful examination after lavage for perforating ocular injury should be made. *Direct pressure on the globe during lavage should be avoided if ocular global laceration is at all suspected* (see sec. **VI.**, below).

3. **Irrigation should be continued** until pH paper reveals that the conjunctival readings are close to normal (pH between 7.3 and 7.7). Once a relatively normal pH is achieved, the patient should be checked again in 5 minutes to ascertain that the pH is not changing again in the direction of acidity or alkalinity, depending on the nature of the burn.

4. **Medications.** While the pH is being stabilized near normal, the **mydriatic–cycloplegics** atropine 1% or scopolamine 0.25% should be instilled to dilate the pupil and prevent massive iris adhesions to the lens (posterior synechiae) as well as to reduce the pain secondary to iridociliary spasm. After irrigation is complete, **antibiotics** such as ciprofloxacin, ofloxacin, tobramycin, or polymyxin–bacitracin ointment should be started to protect against infection. For alkali or more severe acid burns, there is frequently an **immediate rapid increase in intraocular pressure** (IOP) secondary to shrinkage of the collagen

fibers of the sclera. Carbonic anhydrase inhibitors such as acetazolamide 500 mg intravenously (i.v.) or orally (p.o.) stat., should be given.

5. **For pain,** systemic analgesics should be administered. Oxycodone and acetaminophen (Percocet), one tablet p.o. q3h, or meperidine, 50 to 100 mg intramuscularly (i.m.) or p.o. q4h, is effective.

6. **An emergency complete physical examination** should be done not only by the ophthalmologist, but also by an otolaryngologist and an internist, because many toxic chemicals are aspirated or swallowed at the time of original injury and there may be concomitant chemical burns of the respiratory or upper gastrointestinal tract. During irrigation the examiner should always be aware of the possibility of an **acute obstruction of the airway** secondary to chemical burn, inducing laryngeal edema.

7. **Once the immediate emergency situation is controlled,** the burned eye(s) is patched and the patient is admitted unless the burn is mild, in which case therapy may be done on an outpatient basis with initial frequent office visits. Topical antibiotic ointments and drops should be continued q4h to q6h along with the mydriatic–cycloplegics.

E. **Midterm therapy** is used for several days to weeks immediately postburn.

1. **Elevation of IOP** may be noted and is probably due to prostaglandin release. Long-term elevation of pressure is secondary to scarring of outflow channels. Carbonic anhydrase inhibitors such as acetazolamide 250 mg p.o. qid, ethoxyzolamide 50 mg p.o. tid, or dichlorphenamide 50 mg p.o. tid are usually effective in reducing this pressure and should be continued as long as it is elevated more than 22 to 25 mm Hg. A beta-blocker such as timolol 0.50 bid, an alpha-adrenergic agonist such as 0.5% brimonidine bid, and other IOP-lowering drops (see Chapter 10 and Appendix A) may be added if needed. Glycerol 50%, 40 to 60 mL p.o. q12h may be used as an oral hyperosmotic agent for a few days in patients with severely elevated pressure. Mannitol 20% solution i.v., 2.5 mL per kg, may be given for short-term pressure control in those patients who cannot take oral medication. *Cardiac status* should be ascertained before use of any hyperosmotic agent, and long-term carbonic anhydrase inhibitors (with the probably exception of ethoxyzolamide) should be avoided in patients with a history of *renal stones*.

2. **Topical steroids** such as dexamethasone 0.1% or 1% prednisolone q4h should be used to quiet inflammation but only during the first 7 to 10 days after injury to control anterior segment inflammation. After this period, if the corneal epithelium is not 100% intact, particularly in alkali burns, steroids should be withdrawn because of the increased chance of corneal melting and perforation due to collagenolytic enzyme release. **Systemic steroids** such as prednisone 30 mg p.o. bid may be substituted if iridocyclitis is still uncontrolled.

3. **Ca^{2+} chelators ascorbate or citrate** are important in Grade 3 and 4 alkali-burned eyes. Ten percent citrate and 10% ascorbate in artificial tear solution q2h while the patient is awake for 1 week then qid inhibits polymorph activity and inflammatory chemotaxis and may slow or prevent *melting*. These eyes become rapidly scorbutic, thus interfering with collagen synthesis and leading to ulceration. Ascorbate (vitamin C) 2 g p.o. is also given qid until epithelial tissue is healed. Ascorbate should **never** be used in **nonalkali** burn situations, because ciliary body concentration of the drug will enhance rather than inhibit corneal melting. **Tetracycline** 250 mg p.o. qid also chelates Ca^{2+} and thus collagenase should also be used for several weeks.

4. **Therapeutic soft contact lenses** with high water content (Permalens) may be of great benefit in assisting epithelial healing, which in turn will inhibit enzyme release and stromal melting. The lenses may be placed soon after injury and are generally left in place for 6 to 8 weeks.

5. **Topical antibiotics** (drops if a soft contact lens is in place) should be used several times daily initially and then tapered to qid, and

cycloplegia (atropine, scopolamine) should be maintained as long as there are more than mild cells and flare in the anterior chamber.

6. **Dermal injury** should be cared for with the guidance of a dermatologist.

F. **Long-term therapy** depends on the severity of the burn and may vary from an antibiotic and artificial tears to surgical reconstruction of the eye with conjunctival flaps or transplants, mucous membrane transplants, patch grafts, penetrating keratoplasty, and keratoprosthesis.

II. **Thermal injuries** usually involve injury to the lids. Their treatment is similar to that of thermal injury elsewhere in the body.

A. **A contact burn** of the globe may be mild, such as one caused by tobacco ash, or severe, such as one seen with molten metal, which may produce severe permanent burns of the globe itself. Burns can be caused by glass and iron, which have melting points of 1,200°F. Lead, tin, and zinc melt below 1,000°F. After a molten cast of the eye has been removed from under the lids, a permanently opacified globe is often found underneath. **Sympathetic uveitis** may develop in a nonburned contralateral eye.

B. **Therapy.** For partial-thickness lid burn, topical antibiotic ointment with sterile dressings is used, but with minimum burns no dressing is needed. Frequent saline or lubricated dressing, avoidance of early débridement, topical antibiotic qid, prevention of secondary infection, and protection of the globe are critical factors in successful management. Topical steroids such as dexamethasone 0.1% or prednisolone 1% qid may be used to decrease scarring between the lids and globe (symblepharon formation) if the corneal epithelium is intact. Secondary steroid glaucoma should be checked for periodically. Systemic steroids may be used to control secondary iridocyclitis if topical steroids must be limited because of the severity of the corneal burn.

C. **Exposure therapy.** If the eyelids are burned so severely that there is exposure of the globe, topical antibiotic ointment tid should be placed on the lid and globe, and a piece of sterile plastic wrap placed over this to protect the globe from exposure by forming a moist chamber. This same technique of a plastic-wrapped moist chamber may be used to protect patients with exposure secondary to marked exophthalmos, severe conjunctival hemorrhage or chemosis, or traumatic avulsion of the eyelid. The covering film is cut in 10 × 15 cm rectangular pieces and may be gas autoclaved in individual packages. These pieces are large enough to cover the entire orbit from forehead to cheek. When the plastic wrap is applied, antibiotic ointment is applied to the skin around the orbit, and the sterile film is placed over the area to be protected. The film will adhere to the skin by static charge and by adherence to the ointment.

In mild burn cases where **exposure is minimum** and Bell's reflex (phenomenon) is good so that only the inferior conjunctiva is exposed, antibiotic ophthalmic ointments q4h should suffice to protect the globe until surgical repair, if needed, is possible.

III. **Radiation burns: ultraviolet (UV) and infrared**

A. **UV radiation** is the most common cause of light-induced ocular injury. Sources are welding arcs, sun lamps, and carbon arcs. Ultraviolet burns may be prevented by use of ordinary crown glass, regular glass lenses, or special UV-blocking plastics as they absorb the rays.

1. **After exposure** there is a delay of 6 to 10 hours before the burn becomes symptomatically manifest. **Symptoms** may range from mild irritation and foreign body sensation to severe photophobia, pain, and spasm of the lid.

2. **Examination** will reveal varying lid edema, conjunctival hyperemia, and punctate roughening of the corneal epithelium. This punctate pattern is easily seen with fluorescein staining. Because of high absorption in the cornea, UV light rarely damages the lens and does so only if intensity has been extremely high. This radiation does not reach the retina and therefore produces no deep changes within the eye.

3. **Therapy** is a short-acting cycloplegic drop such as cyclopentolate 1% to relieve ciliary spasm and topical antibiotic ointment or drop. A semipressure dressing with the eyes well closed underneath is left on for 24 hours. The patient in pain may need sedatives and analgesics. The patient should be reassured that damage is transient and that all symptomatology will be gone within 24 to 48 hours.

B. **Infrared burns** are also usually of little consequence and produce only temporary lid edema and erythema, but little or no damage to the globe. Therapy is antibiotic ointment bid for 4 to 5 days after injury. Chronic exposure to infrared light is seen in glass blowers and metal furnace stokers improperly protected by industrial goggles. These workers develop cataracts after many years of exposure, but no other anterior segment changes are found, and the posterior segment is not affected. The mechanization of furnaces has made this problem relatively rare.

C. **Ionizing radiation** from cyclotron exposure and beta-irradiation from periorbital therapy of malignancy are the most common causes of radiation burns. The cornea, lens, uvea, retina, and optic nerve may suffer from injury, but also may be protected from it by use of lead screens and leaded glass to absorb x, gamma, and neutron radiation.

   1. **Signs and symptoms** are conjunctival hyperemia, circumcorneal injection, and watery or mucopurulent discharge. The earliest sign of corneal damage is hypesthesia. Radiation keratitis ranges from a punctate epithelial staining to sloughing of large areas of epithelium, and stromal edema with interstitial keratitis and aseptic corneal necrosis. The minimum cataractogenic dose from x-ray is approximately 500 to 800 rad. The younger the lens, the greater the vulnerability to x-ray. A latency period of 6 months to 12 years exists, depending on dosage, but independent of whether gamma rays or neutrons were the source of injury. The uveal tract may undergo vascular dilation with subsequent boggy edema. Intraretinal hemorrhages, papilledema, and central retinal vein thrombosis may rarely be seen after radiation injury.

   2. **Therapy** of radiation injury is symptomatic. Cycloplegics, such as cyclopentolate 1% or scopolamine 0.1% bid, and topical antibiotic ointments or drops, such as ciprofloxacin, ofloxacin, or gentamicin qid, should be used to reduce the pain of ciliary spasm, to prevent synechia formation, and to protect against infection. Topical steroids are rarely indicated and should not be used in the presence of epithelial ulceration. A **therapeutic soft contact lens** (Permalens) with antibiotic eye drops (ointments dislodge the lens) may assist healing of an epithelial defect.

D. **Solar viewing.** Unprotected viewing of the sun as in a solar eclipse or psychotic state can cause irreversible macular burns via focusing of visible and short infrared rays on this retinal area. An immediate loss of visual acuity may become permanent, or there may be return of vision toward normal. There is no specific treatment, and prophylaxis is the key to prevention, e.g., viewing through treated photographic film or indirect viewing via a series of mirrors in combination with treated photographic film.

E. **Laser burns** of an accidental nature are being seen with increasing frequency with industrial use of these machines. The burns are almost always macular, with instantaneous and usually permanent loss of central vision. Prophylactic wearing of absorbing goggles will protect against indirect laser beam scatter, but only avoidance of direct viewing of the beam will prevent the tragic irreversible and untreatable macular burns.

IV. **Electric shock cataract.** After electrical injury is sustained, particularly around the head, a periodic check for cataract formation through dilated pupils should be made, starting a few weeks after injury. The appearance of characteristic vacuoles is a key prognostic factor. The latency period for cataract formation ranges from months to years.

V. Corneal abrasions and foreign bodies

A. **Traumatic corneal abrasions** result in the partial or complete removal of a focal area of epithelium on the cornea, producing severe pain, lacrimation, and blepharospasm. Motion of the eyeball and blinking increase the pain and foreign body sensation.

   1. **Examination** should be made after a drop of topical anesthetic is instilled. The cornea is inspected under magnification, if possible, using a bright handheld light and oblique illumination. Even without fluorescein dye, a corneal abrasion may be detected by noting that an obvious shadow is cast on the iris from a surface defect illuminated with incident light. Identification of these abrasions, however, is infinitely easier if sterile fluorescein strips or drops are used to dye the tear film. A green dye will be seen wherever corneal epithelial cells have been damaged or lost. The presence of a **foreign body under the upper lid** should always be looked for in the presence of a corneal abrasion (see Chapter 1, sec. **II.D.**).

   2. **Differential diagnosis.** Viral keratitis, particularly that resulting from either **herpes** simplex or herpes zoster, may produce a foreign body sensation associated with lacrimation and blepharospasm. Fluorescein staining of the corneal ulcer, however, will usually reveal a diagnostic branching dendritic ulcer, although a nondescript ovoid or map-shaped ulcer similar to that seen after traumatic abrasion may also be secondary to herpetic infection.

   3. **Treatment** involves the instillation of antibiotic ointment such as polymyxin–bacitracin or gentamicin and a short-acting cycloplegic such as cyclopentolate 1% bid. A moderate, two-pad pressure dressing is then placed over the closed lids of the affected eye for 24 to 48 hours. After removal of the dressing, topical antibiotic ointment or drops two to three times a day should be continued for 4 days after the injury as protection against infection.

B. **Contact lens abrasion.** Acute discomfort caused by a contact lens may be due to a foreign body between the lens and the cornea, improper fit, overwear with secondary corneal edema, or damage to the corneal epithelium on inserting or removing the lens.

   1. **Removal of lens.** If the lens is still in place at the time the patient is seen, **topical anesthesia** should be instilled. A **hard contact lens** is removed with a suction cup apparatus or by sliding the lens to the nasal portion of the bulbar conjunctiva by gently pressing two fingers on the globe through the upper lid just lateral to the contact lens, with the patient looking horizontally toward the side of the affected eye. Once the lens has slid over the nasal conjunctiva, finger pressure is applied through the lids at the lower margin of the contact lens so that the upper lens margin is flipped off the globe. The upper lid margin is then slid beneath the contact lens and the lids allowed to close behind the lens. If the lens slides into the upper or lower fornix, the edge of the lid is simply grasped and the patient is asked to look in the direction opposite from that where the lens is located. The upper lid is pressed gently against the globe to block the lens from sliding up and the edge of the lower lid is then slipped under the edge of the contact lens and the lens flipped out of the eye. **Soft lenses** are pinched off the eye between the thumb and index finger.

   2. **The type of fluorescein staining** of the cornea seen after removal of the contact lens may determine the cause of the abrasion. Diffuse mild central staining and haziness indicate contact lens overwear, that the lens is too tight fitting, or that the lens chemical cleaners were not washed off before insertion of the lens. Small irregular abrasions, usually near the limbus, may indicate difficulties with inserting or removing the lens. Irregular linear scratches on the corneal epithelium are indicative of a foreign body trapped between the lens and the cornea. The lens should be examined to see if there are defective edges, cracks, or foreign bodies on the posterior surface.

3. **Treatment** of **hard contact lens** abrasion is the same as for other forms of corneal abrasions. Contact lens wear may begin again 2 days after the cornea has healed. For **soft contact lens** abrasion, a potential *Pseudomonas* infection must be suspected until proven otherwise. The abrasion should be cultured and treated with tobramycin or ciprofloxacin drops q1h for 6 hours and then q3h while the patient is awake until seen by the physician again the next day. If there is an infiltrate present on the first or follow-up examination, the patient should undergo the same treatment as for central microbial ulcers (bacterial, fungal, *Acanthamoeba*) (see Chapter 5).

C. **Recurrent erosion** (see Chapter 5, sec. **VIII.B.4.**). Fingernail or paper cut injuries to the cornea may lead many months to years later to spontaneous ulceration of the corneal epithelium secondary to imperfect healing of basement membrane. Such recurrent erosions may occur, however, without a past history of injury and result in inherited map-dot-fingerprint dystrophy.

1. **Symptoms.** The patient usually awakens in early morning with severe pain, redness, and lacrimation in the affected eye. Fluorescein staining will reveal a nondescript ovoid or triangular ulcer, frequently with a filament of detached epithelium still clinging to it. There may be superficial corneal edema and haze at the site of the abrasion.

2. **Treatment** of the acute erosion is antibiotic ointment and pressure patching for 24 hours. Over the ensuing 2 to 3 months, copious use of artificial tears q2h to q3h and antibiotic or artificial tear ointment at bedtime should be used in an effort to prevent another erosion by lubricating the interface between lid and corneal epithelium. In severe recurrent cases, constant-wear therapeutic soft contact lenses (Permalens, Kontur) with artificial tears may prove successful in resolving and permanently healing the condition.

D. **Corneal foreign bodies.** Foreign bodies embedded in the corneal epithelium may be single or multiple, and easily seen without magnification or barely detectable with slitlamp examination.

1. **Types.** Bits of rust, windblown dirt, glass fragments, caterpillar hairs, and vegetable matter are the most commonly found foreign bodies.

2. **History.** While taking a history of the origin of the foreign body, it is important to note **if the object was propelled** toward the eye with a force that might cause the examiner to suspect intraocular foreign bodies as well. Hammering steel on steel is one such typical situation. The examiner should also note whether the **accident** occurred during the **course of employment.**

3. **Iron foreign bodies** will frequently form **rust rings,** ring-shaped orange stains in the anterior stroma, that will wash out spontaneously with time, leaving a white, nebulous telltale scar.

4. **Treatment.** After topical anesthetic has been instilled, the corneal foreign body may often be removed with a gentle wipe with a moistened applicator. Foreign bodies embedded somewhat more firmly may often be picked off the cornea with the side of the beveled edge of a No. 18 needle attached to a handle or syringe **(Fig. 2.1).** Alternatively, a "golf stick" instrument may be obtained from a commercial medical supply house. The physician should not be unduly concerned about perforating the cornea when using the **side** of a needle or a golf stick to remove the corneal foreign body, because it takes considerable dull pressure to penetrate the stroma. Direct pressure on the cornea with the end of a sharp instrument is contraindicated. Rust rings may be removed either at the time of the initial scraping or, **if healing does not occur** over the rust ring within a few days, it may be rescraped or removed with a handheld, battery-driven rust ring removal burr. If possible, these procedures should be done under magnification with a loupe or slitlamp.

a. **If multiple foreign bodies** are present in the corneal epithelium, such as after an explosion, undue scarring may occur from attempted

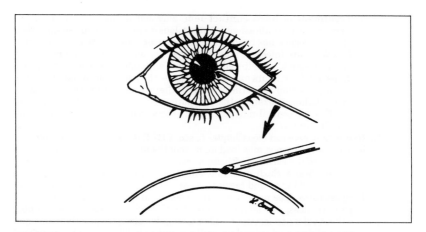

FIG. 2.1. Removal of superficial corneal foreign body. Front and side views illustrate thickness of cornea relative to beveled needle edge. The needle should be moved in a sideways motion to lift or gently scrape off foreign body.

removal of every particle. Most may usually be removed by instilling topical anesthetic and denuding the entire epithelium to within 1 or 2 mm of the limbus with an alcohol- or ether-soaked cotton-tipped applicator. Bowman membrane is thereby spared additional scarring. Limbal foreign bodies may be removed individually leaving an intact rim of corneal epithelium that will provide the source of stem cells from which reepithelialization of the cornea will take place over several days.

b. **After removal of the foreign body or bodies,** a short-acting cycloplegic such as cyclopentolate 1% and broad-spectrum antibiotic ointment such as tobramycin, ciprofloxacin, or ofloxacin should be instilled in the lower cul-de-sac and a moderate pressure patch placed for 24 to 48 hours *(no patch is used for vegetative foreign bodies).* More extensive reepithelialization may take longer to heal, thereby requiring another few days of antibiotic and therapeutic soft contact lens. If penetrating injury is suspected, ointment should not be instilled because the injury may allow it access to the anterior chamber. In this case, a protective metal shield should be placed over the eye and the patient referred for surgical management.

c. **Contraindicated therapy.** It is important to note that **no patient with an acute corneal abrasion or foreign body should be maintained on topical anesthetics.** Topical anesthetics will not only prevent healing, but also will ultimately cause total breakdown of the epithelium, stromal edema, and severe pain, because the anesthetic loses its ability to prevent pain in an eye that has had multiple applications of the drug. Similarly, no eye that has had an epithelial abrasion or foreign body should be treated with a medication containing topical **steroids** because of the greatly increased chance of secondary bacterial, viral, or fungal infection.

5. **Deep corneal foreign bodies** that are suspected of partially penetrating into the anterior chamber should be removed only by an ophthalmologist because there is great danger that an **aqueous leak** will result, with collapse of the anterior chamber. A protective shield should be placed over such an eye and the patient referred for surgical management. *Certain*

deep corneal foreign bodies need not be removed because of their nontoxic nature and because their removal may result in greater scarring than if they were left in situ. These foreign bodies should be buried sufficiently deeply (but not protruding into the anterior chamber) that the epithelium over them heals without difficulty, and the nature of the foreign body should be such that it is inert. An excellent example of this is nonleaded glass, which may be found when a patient has been struck in the glasses, resulting in multiple pieces of shattered glass fragments entering the cornea. Only accessible foreign bodies on the surface should be removed in such a situation. Many such eyes have excellent vision despite an array of inert foreign material scattered throughout the mid- and deep stromal layers of the cornea.

VI. **Corneoscleral lacerations** (see sec. **VIII.H.,** below). Some lacerations are partial thickness, or small, full thickness but self-sealing. If the cornea or sclera has been fully lacerated, the eye will frequently but not always be extremely soft. Intraocular contents may protrude from the wound, making the extent of the injury quite obvious.

   A. **History.** When a perforation or **intraocular foreign body** is suspected, a careful history should be taken to ascertain an exact description of the accident, which may indicate the extent and seriousness of the injury. In children, the most common **causes** of perforating global injuries are knives, pens, pencils, needles, and sharp toys. In adults, industrial accidents are the most common cause of intraocular foreign bodies or global laceration, and include glass fragments, sharp instruments and tools, and small flying metallic and nonmetallic foreign bodies.

   B. **The examination** of the globe should be done most cautiously, with great care taken not to apply pressure that might rupture a partial-thickness laceration or herniate intraocular contents through a full-thickness laceration. If blepharospasm is marked and prevents examination or threatens to herniate intraocular contents, akinesia of the lids may be induced with a **50:50 2% xylocaine–0.75% bupivacaine block.** Subcutaneous (s.c.) and intramuscular (i.m.) anesthetic should be infiltrated lateral to the lateral canthus and just above and below the lateral two-thirds of the orbital rim. The examination should not proceed further without ascertaining visual acuity (at least light perception [LP]) in the affected eye.

   C. **If the wound is large** and if any manipulation in the emergency area may threaten the entire integrity of the globe, **no further examination should be done at this time.** A metallic shield should be placed over the eye and the patient sent to the operating room where, after primary temporary repair, further investigation such as x-ray examination for intraocular foreign body can be carried out.

   D. **Signs of global perforation.** Any one or combination of the following suggests possible perforation of the globe:
   1. Decreased visual acuity.
   2. Hypotony (markedly decreased IOP).
   3. Shallowing or flattening of the anterior chamber or hyphema.
   4. Alteration in pupil size, shape, or location.
   5. Focal iris transillumination.
   6. Corneal, lens, or vitreal track.
   7. Marked conjunctival edema (chemosis) or subconjunctival hemorrhage.

   E. **Perforation may be present even though the eye appears entirely normal.** Any patient with a high index of suspicion for perforating injury should be referred for further evaluation. Similarly, some of the preceding signs, such as lowered IOP, may be present after ocular **contusion without any perforation.** Conjunctival chemosis may also occur without perforation. Anterior chamber shallowing, however, is indicative of an **aqueous leak** through a perforation in the absence of any previous history of disease that might have shallowed the chamber at an earlier time. The instillation of a sterile **fluorescein paper strip** in the lower cul-de-sac will stain the tear film, and any aqueous flow through the cornea will be seen as a bright green stream. Alteration in pupillary shape and location may indicate uveal extrusion through a wound that may not be visible due to posterior location or subconjunctival hemorrhage and chemosis masking the laceration.

F. **Immediate management of global perforation.** After any lifesaving measures necessary to stabilize the patient have been performed, the immediate management of the global injury is as follows:

   1. Determine visual acuity, even if only to ascertain LP or hand motion.

   2. Partial thickness or small, self-sealing full-thickness lacerations should heal with antibiotic ointment and semipressure patching

   3. Full thickness. Tissue adhesive (Dermabond [Ethicon] is not approved by the U.S. Food and Drug Administration [FDA] for ocular use) and a Plano T soft contact lens may seal a small leaking perforation. Use antibiotic (Bausch & Lomb) drops qid and a protective shield until the injury is well healed and the glue dislodges. For surgical cases, place a metal shield over the eye for protection. Cycloplegic or miotic eye drops should **not** be used prior to surgery, because their use may make subsequent repair more difficult or may pull out an iris that is incarcerated in a corneal laceration where it is serving as a plug against a direct opening into the anterior chamber. Topical antibiotics may interfere with cultures taken in the operating room. **No ointments** should be instilled in any eye suspected of having an open wound because ointment may enter the open globe and be irretrievable.

   4. Nausea or vomiting should be suppressed by immediate administration of antiemetics. Any Valsalva maneuver will raise the IOP and thus threaten prolapse of intraocular tissue through the wound.

   5. The patient should not be given anything to eat or drink in anticipation of administration of general anesthesia in the immediate future.

   6. Appropriate sedatives and analgesics as well as **tetanus antitoxin** should be administered.

   7. Obtain appropriate x-rays, ultrasound, computed tomography (CT) scan, and magnetic resonance imaging (MRI) (as indicated in Chapter 1).

G. **Ultimate therapy is surgical repair** under general anesthesia. *Cultures* should be taken in the operating room. Depending on the extent of injury *systemic antibiotic treatment* i.v. may be started as in endophthalmitis (see Chapter 9, sec. **XII.,** and Appendix B) using an aminoglycoside and cephalosporin or, in penicillin-allergic patients, vancomycin replaces cephalosporin. Broad-spectrum topical antibiotics are used q1h to qid as indicated along with a cycloplegic agent (scopolamine). Steroids are used only after infection risk is reduced.

VII. **Intraocular foreign bodies** must always be ruled out whenever periorbital ocular tissue damage or wounds are apparent.

A. **History.** At the time the patient first comes to the emergency area, the physician should ascertain the circumstances of the injury, particularly, how it occurred: Was the patient at work? Were safety glasses in place? Had the patient been drinking? The timing of events is important in that the physician must know the exact time of injury and what activities occurred after the injury, particularly those that might have resulted in increased IOP, such as the lifting of heavy objects. It is also important to note when the patient last ate, because general anesthesia may be anticipated if a perforation is present. The last time the patient had tetanus immunization must be ascertained as well as allergy to tetanus antitoxin in anticipation of the administration of tetanus immunization for injury. The condition of the eye prior to the injury, particularly visual acuity, is critical information, as is the status of the uninjured eye. Questions pertinent to the foreign body include whether it was shot as a missile or simply fell or blew gently into the eye; what its composition is, if known; and if metallic, its magnetic properties. It is also important to ascertain if the foreign body hit the eye as a highly driven missile, what materials were being used at the time, e.g., steel on steel, concrete, wood, brass. Intracranial extension of the injury must also be considered. **Prognosis** for visual outcome correlates mainly with presenting visual acuity, but also with mechanism of injury, afferent pupillary defect, and vitreous hemorrhage.

B. **Foreign bodies are either metallic or nonmetallic,** with the metallic being divided into **magnetic** and **nonmagnetic** foreign bodies. It is extremely important to note if the foreign body is magnetic because this not only indicates the presence of toxic iron content, but also means that the foreign body is amenable to removal from the eye using magnetic devices. The following table indicates the most commonly seen metallic (in order of decreasing toxicity) and nonmetallic foreign bodies and their toxicities:

Metallic		**Nonmetallic**	
Toxic	*Nontoxic*	*Toxic*	*Nontoxic*
Iron	Gold	Vegetable matter	Stone
Copper (bronze,	Silver	Cloth particles	Glass
brass)	Platinum	Cilia	Porcelain
Mercury	Tantalum	Eyelid particle	Carbon
Aluminum			Some plastics
Nickel			
Zinc			
Lead			

It is obvious that every effort should be made to locate and remove those intraocular foreign bodies that have toxic potential. Iron and copper (bronze and brass alloys) can cause electroretinogram (ERG) changes and consequent siderosis (iron deposition in intraocular epithelial cells such as retinal pigment epithelium [RPE]) or chalcosis (copper deposition in basement membranes such as lens capsule or Descemet's membrane). Foreign bodies that are nontoxic may be left in place if their removal would be so difficult that damage to the eye would be greater from surgical manipulation than from leaving them in place.

C. **Techniques by which foreign bodies may be located** include magnified view of the anterior segment, ophthalmoscopy of the posterior segment, x-ray, ultrasound, CT scan, and MRI **(if metal is nonmagnetic).** The first three may be carried out by the emergency room physician. Radiologic views most useful for intraocular foreign body location are the **Waters view,** which moves the shadow of the petrous pyramid away from the region of the eyeball, and Bellow modified lateral view, which superimposes only the shadow of the lateral orbital wall onto the area of the eyeball. Bone-free projections of the anterior segment should be taken using dental x-ray film if an anterior segment foreign body is suspected (see Chapter 1 for the roles of ultrasound, CT scan, and MRI). The physician should be present during any radiologic procedures or communicate ahead of testing because a radiologist or a radiologic technician might be unaware of the potential dangers involved in certain manipulations of the patient that might produce undue pressure on the globe.

D. **The sizes of retained foreign bodies** vary, with the smallest foreign body that may enter an eye being $0.25 \times 1 \times 1$ mm in size and the largest being $3 \times 3 \times 3$ mm and 500 mg in weight. Any foreign body larger than this will usually destroy the globe. Frequently, direct visualization of the foreign body by slitlamp or ophthalmoscopy may be successful; however, hemorrhage or cataract formation may obscure the examiner's view, leaving x-ray, CT, or MRI techniques (see Chapter 1) the only alternatives for locating the foreign body. The decision as to whether a foreign body should be removed from the globe should be made before the particle becomes encapsulated by fibrous tissue. This process of encapsulation takes a few days, however, thereby giving the physician sufficient time to perform necessary diagnostic tests.

E. **Intraocular foreign bodies are retained at different sites** with varying frequencies: in the anterior chamber, 15%; in the lens, 8%; in the posterior segment, 70%; and in the orbit (double perforation), 7%. The eye should be examined for multiple foreign bodies, and the examiner should not be satisfied with the detection of a single foreign body in any one of these sites, although a single foreign body is certainly sufficient grounds for immediate referral for surgical management.

F. **Immediate management** is the same as for global perforation (see sec. **VI.F.,** above).

VIII. **Contusion injuries of the anterior segment.** A direct blow to the eye by a blunt missile such as a clenched fist, squash ball, or champagne cork may produce any one or a combination of the following injuries: hyphema (blood in the anterior chamber), dislocation of the crystalline lens, blowout fracture of the orbital floor or nasal wall, iridodialysis (rupture or tear of the iris from its base on the ciliary body), traumatic pupillary mydriasis (dilation), or traumatic iritis. The most common finding, **subconjunctival hemorrhage,** is the only one of little to no consequence. It requires no treatment and will resolve over 1 to several weeks.

A. **Traumatic hyphema** may be very mild and detectable only with slitlamp examination (microscopic hyphema), revealing multiple red cells floating in the aqueous, or may be severe, with filling of the entire anterior chamber with blood to produce the "eight-ball hemorrhage" and acute secondary glaucoma. Ten percent to 30% of untreated hyphemas rebleed 2 to 5 days after injury when the clot is lysing. Microscopic hyphemas rarely rebleed. Of those eyes that do have a secondary or initial total hyphema, 20% to 50% will end up with visual acuity of 20/40 or less. Approximately 5% to 10% of traumatic hyphemas require surgical intervention, and 7% of patients with a history of such hyphema develop glaucoma in later years, particularly if there has been a recession or partial rupture and posterior dislocation of the iris angle. Dislocation of the lens and vitreous hemorrhage occur in approximately 8% of cases. Retinal hemorrhage occurs in 50% of cases.

1. **Signs and symptoms.** The patient will frequently present with a history of trauma to the eye. Examination may reveal marked decrease in vision with red cells present diffusely throughout the anterior chamber **(microhyphema),** a settled layer of blood present inferiorly, or a complete filling of the anterior chamber so that no posterior segment structures can be seen with the ophthalmoscope. *IOP* may be *increased* due to interference with aqueous drainage by the blood, or the eye may be soft due to decreased aqueous production secondary to ciliary body trauma. Gonioscopy or scleral depression should be avoided. The pupil is often irregular and poorly reactive. Traumatic hyphemas, regardless of severity, are frequently accompanied by such marked *somnolence,* particularly in children, that the examining physician may suspect neurologic complication. The hyphema alone may be sufficient cause for this somnolence, although the presence of concussion or more severe neurologic damage must always be considered.

2. **Therapy.** Cooperative patients with micro or small hyphemas are seen daily for 5 to 10 days to check for glaucoma, vision drop, corneal staining, and rebleed. Treatment is cycloplegia (atropine 1% tid) to the affected eye, antibiotic as indicated qid, steroid drop tid, a shield, and moderate restriction of activity. Uncooperative or unreliable adults or children ideally should be hospitalized for 5 days after the initial bleed. Daily examination under magnification and determination of IOP are important for detecting rebleeding or increase in IOP that may result in iron staining of the cornea. The patient should be on bed rest with bathroom privileges, have his or her head positioned at 30 degrees, and wear a shield (no patch) on

the affected eye. Atropine 1% tid cycloplegia of the affected eye will prevent contraction of the ciliary body and pupil, and subsequent disruption of recently diffusely damaged vessels. Antibiotics and steroids are similar to outpatient care. **Aminocaproic acid (Amicar),** an antifibrinolytic agent, in dosage of 50 mg per kg p.o. or i.v. q4h to a maximum dose of 30 g per 24 hours for 5 days, may reduce rebleeding. Oral prednisone 20 mg bid may be used in place of aminocaproic acid because rebleed data are similar. **Secondary glaucoma** is treated with oral carbonic anhydrase inhibitors, beta-blockers, alpha-adrenergic blockers, and other nonmiotic pressure-lowering drugs (see Appendix A and Chapter 10). IOP may increase during clot lysis or later from red cell debris (erythroclastic glaucoma). Treatment is as for secondary glaucoma (Chapter 10, sec. **XVII.**).
3. **African-American** patients should have sickle cell screening because they may develop optic atrophy after mild increase in IOP over 24 hours. **Hyperosmotic agents** are **contraindicated** because they induce vascular sludging.
4. **Rebleeding** occurs in up to one-third of patients, usually between 3 and 5 days after the initial trauma and almost invariably before the seventh day post-trauma. Rebleeding is more frequent in African-American than white patients. A rebleed is almost invariably more severe than the original hemorrhage and the prognosis for reduced vision, **corneal blood staining,** and **secondary glaucoma** is worse. If there is not immediate resorption of the blood, iron pigment will enter the cornea, particularly if IOP is increased. If the corneal endothelium is unhealthy, blood staining will occur even without increased IOP. It will take many months for this pigment to clear. Clearing occurs from the periphery toward the center so that the visual axis is the last to resorb. Blood staining may be a cause of **deprivation amblyopia** in a very young child, and patching the other eye may be necessary after clearing of corneal staining. Elevated IOP is managed by oral carbonic anhydrase inhibitors and topical nonmiotic pressure-lowering drops. If rebleeding does occur during hospitalization, the physician should start counting time again from day zero at the time of the rebleed and keep the patient hospitalized until the hyphema has totally cleared and there has been **no further rebleeding for at least 7 days.**
5. **Surgical intervention** is indicated in 5% to 10% of patients to prevent secondary glaucoma, optic atrophy, and peripheral anterior synechia formation. Blood staining of the cornea occurs in almost all cases of total hyphema if IOP exceeds 25 mm Hg for at least 6 days. Optic nerve damage may be expected with IOPs of 50 mm Hg or more for at least 5 days or 35 mm Hg for 7 days. Patients with sclerotic vascular disease or hemoglobinopathies are at even greater risk due to reduced ocular tolerance of blood flow impairment. Peripheral anterior synechia formation is usually found in total hyphemas lasting 9 days or more.
B. **Air bag ocular injuries** are due to blunt ocular trauma from bag impact and alkaline chemical keratitis from the Na^+ azide gas used to inflate the bag. Most air bag injuries are self-limited, but all should be evaluated and treated as alkali burns and blunt trauma as described in the sections above.
C. **Iridodialysis** is the disinsertion of the iris base from the ciliary body. It is frequently associated with hyphema. Its presence and location should be noted at the time of initial examination. **No treatment is immediately necessary** for this condition. Whether surgical repair will be necessary may be decided when the effect and extent of the iridodialysis on visual acuity are determined after a suitable recovery period.
D. **Traumatic pupillary mydriasis and miosis.** At the time of the initial examination after blunt contusion of the eye, an abnormal mydriasis (dilation) or miosis (constriction) of the pupil may be present. In addition, the pupil may react only minimally or not at all to light and have an irregular shape.

In the absence of a global rupture or perforation, this deformity is indicative of partial or complete rupture of the iris sphincter, and its presence may be permanent or transient, as is the mydriasis or miosis.

E. **Posttraumatic iridocyclitis** is an inflammatory reaction of the iris or ciliary body or both after blunt trauma to the eye. The patient complains of an aching in the eye, and IOP is low normal in the early posttraumatic period. Cells and flare may be seen in the anterior chamber. Relief is achieved by dilation with cycloplegics such as cyclopentolate 1% tid and topical corticosteroids such as prednisolone 1% qid for 5 to 10 days.

F. **Traumatic angle recession** is a separation or posterior displacement of the tissue at the anterior chamber angle at the site of the trabecular meshwork (area of aqueous drainage from the eye). At least 20% of eyes with a history of traumatic hyphema have some chamber angle recession and therefore should be followed periodically for the development of secondary glaucoma. There is no emergency care needed for angle recession (see Chapter 10, sec. **XVII.B.**).

G. **Luxation and subluxation of the lens.** Traumatic rupture of the zonular fibers holding the lens to the ciliary body may occur after blunt trauma.

1. **If more than 25% of these fibers are ruptured,** the lens is no longer securely held behind the iris. There may be deepening of the anterior chamber uniformly or locally resulting from tilting of the lens posteriorly, or the anterior chamber may shallow if the lens moves anteriorly, particularly if **pupillary block** develops, because the lens entirely occludes the pupil, thereby blocking escape of aqueous humor from the posterior chamber. In addition, the **iris becomes tremulous (iridodonesis).** This can be easily detected with the handheld flashlight while the patient moves the eye back and forth.

2. **Subluxation** of the lens should be particularly suspected in patients who have Marfan syndrome, lues, Marchesani syndrome, or homocystinuria.

3. **Emergency treatment** for luxation is necessary only if there is shallowing of the anterior chamber with pupillary block and secondary glaucoma. Treatment is dilation of the pupil with a strong mydriatic cycloplegic such as atropine 4% to break the pupillary block and allow aqueous to escape from the posterior chamber. The patient should then be referred for evaluation for surgical management.

4. **Surgery** is indicated if the lens is entirely dislocated into the anterior chamber where it may compromise the corneal endothelium by direct abrasion. Miotics such as pilocarpine 2% qid will prevent the lens from falling back into the vitreous cavity. Dislocation of the lens into the **vitreous cavity** is **not** an indication for **emergency therapy,** either medical or surgical. Because relief of secondary open-angle glaucoma associated with a vitreous dislocated lens is unreliable using surgical techniques, surgery should be reserved for those cases in which phacolytic glaucoma from hypermaturation of the cataract will predictably relieve the secondary inflammatory glaucoma.

H. **Contusion cataract.** The presence on the anterior lens capsule of a **circle of iris pigment (Vossius ring)** may be noted after pupillary dilation. A Vossius ring is benign in itself, but is diagnostic of previous blunt trauma. Contusion cataracts in the form of anterior cortical vacuoles, anterior nodular plaques, posterior cortical opacification, wedge-shaped and generalized opacification, and total lens swelling may occur as an immediate or long-term result of blunt injury to the eye. Treatment is surgical removal when visual impairment becomes significant.

I. **Scleral rupture.** Intact conjunctiva may mask a significant scleral rupture. The most **common sites of rupture** after blunt trauma are in a circumferential arc parallel to the corneal limbus at the insertion of the rectus muscle opposite the site of impact, or at the equator of the globe. The most common site to be ruptured is the supranasal quadrant near the limbus.

1. **Rupture should be suspected** if the anterior chamber is filled with blood and the eye is soft, or if there is marked hemorrhagic chemosis of the conjunctiva out of proportion to other evidence of injury.
2. **Management** is the same as corneoscleral laceration in terms of immediate management, with ultimate therapy being surgical repair.

IX. **Contusion injuries of the posterior segment** (see Chapter 8, sec. **X.** and Chapter 9, sec. **XVIII.**).

A. **Trauma to the choroid.** A typical small choroidal hemorrhage is a round, dark red-blue mound with pinkish edges, located at the equator or adjacent to the disk. It takes many weeks to resorb and leaves areas of pigmentary alteration. Massive subchoroidal hemorrhage is often associated with profound secondary glaucoma. If it is recognized early enough, sclerotomy may be attempted. Choroidal tears appear to result from contrecoup mechanisms producing a yellow-white crescentic scar concentric with the optic disk and usually temporal to it. There may be multiple scars parallel to each other.

B. **Traumatic choroiditis.** Chorioretinitis sclopetaria refers to direct choroidal and retinal trauma from a propelled object wound in the orbital area. A peculiar syndrome secondary to trauma, usually of the perforating type that involves the lens, is **pseudoretinitis pigmentosa.** There is a selective loss of the photoreceptor layer, extinguished ERG, and migration of pigment into the retina.

C. **Ciliochoroidal (uveal) effusion.** There is a collection of fluid in the potential space of the suprachoroid that is external to the main layers of the choroid and ciliary body and internal to the sclera. *Effusion* is considered a better term than *edema* or *detachment* because the fluid is contained within the expansion zone of the uveal tract. Fluid collection is limited anteriorly by the scleral spur and posteriorly by the attachment of the choroid at the optic disk. Where large veins, arteries, or nerves course through the suprachoroid, the lamellae are compacted. Significant landmarks are the vortex veins and the anterior ciliary arteries. There are three types of collections of suprachoroidal fluid according to the clinical appearance: annular, lobular, and flat.

1. **The annular type** involves the ciliary body and peripheral choroid.
2. **Lobular effusions** are hemispheric. Valleys separating them superiorly and inferiorly are created by the vortex veins.
3. **Flat detachments** are most often in isolated peripheral choroidal areas.
4. **A ciliochoroidal effusion** is likely to occur after surgery or trauma and is the second most common lesion of the ciliary body to be confused with malignant melanoma. It is difficult to differentiate ring malignant melanoma from annular choroidal detachment. Acute myopia may develop from ciliary body effusion. Whenever suprachoroidal edema develops without clear traumatic or surgical antecedent, a systemic or focal vascular disease, inflammatory focus, or malignancy must be considered. Scleritis sufficient to produce suprachoroidal edema need not cause signs of choroidal inflammation. Suprachoroidal effusion has been seen in toxemia of pregnancy and can be treated by treating the general disorder. A positive phosphorus-32 test may be obtained. Provided that retinal detachment does not result, the prognosis in suprachoroidal effusion from inflammation is good.
5. The **uveal effusion syndrome** may be seen after contusion, intraocular surgery, in chronic uveitis, with arteriovenous fistulas, hypotony or leak, abnormally thick sclera, and idiopathically. Depending on etiology, it is an insidious, progressive, uni- or bilateral, nonrhegmatogenous retinal detachment with dependent fluid, flat peripheral effusion, occasional retinal exudates, and localized areas of RPE hypertrophy and hyperplasia. Treatment is aimed at the specific etiology. The contusion and idiopathic forms respond poorly to steroids, but prostaglandin inhibitors, e.g., celecoxib 200 mg p.o. bid, may be useful.

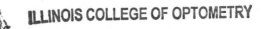

X. Shaken baby syndrome (SBS child abuse) is characterized by traumatic intracranial hemorrhages, occult bone fractures, and retinal hemorrhages in children usually under 3 years old. The damage may be from violent shaking alone, but infants may show signs of impact injury. Other eye findings are extraocular muscle palsies, retinal scars, edema, pigment atrophy, and disk edema. Anterior segments are usually uninvolved. Nonreactive pupils and midline shift correlate with high mortality; ventilation support correlates with poor vision.

3. EYELIDS AND LACRIMAL SYSTEM*

Peter A.D. Rubin

I. **Eyelids.** The eyelids protect the eye by preventing contact with foreign materials and by preventing excessive drying of the cornea and conjunctiva. The palpebral fissure must be wide enough to allow light to enter the pupil and should close sufficiently to provide protection and moisture to the globe. The lid contours and palpebral fissures should be symmetric to avoid cosmetic deformity.

   A. **Eyelid anatomy.** The eyelids are lamellar structures covered on their outer surfaces by skin and on their inner surfaces by conjunctiva. Between the skin and conjunctiva are the fibrous tarsal plates, the orbital septum, the upper lid elevators (levator muscle, levator aponeurosis, and Müller muscle), and the lower lid retractors (inferior rectus fascia and inferior tarsal muscle). The levator muscle is innervated by the third cranial nerve, whereas Müller muscle and the inferior tarsal muscle are innervated by sympathetic nerves. The lids and palpebral fissures are maintained in a stable position by periosteal attachments provided by the medial and lateral canthal tendons. The palpebral fissure is closed by the orbicularis muscle, which is innervated by the seventh cranial nerve.

   B. **Congenital and developmental eyelid anomalies**

      1. **Ptosis.** Most congenital ptosis is caused by a deficiency of the striated fibers in the levator muscle. Many cases of congenital ptosis are associated with other developmental abnormalities such as blepharophimosis and epicanthus. Congenital ptosis will be discussed with other eyelid malpositions (see sec. **I.C.1.**, below).

      2. **Blepharophimosis and epicanthus.** Blepharophimosis is a generalized narrowing of the palpebral fissure. This abnormality is frequently associated with congenital ptosis and epicanthus. Epicanthus is a semilunar fold of skin that crosses the medial canthus. Blepharophimosis and epicanthus should usually be repaired prior to surgical correction of ptosis.

      3. **Colobomas** are usually full-thickness defects in the medial portions of the upper lids. Colobomas are often associated with other congenital defects such as facial dermoids. Unless exposure keratopathy occurs, surgical repair of most colobomas can be delayed until the child is several years old.

      4. **Ankyloblepharon** is an abnormal fusion of the upper and lower eyelid margins, usually near the lateral canthus. The fused lids may be surgically divided if the attachment is cosmetically disfiguring.

      5. **Ectropion and entropion** are both uncommon congenital disorders (see secs. **D.** and **E.**, below). Congenital ectropion is usually minimal and may be associated with blepharophimosis. Congenital entropion is quite unusual but is frequently confused with epiblepharon.

      6. **Epiblepharon** is a relatively common condition in which a prominent skin fold is present in front of the tarsus, usually near the medial margin of the lower lid. The lashes may be rotated inward without actual rotation of the eyelid margin (entropion). Surgical correction is seldom required, because epiblepharon usually resolves spontaneously.

   C. Ptosis is a malposition of the upper eyelid in which the lid margin is abnormally low because of insufficient upper eyelid retraction. Evaluation of a patient with ptosis should include measurement of palpebral fissure heights, distance from the pupillary light reflex to the upper eyelid margin (marginal reflex distance and levator function, excursion of the upper eyelid margin from downgaze to upgaze, while fixating the brow in a stable position). Complete ptosis

*Updated from Grove AS. Eyelids and lacrimal system. In: Pavan-Langston D. *Manual of ocular diagnosis and therapy,* 4th ed. Boston: Little, Brown, 1996:45–52.

evaluation should also include assessment of the protective mechanisms of the globe, including Bell phenomenon, corneal sensation, and baseline tear production (Schirmer test). The positions of the eyelid folds and any abnormalities of the extraocular muscles should be documented. The type of ptosis should be carefully established by history, because the treatment of congenital ptosis is usually different from that for acquired ptosis. Both congenital and acquired ptosis must be distinguished from pseudoptosis, a condition in which the upper eyelid appears to be low but lid elevation is adequate. Pseudoptosis of the lid margin may be due to descent of the brows (brow ptosis) or excessive skin and fat of the upper eyelid mechanically lowering the upper eyelid margin (dermatochalasis).

1. **Congenital ptosis** is usually unilateral, although approximately one-fourth of the cases involve both upper eyelids. It may be associated with other abnormalities:
   a. **Blepharophimosis–epicanthus inversus–ptosis syndrome.**
   b. **Marcus Gunn "jaw-winking" syndrome,** a synkinesis in which the ptotic eyelid is elevated with movement of the mandible.
   c. **Extraocular muscle palsies,** particularly those involving the superior rectus and inferior oblique muscles ipsilateral to the ptosis.
   d. **Treatment** of congenital ptosis usually requires resection of part of the weak levator muscle and aponeurosis, or suspension of the lids from the frontalis muscle (brow).

2. **Acquired ptosis** is frequently associated with good levator muscle function and may be categorized according to etiology.
   a. **Involutional** ptosis is the most common ptosis encountered, often involves both upper lids of older patients, and may occur following cataract extraction. This is the most common form of acquired ptosis and is caused by stretching of the levator aponeurosis or disinsertion of the levator muscle from its insertion onto the tarsus.
   b. **Myogenic** ptosis may be associated with a variety of muscular disorders, including myasthenia gravis, oculopharyngeal muscular dystrophy, and progressive external ophthalmoplegia.
   c. **Neurogenic** ptosis can be caused by deficient innervation of the third cranial nerve to the levator muscle or deficient sympathetic innervation to Müller muscle.
   d. **Traumatic** ptosis may result from lacerations of the levator muscle or aponeurosis and may sometimes follow severe blunt trauma with eyelid edema.
   e. **Mechanical** ptosis may be associated with lid tumors such as neurofibromas and may result from scars or foreign bodies.
   f. **Treatment** of acquired ptosis involves correcting the cause of the ptosis, typically repair of the levator aponeurosis (tendon) if possible. If levator function is not good, this involves a larger resection of the levator aponeurosis, including the distal levator muscle; in more severe cases, the levator aponeurosis may be suspended from the frontalis muscle if levator function is poor.

3. **Pseudoptosis** is a condition in which the upper eyelid appears to be abnormally low without insufficiency of the lid retractors. Causes of pseudoptosis include:
   a. Epicanthus and facial asymmetry.
   b. Excessive upper eyelid skin, as found in dermatochalasis (very common).
   c. Contralateral palpebral fissure widening.
   d. Palpebral fissure narrowing associated with adduction in Duane retraction syndrome.
   e. Hypertropia or contralateral hypotropia.
   f. Enophthalmos or contralateral exophthalmos.

D. **Ectropion** is a malposition of the eyelid in which the lid margin is rotated away from the globe. The lower lid is involved much more commonly than the upper lid. Ectropion sometimes leads to exposure keratopathy and conjunctival hypertrophy. Tearing may result from eversion of the lacrimal punctum if the ectropion involves the medial lid.

1. **Congenital ectropion** is quite uncommon, although it may be found with blepharophimosis. Treatment is rarely required because the eversion is usually minimal.

2. **Acquired ectropion** is categorized on the basis of etiology.
    a. **Involutional** ectropion is relatively common and is a frequent cause of tearing **(epiphora)**. This abnormality is caused by attenuation of the lower eyelid retractors, the orbicularis muscle, and the canthal tendons. Treatment involves horizontal eyelid shortening and canthal suspension. If punctal eversion is the most significant feature, conjunctival shortening and a punctoplasty may reduce tearing.
    b. **Paralytic** ectropion usually results from seventh nerve injury, with resulting drooping of the lower lid and widening of the palpebral fissure. Treatment may require tarsorrhaphy, horizontal lid shortening, canthoplasty, or suspension of the upper cheek. A flaccid brow and upper lid may be surgically elevated if they partially cover the palpebral fissure.
    c. **Mechanical** ectropion may be caused by abnormalities that push or pull the lid away from the eye. Treatment usually involves treatment of the underlying abnormality.
    d. **Cicatricial** ectropion occurs when the anterior lamella of the eyelid (skin and orbicularis muscle) is contracted by a variety of possible causes (e.g., burns, tissue loss, traumatic scars, or inflammation). Linear and circumscribed scars may respond to massage or relaxing operations. More extensive cicatricial ectropion usually requires a skin graft.

E. **Entropion** is a malposition of the eyelid in which the lid margin is rotated toward the globe. Entropion is functionally important because inturned lid margins may damage the cornea and produce keratitis or ulceration. Related conditions that should be differentiated from entropion are epiblepharon, trichiasis, and distichiasis.

1. **Congenital entropion** is rare and is usually associated with other abnormalities such as tarsal hypoplasia or microphthalmia. Congenital entropion may be confused with epiblepharon, a mild deformity that usually resolves spontaneously. Depending on severity, this condition may be treated similarly to acquired entropion.

2. **Acquired entropion** is a common disorder that is usually either involutional, as a result of aging, or cicatricial, resulting from tarsoconjunctival shrinkage.
    a. **Involutional** entropion usually involves the lower lid and is caused by degenerative changes similar to those that cause involutional ectropion. With aging, atrophy of the orbital tissues can lead to a relative enophthalmos and a tendency for inward rotation of already attenuated eyelid structures. Treatment should be directed toward correction of those abnormalities that are most prominent. Penetrating pretarsal cautery or three Quickert lid eversion sutures may temporarily correct a moderate entropion, but may be followed by recurrence. Many operations have been devised for correction of involutional entropion. The most physiologic procedures are those that restore the action of attenuated eyelid retractors and that tighten a lax lower lid.
    b. **Spastic** entropion is a temporary or intermittent accentuation of involutional changes caused by irritation and vigorous lid closure. Treatment can be directed toward removing the cause of irritation or treating the underlying involutional abnormalities.
    c. **Cicatricial** entropion is usually the result of tarsoconjunctival shrinkage. This may be caused by a wide variety of disorders, including trachoma, Stevens-Johnson syndrome, pemphigus, ocular pemphigoid, and mechanical, thermal, or chemical injury. Cicatricial changes are often accompanied by trichiasis, reduced tear production, mucosal epidermalization, and punctal occlusion. Treatment may consist of marginal

rotation of the lid margin and grafts of mucosa or other tissue to replace contracted tarsus and conjunctiva.

F. **Blepharospasm** is a disorder of unknown cause that involves involuntary closure of the eyelids. The severity of this closure ranges from mild increased frequency of blinking to severe spasms that completely occlude the eyes. Essential blepharospasm, in which the eyelids are chiefly involved, is distinguished from conditions such as Meige's disease, in which lower face and neck muscles also spasm, and hemifacial spasm, which may be caused by facial nerve compression. Excision of facial muscles (myectomy) and nerves (neurectomy) has been used in the past as treatment for severe cases of essential blepharospasm. Currently, **botulinum toxin injections** are considered the most effective treatment for the majority of patients with this condition. Multiple small amounts of the toxin are injected into the muscles around the eyelids. Blepharospasm is usually relieved within several days, but the effect is temporary and additional injections are often necessary within 3 months. Side effects include ptosis, double vision, and drying of the eyes from inability to close the lids (see Chapter 12, sec. **XII.**).

G. **Eyelash disorders.** The eyelashes normally emerge from the lid margin anterior to the mucocutaneous junction and are directed away from the surface of the eye. In a number of conditions the lashes either arise abnormally posterior or are directed toward the eye (Table 3.1).

1. **Distichiasis** is an abnormality in which extra lashes arise from the lid margin behind the mucocutaneous junction, frequently from the meibomian gland orifices. These lashes are usually small and cause few symptoms, but occasionally they may produce severe corneal damage. Treatment is not required in mild cases. If the eye is being injured, the lashes may be destroyed with cryotherapy, electrolysis, or surgery.

2. **Trichiasis** is an acquired condition in which the lashes are directed posteriorly, toward the surface of the eye. Although the lid margin is not necessarily inverted, trichiasis can occur in association with entropion. Trichiasis often accompanies chronic blepharoconjunctivitis or cicatricial conjunctivitis. Electrolysis is usually effective in treating focal areas of abnormal lashes. Surgical excision of the lashes and replacement with a mucous membrane graft may be used to treat severe cases of trichiasis in which retention of some normal lashes is desired.

TABLE 3.1. DIFFERENTIAL DIAGNOSIS OF EYELASHES DIRECTED AGAINST THE GLOBE

Term	Features
Distichiasis	Eyelashes emerging from meibomian gland orifices
Congenital	Fine pigmented cilia
Acquired	Cilia often nonpigmented, stunted
	Associated conditions: severe ocular surface inflammation, i.e., erythema multiforme major (Stevens-Johnson syndrome); ocular cicatricial pemphigoid; severe, longstanding blepharitis
Epiblepharon	Congenital fold of pretarsal skin applies cilia of normal origin against the globe
Trichiasis	Cilia emerge from their normal anterior lamellar location
	Associated with cicatrizing processes of the conjunctiva
Entropion	Abnormal rotation of the entire eyelid margin toward the globe
	Etiologies: congenital, spastic, involutional, cicatricial

(Updated from Grove A. Lids and lacrimal system. In: Pavan-Langston D. *Manual of ocular diagnosis and therapy,* 4th ed. Boston: Little, Brown, 1996.)

H. **Eyelid tumors.** The first priority in treating any tumor of the eyelids is to establish the diagnosis. Except for inflammatory lesions such as chalazia, any tissue removed from the eyelids should be examined histologically. Treatments such as cauterization that destroy tissue and make histologic evaluation impossible should be avoided. In the case of a small skin lesion, excisional biopsy can be performed with removal of all clinical evidence of the tumor. If a benign tumor is suspected, the margins of the incision may be within 1 or 2 mm of the lesion. If a malignant tumor is suspected, 3 to 5 mm of clinically uninvolved tissue should be removed with the lesion. When a tumor is histologically malignant, the pathologist should be asked to examine all margins of the specimen, including the deep surface, for evidence of tumor that has been cut across. If the tumor is found to have been transected, additional tissue should usually be removed. The management of each kind of tumor should obviously depend on its individual growth characteristics and on the requirements for reconstructing functional eyelids. The most common benign and malignant tumors of the eyelids are listed below:

Benign tumors	Malignant tumors
Keratoses	Basal cell carcinomas
Nevi	Squamous cell carcinomas
Epithelial, sebaceous, and	Malignant melanomas
sudoriferous cysts	Sebaceous cell carcinomas

1. **Basal cell carcinomas** are by far the most common malignant tumors of the eyelids. These tumors most frequently arise on the sun-exposed lower lids and medial canthal areas. Most basal cell carcinomas are nodular with a pearly surface and telangiectatic vessels. Some are flat and leathery and are described as morpheaform or sclerosing basal cell carcinomas. This latter type of tumor is particularly likely to be infiltrative. Treatment usually consists of histologically confirmed surgical excision. Although cryotherapy and radiation are sometimes used to destroy basal cell carcinomas, their use does not provide microscopic confirmation of complete tumor excision. Metastatic spread of basal cell carcinomas is exceedingly uncommon. Concern that the tumors may invade into the orbit occur when the tumor is located adjacent to the bony orbital rim in the region of the medial or lateral canthi, hence it is critical that the deep margins are carefully assessed during the primary excision of these tumors to ensure that the entire tumor is excised.

2. **Squamous cell carcinomas** usually arise among older patients and commonly develop from actinic keratoses. Differentiation from benign keratoacanthomas is sometimes difficult. Treatment of these potentially metastasizing tumors should consist of wide surgical excision that is histologically confirmed to be adequate by careful examination of all margins.

3. **Malignant melanomas** of the eyelids are uncommon and may extend from melanomas of the conjunctiva. These potentially metastasizing tumors may occur de novo or may evolve from preexisting nevi or from areas of acquired melanosis. The histologic feature of greatest prognostic importance seems to be the tendency toward vertical growth (deep invasion below the epithelial surface). Conjunctival melanomas that grow deeply tend to be more likely to metastasize than those that grow peripherally. Complete wide excision is the most common therapy, and radical surgery such as exenteration may be advised if there is extensive conjunctival disease or evidence of orbital invasion.

4. **Sebaceous cell carcinomas** arise most often from the meibomian glands within the tarsal plates. These highly malignant tumors may also develop from the sebaceous glands of the eyelashes, the caruncle, and the eyebrow. Their growth may mimic **chalazia** and the contents of a presumably recurrent chalazion should always be examined histologically. Fat stains

should be performed on fresh tissue whenever sebaceous carcinoma is suspected. These tumors may be multifocal and can spread peripherally by intraepithelial or pagetoid growth. Metastasis and orbital extension frequently occur. Treatment consists of wide surgical excision, with histologic confirmation of complete removal. Because of insidious intraepithelial growth, multiple areas of excision or exenteration may be required.

I. **Eyelid inflammation and degeneration.** The most common inflammations of the eyelids are those involving the lashes and the lid margins (blepharitis) and those that arise within the meibomian glands as an acute lesion (hordeolum) or evolve into a chronic lesion (chalazion). Diffuse inflammatory eyelid atrophy (blepharochalasis) should be distinguished from involutional degeneration of the eyelids (dermatochalasis).

1. **Blepharitis** is the most common inflammation of the eyelid and may present as anterior, posterior, or both forms.

   a. **Anterior blepharitis (AB)** involves the lashes and anterior lid margin. Seborrheic AB shows inflammation and flaking of the skin with oily scruff (cuffing) at the base of the lashes, and often lash loss or misdirected growth. Eczematous AB has dry, roughened, flaking skin with some inflammation, whereas bacterial AB has inflammatory, purulent changes and discharge. The meibomian glands and tarsus are not primarily involved.

   b. **Posterior blepharitis (PB)** is frequently associated with acne rosacea. Malar and nasal bridge skin findings are tiny telangiectasia and often slightly raised, rough macules. Lid margin telangiectasia is common. Meibomitis causes stenosis of the orifices with bloating of the glands beneath the inferior tarsal conjunctiva, injection, and cyst formation. Early on, oil can still be expressed from the glands by pressure on the lids, but chronic meibomitis causes scarring and lid thickening with lash loss, loss of tear film surface oil, and tear film destabilization.

   c. **Treatment** of **AB** *eczematous* and *seborrheic* disease is steroid antibiotic ointment and lid hygiene with warm compresses bid to tid and baby shampoo scrubs with lathered fingertips daily. In addition, antiseborrheic shampoo applied to the scalp qd is useful for seborrhea. Therapy is essentially life-long. *Bacterial* AB is treated with topical antibiotic ointment or drops (bacitracin ointment, Polytrim, drops bid to qid for 10 days) along with warm compresses. Two or three forms of AB may occur together; adjust treatment accordingly.

   d. **Treatment** of **PB** includes lid hygiene plus doxycycline or minocycline 100 mg p.o. qd for 3 weeks, then 50 to 100 mg p.o. qd for 3 months or indefinitely if needed. For pregnant women or children under 10 ears, erythromycin 250 mg p.o. qd may be used instead. The facial rosacea will benefit from the antibiotic, but may need additional treatment with metronidazole 0.75% cream or ointment bid for 6 months to the involved facial area (see Chapter 5, secs. **III.D.3.A** and **VII.H.**).

2. **Hordeolum** is a focal acute infection arising within the meibomian glands or other glands at the eyelid margins. These lesions are commonly caused by *Staphylococcus* and usually respond to conservative therapy. Treatment with warm, moist compresses and topical antibiotics usually produces resolution of the inflammation (see Chapter 5, secs. **III.B.** and **D.**).

3. **Chalazion** is a focal chronic inflammation of a meibomian gland. It is a common disorder that may occur as the result of a chronic hordeolum. Treatment with warm compresses is effective in most cases, with topical antibiotics used to prevent secondary spread of infection. If the lesion fails to resolve with compresses, incision and curettage through the conjunctiva may be necessary in some instances to facilitate resolution of the lesion. Recurrent lesions should be examined histologically because of the possibility that a malignancy such as sebaceous cell carcinoma may be present.

4. **Dermatochalasis** is a redundancy of the skin of the eyelids that is often accompanied by herniation of fat through the orbital septum. This condition usually occurs as an involutional change among older or middle-aged people.

A familial predisposition is common, although there is no sex predilection. The excessive skin may cause a pseudoptosis, although a true involutional ptosis may be present. Treatment is blepharoplasty with optional fat excision and repair of acquired ptosis, if present.

5. **Blepharochalasis,** unlike dermatochalasis, is a very rare condition that results from repeated idiopathic episodes of eyelid edema and inflammation. These acute attacks occur most frequently among younger individuals and are more common among women than men. The inflammation often results in wrinkling of the skin, atrophy of fat, and ptosis. Treatment of acute attacks is usually not necessarily because they are self-limited, although systemic steroids may be of some value. The chronic atrophic changes may respond to blepharoplasty and to repair of the acquired ptosis.

J. **Eyelid trauma.** Injuries to the globe may be relatively occult and may be overshadowed by obvious lid damage. Therefore, the eye should be carefully examined and the visual acuity should be documented before injured eyelids are treated. During lid repairs the globe should be protected to prevent additional injury. The possible occurrence of orbital fractures or of embedded foreign bodies should always be considered. If necessary, x-rays and computed tomography scan may be used to evaluate these possibilities.

1. **Burns** of the lids may be chemical, thermal, or electrical (see Chapter 2, secs. **I.** and **II.**). The first priority is to treat associated ocular injury. Lid retraction and cicatricial ectropion may result from burns and require skin grafting or other surgical repair after a period of time.

2. **Lacerations** of the eyelids may be repaired primarily even as long as 12 to 24 hours after injury, because of their rich vascular supply and the rarity of infections. Treatment should involve minimum débridement and retention of as much tissue as possible. The wound should be explored to rule out foreign bodies, and all tissues should be replaced in their anatomic positions. The tarsus should be separately approximated by sutures tied away from the surface of the eye. Tissue loss can be replaced by lid advancement or a skin graft. When the deep tissues of the upper eyelid are involved by a laceration, the levator aponeurosis should be examined and repaired if it is damaged.

II. **Lacrimal system.** The tear film is composed of mucin, oil, and watery lacrimal fluid. The mucin component is the product of the conjunctival goblet cells, whereas oil is secreted by the sebaceous meibomian glands within the tarsal plates and by the glands of Zeis and Moll, which lie near the lid margins. The bulk of the tear film is made up of lacrimal fluid from the main lacrimal gland and from the accessory lacrimal glands of Krause and Wolfring (see Chapter 1, secs. **II.J.** and **K.** for the **clinical tests** used to measure tear film adequacy, including tests of secretion). The lacrimal secretions are distributed over the surface of the eye by gravity, capillary action, and the eyelids. Tears leave the eye by evaporation and by flow through the lacrimal excretory system, composed of the puncta, the canaliculi, the lacrimal sac, and the nasolacrimal duct.

A. **Lacrimal excretory anatomy and physiology**

1. **Puncta.** The puncta are small openings approximately 0.3 mm in diameter that lie at the edge of each eyelid. Each upper punctum is approximately 6 mm temporal to the medial canthal angle among adults; the lower punctum is slightly more temporal than the upper.

2. **Canaliculi.** The canaliculi are composed of short vertical segments that begin at the puncta, and horizontal segments approximately 8 mm long that empty into the lacrimal sac. The upper and lower canaliculi usually empty into a common canaliculus (sinus of Maier) before communicating with the sac. In approximately 10% of patients, the upper and lower canaliculi open separately into the lacrimal sac.

3. **Lacrimal sac.** The sac is a cystic structure lined with columnar epithelium. The medial canthal tendon passes in front of the sac, and the lacrimal diaphragm and Horner muscle (the deep head of the pretarsal muscle) pass behind the sac.

4. **Nasolacrimal duct.** This duct is a vertically oriented tube that is continuous with the lower end of the sac. It passes through the bony nasolacrimal

canal to drain into the nose beneath the inferior turbinate via the nasal os-
tium. At the junction between the duct and the nasal fossa, a mucosal fold
(valve of Hasner) may be found.

5. **Lacrimal excretion.** Passage of tear fluid from the surface of the eye
through the excretory system depends on the anatomic patency of each segment of the pathways. For fluid to enter the system, the puncta must be
in anatomic apposition to the tear film meniscus on the surface of the eye.
Entrance of tears into the canaliculi is aided by capillary action. Movement
of fluid through the pathways is aided by a **lacrimal pump** mechanism.
This pumping action results from eyelid blinking, during which the muscles
and diaphragm around the lacrimal sac move to create internal pressure
changes and propel tears. The patency and function of the excretory system
can be evaluated by dye tests, irrigation, and dacryocystography.

B. **Congenital and developmental lacrimal anomalies**
1. **Nasolacrimal duct obstruction** is the most common congenital abnormality of the lacrimal system. As many as 30% of newborn infants are believed
to have closure of the duct at birth. This obstruction is usually located at the
nasal mucoperiosteum, near the site of the valve of Hasner. In most cases,
this obstruction is transient, and patency occurs within 3 weeks of birth.
Tears and mucus may accumulate in the lacrimal sac, causing distention of
the sac and sometimes leading to dacryocystitis. Treatment of a distended
sac in an infant consists of sac massage and application of topical antibiotics.
In the absence of an acute infection, if the obstruction is not relieved by the
first birthday, nasolacrimal duct probing and irrigation is usually curative.
2. **Punctal and canalicular** abnormalities include absence, stenosis, duplication, and fistulization. Imperforate or absent puncta can sometimes be
opened by a sharply pointed dilator and a microscope. Fistulas can be surgically excised. Absent canaliculi can be bypassed by performing a conjunctivodacryocystorhinostomy with insertion of a glass or plastic tube into the
nose.
3. **Diverticula** may arise from the lacrimal sac, the canaliculi, or the nasolacrimal duct. These cystic outpouchings may accumulate fluid and therefore simulate a mucocele of the lacrimal sac. They may become infected and
mimic dacryocystitis. Chronic epiphora, however, is usually not a prominent
symptom of diverticula. Treatment is surgical excision.

C. **Lacrimal sac tumors.** Neoplasms of the lacrimal sac are unusual and therefore may go undiagnosed for a long time because they are confused with inflammations and other causes of nasolacrimal obstruction. Tumors of the sac
typically cause **epiphora** with a subcutaneous mass superior to the medial
canthal tendon. Blood may reflux from the puncta and saline irrigation may
pass into the nose, despite a history suggestive of dacryocystitis. Squamous
papillomas are the most common benign tumors of the sac, whereas epidermoid carcinomas are the most frequent malignancies. Treatment of lacrimal
sac tumors usually requires dacryocystectomy. Removal of the medial canthal
tissues and adjacent bone may be necessary to eradicate malignant epithelial
lesions. Lymphoid tumors frequently respond to radiation therapy.

D. **Lacrimal inflammations and degenerations.** Acquired obstructions of the
lacrimal excretory system may result from infections, other inflammations, and
involutional changes.
1. **Dacryocystitis** is an infection of the lacrimal sac that usually results from
obstruction of the nasolacrimal duct. Dacryocystitis usually produces localized pain, edema, and erythema over the lacrimal sac. This clinical pattern
must be distinguished from acute ethmoid sinusitis, although purulent discharge from the puncta almost always indicates an infection within the sac.
Irrigation and probing should usually not be performed during an acute
infection. This disorder usually responds to warm, moist compresses, together with topically and systemically administered antibiotics. A distended
lacrimal sac should be incised and drained only if the infection does not respond to conservative therapy or if an abscess begins to point.

2. **Lacrimal sac obstructions** are uncommon and generally result from dacryoliths. Solid concretions within the sac may be caused by infection with *Actinomyces israelii (Streptothrix)*. Although such infections sometimes respond to irrigation with antibiotics, the sac must frequently be opened and a dacryocystorhinostomy performed.

3. **Nasolacrimal duct obstruction** usually occurs among older individuals and is commonly idiopathic. Most such involutional cases are probably the result of mucosal degeneration with stenosis. The most common sequelae of duct obstruction are epiphora and a mucocele of the sac. Dacryocystitis often follows a chronic mucocele. Probing of obstructed nasolacrimal ducts among adults rarely restores patency. Partial obstruction may respond to intubation of the entire excretory system with Silastic tubing. A dacryocystorhinostomy may be considered in cases in which the canaliculi are patent. Such an operation is usually not indicated unless tearing and mucous discharge are extremely bothersome, or unless the patient suffers repeated attacks of dacryocystitis. It is possible that a duct obstruction may result from a mass within the nose. Therefore, the nasal fossa should always be examined before a dacryocystorhinostomy is performed.

4. **Punctal and canalicular obstructions** may occur in association with conjunctival disorders such as Stevens-Johnson syndrome, pemphigus, ocular pemphigoid, and mechanical, thermal, or chemical injury. Systemic chemotherapy (e.g., 5-fluorouracil or docetaxel [Taxotere]) that is preferentially concentrated in the tear film is caustic to the canalicular epithelium and may result in canalicular or punctal occlusion. Canaliculitis may sometimes result from infections caused by *A. israelii*. Stenotic or obstructed puncta can be dilated and incised if necessary. If canalicular stenosis can be opened by probing, Silastic tubing can sometimes be passed through the entire excretory system into the nose to maintain patency. In cases of complete and irreversible punctal or canalicular stenosis when epiphora is severe, the obstruction can be bypassed by performing a conjunctivodacryocystorhinostomy with insertion of a glass or plastic tube into the nose (Jones tube).

E. **Lacrimal trauma.** Although the lacrimal excretory system may be obstructed by trauma to any of its components, the most common injuries are lacerations of the canaliculi or puncta and nasolacrimal duct obstructions associated with medial orbital fractures (see Chapter 4, sec. **VIII.**).

1. **Lacerations** of the canaliculi usually need not be repaired as emergencies. Because of the rich vascular supply and the infrequency of infections near the eyelids and medial canthus, primary repair can sometimes be delayed for as long as 12 to 36 hours after injury. Such a delay may actually be beneficial because transected canaliculi can occasionally be better identified after a period of time, and because nighttime surgery may be avoided. If only one canaliculus is severed, it should be repaired, but unnecessary damage to the uninjured canaliculus should be carefully avoided. In many individuals, no significant tearing occurs even after complete obstruction or loss of a single canaliculus. A wide variety of sutures, wires, and tubes have been described for the support of lacerated canaliculi during surgical approximation and healing. If possible, these supports should remain within the canaliculus 6 to 8 weeks after injury.

4. ORBITAL DISORDERS*

Peter A.D. Rubin

The orbits are bony cavities located on each side of the nose. Each orbit contains a complex structure of soft tissues including the globe, optic nerve, extraocular muscles, fat, fascia, and vessels. Orbital disorders are associated with a wide variety of local and systemic diseases, and their treatment requires a thorough knowledge of regional anatomy, radiology, neurology, and endocrinology.

    I. Orbital anatomy. Each bony orbit is pear-shaped, tapering posteriorly toward the apex and the optic canal. The medial orbital walls are nearly parallel and are approximately 25 mm apart in the average adult, whereas the lateral orbital walls are perpendicular.

        A. Orbital walls. The surfaces of each orbit (roof, lateral wall, medial wall, and floor) are composed of seven bones: ethmoid, frontal, lacrimal, maxillary, palatine, sphenoid, and zygomatic. The thinnest of these surfaces are the lamina papyracea over the ethmoid sinuses (along the medial wall) and the maxillary bone over the infraorbital canal (along the orbital floor).

        B. Orbital apertures

            1. The ethmoidal foramen is located in the medial orbital wall, at the junction of the ethmoid and frontal bones, through which pass the anterior and posterior ethmoidal arteries.

            2. The superior orbital fissure is located between the greater and lesser wings of the sphenoid, through which pass most of the orbital veins, some sympathetic fibers, the third, fourth, and sixth cranial nerves, and the ophthalmic division of the fifth cranial nerve.

            3. The inferior orbital fissure is located at the lower portion of the orbital apex, through which pass some orbital veins, the zygomatic nerve, and the maxillary division of the fifth cranial nerve.

            4. The zygomaticofacial and zygomaticotemporal canals are located in the lateral orbital wall, through which pass vessels and branches of the maxillary nerve.

            5. The nasolacrimal canal is formed by the maxilla and lacrimal bone, through which passes the nasolacrimal duct between the lacrimal sac and the inferior nasal meatus.

            6. The optic canal is located in the lesser wing of the sphenoid, through which pass the optic nerve, the ophthalmic artery, and sympathetic nerves. This canal is 5 to 10 mm long and is separated from the superior orbital fissure by the bony optic strut. The orbital end of the canal is the optic foramen, which normally measures 6.5 mm or smaller in diameter.

    II. Orbital evaluation (see Chapter 1, II,J,K). The evaluation and diagnosis of an orbital abnormality is guided by considering the most common disorders that occur among children and adults (see sec. **III.**, below). A clinical history should include questions about the presence of malignant tumors or thyroid disease that might involve the orbit. Evaluation of the orbits should be preceded by a careful ophthalmic examination.

        A. X-rays provide a simple method of studying the orbital bones, but their use is limited because of poor soft tissue definition.

        B. Ultrasonography is a sensitive technique for evaluating intraocular details and for visualizing many orbital lesions. However, the sound waves cannot penetrate bone, and some orbital masses may not be detected unless

---

*Updated from Grove AS. Eyelids and lacrimal system. In: Pavan-Langston D. *Manual of ocular diagnosis and therapy*, 4th ed. Boston: Little, Brown, 1996:45–52.

the waves strike a perpendicular surface. This is occasionally a helpful adjunctive imaging modality. Color Doppler, a specialized type of ultrasound permits detection of blood flow, which is useful in the assessment of vascular orbital lesions.

C. **Computed tomography (CT)** uses thin x-ray beams to obtain tissue density values, from which detailed cross-sectional images of the body are produced by a computer. Newer, rapid spiral CT permits acquisition of an orbital CT in less than 30 seconds. These continuously acquired scans (spiral CT) can be reformatted with minimal artifact, thus obviating the need for both direct and axial scans. CT simultaneously visualizes orbital and intracranial structures including soft tissues, bones, and many foreign bodies. Vessels may be seen most clearly after intravenous injection of contrast material. CT is the most useful single imaging technique for orbital evaluation.

D. **Magnetic resonance imaging (MRI)** is a method of visualizing thin anatomic sections by exposing patients to a magnetic field and then recording the radiofrequency emissions from protons (which are the nuclei of hydrogen atoms). The advantages of MRI include the lack of ionizing radiation (as used in x-rays and CT) and the ability to distinguish among certain vascular and neurologic abnormalities. A disadvantage is that bone does not give magnetic resonance signals; therefore most orbital lesions may be better evaluated by CT scans. MRI is the imaging modality of choice if one needs to assess intracranial disease or one is assessing pathology and the cranioorbital junction (e.g., optic nerve tumors). Magnetic resonance angiography provides a noninvasive view of vascular anomalies.

E. **Arteriography** is performed by injection of radiopaque dye into the carotids to visualize the orbital and intracranial arteries. It has a low, but significant, risk of serious neurologic and vascular complications. Maximum information can be obtained from arteriography through the use of selective internal and external carotid injections, magnification, and radiographic subtraction.

III. **Incidence of orbital abnormalities.** It is useful to group orbital disorders into those that most commonly occur during childhood through the second decade of life, and those that are found predominantly among adults.

A. **Common orbital abnormalities among children**
   1. Orbital cellulitis.
   2. Idiopathic inflammation ("pseudotumor").
   3. Dermoid and epidermoid cysts.
   4. Capillary hemangioma.
   5. Lymphangioma.
   6. Rhabdomyosarcoma.
   7. Optic nerve glioma.
   8. Neurofibroma.
   9. Leukemia.
   10. Metastatic neuroblastoma.

B. **Common orbital abnormalities among adults**
   1. Thyroid eye disease.
   2. Idiopathic inflammation ("pseudotumor").
   3. Metastatic neoplasms.
   4. Secondary neoplasms.
   5. Cavernous hemangioma.
   6. Lymphangioma.
   7. Lacrimal gland tumors.
   8. Lymphoma.
   9. Meningioma.
   10. Dermoid and epidermoid cysts.

IV. **Exophthalmos** is one of the most common clinical manifestations of an orbital abnormality. *Exophthalmos* is defined as an abnormal prominence of one or both eyes, usually resulting from a mass, a vascular abnormality, or an inflammatory process. Among adults, the usual distance from the lateral orbital rim to the corneal apex is approximately 16 mm; it is uncommon for a cornea to protrude more than 22 mm beyond the orbital rim. **An asymmetry of more than 2 mm between the eyes is suggestive of unilateral exophthalmos.**

A. **Unilateral exophthalmos** among children is most commonly caused by orbital cellulitis as a complication of either ethmoid sinus disease or a respiratory infection. Among adults, prominence of one eye is most commonly due to thyroid eye disease.

B. **Bilateral exophthalmos** among children may be caused by leukemia or by metastatic neuroblastoma. Among adults, bilateral exophthalmos is most often caused by thyroid eye disease.

C. **Pseudoexophthalmos** is either the simulation of an abnormal prominence of the eye or a true asymmetry that is not caused by a mass, a vascular abnormality, or an inflammatory process. Causes of pseudoexophthalmos are as follows:

1. Enlarged globe.
   a. Myopia.
   b. Trauma.
   c. Glaucoma.
2. Asymmetric orbital size.
   a. Congenital.
   b. Postradiation.
   c. Postsurgical.
3. Asymmetric palpebral fissure.
   a. Contralateral ptosis.
   b. Lid retraction.
   c. Facial nerve paralysis.
   d. Lid scar, ectropion, entropion.
4. Extraocular muscle abnormalities.
   a. Postsurgical muscle recession.
   b. Paralysis or paresis.
5. Contralateral enophthalmos.
   a. Contralateral orbital fracture.
   b. Contralateral small globe.
   c. Contralateral cicatricial tumor (especially metastatic breast carcinoma). *Even if a patient is found to have pseudoexophthalmos, it is appropriate to examine the orbits carefully and possibly to obtain an orbital CT to serve as a reference for future examinations.*

V. **Orbital inflammations.** Inflammations of the orbit are responsible for more cases of exophthalmos than are neoplasms. Among adults, thyroid eye disease causes more unilateral and bilateral exophthalmos than any other disorder. Among children, orbital cellulitis probably produces exophthalmos more often than any neoplasm. Pseudotumors are idiopathic inflammations that resemble neoplasms and are often associated with exophthalmos and pain. The orbit is a common site of occurrence for a wide variety of other inflammatory disorders related to infections, trauma, and systemic disease.

A. **Thyroid eye disease or ophthalmic Graves' disease** has been defined as multisystem disease of unknown etiology characterized by one or more of three pathognomonic clinical entities: hyperthyroidism with diffuse thyroid hyperplasia, infiltrative dermopathy, and infiltrative ophthalmology. Histopathologic changes seen within the orbital tissues, which are not diagnostic include: a polytypic infiltrate, increased fibroblastic activity, glycosaminoglycan deposition, edema, and fibrosis.

1. **Ophthalmic Graves' disease** includes any of the orbital manifestations of this disorder. Thyroid eye disease appears in 30% to 70% of patients with Graves' thyroid disease. Females are affected approximately four times more commonly than males. Orbitopathy may appear before, during, or after thyroid disease and is directly correlated with the level of endocrine dysfunction. Up to 25% of patients present initially to an ophthalmologist prior to detection of systemic disease. The most common finding

among patients with thyroid eye disease is widening of the palpebral fissure, termed lid retraction. Lid "lag," or upper eyelid trailing behind the globe on downgaze, is another subtle finding of thyroid eye disease. The orbitopathy seems to be most severe in patients who are smokers, thus patients with signs of orbitopathy are given yet another compelling reason to eliminate smoking. The defining features on the clinical examination include: proptosis, eyelid retraction, restrictive myopathy with diplopia, and compressive optic neuropathy.

2. The **orbitopathy** exhibits great heterogeneity and has been subclassified:

Type I orbitopathy
Symmetric proptosis
Symmetric eyelid retraction
Minimal orbital inflammation
Minimal extraocular muscle (EOM) inflammation/restriction
Occurs more often in women
EOM moderately or diffusely enlarged

Type II orbitopathy
EOM myositis
Restrictive myopathy
Hypotropia, esotropia
Compressive neuropathy
Incidence in males similar to that in females

3. **Thyroid tests** are usually abnormal among 90% of patients with ophthalmic Graves' disease. Some patients, however, will be euthyroid by all tests, so that the diagnosis of Graves' disease is established by clinical features alone.

   a. **Initial screening tests.** Thyroid stimulating hormone is the single best screening test to evaluate for Graves' disease. Effected patients will typically have abnormally low levels.

4. **Anatomic tests** allow the clinician to visualize characteristics, but not pathognomonic changes in orbital anatomy with Graves' disease.

   a. **CT** shows enlarged EOM, typically sparing the tendons. The inferior rectus muscle is most commonly involved, followed by the medial rectus and superior rectus. It is rare to see lateral rectus enlargement alone in the setting of thyroid eye disease.

5. **Treatment.** Most patients can be effectively managed with local measures including: lid taping, lubrication, and sunglasses. Medical antiinflammatory treatment (prednisone) is reserved for more severe cases of inflammation or optic neuropathy, and should be viewed as a temporary modality (<6 weeks). For patients who initially respond to steroids, but cannot be successfully tapered, low-dose radiotherapy should be contemplated. *Surgery* is ideally pursued when the patient exhibits clinical stability for greater than 6 months. However, in case of severe inflammation or optic neuropathy, surgery may need to be performed more urgently. The order of surgery is orbital decompression (expansion of the bony orbit) to reduce proptosis and decrease orbital apical congestion, followed by strabismus surgery to address the restrictive strabismus and diplopia, followed by eyelid surgery to address eyelid retraction and secondary ocular surface exposure, as well as to improve the cosmetic appearance of the eyelids. The surgery needs to be tailored to the individual needs of the patient.

B. **Pseudotumors (pseudotumor oculi).** Orbital inflammations of unknown etiology are collectively described as pseudotumors. Patients with pseudotumors typically have orbital pain, exophthalmos, restricted eye movement, and impaired vision.

   1. **Tolosa-Hunt syndrome** is a variant of pseudotumor in which a steroid-sensitive granuloma is localized either in the cavernous sinus or near the

superior orbital fissure and optic canal. Gnawing pain may precede the ophthalmoplegia. The bilateral orbital inflammation among adults increases the likelihood of a systemic vasculitis or lymphoproliferative disorder (see Chapter 9 for immune vasculitis workup). Among children, however, nearly one-half of the cases of orbital pseudotumor are bilateral and few are associated with systemic disease.

2. **Treatment.** Oral steroids usually produce rapid and dramatic resolution of pseudotumor symptoms. Despite an initial excellent response to steroid therapy, patients should be slowly tapered off of steroids over 4 to 6 weeks to prevent recurrence of the inflammation. In patients with recurrent or recalcitrant inflammation, a systemic work-up and orbital tissue biopsy may be indicated to search for a more specific cause of the inflammation (e.g., Wegener granulomatosis). Non-specific, steroid-dependent inflammations tend to respond well to low dose orbital irradiation. Although pseudotumors can simulate neoplasms, secondary inflammatory responses caused by actual tumors can also subside after steroid therapy.

C. **Cellulitis.** Orbital cellulitis is probably the most common cause of exophthalmos in early childhood and is usually the result of extension of infection from the adjacent sinuses (see Table 4.1).

1. **Clinical signs** of orbital cellulitis include fever, pain, soft tissue edema, and restricted eye movements. Orbital CT usually shows opacification of the involved sinus without bone destruction.

2. **The most common organisms** that cause orbital cellulitis are *Staphylococcus aureus, Streptococcus,* and *Haemophilus influenzae.* Cavernous sinus thrombosis can very rarely result from cellulitis and is usually manifested by ophthalmoplegia with pupillary abnormalities and by the development of diffuse neurologic disturbances.

3. **Treatment.** Cultures should be obtained from the nasopharynx and conjunctiva. Initial treatment consists of systemic administration of penicillinase-resistant drugs such as methicillin or other appropriate antibiotics (see Appendix B). Surgical drainage of the affected sinus should be deferred if possible until the acute inflammation has subsided. Orbital surgery is not necessary unless an abscess cavity is present. If cavernous sinus involvement is suspected, a lumbar puncture may reveal acute inflammatory cells and may yield a positive cerebrospinal fluid (CSF) culture.

TABLE 4.1. CAUSATIVE ORGANISMS OF ORBITAL AND PERIORBITAL INFECTION

Bacteria	Viral
In adults: Staphylococci, Streptococci, anaerobes; Gram-negative rods occur less commonly In children: adult forms plus *Hemophilus influenzae* Rare: tuberculosis, Lyme disease; syphilis	Herpes simplex (usually limited to the eyelids and cornea) Herpes zoster (usually limited to the skin, but may affect the optic nerve and ciliary ganglion) Adenovirus, Epstein-Barr virus, mumps (may present as a viral dacryoadenitis) Molluscum contagiosum

Fungi	Parasites (rare in the United States)
Aspergillus *Rhizopus* sp. (*Mucor*) *Cryptococcus* (spread from meninges along optic nerve sheath) Other	*Echinococcus* *Taenia solium*

D. **Phycomycosis.** The most common and most virulent fungal diseases involving the orbit are caused by organisms of the class Phycomycetes.

   1. **The most common fungal genera** causing phycomycosis are *Mucor* (mucormycosis) and *Rhizopus*. These fungi usually extend from the sinuses or the nasal cavity and commonly grow among patients with metabolic acidosis and disabling systemic illness. The most common factors that predispose to such infections are diabetes, renal failure, malignant tumors, and therapy with antimetabolites or steroids.

   2. **Treatment.** Diagnosis is made by biopsy of the involved tissues and the finding of nonseptate branching hyphae. Any underlying metabolic abnormality should be corrected, if possible. Infected tissues should be surgically excised and appropriate antibiotics used to control growth of the fungi (see Table 9.7).

VI. **Orbital tumors**

A. **Dermoids, epidermoids, and teratomas.** These tumors, most of which are benign, are usually considered to be developmental growths (choristomas) rather than neoplasms. Although choristomas are usually cystic, a solid component is often present and the lesions may be completely solid.

   1. **Dermoids** contain one or more dermal adnexal structures such as hair follicles and sebaceous glands. The cystic component is lined with keratinizing epidermis. Treatment is surgical excision, with special care to avoid leaving potentially irritating cyst contents within the orbit.

   2. **Lipodermoids** are solid tumors usually found beneath the conjunctiva adjacent to the superior temporal quadrant of the globe. Unless these lesions enlarge dramatically, they should be observed without surgery, because excision may be complicated by ptosis, restricted ocular motility, or damage to the globe.

   3. **Epidermoids** contain epidermal tissues without adnexal structures. These lesions are almost always cystic, in which case the cavity may contain cholesterol crystals and epithelial debris such as keratin. Treatment is surgical excision.

   4. **Teratomas** are rare tumors that arise from multiple germinal tissues including ectoderm and either endoderm or mesenchyme or both. Although exenteration is sometimes performed because of fear of malignancy, cystic teratomas can sometimes be removed with preservation of the eye.

B. **Vascular tumors.** Hemangiomas and lymphangiomas are usually considered to be developmental growths (hamartomas) rather than neoplasms. Hemangiomas are among the most common benign tumors of the orbit and can be grouped into two major types: capillary hemangiomas (occurring among children) and cavernous hemangiomas (occurring among adults).

   1. **Capillary hemangiomas** usually arise as enlarging red nodules during the first month after birth. The skin near the eyelids is often dimpled and elevated, accounting for the description of "strawberry birthmark." Because spontaneous regression and disappearance usually follow initial growth, treatment is usually not necessary. Marked refractive errors may be associated with eyelid and orbital hemangiomas among children, and efforts should be made to combat amblyopia. If significant ocular dysfunction or cosmetic deformity occurs, tumor size may be reduced by steroid injection, low-dose radiation, and surgery in severe cases.

   2. **Cavernous hemangiomas** are the most common benign tumors of the orbit among adults, although they are rarely clinically evident during childhood. Symptoms usually result from a retrobulbar mass within the muscle cone that appears during the second to fourth decades of life. Complete surgical excision by a lateral orbitotomy is usually possible because of the thick capsule around the cavernous hemangioma.

   3. **Lymphangiomas** are uncommon tumors that often enlarge because of spontaneous internal hemorrhage into delicate vascular spaces. Exophthalmos may be caused by blood-filled "chocolate cysts," which must be distinguished from a malignancy such as rhabdomyosarcoma. Treatment

is usually not necessary because blood-filled cysts commonly resolve spontaneously. Aspiration and drainage of blood may be required if the optic nerve or eye is severely compressed.

C. **Neural tumors and meningiomas.** The most common tumors of neural origin involving the orbit are optic nerve gliomas and plexiform neurofibromas. Both of these abnormalities frequently occur in the neurofibromatosis syndrome (von Recklinghausen's disease) and are sometimes considered to be developmental lesions (hamartomas) rather than neoplasms.

  1. **Optic nerve gliomas** are well-differentiated tumors, approximately one-fourth of which are found among patients with neurofibromatosis. Therefore, the presence of café-au-lait spots in a child with exophthalmos and optic nerve abnormalities should increase the likelihood that an optic nerve glioma is present. These findings, together with an enlarged optic canal on x-rays, are virtually pathognomonic of this tumor. CT and MRI scans are usually performed if intracranial extension is suspected. Treatment is controversial, but it is reasonable to biopsy a suspected optic glioma and to excise the tumor when the optic canal is enlarged and vision is poor.

  2. **Neurofibromas** are usually plexiform, highly vascular, infiltrative tumors that involve the lateral portion of the upper eyelid and the anterior orbit. Progressive ptosis and sphenoid dysplasia frequently accompany plexiform neurofibromas. Because complete excision of plexiform tumors is usually impossible, surgery should usually be limited to debulking, eyelid reconstruction, and ptosis correction.

  3. **Meningiomas** arise from arachnoidal villi and usually originate intracranially, in which case they may secondarily extend into the orbit through bone or along the optic canal. Primary orbital meningiomas that arise from the optic nerve sheath are less common than intracranial meningiomas. Complete excision should be attempted, although this is seldom possible in the case of intracranial tumors because of their extensive growth.

D. **Rhabdomyosarcomas** are the most common primary orbital malignant tumors among children. Approximately 90% of these lesions occur in patients under 15 years of age. Imaging studies may demonstrate bone destruction, which would help to establish the diagnosis of rhabdomyosarcoma, because other primary orbital tumors seldom destroy the orbital walls. The neck should be examined to rule out lymph node metastases, and chest x-rays as well as bone marrow aspirates should be obtained to rule out distant metastases. The diagnosis should be established by biopsy. High-dose radiation therapy combined with systemic chemotherapy has replaced exenteration and may cure more than one-half of patients with rhabdomyosarcomas.

E. **Lacrimal gland tumors.** Approximately one-half of all lacrimal gland tumors arise from epithelial tissue, and most of these are nonmetastasizing benign mixed tumors. Most nonepithelial tumors are inflammatory and lymphoid lesions.

  1. **Benign mixed tumors** are nonmetastasizing epithelial tumors that tend to recur and may undergo frankly malignant degeneration unless they are completely removed. Symptoms usually occur during the fourth and fifth decades of life. The tumors usually grow slowly and may produce smooth deformities in the adjacent orbital bones. When a benign mixed tumor is suspected, the entire lesion should be excised if possible. Incisional biopsy may allow tumor cells to spill into the orbit and can lead to infiltrative recurrent tumor, which requires extensive surgery for removal.

  2. **Malignant epithelial tumors** are all highly aggressive and frequently lethal. Adenoid cystic carcinomas (cylindromas) are the most common malignant tumors of the lacrimal gland. Most malignant epithelial tumors arise de novo, but occasionally benign mixed tumors may undergo malignant transformation. All of these malignant tumors should be treated by

radical surgery (exenteration and removal of involved bone) unless they have already metastasized or have invaded beyond possible excision.

3. **Nonepithelial tumors** of the lacrimal gland are usually inflammatory, in which case they may be idiopathic pseudotumors, lymphoepithelial lesions, or sarcoid granulomas. Malignant lymphomas and lymphosarcomas occasionally involve the lacrimal gland. Malignant lymphoid tumors are usually treated by local radiation or by systemic chemotherapy.

F. **Lymphoproliferative tumors.** Both benign and malignant lymphoid tumors of the orbit occur much more frequently among adults than among children. Reactive lymphoid hyperplasia is an idiopathic benign process that must be distinguished from malignant lymphoma. Biopsy is almost always necessary to establish the diagnosis of these lesions. Evaluation of patients with orbital lymphoid tumors should include a general physical examination to detect manifestations of systemic lymphoma. The treatment of malignant lymphoid tumors is usually radiation therapy, although systemic chemotherapy may be used if disseminated disease is present.

G. **Metastatic tumors.** Among children, neuroblastoma and Ewing sarcoma are the most common distant tumors that metastasize to the orbit. Most neuroblastomas occur among patients younger than 7 years of age and may produce bilateral exophthalmos with eyelid ecchymosis. Among adults, breast and lung malignancies metastasize to the orbit much more commonly than any other lesions. Metastatic breast carcinoma may arise in the orbit many years after primary cancer surgery. Rarely, breast metastases to the orbit elicit fibrosis that causes cicatricial enophthalmos. Treatment of metastatic tumors is usually palliative, using radiation and sometimes chemotherapy. Breast tumors should be assayed for estrogen receptor activity, so that the possible usefulness of adjunctive hormone therapy can be determined. Some metastatic tumors such as carcinoids should be treated by wide excision, because patients with slowly growing primary lesions may survive for long periods of time.

VII. **Congenital and developmental orbital anomalies.** Most nonneoplastic congenital and developmental orbital abnormalities are uncommon and are so obvious that they do not present a diagnostic problem. Some disorders, such as meningoencephaloceles, may resemble enlarging neoplasms. Other conditions, such as neurofibromatosis, may be associated with true neoplasms. Although choristomas (e.g., dermoids) and hamartomas (e.g., hemangiomas) are believed to be developmental in origin, they often produce initial symptoms during adult life and are usually grouped with the general category of orbital tumors.

A. **Microphthalmos and anophthalmos.** In most cases in which a child is born with a unilateral small orbit and no visible eye, a small microphthalmic globe is present within the orbital soft tissues. Microphthalmos is sometimes associated with an orbital cyst. All children with congenitally small or absent eyes have hypoplastic orbits. If possible, surgery should be avoided and the socket should be expanded using progressively larger conformers.

B. **Craniostenosis.** Premature closure of the cranial sutures results in craniostenosis. The most common facial–orbital syndromes associated with craniostenosis are Crouzon's disease (frequently including hypertelorism and exophthalmos) and Apert syndrome.

C. **Meningocele and encephalocele.** Congenital dehiscences of the skull may permit herniation of intracranial contents into the orbit. A meningocele consists of herniated meninges and CSF. If brain is also found within the herniated meninges, the defect is an encephalocele. Defects in the greater wing of the sphenoid may occur in patients with neurofibromatosis and may produce pulsating exophthalmos.

D. **Choristomas** are developmental growths that arise from tissues not normally found at the involved location, such as dermoids, epidermoids, and teratomas.

E. **Hamartomas** are developmental growths that arise from tissues usually found at the involved location, such as hemangiomas, lymphangiomas, and many neurofibromas. Some investigators consider optic nerve gliomas to be hamartomas; others consider them to be true neoplasms. Neurofibromatosis (von Recklinghausen's disease) is a disseminated hamartoma syndrome or phakomatosis, of which the orbital manifestations may include plexiform neurofibromas, dysplasia of the orbital walls, and optic nerve gliomas.

VIII. Orbital trauma. Facial trauma can damage the orbital bones and adjacent soft tissues. Fractures may be associated with injuries to the orbital contents and brain, paranasal sinus injuries, nasolacrimal damage, CSF leaks, carotid–cavernous sinus fistulas, and embedded foreign bodies (see Chapter 2, secs. **VIII.** and **IX.**).

A. Orbital trauma evaluation. *Rule out:*
Ruptured globe
> Emergent surgical repair

Orbital compartment syndrome
> Orbital soft tissue decompression (lateral canthotomy and cantholysis)

Traumatic optic neuropathy
> Direct or indirect trauma
> Megadose of intravenous steroids
> ? Surgery: optic canal or sheath decompression

B. Soft tissue injuries. Because the eye may be seriously damaged even without actual penetration, the visual acuity should be measured and a thorough ophthalmic examination conducted in any patient who has suffered orbital trauma. Partial or complete visual loss may result from direct damage or secondary compression to the optic nerve or from interruption of its vascular supply. Injuries to the motor nerves or to the levator and extraocular muscles may cause ptosis and limitation of ocular motility. The eyelids, canthi, and lacrimal system may be lacerated or avulsed. Exophthalmos may be caused by orbital hemorrhage following trauma. Injuries to the eye should be treated as the first priority, after which damage to the eyelids and lacrimal apparatus can be repaired.

C. "Orbital compartment syndrome (OCS)." From an orbital perspective, the presence of vision-threatening elevated intraorbital pressure, termed "orbital compartment syndrome," may occur from orbital hemorrhage, emphysema, or profound edema. Clinical signs include decreased vision, limited extraocular motility, afferent pupillary defect, proptosis, elevated intraocular pressure (IOP), or even central retinal artery pulsations (implying that IOP is higher than diastolic pressure). In such severe cases, where the elevated intraorbital pressure may result in impaired perfusion of the globe and optic nerve, emergent intervention of lateral canthotomy and inferior cantholysis are typically curative. Drainage or aspiration of an orbital hemorrhage is seldom necessary. OCS may be summarized as:

> *Orbital compartment syndrome: EMERGENCY!*
> Etiology
>> Hemorrhage
>> Emphysema
>> Inflammation
>> Noninfectious (pseudotumor)
>> Infectious (cellulitis/abscess)
>
> Signs
>> Optic neuropathy: decreased vision, dyschromatopsia, afferent pupillary defect
>> Tight orbit, lids
>> EOM dysfunction
>> Increased IOP
>> Decreased retinal perfusion, central retinal artery occlusion
>> Venous stasis, central retinal vein occlusion

> Diagnostic test
> > CT imaging
> Treatment
> > Immediate canthotomy, inferior cantholysis
> > Osmotic agents (mannitol)
> > Intravenous steroids
> > Ice compresses

D. Orbital fractures. Fractures of the orbital roof may involve the paranasal sinuses or cause cerebrospinal rhinorrhea. Fractures at the orbital apex may injure the optic nerve. They should be evaluated by tomography of the optic canal if there is no significant acute visual loss. Emergency surgical decompression of the optic canal in the setting of indirect traumatic optic neuropathy is controversial, with advocates of no intervention, high-dose steroids, or steroids and optic canal decompression. Carotid–cavernous sinus fistulas should be suspected if prolonged conjunctival vascular congestion or bruits are found after orbital injury. Other important fractures, because of their possible effect on ocular and orbital function, are those that involve the medial wall and floor of the orbit.

1. **Medial orbital fractures** usually result from trauma to the nose or medial orbital rim. The lacrimal secretory system (especially the naso-lacrimal duct) may be damaged, and the medial rectus muscle may be entrapped within fractures of the lamina papyracea. Dacryocystorhinos-tomy may be required if the nasolacrimal duct is obstructed. Surgical exploration of the medial orbit may be indicated if mechanical restriction of ocular motility is present.

2. **Orbital floor fractures** may be direct, in which the inferior orbital rim is involved, or indirect, in which the rim remains intact. Indirect fractures are frequently referred to as blow-out fractures because they are produced by the transmission of forces through the orbital soft tissues by a nonpenetrating object such as a fist or ball. These fractures generally occur in the thin bone over the infraorbital canal and may be complicated by entrapment of the inferior rectus or inferior oblique muscles and surrounding orbital fibroadipose tissue. *Coronal orbital CT* is the preferred imaging modality to demonstrate the full extent of defects as well as details of the extraocular muscles. Urgent surgery is indicated if there is minimal edema and marked limitation of extraocular movement associated with diplopia within 20 degrees of primary position and pain with extraocular movements. These relatively unusual cases are termed "white-eyed blow-out," occur more frequently in children, and will not improve spontaneously.

3. In other **equivocal cases,** it is difficult to distinguish between orbital contusion (which resolves spontaneously) versus orbital soft tissue entrapment (which will not spontaneously improve). In such cases, forced ductions of the globe help distinguish between these possibilities. The primary orbital indications for surgery of orbital fractures are visually significant entrapment, manifest enophthalmos (>2 mm), and large internal orbital fracture (greater than 50% of the floor and medial wall) that will likely result in late enophthalmos, or in the setting of a panfacial fracture. Clinicians should bear in mind that most internal orbital fractures are small and are not associated with soft tissue entrapment, thus only the minority of patients will require surgery. In cases where more than just the internal orbit is fractured (e.g., zygomatic complex fracture, Le Fort II and III fracture, and nasoorbital ethoidal fracture), patients are best served by using a team approach combining the expertise of oculoplastics as well as the expertise of other surgeons operating in this area (ear, nose, and throat; plastics; and oral maxillofacial).

E. **Intraorbital foreign bodies** can usually be localized by conventional x-rays if they are radiopaque. Many wooden or vegetable matter foreign bodies, however, cannot be visualized by x-rays and may require CT for visualization. If an infection occurs after a penetrating injury, a retained foreign body should be suspected. A fistula tract may be produced that can be surgically followed into the orbit. Wounds caused by intraorbital foreign bodies should be cultured and antibiotics administered. Foreign bodies should be removed if they are composed of vegetable matter, if they have sharp edges, or if they are anterior in the orbit. They can often be left in place if they are inert with smooth edges and located in the posterior orbit (see Chapter 2, sec. **VII.**).

5. CORNEA AND EXTERNAL DISEASE

Deborah Pavan-Langston

I. Normal anatomy and physiology
   A. Conjunctiva: anatomy
      1. **Gross anatomy.** The conjunctiva is a thin, transparent mucous membrane lining the inner surface of the eyelid (palpebral conjunctiva) and covering the anterior sclera (bulbar conjunctiva). The palpebral portion is designated as marginal, tarsal, and orbital and merges with the conjunctiva of the superior and inferior fornices in loose folds. The bulbar conjunctiva is adherent to the underlying Tenon capsule and therefore to sclera, with the tightest adhesion occurring in a narrow band at the corneoscleral limbus. A delicate vertical crescent, the semilunar fold (plica semilunaris), separates the bulbar conjunctiva from the lacrimal caruncle at the medial canthus. The conjunctiva tends to be a mobile tissue and is capable of great distention with edema fluid, as is often seen with trauma or inflammation.
      2. **Microscopically,** the conjunctiva is composed of (a) an anterior stratified columnar epithelium that is continuous with the corneal epithelium, and (b) a lamina propria composed of adenoid and fibrous layers. The epithelium is from two to seven layers thick and contains numerous unicellular mucous glands (goblet cells) that secrete the inner mucoid layer of the tear film. Although the healthy epithelium is never keratinized, it may become keratinized in certain disease states. The lamina propria is composed of connective tissue housing blood vessels, nerves, and glands. The accessory lacrimal glands of Krause are located deep in the substantia propria in the superior and inferior fornices. The accessory lacrimal glands of Wolfring are situated near the upper margin of the superior tarsal plate. The adenoid layer of the lamina propria, which develops particularly after 3 months of age, contains lymphocytes enmeshed in a fine reticular network without the presence of true lymphoid follicles. The fibrous layer of the lamina propria surrounds the smooth palpebral muscle of Müller.
      3. The **blood supply** of the palpebral conjunctiva originates from peripheral (bulbar and fornix) and marginal arterial arcades of the eyelid. Within 4 mm of the limbus the vascular supply is derived from the anterior conjunctival branches of the anterior ciliary arteries (superficial plexus), which anastomose with the posterior conjunctival vessels from the peripheral arcade. Conjunctival vessels move with the conjunctiva and constrict with instillation of 1:1,000 epinephrine—a point of differentiation from the deeper episcleral and ciliary vessels.
      4. **Innervation** of the bulbar conjunctiva is via the sensory and sympathetic nerves from the ciliary nerves. The remaining palpebral and fornix conjunctiva is innervated by the ophthalmic and maxillary divisions of the trigeminal nerve (cranial nerve V).
      5. **Lymphatic** drainage of the conjunctiva parallels that of the lid, with lateral drainage to the preauricular nodes and medial drainage to the submandibular nodes.
   B. Cornea
      1. **Gross anatomy.** The cornea represents the anterior 1.3 cm^2 of the globe and is the main refracting surface of the eye. Although the cornea is continuous with the sclera at the limbus, the anterior corneal curvature (radius equal to 7.8 mm) is greater than that of the sclera, with the central 4-mm optical zone almost spherical and the periphery gradually flattening toward the scleral curve. The horizontal diameter of the anterior

surface of the cornea (11.6 mm) is longer than the vertical diameter (10.6 mm), so that the anterior aspect of the cornea forms a horizontal ovoid. Viewed from the posterior surface, the cornea is circular (with a diameter of 11.6 mm). A corneal diameter greater than 12.5 mm is termed *megalocornea;* a corneal diameter less than 11.0 mm is termed *microcornea.* The height of the cornea from the basal plane of the visible limbus to the apex is 2.7 mm. The central thickness of the cornea is 0.52 mm, which increases to 0.70 mm in the far periphery.

2. **Microscopically,** the cornea consists of five strata: the epithelium and its basement membrane, Bowman's layer, stroma, Descemet's membrane, and endothelium.

   a. The corneal **epithelium** is a uniform five- to six-layer structure 50 to 100 μm thick and is composed of (a) a basal cell layer of replicating cylindric cells, 18 μm high and 10 μm wide, (b) a wing cell layer with superior convex–inferior scalloped cells interdigitating between the apices of the basal cells, and (c) surface cells composed of flat cells in two or three layers culminating in a smooth corneal surface that is studded with ultrastructural microplicae and microvilli. Corneal **nerves** passing from the corneal stroma through Bowman's layer terminate freely between the epithelial cells, thus accounting for the great sensitivity of the cornea. The epithelium is firmly attached to the underlying Bowman's layer by a continuous basement membrane that is a very important source of firm epithelial adhesion.

   b. **Bowman's layer** is a homogeneous condensation of the anterior stromal lamellae continuous with the corneal stroma. Its termination at the corneal periphery marks the anterior margin of the corneoscleral limbus.

   c. The **stroma** represents 90% of the corneal thickness, with bundles of collagen fibrils of uniform thickness enmeshed in mucopolysaccharide ground substance. These bundles form 200 lamellae arranged parallel to the corneal surface but with alternate layers crisscrossing at right angles. This regular lattice structure, coupled with the deturgescent state of the stroma, has been credited with providing the extreme transparency of the cornea necessary for optical clarity.

   d. **Descemet's membrane** is the basement membrane of the endothelial cells and can be easily stripped from the stroma. When torn or traumatized, the ends will tend to retract, indicating an inherent elasticity. Gradual thickening of this layer with age is noted, with the thickness approximately 3 to 4 μm at birth but increasing to 10 to 12 μm in adulthood. Peripheral dome-shaped excrescences of Descemet's membrane (Hassall-Henle warts) occur in persons over age 20 years. Histologically, the membrane is a homogeneous glass-like structure, but ultrastructurally is composed of stratified layers of very fine collagenous filaments in the anterior layer (anterior banded layer) with an amorphous posterior layer that increases with age.

   e. The **endothelium** is a single layer of approximately 500,000 polygonal cells, 5 to 18 μm in size, that spread uniformly across the posterior surface of the cornea. Although mitotic activity can be seen in very young endothelial cells in the adult, repair most often occurs by amitotic enlargement of the central endothelial cells. These cells maintain deturgescence and contribute to the formation of Descemet's membrane.

3. The **blood supply** of the cornea arises predominantly from the conjunctival, episcleral, and scleral vessels that arborize about the corneoscleral limbus. The cornea itself is avascular.

4. The **innervation** of the cornea is that of a rich sensory supply mostly via the ophthalmic division of the trigeminal nerve. This innervation is via the long ciliary nerves that branch in the outer choroid near the ora serrata region. These nerves pass via the sclera into the middle third of the cornea as 70 to 80 large nerve trunks that lose their myelin sheaths approximately 2 to 3 mm from the limbus, but can be visualized as fine

filaments beyond. There is significant dichotomous and trichotomous branching, and the subsequent passage of nerve fibers through Bowman's layer ends freely between the epithelial cells.

C. **Physiology: precorneal tear film**

1. The **physiology** of the cornea and conjunctiva is best introduced in a discussion of the **precorneal tear film.** This film, which is 6 to 10 μm thick, is composed of three layers: (a) superficial lipid layer, (b) middle aqueous layer, and (c) inner mucous layer. The normal tear volume in the conjunctival sac is about 3 to 7 μL and can increase to the conjunctival sac capacity of 25 μL before overflow occurs. Tear flow rate is approximately 1 μL/per minute and comes from the secretion of the main and accessory lacrimal glands. After their release in the superotemporal region, the tears are distributed by the blinking action of the lids with the tear meniscus forming superior and inferior marginal tear strips before draining into the lacrimal puncta located near the medial canthus. With a pH of 7.6 and an osmolarity comparable to sodium chloride 0.9%, there is a low glucose concentration and an electrolyte distribution similar to plasma, with the exception of a slightly greater potassium content. Oxygen dissolves readily in the tear film, and the dissolved protein content of the tear film includes immunoglobulins and lysozyme. These characteristics allow the tear film to provide a smooth surface for refraction, to mechanically wash and protect the cornea and conjunctiva, to provide oxygen exchange for the epithelium, to lubricate the surface during a blink, and to provide bacteriostasis.

2. **Corneal function.** The primary physiologic function of the cornea is to maintain an optically smooth surface and a transparent medium while protecting the intraocular contents of the eye. This duty is fulfilled by the effective interaction of the epithelium, stroma, and endothelium. The epithelium, endothelium, and Descemet's membrane are transparent because of the uniformity of their refractive indices. The transparency of the stroma is conferred by the special physical arrangement of the component fibrils. Although the refractive index of collagen fibrils differs from that of the interfibrillar substance, the small diameter of the fibril (300 Å) and the small distance between them (300 Å) provide a separation and regularity that causes little scattering of light despite the optical inhomogeneity. The relative state of deturgescence is provided by the barrier functions of the epithelium and endothelium as well as by the dehydrating function of the endothelium. Disturbance of this equilibrium, such as occurs in corneal edema, will increase light scattering and the opacity of the stroma.

   a. The **anterior epithelial surface** with its microplicae and microvilli provides the scaffold for a smooth and continuous precorneal tear film. In addition, the epithelium serves as a relatively impermeable barrier to water-soluble materials. The epithelium also provides an effective barrier to many infectious agents. The epithelium is the most mitotically active layer of the cornea, and because of its high cellular density consumes considerable glucose and oxygen. The major source of oxygen for the epithelium is atmospheric oxygen dissolved in the tear film, which explains the sensitivity to hypoxia that occurs with improperly fitted or overworn contact lenses. Glucose for the epithelium is obtained from the aqueous humor by diffusion through the corneal stroma. The substance is either used or stored as glycogen. Epithelial metabolism occurs through the hexose monophosphate shunt or tricarboxylic acid cycle in the presence of oxygen, or via the anaerobic glycolysis pathway in the absence of oxygen. With these metabolic capabilities, the turnover of the epithelium is rapid, occurring approximately once every 7 days, and explains the ability of the epithelium to heal itself rapidly.

   b. **Stroma.** There is little turnover of the stromal matrix, and the keratocytes may survive as long as 2 years under normal conditions.

Glucose is obtained from the aqueous humor and oxidized via the Embden-Meyerhof tricarboxylic acid cycle. Interaction of the interfibrillar substances, particularly the acid mucopolysaccharides, generates a swelling pressure for the stroma both in vivo and in vitro. This tendency to imbibe fluid results in light scattering if it is not kept in check by the dehydrating function of the endothelium.

c. **Endothelium.** The major function of the endothelium is the maintenance of proper corneal hydration. The endothelium requires oxygen and glucose to maintain the metabolically active process, but the exact nature of the endothelial pump is not completely clear. Impairment of the pump function can occur in dystrophic conditions (Fuchs dystrophy), injury (postsurgical or traumatic), and in some inflammatory conditions (anterior segment necrosis).

II. **Acute traumatic conditions**

A. **Abrasions and lacerations.** (see Chapter 2, secs. **V.** and **VI.**).

B. **Perforations**

1. **Etiologically,** corneal perforation can result from any corneal ulceration, either infectious (bacterial, fungal, or viral), inflammatory (rheumatoid arthritis or collagen disease), posttraumatic (burn), or trophic defects of degenerations, neurotrophic ulcer, or postherpetic ulcer. Use of topical *nonsteroidal antiinflammatory drugs (NSAIDs)* such as diclofenac in at-risk patients may trigger or worsen thinning and perforation.

2. **Treatment.** Occasionally, these perforations will seal with a small knuckle of iris and rarely can be self-sealing, but they usually result in partial or complete loss of the anterior chamber. Thus, they represent an urgent situation to be treated in most cases. Small, noninfectious perforations can often be splinted by use of a therapeutic *soft contact bandage lens* (Permalens, Kontur). Such treatment will sometimes allow healing of the perforation, but often is a stabilizing or interim treatment that requires further definitive therapy. *Medical adhesive* is of great use in helping to seal small perforations. **Cyanoacrylate tissue adhesive** (Dermabond Ethicon; not U.S. Food and Drug Administration [FDA] approved for ocular use) can successfully seal a perforation without excess ocular toxicity. It is essential that epithelium and necrotic stroma be débrided to allow firm adhesion of the cyanoacrylate glue to surrounding healthy basement membrane. A thin application of this glue will often remain intact for several months and is tolerated by the patient if covered with a continuously worn soft contact lens (Plano T). Healing of the corneal defect will often occur beneath the glue. Even if spontaneous healing of the leak is not expected, the glue will provide adequate time to obtain corneal donor material if keratoplasty becomes necessary. It is essential to observe the patient closely to ensure that the anterior chamber has reformed and there is no associated superinfection. Topical antibiotic coverage is advisable after gluing and with the use of a soft contact lens. When contact lens or adhesive therapy is inadequate, *surgical patch grafting* will usually be successful. For moderate-size perforations, a small lamellar button may be sutured into the débrided defect. In the event of large central perforations, it may be preferable to perform penetrating keratoplasty.

C. **Burns.** Anterior segment burns may be chemical, thermal, radiation, or electric (see Chapter 2, secs. **I.–IV.**).

D. **Subconjunctival hemorrhage** may be induced with major, minor, or no detectable trauma to the front of the eye. Occasionally, a patient will wake up with a "spontaneous" hemorrhage. Clinically, it presents as a striking flat, deep-red hemorrhage under the conjunctiva and may become sufficiently severe to cause a dramatic chemotic "bag of blood" to protrude over the lid margin. Occasionally, pneumococcal or adenoviral conjunctivitis may be associated, in which case there will be discomfort and discharge. In the absence of infection or significant trauma to the eye, **treatment** is unnecessary. The patient should be reassured that the blood will clear over a 2- or 3-week period.

III. **Conjunctival infection and inflammation**

    A. **Conjunctivitis** is an inflammation of the conjunctiva characterized by vascular dilation, cellular infiltration, and exudation. The differential features of bacterial conjunctivitis versus those caused by virus, allergy, or toxic factors are listed in **Table 5.1. Floppy eyelid syndrome** is an often-overlooked cause of *chronic conjunctivitis.* Unrecognized eversion of the "loose" upper lid during sleep is associated with papillary conjunctivitis and red eye. Treatment is horizontal lid shortening.

    B. **Bacterial conjunctivitis** can be acute or chronic. The **acute** stage classically is recognized by vascular engorgement and mucopurulent discharge, with the associated symptoms of irritation, foreign body sensation, and sticking together of the lids. Occasionally, a severe reaction with purulent conjunctivitis and corneal involvement can occur. The **chronic** infection is more innocuous in its onset, runs a protracted course, and is often associated with involvement of the lids or lacrimal system by low-grade inflammatory reaction. A wide variety of bacterial organisms can infect the conjunctiva. Although the bacterial etiology is often clinically apparent, the identity of the causative organism may not be obvious. Certain clinical features determined by the pathogenicity of the infectious agent, however, may provide an accurate clinical diagnosis.

        1. **Acute bacterial conjunctivitis**

            a. *Staphylococcus aureus* is probably the single most common cause of bacterial conjunctivitis and blepharoconjunctivitis in the Western world. The aerobic Gram-positive coccus is often harbored elsewhere on the skin or in the nares. It may affect any age group. Although usually not aggressively invasive, the organism is very toxigenic and can provide corneal infiltrates, eczematous blepharitis, phlyctenular keratitis, and angular blepharitis.

            b. *Staphylococcus epidermidis* is usually considered an innocuous inhabitant of the lids and conjunctiva, but in some instances it can cause blepharoconjunctivitis. The organism is capable of producing necrotic exotoxin and has been shown to colonize eye cosmetics, with subsequent production of blepharoconjunctivitis.

            c. *Streptococcus pneumoniae* (pneumococcus) is an aerobic encapsulated Gram-positive diplococcus that is often present in the respiratory tracts of asymptomatic carriers. This organism more commonly affects the conjunctiva of children and can run a self-limiting course of 9 to 10 days.

            d. *Streptococcus pyogenes* is an aerobic Gram-positive coccus. Although an infrequent cause of conjunctivitis, the organism is invasive and toxigenic, and thus is capable of producing a pseudomembranous conjunctivitis. The pseudomembrane consists of a fibrinous layer entrapping inflammatory cells and is attached to the conjunctival surface. Removal of this pseudomembrane is possible with minimal bleeding of the underlying tissue.

            e. *Haemophilus influenzae (H. aegyptius,* Koch-Weeks bacillus) is a fastidious aerobic Gram-negative pleomorphic organism often seen as a slender rod or a coccobacillary form. It is frequently isolated from upper respiratory tracts of healthy carriers and most commonly causes conjunctivitis in children rather than in adults. It is a toxigenic organism and can be accompanied by patchy conjunctival hemorrhages during an acute infection. An untreated case can last for 9 to 12 days, occurring as a self-limited infection, but occasionally can be part of a more ominous periorbital cellulitis associated with respiratory infection that can lead to bacteremia in young children. Accompanying the acute infection and probably a manifestation of the toxigenic potential is the presence of *inferior corneal limbal infiltrates.*

TABLE 5.1. CLINICAL FEATURES OF CONJUNCTIVITIS

Sign	Bacterial	Viral	Allergic	Toxic	TRIC
Injection	Marked	Moderate	Mild/Moderate	Mild/Moderate	Moderate
Hemorrhage	+	+	–	–	–
Chemosis	++	+/–	++	+/–	+/–
Exudate	Purulent Mucopurulent	Scant/watery	Stringy/white	–	Scant
Pseudomembrane	+/– *Streptococcus Corynebacterium*	+/–	–	–	–
Papillae	+/–	–	+	+	–
Follicles	–	+	–	+ (Medication)	+
Preauricular node	+	++	– (Except vernal)	–	+/–
Pannus	–	–		–	+

TRIC, trachoma-inclusion conjunctivitis; ++, strongly positive; +, positive; +/–, sometimes positive; –, negative.

f. *Moraxella lacunata* is an aerobic Gram-negative diplobacillus once considered the most common cause of **angular blepharoconjunctivitis**. Although angular blepharoconjunctivitis is now more commonly the result of staphylococcal infection, *Moraxella* sp can produce an acute conjunctivitis that occasionally results in a chronic conjunctivitis with follicular reaction.

2. **Hyperacute conjunctivitis (acute purulent conjunctivitis)**

    a. *Neisseria* sp (gonococcus, meningococcus) are Gram-negative diplococci. Like *Haemophilus* sp, *Streptococcus* sp, and *Corynebacterium diphtheriae* are aggressively invasive bacteria that can produce a severe conjunctivitis that is often bilateral. Occurring in the child as an infection from the maternal genital tract, in adolescents via fomite transmission, or in via inoculation from infected genitalia, the conjunctivitis can start as a routine mucopurulent conjunctivitis that rapidly evolves into a severe inflammation with copious exudate and marked chemosis and lid edema. This clinical appearance demands laboratory confirmation, immediate therapy, and occasionally, hospitalization.

    b. **Neonatal conjunctivitis (ophthalmia neonatorum).** Conjunctivitis of the newborn deserves special mention because of the severity and threatening potential of this condition. Conjunctivitis caused by *Neisseria* sp usually becomes symptomatic in the newborn 2 to 4 days following inoculation of the conjunctival mucosa at the time of birth. Clinically, a yellow purulent discharge with prominent lid edema and conjunctival chemosis appears. This condition needs to be distinguished from the neonatal conjunctivitis caused by inclusion conjunctivitis agents, chemical keratoconjunctivitis, nasolacrimal obstruction with other bacterial superinfection, or trauma. The differential points in diagnosis are listed in **Table 5.2** (see sec. **III.C.2.** and Chapter 11, sec. **II.B.**).

3. **Chronic bacterial blepharoconjunctivitis**

    a. *S. aureus* is the most common cause of chronic bacterial conjunctivitis or blepharoconjunctivitis, with *S. epidermidis, Propionibacterium acnes, Corynebacterium* sp, and the yeast *Pityrosporium* being other etiologic agents. Often this conjunctivitis is associated with **rosacea** of the skin, a low-grade inflammation of the lid margins, and colonization of the meibomian orifices and lash follicles with *Staphylococcus*. **Anterior blepharitis** has crusty, red, thickened lids with prominent blood vessels, and **posterior blepharitis** (meibomitis) has inspissated oil glands with fluorescein staining along the palpebral conjunctival margin. *Staphylococcus* can produce a variety of exotoxins, which probably accounts for the clinical manifestations. An ulcerative blepharitis

TABLE 5.2. NEONATAL CONJUNCTIVITIS

Agent	Onset	Cytology	Culture
Neisseria	2–4 d	Gram-negative intracellular diplococci	Blood + chocolate agar (37°C, 10% CO_2)
Other bacteria	1–30 d	Gram-positive or gram-negative organisms	Blood agar
Inclusion blenorrhea (TRIC)	2–14 d	Giemsa-positive intracytoplasmic inclusions	Negative
Chemical	1–2 d	Negative	Negative or normal flora

TRIC, trachoma-inclusion conjunctivitis.

can occur as well as an eczematoid scaling, and sometimes weeping inflammation of the lids occurs. **Eczematoid** blepharitis is usually distinguishable from the less severe seborrheic blepharitis, which is often accompanied by scaling and greasy deposits on the eyelid, as well as from frequently associated seborrheic dermatitis. An **angular blepharoconjunctivitis** with maceration of the tissue at the lateral canthus, at one time most commonly associated with *Moraxella* sp, is now most commonly produced by *Staphylococcus.* The cornea also can be involved, with an inferior superficial punctate keratitis or by limbal infiltrates. **Marginal corneal ulcers** can be produced by chronic staphylococcal blepharoconjunctivitis.

  b. Chronic conjunctivitis can also be produced by Gram-negative rods including *Proteus mirabilis, Klebsiella pneumoniae, Serratia marcescens,* and *Escherichia coli.* Gram-negative diplobacilli *(M. lacunata)* can produce a chronic blepharoconjunctivitis (angular conjunctivitis) as previously mentioned and may be present with a chronic follicular reaction.

  c. Parinaud ocular glandular syndrome (catscratch disease, bartonellosis) is a febrile illness caused by the bacillus, *Bartonella henselae,* and is usually contracted through cat or flea exposure. Eye findings include unilateral conjunctival redness, often with epithelial ulceration, foreign body sensation, epiphora, mild lid swelling, serous to purulent discharge, and the disease hallmark: *regional lymphadenopathy.* Neuroretinitis and focal chorioretinitis are not uncommon (2%) (see sec. **III.D.4.,** below).

C. Laboratory diagnosis in bacterial conjunctivitis is not routine. However, when clinical findings are insufficient to diagnose confidently the etiology of an infection, or in those situations in which the reaction is severe or has not responded to routine therapy, conjunctival scrapings for microscopic examination and cultures are indicated. These should also be performed in cases of neonatal conjunctivitis, hyperacute conjunctivitis, and chronic recalcitrant conjunctivitis.

  1. Conjunctival cultures should be taken prior to the use of topical anesthetics, because these agents and their preservatives will reduce the recovery of certain bacteria. Cultures are taken by moistening a sterile alginate *(not cotton)* swab with sterile saline and wiping the lid margin or conjunctival cul-de-sac. The culture medium is then inoculated directly with the swab tip. Inoculation of solid media can be made in the shape of the letter *R* for the right lid and *L* for the left lid margin. On the same plate, a conjunctival culture may be inoculated at a different site using a zigzag pattern. In this way, the site of culture may be distinguished by the pattern of growth on the plate. After inoculating solid media, the tip of the applicator may be broken off and dropped into a tube of liquid culture medium if it is available.

  2. For **bacterial isolation** and **identification,** the most widely used and generally available **media** are blood agar and chocolate agar. Meat broth has a significantly higher growth rate for most common organisms, but must be secondarily plated for identification. Chocolate agar is well suited for growth of any organism that can be isolated on blood agar and has the added advantage of isolating *Haemophilus,* the fastidious *Neisseria* organisms, and fungi. Thayer-Martin medium is a chocolate agar medium containing vancomycin, colistimethate, and nystatin, and is of use in culture and isolation of gonococcus. Thioglycolate medium is a commonly used medium in cultivating anaerobic organisms from ocular infection. Liquid Sabouraud medium may be useful in isolating fungal organisms when solid agar medium has failed. **Table 5.3** summarizes the culture media of use in specific ocular infectious states. Cultures for *B. henselae* (catscratch disease) are difficult. Diagnosis is usually based on polymerase chain reaction (PCR) testing on local tissue biopsy and serology.

TABLE 5.3. CULTURE MEDIA

General Media	Bacterial	Fungal	Parasitic	Viral
Blood agar plate	Good recovery (37°C)	Good recovery (room temperature)		
Chocolate agar plate	Especially *Haemophilus*, *Neisseria*, fungus			
Sabouraud		Good recovery (broth or agar)		
Chopped-meat broth	Good recovery (37°C)	Good recovery		
Thioglycolate broth	Microaerophilic species			
Special media (Lowenstein-Jensen, Thayer-Martin)	Mycobacteria, *Neisseria*			
Page medium to *Escherichia coli* plates			Good for *Acanthamoeba*	
Viral carrier medium (minimal essential medium, Hank balanced salt solution) to human cell tissue culture				Good for herpes simplex, herpes zoster, adenovirus, pox

TABLE 5.4. CYTOLOGIC FEATURES OF CONJUNCTIVITIS

Cell	Bacterial	Viral	Allergic	TRIC
Polymorphonuclear				
Neutrophil	+	+ (Early)	−	+
Basoeosinophil	−	−	+	
(occasional)				
Mononuclear				
Lymphocyte	−	+	−	+
Plasma cell	−	−	−	+
Multinuclear	−	+	−	−
Inclusion				
Cytoplasm	−	+ (Pox)	−	+
Nucleus	−	+ (Herpes)		
Organism	+	−	−	−

TRIC, trachoma-inclusion conjunctivitis (group); +, present; −, absent.

3. **Scrapings for microscopic examination** are made after cultures have been taken. Local anesthetic is instilled. A platinum spatula is flamed and allowed to cool to room temperature. The spatula can then be used to scrape gently the involved conjunctival surface, and the material obtained can be spread in a thin layer on a precleaned glass slide. If possible, two or three such slides are made and stained for microscopic examination **(Table 5.4).** Because scrapings are only about *70% reliable* and may be traumatic to the patient, cultures take priority and, in appropriate situations, scrapings are omitted.

4. **Stains** most useful for identifying organisms and inflammatory cell type are the Gram, Giemsa, or Wright stain. The Hansel stain is also a useful technique for rapid identification of any eosinophilic response. The Giemsa and Wright stains are most useful in revealing the condition and character of epithelial cells and inflammatory cells. The Giemsa stain is most effective in showing the presence or absence of viral cytoplasmic or intranuclear inclusion bodies and in outlining the morphology of bacteria. The Gram stain is useful in revealing whether an organism is Gram positive or negative; it also provides some information about the morphology of the organism.

5. The **cytologic features** of each type of conjunctivitis are helpful in diagnosis. As a rule, a *polymorphonuclear leukocyte* response occurs with bacterial conjunctivitis (with the exception of diplobacillus). Acute Stevens-Johnson syndrome may produce a polymorphonuclear response, as will the early stages of a viral infection. A mixed outpouring of polymorphonuclear leukocytes and lymphocytes is commonly noted with adult and neonatal inclusion conjunctivitis. Such a mixed response with the added presence of plasma cells and macrophages (Leber cells) are almost diagnostic of trachoma. Chemical conjunctivitis can also produce a polymorphonuclear response. A predominantly *lymphocytic* response is most commonly seen in viral infections, but can also be seen in drug-induced toxic follicular conjunctivitis. Numerous **eosinophils** are indicative of vernal conjunctivitis or allergic conjunctivitis. The appearance of eosinophils and polymorphonuclear leukocytes in conjunction with a hyperacute conjunctivitis may be indicative of early erythema multiforme, particularly if associated with systemic symptoms. *Basophils,* rarely seen in conjunctival scrapings, are equivalent in interpretation to eosinophilic reaction. *Epithelial cells* may demonstrate cytoplasmic *inclusions* that, if basophilic, suggest inclusion conjunctivitis and, if

eosinophilic, suggest pox virus. Pink intranuclear inclusions on Giemsa stain are diagnostic of herpesvirus infection (either simplex or zoster). Multinucleate giant cells are suggestive of a viral disorder.

6. When **organisms** are identified, Gram-positive cocci in pairs or chains may indicate *S. pyogenes.* The Gram-negative diplococci, appearing within polymorphonuclear leukocytes and having the "coffee bean" shape, indicate *Neisseria* sp. Large Gram-negative diplobacilli characterize *Moraxella* sp. *H. influenzae* is a pleomorphic organism variably appearing as Gram-negative coccobacillus or slender rods. Gram-negative rods may also be noted, but are difficult to differentiate as to species.

D. **Treatment of bacterial conjunctivitis and blepharitis** (see Chapter 3, sec. **I.1.**).

1. **Acute mucopurulent conjunctivitis**

   a. **Topical antibiotic therapy.** Acute mucopurulent conjunctivitis will typically respond to topical antimicrobial therapy in solution or ointment form. If treatment is based on clinical diagnosis alone, topical antibiotics should be broad spectrum, i.e., anti-*Staphylococcus* sp, *Streptococcus* sp, and anti-Gram-negative organisms such as *Moraxella, Serratia, Haemophilus,* and *Pseudomonas.* Erythromycin or bacitracin ointment or sodium sulfacetamide 10% to 15% solution or ointment effectively covers only the more common Gram-positive infections. About 50% of staphylococci are resistant to the sulfonamides. There has been a significant increase in resistance to ciprofloxacin and cefazolin. Neomycin–polymyxin–bacitracin (Neosporin, Ocutricin, AK-Spore) is a very effective broad-spectrum antimicrobial (Gram-positive and negative organisms are covered), but there is a 6% to 8% allergic sensitivity to neomycin. Polymyxin B–bacitracin (Polysporin, AK Poly-Bac) ointment and polymyxin B–trimethoprim drop (Polytrim) have excellent broad-spectrum coverage. Gentamicin (generics), tobramycin (Tobrex), netilmicin (Nettacin) drops or ointment are very good broad-spectrum agents, but are usually reserved for suspected Gram-negative organisms. They are poorly effective against *Streptococcus* sp, and there is increasing incidence of resistance to *Staphylococcus* sp. The **quinolones,** ciprofloxacin (Ciloxan), ofloxacin (Ocuflox), levofloxacin (Quixin), and norfloxacin (Chibroxin), have very broad and potent Gram-positive and negative antibacterial activity with low, but unfortunately increasing, Gram-positive and -negative rates of resistance. The first two are also approved for corneal ulcers and the latter are pending approval.

   b. **Systemic therapy.** For particularly *acute* staphylococcal blepharitis, oral dicloxacillin or, if penicillin allergy exists, erythromycin are very effective adjuncts (see Appendix B).

   c. **Local measures** are of great value in treatment, particularly when blepharitis is present and chronic. Warm wet compresses improve circulation, mobilize meibomian secretions, and help cleanse crusting deposits of the lashes. Thick or inspissated lid secretions may require the physician to express the lids between cotton-tipped applicators after topical anesthesia, followed by daily lid margin scrubs with commercial cleansing pads (Eye Scrub, Lid Wipes SPF) or baby shampoo scrubs (using fingertips) performed by the patient. Seborrheic blepharitis is often improved by use of ***dandruff shampoo*** to the scalp and eyebrows. Daily application of ***steroid*** ointment to lid margins for 10 to 14 days often controls the pronounced lid inflammation.

2. **Hyperacute bacterial conjunctivitis** (acute purulent conjunctivitis) is a more serious situation and demands more vigorous therapy. After the patient is examined and the necessary cultures and scrapings are obtained, it is important to institute treatment prior to obtaining the culture results.

   a. **Systemic therapy** is indicated for *Neisseria gonorrhoeae, N. meningitidis,* and *H. influenzae,* and is far ***more critical than topical*** *therapy.* Because more than 20% of *N. gonorrhoeae* cases are resistant, *penicillin and tetracycline are no longer adequate as first-line treatment.* Recommended therapy that covers antimicrobial-resistant strains is any of the following: (a) norfloxacin 1.2 g orally (p.o.) qd for 5 days or other quinolone (for penicillin-allergic patients); (b) cefotaxime intravenously (i.v.) or intramuscularly (i.m.) or 50 mg per kg, or ceftriaxone 125 mg i.m., q8 to 12h all for 7 days; or (c) spectinomycin 2 g i.m. for 3 days. All of the above regimens should then be followed by a 1-week course of either doxycycline 100 mg p.o. bid or erythromycin 250 to 500 mg p.o. qid. An alternative combination is ceftriaxone 1 g or 50 mg per kg i.v. once on an outpatient basis, followed by a week of doxycycline or erythromycin p.o. Doses are adjusted per Appendix B, in consultation with a pediatric or infectious disease consultant. For patients who may only be treated with oral medication, norfloxacin, levofloxacin, or other quinolone, and cefaclor with probenecid are recommended (see Appendix B).

  b. Prophylactic therapy for intimate contacts of *N. gonorrhoeae* patients is 1 g of ceftriaxone i.v. once or, for *N. meningitidis,* rifampin 600 mg p.o. q12h for 4 days. Isolation of *H. influenzae* in children warrants therapy with ampicillin 100 to 200 mg per kg i.m. or i.v. for 7 to 10 days or 50 to 100 mg per kg q6 to 8h p.o. for 10 to 14 days; neonates receive 50 to 200 mg per kg q12h i.m. or i.v. for 10 days (see Appendix B). Adult dosage is 2 to 4 g p.o., i.m., or i.v. q6 to 8h for 10 to 14 days. If the *Haemophilus* strain is *ampicillin resistant* or the patient is *penicillin allergic,* a quinolone, e.g., levofloxacin or norfloxacin, in the dosages described in Appendix B, is given for 10 to 14 days. The *quinolones should not be used in neonates* or children without consultation with a pediatrician or infectious disease consult.

  c. Topical bacitracin or erythromycin ointment is instilled every 2 hours for the first 2 to 3 days for *N. meningitidis, Streptococcus* sp, *C. diphtheriae,* and *N. gonorrhoeae* in the neonate, child, or adult, and then five times daily for 7 days. *Haemophilus* or *Moraxella* infections are treated with topical ciprofloxacin, ofloxacin, gentamicin, or tobramycin in the same dosage schedule as that for *Neisseria.* Frequent *irrigation* with sterile saline is very therapeutic in washing away infected debris.

3. **Chronic conjunctivitis** and **blepharitis** (see secs. III.C., above, and VII.I., below, and Chapter 3 for anterior and posterior blepharitis review) are especially common in patients with acne **rosacea.** It is rarely cultured and only if there is no response to standard treatment, and is then re-treated in accordance with the sensitivities obtained after the pathogen is cultured. The presence of recalcitrant blepharitis or meibomitis in association with chronic staphylococcal conjunctivitis requires not only topical treatment with bacitracin or erythromycin, but also intensive *hygiene of the lid margins.* This hygiene may be initiated in the office by expression of the lid meibomian glands (using topical anesthesia) with cotton-tipped applicators. Daily lid hygiene with 5-minute warm compresses and lid margin massage with Eye Scrub or baby shampoo by the patient using the lathered fingertips are important in completely eradicating the inflammation. *Certain antibiotics* inhibit the abnormal fatty acid metabolism, which invites lid margin inflammation. Doxycycline 100 mg p.o. qd for 1 month, then 50 to 100 mg qd 3 to 6 *months* with a meal; or (less convenient) tetracycline 250 mg p.o. qd on an empty stomach; erythromycin 250 mg p.o. qd; or minocycline 100 mg qd, in the same multimonth regimen, is generally very effective. Daily hand and face scrubs with pHisoHex for 2 to 3 weeks and then three to four times weekly will lower the facial germ count and reduce acneiform eruptions and styes. Metronidazole 0.75% gel (Metro Gel) bid to the facial skin for 6 months is highly effective adjunctive

therapy. Infectious **eczematoid dermatitis** occurring with staphylococcal blepharitis is an indication for erythromycin or bacitracin ointment bid for 10 days, or antimicrobial–steroid combination. Sulfacetamide–prednisolone combinations are particularly effective. Acne **rosacea** patients should use steroids with caution, however, because they are more prone to corneal ulceration with these drugs. Sterile **corneal marginal infiltrates** and ulcerations that occur with chronic staphylococcal blepharoconjunctivitis also respond to topical steroids, usually within 4 or 5 days. **Phlyctenular keratoconjunctivitis** will resolve on treatment with topical antibiotic–steroid agents qid for 10 to 14 days (see sec. **VII.H.,** below; for chalazia, see Chapter 3, sec. **I.I.3.**).

    4. Catscratch fever (Parinaud ocular glandular syndrome, bartonellosis) responds well to doxycycline 100 mg p.o. Erythromycin p.o. is effective in children and may be combined with rifampin 300 mg p.o. bid for more severe infections. Duration of treatment is 2 to 4 weeks in immunocompetent patients and 4 months in immunocompromised patients (see sec. **III.B.3.c.,** above).

IV. Corneal infections and inflammation (keratitis and keratoconjunctivitis)

  A. Superficial keratitis includes inflammatory lesions of the corneal epithelium and adjacent superficial stroma. Although some of the changes described in this section can be produced by noninflammatory conditions and therefore would more appropriately be considered keratopathy, they are considered here because of their diagnostic importance. The etiologies of this clinical condition include numerous *infective, toxic, degenerative, and allergic* conditions that can often be characterized by the morphology and distribution of the lesions produced. These conditions may occur with bacterial, viral, and fungal infections. Degenerative states resulting from dry eye, neurotrophic defects, or in association with systemic disease can also produce ulceration of the cornea. When accompanied by infiltration or significant ocular anterior chamber reaction, infection must be excluded or diagnosed and treated.

    1. Morphologically, the lesions include punctate **epithelial erosions** that are focal defects in the corneal epithelium, best visualized by rose bengal and fluorescein staining and slitlamp biomicroscopy. Punctate **epithelial keratitis** is characterized by focal inflammatory infiltration of the epithelium, resulting in minute opaque epithelial lesions observed in focal illumination or with the slitlamp. Although they may occur without staining, they often do stain with rose bengal or fluorescein because of associated punctate epithelial erosion. Punctate **subepithelial infiltrates** are nonstaining focal areas that occur as semiopaque spots in the superficial stroma.

    2. Identification of the morphology and distribution of the lesions is greatly enhanced by the use of vital *clinical stains,* most notably rose bengal and fluorescein. **Rose bengal** stains dead or degenerating cells and presently is available as sterile paper strips (wet with saline). Prior instillation of proparacaine 0.5% will relieve the smarting sensation produced by rose bengal, but tetracaine and cocaine should be avoided, because they will often produce an artifactual rose bengal staining pattern. Rose bengal is also an excellent stain for mucus and filaments. Fluorescein from a 2% solution or from a Fluri-strip wet with saline will stain epithelial defects or bared basement membrane, and is also used when highlighting corneal filaments.

    3. The **distribution** of the epithelial and subepithelial lesion is of *diagnostic value.* Figure 5.1 summarizes the **six** clinical patterns and their respective etiologies. *Diffuse* and nonspecific *punctate epithelial erosions* may occur with early bacterial or viral infections of many types. Breakdown of microcystic areas of epithelial edema can also produce this pattern, and such areas of edema will also demonstrate areas of

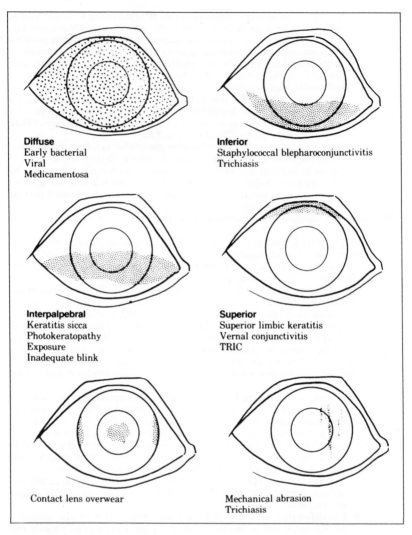

FIG. 5.1. Staining patterns of the cornea and conjunctiva in various disease states. TRIC, trachoma-inclusion conjunctivitis.

negative staining in the fluorescein film corresponding to intact epithelial microcysts. Any toxic reaction to topical medications, chemicals, or aerosol sprays can produce this pattern. Mechanical trauma from a foreign body or eye rubbing must also be considered. The epithelial erosions secondary to molluscum contagiosum of the lids will occur in areas *contiguous* to the lesion. *Inferior* punctate epithelial erosions frequently result from staphylococcal blepharitis or blepharoconjunctivitis and are often accompanied by epithelial keratitis and subepithelial infiltrates. Trichiasis or incomplete lid closure *(exposure keratopathy)* can produce this distribution of erosion, and the pattern is also occasionally seen in dry eye patients. The *interpalpebral* distribution is typical of keratitis sicca, ultraviolet radiation exposure, chronic exposure, or incomplete blinking. Conjunctival staining usually will accompany the corneal lesion. Episodic recurrent erosions frequently will occur in the inferior area or interpalpebral area. The *superior* distribution of epithelial erosion is typical of superolimbic keratoconjunctivitis, but can also be seen in vernal conjunctivitis and with trachoma. Corneal epithelial filaments consisting of coiled epithelial remnants and adherent mucous strands may be associated with any of these patterns, but most typically appear with superolimbic keratoconjunctivitis or keratoconjunctivitis sicca. *Central* lesions, with or without some peripheral punctate, suggest contact lens malfit or overwear, and *linear* lesions suggest a foreign body on the lid rubbing the cornea.

4. The **etiology** of **punctate epithelial erosion** is often local desiccation. Instability of the tear film results in focal dry spots and epithelial breakdown. Epithelial membrane damage from detergent chemicals, liquid solvents, quaternary amines, and a variety of drugs also results in erosions. Superficial viral and chlamydial infections can produce focal erosions, as can the epithelial hypoxia of contact lens overwear. **Punctate epithelial keratitis** with minute focal opacities is typical of viral keratitis, especially that associated with epidemic keratoconjunctivitis of adenovirus, but may also be seen with staphylococcal and chlamydial infections. The infiltrates also occur with vaccinia, Reiter syndrome, and acne rosacea. The coarse, granular infiltrates of punctate epithelial keratitis are quite characteristic of Thygeson superficial punctate keratitis.

5. **Nonstaining punctate subepithelial infiltrates** in the superficial stroma are sometimes seen after such entities as adenoviral, herpes simplex, herpes zoster, Epstein-Barr viral, vaccinial, chlamydial, Reiter, Lyme disease, and rosacea keratitis. Staphylococcal infection must be considered when this pattern appears in a marginal infiltrate distribution. Inferior peripheral limbal infiltrates can accompany acute *H. influenzae* conjunctivitis.

B. **Bacterial corneal ulcers**
1. **Central ulcer.** Predominant causes of central bacterial keratitis are *Staphylococcus,* e.g., *S. aureus, and S. epidermidis*; *Streptococcus,* such as *S. pneumococcus* and groups A–G *Streptococcus*; other **Gram-positive organisms,** such as *Bacillus and Propionibacterium* sp; the **Gram-negative organisms Haemophilus, Pseudomonas,** and *Moraxella*; and other **Enterobacteriaceae (*Proteus, Serratia, E. coli*,** and *Klebsiella*).** Mycobacterium chelonae* keratitis may follow laser-assisted in situ keratomileusis (LASIK) surgery. Gram-negative diplococci are an uncommon cause of corneal ulceration except in inadequately treated cases of hyperacute gonococcal conjunctivitis. Infection of the cornea usually tends to occur after injury to the epithelium or in compromised hosts, except for *Neisseria* and *Corynebacterium,* which may invade intact epithelium. Stromal infiltration in an area of an epithelial defect with surrounding edema and folds associated with endothelial fibrin plaques or anterior chamber reaction is usually indicative of microbial infection. Staphylococcal ulcers are often more localized, whereas pneumococcus may produce a shaggy undermined edge of an ulcer that is associated with a hypopyon. A destructive keratitis with rapid necrosis and adherent mucopurulent discharge is highly suggestive of *Pseudomonas, Streptococcus,* or anaerobic infection. **Infectious crystalline keratopathy** is an indolent, noninflammatory branching crystalline growth commonly associated with *Streptococcus viridans,* but also reported with *Peptostreptococcus* sp, *S. epidermidis, H. influenzae,* and two fungal species. There is also often a history of local ocular trauma, contact lens use, steroid use, and/or chronic antibiotic administration. Response to antibiotic therapy is very slow and may fail. Surgical

intervention with neodymium:yttrium, aluminum, garnet (Nd:YAG) **laser disruption,** e.g., 3.2 mJ × 30, creates diffuse haze of the protective glycocalyx matrix within the intrastromal crystals making the bacteria drug-susceptible. This should be considered before more extensive surgical steps are taken.

2. **Marginal ulcers.** Ulceration with superficial white infiltrates in the corneal periphery is seen most commonly with *staphylococcal* bacterial disease. There is concurrent blepharoconjunctivitis. The ulceration may be caused by hypersensitivity reaction, because culture of the ulcer is often sterile. The ulceration must be distinguished from Mooren ulcer and the peripheral ulceration seen with collagen vascular diseases such as rheumatoid arthritis. *Moraxella* sp has been described as producing ulcers that extend to the limbus, especially inferiorly.

3. **Laboratory tests** are similar to those for hyperacute conjunctivitis (see sec. III.C., above) apply also to bacterial corneal disease.

   a. **Cultures** are performed after instillation of topical proparacaine 0.5% (tetracaine, benoxinate, and cocaine are more likely to interfere with recovery of the organisms) and should obtain as much material as feasible, particularly from the deeper areas and the margin of the ulcer, using a sterile broth or saline-moistened calcium alginate or dacron–rayon swab. *Organism recovery is much higher when alginate swabs are used* rather than spatulas. Cultures are done on meat broth, blood agar plates (at room temperature and 38°C), chocolate agar, thioglycolate broth, and Sabouraud agar–broth (fungus), and Page medium *(Acanthamoeba),* if suspected. Scrapings taken from a nonnecrotic area may be examined microscopically with Gram and Giemsa stains. Because 30% to 40% will be negative even if infection is present, these scrapings may be judiciously omitted.

   b. **Corneal biopsy** is often diagnostic in cases that progress despite seemingly adequate treatment; even if an organism has been identified, another may have been missed. In the minor operating room or at the slitlamp, after local anesthesia (drops or xylocaine block), a 2 to 3 mm sterile disposable dermatologic trephine is advanced to partial depth into the anterior corneal stroma, taking both clinically infected and adjacent clear cornea. The base is then undermined with a surgical blade to complete the lamellar keratectomy.

4. **Initial treatment** is based on clinical impression and results, if any, of the scraping. Coverage should be broad, intensive, and amenable to change when final culture and sensitivity reports are available. Contact lens wearers with central corneal ulcers should particularly be covered for *Pseudomonas* (tobramycin, netilmicin, and/or a quinolone). Antibiotic treatment of infectious corneal ulcers must be aggressive using fortified solutions, and patients should be kept under close observation to prevent serious scarring or frank perforation. Initial antibiotic therapy may be guided by the results of the Gram stain of the corneal scraping, but broad-spectrum therapy should be used (**see Tables 5.5, 5.6, and 5.7 and Appendix B** for detailed lists of drug indications, dosage, and routes of administration).

   a. **Gram-positive cocci.** In mild to moderate infections, frequent topical therapy alone may be used, but it may be advisable to give subconjunctival therapy as well in severe infections, or apply a collagen contact lens soaked 10 minutes in fortified antibiotic solution (see sec. **IV.B.6.**).

      (1) **Coupled fortified cephalosporin–aminoglycoside therapy** is common. Topical cefazolin solution, 100 mg per mL, should be used *q1min for 5 doses to achieve high stromal levels quickly* and then q60min 24 hours per day or 16 times per day with a polymyxin–bacitracin ointment HS depending on severity of disease. Tobramycin is often effective against *Staphylococcus,* but poorly effective against pneumococcus or other *Streptococcus.* Fortified drops of one of these aminoglycosides are used in

TABLE 5.5. INITIAL TOPICAL ANTIBIOTIC THERAPY OF BACTERIAL KERATITIS BASED ON GRAM-STAIN FINDINGS[a]

Bacterial Type	Drugs of Choice (Fortified)	Alternative Drugs (Fortified and Nonfortified)
Gram-positive cocci	Cefazolin, 100 mg/mL	Vancomycin, 25 mg/mL Bacitracin, 10,000 units/mL Ciprofloxacin,[b,c] ofloxacin,[b,c] or levofloxacin[b,c]
Gram-positive bacilli (filaments)	Penicillin G, 100,000 units/mL	Vancomycin, 25–50 mg/mL Bacitracin, 10,000 units/mL
Gram-positive rods	Tobramycin, 14 mg/mL	Gentamicin, 14 mg/mL
Gram-negative cocci	Ceftriaxone, 50 mg/mL[d]	Ofloxacin,[b,c,d] levofloxacin,[b,c,d] or ciprofloxacin[b,c,d]
Gram-negative bacilli	Tobramycin, 14 mg/mL Amikacin, 10 mg/mL Ticarcillin, 6 mg/mL	Gentamicin, 14 mg/mL Polymyxin B, 50,000 units/mL Ciprofloxacin,[b,c] ofloxacin,[b,c] or levofloxacin[b,c]
No organisms seen, but bacteria suspected[e]	Cefazolin, 100 mg/mL, plus tobramycin 14 mg/mL	Gentamicin, 14 mg/mL, or amikacin, 10 mg/mL, plus vancomycin, 25 mg/mL, or bacitracin, 10,000 units/mL

[a]See also Table 5.7 for dosage and preparation of fortified drops and subconjunctival doses, and Appendix B for expanded drug dosage list and organism-susceptibility guide. Subconjunctival and systemic therapy use is based on extent of disease (see Table 5.7).

[b]Drops available as commercial ophthalmic preparations.

[c]Not available in fortified form. Commercial strength only. Systemic therapy should be used in addition to local treatment for *Neisseria* or *Hemophilus* infection (see sec. **III.D.2.**).

[d]Not U.S. Food and Drug Administration approved for topical therapy of *Neisseria*.

[e]Small to medium peripheral infiltrates may be treated with a quinolone (ofloxacin, levofloxacin, ciprofloxacin).

TABLE 5.6. SUBSEQUENT THERAPY FOR CULTURE-IDENTIFIED
BACTERIAL ULCERS[a]

Organisms	Topical	Subconjunctival[b]
Pseudomonas	Tobramycin, 14 mg/mL, or amikacin, 10 mg/mL, and a quinolone	Tobramycin, 40 mg (1 mL), amikacin, 25 mg, or ticarcillin, 100 mg
Staphylococcus	Cefazolin, 100 mg/mL, vancomycin[c], 25–50 mg/mL, or bacitracin, 10,000 units/mL and/or a quinolone	Cefazolin, 100 mg, oxacillin, 100 mg, or vancomycin, 25 mg
Proteus, Enterobacter, Escherichia coli, Klebsiella, Acinetobacter	Tobramycin, 14 mg/mL, gentamicin, 14 mg/mL, amikacin, 10 mg/mL, or ceftriaxone, 50 mg/mL, and/or a quinolone	Tobramycin amikacin, 25 mg, or carbenicillin, 100 mg

[a]See Appendix B for parenteral use of these and other drugs and organism-susceptibility guide. See Table 5.7 for method of preparation of fortified drops and subconjunctival doses.
[b]Uncooperative patient or pending of actual scleral involvement. Add systemic antibiotics.
[c]Methicillin-resistant organisms.

the same regimen as cefazolin to cover any Gram-negative organisms that may be revealed only by culture. Vancomycin (14 to 25 mg per mL) or bacitracin (10,000 units per mL) is effective in Gram-positive coccal and bacillus infections, and especially *methicillin-resistant Staphylococcus,* where cephalosporins would fail. Drops are tapered over a 1- to 2-week period to qid for 3 weeks more as indicated. For *methicillin-resistant organisms,* vancomycin is the drug of choice.

(2) **Single-agent broad-spectrum drops** of the quinolones, (ciprofloxacin, ofloxacin, levofloxacin, or norfloxacin) are commercially available. More severe ulcers should probably be treated at least initially with double agents (sec. **IV.B.**), but either quinolone may be substituted when the situation is under control and organism(s) known. Organisms covered are similar to those for cefazolin or vancomycin and an aminoglycoside, and include the microbes listed in sec. **III.B.1.,** above.

(3) **Subconjunctival therapy** is usually used only in severe cases, or for uncooperative or unreliable patients. Because a 10% cross sensitivity between cephalosporins and penicillin has been reported in *penicillin-allergic patients,* it is usually safer to proceed with vancomycin therapy. Subconjunctival injections are *painful* and are best preceded by topical anesthetic (or general anesthetic when treating children) and adequate postinjection analgesics.

b. **Gram-negative cocci** (*N. meningitidis, N. gonorrhoeae*) and *Haemophilus* require *systemic* and *topical* therapy and are discussed under hyperacute conjunctivitis (see sec. **III.D.2.,** above). Topical therapy should be q1h for 2 to 4 days with taper over 2 to 4 weeks.

c. **Gram-positive rods.** These uncommon agents of ocular infection usually respond to systemic penicillin (see Appendix B). *Bacillus* sp are susceptible to moderate doses of penicillin; clostridial organisms require higher doses. *Bacillus cereus* infections may be extremely hard to treat, even using gentamicin, ofloxacin, norfloxacin,

TABLE 5.7. PREPARATION OF ANTIBIOTICS FOR FORTIFIED TOPICAL AND SUBCONJUNCTIVAL USE

Antibiotic (i.m. or i.v. Formulation)	Commercial Solution	Fortified Topical Drops			Subconjunctival		
		Diluent[a] (mL) Added to 1.0 mL Commercial Solution	Final Concentration	Shelf Life (4°C)[b] (d)	Volume of Diluent (mL) Added to 1.0 mL Commercial Solution	Final Concentration	Final Dose
Amikacin	100 mg/1 mL	9.0	10 mg/mL	30	1.0	50 mg/mL	25–50 mg
Bacitracin	50,000 units/5 mL	—	10,000 units/mL	7	—	10,000 units/mL	5000 units
Carbenicillin	1.0 g/10 mL	24.0	4 mg/mL	3	—	100 mg/mL	100 mg
Cefamandole	1.0 g/7.5 mL	—	133 mg/mL	4	0.3	100 mg/mL	100 mg
Cefazolin	1.0 g/10 mL	2.0	33 mg/mL	10	—	—	—
Cefazolin	1.0 g/7.5 mL	—	133 mg/mL	10	0.3	100 mg/mL	100 mg
Ceftriaxone	1.0 g/7.5 mL	—	133 mg/mL	10	0.3	100 mg/mL	100 mg
Chloramphenicol	1.0 g/10 mL	19.0	5 mg/mL	7	—	100 mg/mL	100 mg
Gentamicin	80 mg/2 mL	1.8	14 mg/mL	30	—	40 mg/mL	20–40 mg
Penicillin G potassium	1 million units/mL	9.0	100,000 units/mL	7	—	1 million units/mL	1 million units
Polymyxin B	500,000 units/20–50 mL	—	10–25,000 units/mL	3	—	10,000 units/mL	10,000 units/mL
Ticarcillin	1.0 g/10 mL	16.0	6 mg/mL	14	—	—	—
Tobramycin	80 mg/2 mL	1.8	14 mg/mL	30	—	40 mg/mL	20–40 mg
Vancomycin	500 mg/10 mL	1.0	25 mg/mL	14	—	50 mg/mL	25 mg

i.m., intramuscular; i.v., intravenous.

[a]With the exception of carbenicillin and vancomycin (sterile water for injection only) and bacitracin (normal saline for injection only), diluent may be sterile water or saline for injection (USP), or sterile artificial tears using the original tears bottle to administer the reconstituted drug solution.

[b]Freezing extends expiration time to 12 weeks for aminoglycosides, cephalosporins, and vancomycin; 4 weeks for ticarcillin.

(Adapted from Pavan-Langston D, Dunkel E. Antibiotics. In: *Handbook of Ocular Drug Therapy and Ocular Side Effects of Systemic Drugs*, Boston: Little, Brown, 1991.)

ciprofloxacin, or clindamycin. **Topical drops** and **subconjunctival** injections are used q1h. Tetracycline topically and orally is a useful adjunctive.

d. **Gram-negative rods**

(1) **Topical** therapy initially should be fortified tobramycin ophthalmic solution q1min for 5 doses, then q60min for 3 to 6 days before starting slow taper. Important adjunctive therapy is topical ticarcillin 6 mg per mL, or carbenicillin 4 mg per mL, q60min. Treat *Pseudomonas* at least 1 month or rebound infection may occur. **Aminoglycoside-resistant** strains are increasing. If *Pseudomonas* is gentamicin-resistant, a quinolone drop should be coupled with ticarcillin or carbenicillin, as above. If the strain is **quinolone-resistant,** *amikacin* is often effective.

(2) **Subconjunctival therapy,** if used, should include tobramycin or amikacin 40 mg, and carbenicillin 100 mg, each injected in a different area of the conjunctiva.

e. **Anaerobic Gram-positive filaments** *(Actinomyces, Nocardia [formerly Streptothrix])* are sensitive to penicillins and tetracyclines.

f. *Mycobacterium chelonae* ulcers are treated with a combination of topical amikacin (50 mg per mL, commercial ciprofloxacin, and either clarithromycin (10 mg per mL) or azithromycin (2 mg per mL) hourly around the clock to start with, then taper over weeks. Oral doxycycline 100 mg bid is additive therapeutically.

g. **When no organisms are identified,** but bacterial etiology is strongly suspected on clinical grounds:

(1) **Topical** therapy should be with fortified cefazolin q1min for 5 doses, then coupled with tobramycin 14 mg per mL q60 min, for 3–6 days before taper over 4–6 weeks. Use vancomycin in severe cases and suspected methicillin-resistant or penicillin-allergic patients.

(2) **Subconjunctival therapy,** if used, should be cefazolin 100 mg, plus tobramycin 40 mg, until culture results are available. A fortified-antibiotic-soaked collagen lens (see sec. **IV.B.6.**) may also be effective adjunctively.

h. **Systemic antibiotics** are used if there is scleral extension of the infection or a threatened perforation. Levofloxacin 500 mg p.o. q24h or ofloxacin 200 to 400 mg p.o. q12h for 7 days both have excellent aqueous and vitreous penetration after oral dosing. A cephalosporin or vancomycin and an aminoglycoside may also be used p.o. or i.v., with doses given as in Appendix B. In cases of *vancomycin resistance,* which is an emerging problem, linezolid 600 mg i.v. or p.o. q12h may be indicated. Tables 5.5, 5.6, 5.7, and Appendix B summarize the recommended therapy. Therapy may be refined when culture and sensitivities return.

i. The **antibiotic regimen is altered,** if necessary, when final culture and sensitivity information is available. Fortified vancomycin and bacitracin are used if *methicillin-resistant staphylococci* are recovered. In the event that a suspected Gram-negative coccus infection was initially treated with penicillin and the subsequent culture results disclose *Acinetobacter* sp, penicillin should be discontinued because these organisms are often not sensitive to penicillin.

5. **Other treatment modalities**

a. **Dilation.** Long-acting cycloplegics such as atropine 1% or scopolamine 0.25% should be used if significant anterior chamber reaction is present. Initial instillation is usually required at least three times a day. If significant synechiae are forming at the pupillary margin, one or two doses of topical 2.5% phenylephrine are often indicated to ensure mobility of the pupil.

b. **Corticosteroid** use in treatment of infectious corneal ulcers is less controversial than in past years. It is probably unwise to use steroids until at least 24 to 48 hours of antibacterial treatment has been completed, or until the etiologic agent has been identified and shown to be sensitive to the antibiotics being used. Corticosteroid use is *contraindicated if fungus* is at all suspected. Low-dose topical corticosteroids (e.g., prednisolone 0.12% qid) have a place in limiting the inflammatory reaction once the clinician is satisfied that the antibiotic treatment is effective.

6. **Collagen shields** (Surgilens, Bausch & Lomb), are contact lenses initially developed to enhance corneal epithelial healing after surgery, trauma, or dystrophic erosions and filaments, but are also used as effective high-dose drug delivery systems (the lenses are not FDA approved as drug delivery systems). The lenses come in two sizes and dissolve spontaneously over 24 to 72 hours. Soaking the lenses in antibiotics, such as tobramycin 40 mg solution for 10 minutes, results in a 30-fold increase in antibiotic penetration into the aqueous compared to subconjunctival injection or a regular therapeutic soft contact lens (TSCL) and q1h drops. The high level of drug may be maintained with q4h drops using the collagen shields.

7. **Special pediatric considerations.** Subconjunctival therapy is usually not feasible unless the child is under general anesthesia at the time of a corneal culture and scraping. Should systemic medication be considered necessary, it is best done with the consultation of a pediatrician or internist. See Appendix B for dosages and organism indications.

C. **Chlamydial (trachoma-inclusion conjunctivitis) organisms** are intracellular "parasites" but not true viruses, having enzyme systems similar to bacteria. They can produce acute inflammatory diseases of the conjunctiva and cornea that will often progress to a more chronic follicular conjunctivitis. Infection with inclusion conjunctivitis usually takes different forms in children and adults.

1. **Neonatal inclusion conjunctivitis (inclusion blennorrhea)** has an acute onset 5 to 12 days after birth, presenting as an acute conjunctivitis with purulent discharge.

   a. **Diagnosis** of this *Chlamydia trachomatis* infection is facilitated by the presence of **intracytoplasmic inclusion bodies** apparent in epithelial cells obtained by conjunctival scraping. Giemsa stain is the most effective method for demonstrating the individual elementary bodies or larger initial bodies as basophilic inclusions with, at times, small eosinophilic opacities. It is obviously important to distinguish this infection from *N. gonorrhoeae*. Although the infection can resolve without sequelae, a membranous conjunctivitis may develop and result in conjunctival scarring, and a definite keratitis may supervene with superficial corneal vascularization.

   b. **Treatment** is **systemic antibiotics** with the topical being adjunctive. Erythromycin 12 mg per kg p.o. daily in four divided doses for 2 to 3 weeks is the preferred therapy in newborns. Sulfisoxazole is the alternative drug (see Appendix B). *Children under 8 years of age should not receive systemic tetracyclines.* In infants, the usual topical treatment is sulfacetamide 10% or erythromycin ointment qid for at least 3 weeks. Because the condition is acquired by the presence of *Chlamydia* in the birth canal, it should be assumed that the parents are infected and probably require treatment with systemic tetracycline to eliminate the source of the infection. If the mother is *breast-feeding,* erythromycin 250 mg p.o. qid, or sulfonamides 500 mg p.o. qid should be used for 21 days (see sec. **IV.C.2.b.,** below).

2. **Adult inclusion conjunctivitis** usually presents as an acute follicular conjunctivitis with mucopurulent discharge occurring after an incubation period of 4 to 12 days. The disease usually occurs in sexually active young adults, but may occur in senior citizens as well, often after having acquired a new sexual partner in the preceding 2 months. The acute conjunctivitis

often evolves into a chronic follicular conjunctivitis. An epithelial keratitis may develop, as well as marginal and more central corneal infiltrates accompanied by superficial vascularization as an *inferior* limbal pannus. Iritis has been reported later in the condition, as well as Reiter syndrome.

a. **Diagnosis** by Giemsa-stained scraping of the epithelium is less likely to show inclusion bodies, but these may be seen in a number of patients with the acute disease. Microtrak assay of scrapings is far more reliable diagnostically, but any culture or immune laboratory test may still have false positives or negatives.

b. **Treatment.** Systemic azithromycin is more effective and efficient than either erythromycin or tetracycline and is given as 1 g p.o. for 2 days. Alternative first-line therapies are doxycycline 100 mg p.o. bid with a meal, or tetracycline 250 to 500 mg p.o. qid 30 minutes before meals or 2 hours after meals for 21 days. Erythromycin or sulfonamides are also effective, as are the quinolones ofloxacin and ciprofloxacin (but not norfloxacin) in bid dosing. Topical antibiotics are relatively ineffective in treating the eye disease, but may modify a conjunctivitis. Because the condition may be associated with an asymptomatic venereal infection *partners* should also be *treated systemically* and the possibility of *other venereal disease* must be excluded. Tetracyclines should not be used in women who are pregnant or breast-feeding. Azithromycin 1 g p.o. qd for 2 days, erythromycin 250 mg p.o. qid, or sulfisoxazole 500 mg p.o. qid for 21 days, are effective alternatives. High-dose amoxicillin may be used in pregnancy (Appendix B).

3. **Trachoma.** The initial manifestation of trachoma is a chronic follicular conjunctivitis that is classically more marked on the upper tarsal plate, with progressive disease scarring of the conjunctiva occurring on the superior tarsal conjunctiva as fine linear scars and often as a transverse band of scar **(Arlt line).** When marked, this scarring can lead to entropion and trichiasis, with secondary ocular surface breakdown, including corneal ulceration. Primary corneal involvement occurring with the conjunctivitis can include an epithelial keratitis, marginal and central corneal infiltrates, and superficial vascularization. This is usually more pronounced on the upper half of the cornea and can appear as a fibrovascular pannus. Follicle formation at the limbus regresses to sharply defined depressions **(Herbert pits)** at the base of the pannus.

a. **The disease,** as classically described by **MacCallan,** considers the *conjunctival* changes according to the following classification:

(1) **Trachoma I.** Immature follicles on the upper tarsal plate including the central area, but without scarring.

(2) **Trachoma II.** Mature (necrotic or soft) follicles on the upper tarsus obscuring tarsal vessels, but without scarring.

(3) **Trachoma III.** Follicles present on the tarsus and definite scarring of the conjunctiva.

(4) **Trachoma IV.** No follicles on the tarsal plate but marked scarring of the conjunctiva. This infection is not commonly seen in developed countries, but only the United Kingdom and some parts of Europe are totally free of endemic disease.

b. **Treatment.** Azithromycin 1 g p.o. qd for 2 days is efficient, effective, but expensive therapy. Individual patients with trachoma will also respond to a 3-week course of either tetracycline or erythromycin p.o. in full dosages (250 mg qid). Clinical response may be slow, and prolonged treatment may be required. When large groups are treated, topical tetracycline or erythromycin ointments may be given twice daily for 2 months. When systemic treatment is used, tetracycline should be used in preference to oral sulfonamides due to the lower incidence of side effects with tetracycline (see secs. **IV.C.1.** and **C.2.,** above, for further therapy information).

D. Herpes simplex virus (HSV) keratoconjunctivitis and iritis. Ocular infections with herpesvirus represent a challenge to diagnosis and treatment. **Primary ocular herpes** is rare and usually occurs as an acute follicular keratoconjunctivitis with regional lymphadenitis, with or without vesicular ulcerative blepharitis or cutaneous involvement. The keratitis can occur as a coarse punctate or diffuse branching epithelial keratitis that does not usually involve the stroma. The condition is self-limited, but the virus establishes a latent infection in the trigeminal ganglion. It may *reactivate* under various forms of physical stress (recent fever, flu, or surgical or dental procedures), with the prostaglandin analog latanoprost used in glaucoma therapy, as well as with any form of ocular laser treatment, and cause recurrence of the disease in a host who has both competent cellular and humoral immunity. **Recurrent disease** of the anterior segment may occur as one or a combination of the following: epithelial infectious ulcers, epithelial trophic ulcers, stromal interstitial keratitis (IK), stromal immune diskiform keratitis, and iridocyclitis. Management of this disease, with its chronic recurring and often progressive nature, can be difficult and must be tailored to minimize permanent ocular damage.

1. **Epithelial infection.** Dendritic or geographic ulceration of the cornea is caused by live virus present in intracellular and extracellular locations, particularly in the basal epithelium. The use of steroids in purely infectious epithelial disease serves only to make the ulceration spread and to prolong the infectious phase of the disease. Fluorescein or rose bengal staining make the ulcers easier to see.

   a. **Topical antiviral chemotherapy** with topical *trifluridine 1%* solution nine times a day for 5 days, then five time per day for 9 to 21 days, *or vidarabine 3%* ointment four to five times a day arrests viral replication until infected cells slough from the eye. *Idoxuridine* 0.1% drops are given hourly by day and q2h at night or as just antiviral ointment at bedtime. With treatment, the infectious epithelial disease resolves 80% to 90% of the time without complication and without the need for antiinflammatory drugs. **Limbal ulcers** are more resistant to healing, but eventually close without much scarring. HSV infections in *human immunodeficiency virus-positive (HIV positive)* patients show a predilection for peripheral versus central involvement, moderately prolonged course with mean healing time of 3 weeks with topical antivirals, rare stromal involvement, and tendency to frequent recurrence (more than two times per year). With prolonged treatment, the antivirals can produce a **toxic** punctate keratopathy, retardation of epithelial healing, superficial stromal opacification, follicular conjunctivitis, or lacrimal punctal occlusion.

   b. **Systemic antiviral acyclovir.** A dosage of 400 mg p.o. tid for 14 days delivers high-titer therapeutic doses in tear film and aqueous for treatment of acute infectious epithelial HSV in those patients for whom topical therapy is difficult (those with severe arthritis or in children). Pediatric dosing ranges from 20 to 40 mg/kg/day. Post-HSV *keratoplasty* dosage of 400 mg bid for 12 to 18 months is indicated therapy and may successfully prevent recurrent infection and graft rejection. Both *epithelial and stromal recurrences* are inhibited by 400 mg bid. This **long-term prophylaxis** is recommended for use in patients at risk of recurrent epithelial or stromal disease more than two times yearly. Treatment is usually given for 1 year, but may go significantly longer (genito-urinary HSV prophylaxis goes for 5 years or longer). Acyclovir is equivocally effective in iritis and not generally used.

   c. **Systemic antiviral famciclovir** and **valacyclovir** are highly effective alternatives to acyclovir. In *acute* first infections, dosage is famciclovir 250 mg p.o. tid for 7 days or valacyclovir 1 g p.o. bid for 7 days. For *recurrent* infection, the dosage is famciclovir 125 mg p.o. bid or valacyclovir 500 mg p.o. bid for 7 days. For *long-term* *suppression* dosages are 125 mg p.o. qd to bid and 500 mg p.o. qd to bid, respectively. Valaciclovir should *not* be used long term in *immunosuppressed* patients because of myelosuppression.

   d. Acyclovir 3% ophthalmic ointment, applied five times a day, is available outside of the United States.

2. **Epithelial sterile trophic ulceration (metaherpetic, postinfectious, persistent epithelial defect).** An indolent linear or ovoid epithelial defect with heaped-up borders can occur at the site of a previous herpetic ulcer and be confused with infectious geographic ulcer. These persistent epithelial defects are mechanical healing problems similar to recurrent traumatic erosion and are caused by damage to the basement membrane sustained during the acute infectious epithelial stage. Damaged basement membrane heals extremely slowly over 8 to 12 weeks. During this period, epithelial cells are unable to maintain their position after migrating across the bed of the ulcer.

   a. Because of the mechanical nature of the problem, **treatment** is designed to protect the damaged basement membrane. Ointments and artificial tears may affect healing, but often a high-water-content plano therapeutic soft contact lens (TSCL) (Permalens, Kontur) worn for 2 to 6 months is needed (see sec. **XI.,** below). Patching, lid taping, partial tarsorrhaphy, or, infrequently, a surgically placed conjunctival flap are alternatives. Stromal inflammatory disease may interfere with the healing of the basement membrane. Mild corticosteroid such as 1/8% prednisolone bid to qid is useful. Antibiotic solution once or twice a day should be used when treatment includes continuously worn therapeutic contact lenses, along with frequent lubrication with artificial tears for several months even after the lens has been removed.

   b. If active **corneal thinning** (melting) occurs, sealing off the ulcer with **cyanoacrylate tissue adhesive** (Dermabond; not FDA approved for ocular use) should be considered. With the patient under topical anesthesia, the physician débrides and dries the ulcer and periulcer area of debris and loose cells with Weckcell sponges, and applies the liquid adhesive in short strokes or concentric spots. It polymerizes almost instantly to the tissue. Sterile saline is dripped on the eye to complete polymerization, a *Plano-T* TSCL is applied, and antibiotic drops are given bid. If needed for inflammation, steroids may now be used with greater safety. The cornea should heal and dislodge the glue in 1 to 3 months, usually leaving the eye quiet but scarred, and it is hoped that it will be amenable to transplant if vision is significantly compromised.

3. **Stromal IK, immune rings, and limbal vasculitis** result from antigen–antibody complement-mediated immune reaction in the stroma. Viral IK presents as *necrotic,* blotchy, white infiltrates that may lie under ulcers or appear independently. Immune rings are gray anterior stromal Wessley rings, and limbal vasculitis is a local Arthus reaction. These lesions must be distinguished from secondary bacterial or fungal infections, which are usually much less indolent. After several weeks of smoldering inflammation, dense leashes of stromal vascularization may begin to advance into the cornea.

   a. Therapy is suppression of immune damage. If the inflammatory infiltrates do not involve the visual axis or there is no active necrosis or neovascularization, steroid therapy may be avoided because the process often burns itself out spontaneously in weeks to months and, with the exception of limbal vasculitis, scars form despite steroid therapy. The vascularization regresses to leave ghost vessels. Treatment may be limited to **lubricants.**

   Generally, if **corticosteroids** have *never been used* in an eye, the clinician should try to do without them, because subsequent recurrences will then require reinitiation of steroids and treatment is prolonged over a taper period. If the inflammatory reaction is moderate to severe, however, if steroids have been used previously, if the visual axis is threatened, or if there is active necrosis or neovascularization, the use of steroids will speed resolution of the inflammation and decrease formation of scar tissue and deep vessel invasion that could later compromise success of surgery. The **corticosteroid dosage** is whatever controls the disease and may range from dexamethasone 0.1% q3h to prednisolone 0.12% every other day. Once hyperemia and edema begin to decrease, steroids should be tapered downward over several weeks to several months. *Prophylactic antiviral agents* such as trifluridine qid or acyclovir 400 mg p.o. bid should be used, and daily *antibiotics* continued until steroid dose is reduced to the equivalent of prednisolone 1% bid unless the patient is prone to infectious recurrences.

4. **Diskiform keratitis** results from a delayed hypersensitivity reaction characterized by sensitized T lymphocytes and macrophages reacting to viral antigen in the cornea. Clinically there is a focal or diffuse, nonnecrotic disk-shaped area of stromal edema often with focal keratic precipitates **(endotheliitis).** With progressive severity, more diffuse edema with folds in Descemet's membrane, neovascularization, and iritis may appear.

    Therapeutically, the same rules apply to treatment of diskiform keratitis as to viral IK (see sec. **IV.D.3.,** above).

5. **If diskiform stromal disease** is present with an HSV-**infected epithelial ulcer,** gentle débridement of the epithelium and full antiviral therapy should be started a day or two before steroids. If the ulcer progresses despite antiviral therapy, steroid dosage should be reduced until the ulcer is under control and is healing. If diskiform keratitis is combined with **trophic ulceration,** control of underlying stromal edema with low-dose topical steroids and the application of a TSCL will aid healing. A **persistent epithelial defect** carries the added risk of collagenase release, and steroids may enhance **melting,** with ultimate corneal perforation. Cyanoacrylate adhesives (see sec. **II.B.,** above) or surgical intervention by conjunctival flap or penetrating keratoplasty may be necessary before perforation actually occurs.

6. **Iridocyclitis, retinitis,** and occasionally **panuveitis** may occur with herpes simplex infection. Intraocular inflammation may occur without concomitant keratitis, but almost invariably accompanies active keratitis. Uveitis in an eye with previous herpetic keratitis should be considered herpetic until proved otherwise. Therapy is discussed in Chapter 9, sec. **VIII.A.2.** Prophylactic antivirals and antibiotic agents should be used with topical steroids. If ulcerative keratitis supervenes, particularly if the cornea is melting, **systemic steroids** such as oral prednisone 60 to 80 mg per day, may be substituted for part or all of the topical steroid regimen.

7. **Oral antivirals** will have no effect on active immune keratitis, but acyclovir 400 mg p.o. bid for 1 year inhibits recurrence of stromal inflammation. Famciclovir 125 mg p.o. bid or valacyclovir (in the nonimmunosuppressed patient) 500 mg p.o. qd for 1 year are alternatives.

8. **Steroid tapering.** Special comment should be made regarding the gradual reduction and termination of steroid treatment. Because too rapid a steroid taper or abrupt cessation of treatment can often be accompanied by recrudescence of the inflammation, it is essential to carefully control the steroid dose. The rule of thumb is ***never taper steroids by more than 50% at any given time.*** Each level should be maintained for several days or, at lower doses, for several weeks depending on the severity of inflammation at the initiation of treatment and the therapeutic response. One method uses progressively decreasing strengths of glucocorticoid such that, from the dexamethasone 0.1% or prednisolone 1% daily, tapered from four times down to once, prednisolone 0.12% solution can

be used qid with gradual reduction to tid, bid, once a day, every 2 days, and so forth, until cessation of treatment. Occasionally, patients will require chronic low-dose (once or twice weekly) prednisolone to maintain a quiet eye. Coverage with antiviral medication need not be continued after reduction to less than 1% prednisolone bid except in patients with epithelial HSV infection within 6 months.

9. **Penetrating keratoplasty (corneal transplant)** of the herpes simplex scarred eye has about 85% 5-year success rate on first procedure in the *quiet* eye. Emergency surgery on inflamed eyes has a success rate of between 40% and 60%. Interrupted 10-O sutures, intensive topical steroids for several weeks, and acyclovir 400 mg p.o. bid for 12 to 18 months are factors favoring success. Antivirals are also critical if steroids are being used to treat an allograft rejection. See also sec. **IX.B.4.,** below, for management of graft rejection.

E. **Herpes zoster ophthalmicus.** Herpes zoster is an acute infection of a dorsal root ganglion by the varicella-zoster virus (VZV, chickenpox) characterized by severe pain and vesicular skin lesions distributed over the sensory dermatome innervated by the affected ganglion. Regional lymphadenopathy with dermatomal pain is common. The ophthalmic (trigeminal ganglion, Vth cranial nerve) form of the disease usually presents as a combination of two or more of the following: conjunctivitis, episcleritis, scleritis, keratitis, iridocyclitis, and glaucoma. Chorioretinitis, V^1 dermatomal vesicular dermatitis, extraocular muscle palsies, retinitis, and optic neuritis may also be seen (see Chapter 9, sec. **VIII.A.3.**). Herpes zoster is increasing in frequency due to the acquired immunodeficiency syndrome (AIDS) epidemic and aging population, but may *soon decrease due to* **vaccination of adults** *(Varivax) to reboot the immune system.*

1. **Conjunctivitis, episcleritis,** and **scleritis** occur in about half of the cases. Conjunctival involvement is common and may occur as watery hyperemia with petechial hemorrhages, follicular conjunctivitis with regional adenopathy, or severe necrotizing membranous inflammation. Scleritis or episcleritis may be diffuse or focal nodular. On resolution, scleritis can leave scleral thinning and staphyloma.

2. **Keratitis** occurs acutely in about 40% of all patients and may precede the neuralgia or skin lesions. Keratitis may occur as a fine or coarse punctate epithelial keratitis with or without stromal edema, or as actual vesicle formation with ulceration in a *dendritiform* pattern that can be mistaken for herpes simplex keratitis. VZV DNA is present from 2 to 34 days after acute onset, especially in patients over 66 years old (HIV negative). Delayed mucoid plaques resembling dendrites may occur months later and also contain VZV DNA. *Corneal sensation* is usually greatly reduced in herpes zoster keratitis due to ganglion damage. Trophic neuroparalytic ulcers may occur with melting and corneal perforation if the epithelial defect persists. Stromal keratitis, either immune diskiform or white necrotic IK, may occur with or independent of epithelial disease.

3. **Iridocyclitis** is a frequent occurrence (50%) and may appear independent of corneal activity. After resolution of the acute perineuritis and vasculitis, there may be focal or sector atrophy of the iris. Hypopyon, hemorrhage into the anterior chamber (anterior segment necrosis), and phthisis bulbi may result from zoster vasculitis and ischemia.

4. **Glaucoma** may occur acutely or months later due to inflammatory trabeculitis. In later stages, synechial closure of the angle may also occur (see Chapter 10, sec. **XVIII.**).

5. **Therapy.** Systemic antivirals (famciclovir, valacyclovir, and acyclovir) decrease acute pain, stop viral progression, and significantly reduce the incidence and severity of keratitis and iritis if started within 72 hours of rash onset. Inhibition of **postherpetic neuralgia (PHN)** is established for famciclovir and valacyclovir. Systemic steroids are currently controversial because of the increased incidence of zoster in HIV-positive patients.

The following regimen is presently recommended for ocular management. Therapy is most effective if started within 72 hours of onset of rash using both *antiviral* and *tricyclic antidepressant (TCA) therapy.* If used in acute disease, the latter greatly inhibits development of PHN.

a. **Antiviral famciclovir** (Famvir) 500 mg p.o. tid for 7 days or **valacyclovir** (Valtrex) 1 g p.o. tid for 7 days are equal to acyclovir in acute disease and better in *reducing late neuralgia.* **Acyclovir** (Zovirax) 800 mg tablet p.o. five times a day (4,000 mg per day total) for 7 days in the immunocompetent patient, or in the immunosuppressed patient, 5 to 10 mg per kg or 500 mg per m^2 i.v. q8h for 5 to 7 days, followed by 2 to 3 weeks of oral dosing is recommended. **Brivudine** 125 mg qd for 7 days is as effective as the above acyclovir regimen, but currently is available only in Europe.

b. **TCAs** are highly effective in inhibiting acute and long-term pain. Desipramine, imipramine, amitriptylene, or other TCA dosage *is started during acute illness* at 10 to 25 mg p.o. HS with increase over 1 to 2 weeks to 50 mg bid for 2 to 4 months, if tolerated. These same dosages are used for long-term therapy of PHN if it does develop.

c. **Topical steroids** are prescribed only if needed for corneal **diskiform** immune edema or **iritis,** e.g., 1/8% (.012%) prednisolone qd to qid with gradual taper. Use cycloplegia and steroids for iritis.

d. **Vidarabine** 3% antiviral ointment is prescribed 5 id for 7 to 14 days for recurring dendritic ulcers if they persist without therapy. Alternatives are trifluridine drops or p.o. antivirals. Response is variable.

e. **Topical antibiotic** is prescribed if epithelium is ulcerated or topical steroids are in use.

f. **Lateral tarsorrhaphy** can be performed if cornea is anesthetic, with frequent artificial tear lubrication to prevent neurotrophic ulceration.

g. **TSCLs** are used if epithelium is unhealthy or has sterile trophic ulceration; antibiotic drops bid for prophylaxis and artificial tears for lubrication are prescribed. Neovascular pannus may heal ulcerated corneas and should not be blocked with steroid therapy. Nerve growth factor improved sensitivity and healed ulcers in human studies.

h. Cyanoacrylate **tissue adhesive** (glue, Dermabond, not FDA approved for the eye) is used if there is corneal ulcer melting (thinning). Cover with a soft contact lens, and administer prophylactic antibiotics and lubricants (see sec. **IV.D.2.,** above).

i. For **secondary glaucoma** beta-adrenergic blockers, adrenergic agonists, antiprostaglandins, carbonic anhydrase inhibitors, and other nonmiotic agents are used to control pressure. Mydriatic cycloplegics prevent synechiae (see Chapter 10).

j. **Nonnarcotic or narcotic analgesics for neuralgia** during the first 10 to 30 days should be used to control pain. Patients *over 55 years* or those presenting *with severe pain at onset* regardless of age are at greatest risk for permanent or prolonged neuralgia. Young patients rarely have sustained pain; 85% of neuralgias resolve spontaneously over several months.

k. **PHN** is often relieved by TCAs, such as in sec. **IV.F.5.b.** above. Therapy may last for years. The anticonvulsant, *Gabapentin (Neurontin)* 300 mg up to 600 mg p.o. qid, is one of the most effective anti-PHN therapies available and may be coupled with all other anti-PHN treatments. *Capsaicin* 0.025% (Zostrix) topical skin cream qd to bid depletes substance P, a tachykinin involved in pain transmission, from the sensory peripheral neurons. Use only after the skin has healed, *discontinue if too irritating,* and avoid the area near the eyes. Pain relief will be noted in 2 to 6 weeks in 50% of patients. Therapy is usually 3 to 5 months, but may be restarted if pain returns. *Lidocaine patches* (Lidoderm) 12 hours out of each 24 hours are very effective in controlling dermal pain. *Oxycodone* 10 to 20 mg p.o. q12h may be added as a slow-release narcotic analgesic if needed despite all other therapy. There is *no successful surgical relief* known.

l. **Penetrating keratoplasty (corneal transplant).** Corneas sufficiently scarred by herpes zoster to warrant keratoplasty for restoration of sight are usually sufficiently anesthetic and susceptible to repeated inflammatory reaction and nonhealing that they are a poor risk for surgical rehabilitation. Corneas with partial sensation are reasonable candidates for keratoplasty. If done, a lateral tarsorrhaphy should also be done and copious postoperative lubrication used. Although not visually effective, the **conjunctival flap** is a safer procedure to perform against progressive melting defects if tissue adhesive has not aided healing.

m. **Bell's palsy** or **Ramsay Hunt syndrome.** Acute VII and VIII cranial nerve paralysis should be treated with full p.o. antiviral therapy and prednisone 40 to 60 mg per day for 14 days (see sec. **V.E.,** below).

F. **Varicella or chickenpox virus** is the same organism that causes VZV, and is morphologically indistinguishable from HSV. It is decreasing greatly in incidence due to early vaccination of infants (Varivax).

1. The **most common clinical manifestation** of the virus, **chickenpox,** is a contagious disease, predominantly of children, transmitted by droplet infection and characterized by fever and papulovesicular rash that is usually self-limiting and uncomplicated. The infectious period is from 2 days prerash until crusting. **Vesicular lesions** may appear along the lid margin and **eyelids** during an episode of chickenpox and rarely may appear on the conjunctiva. Usually unilateral, small, papular lesions that can be contiguous with the lid margin, commonly occurring at the **limbus,** may resolve or form a punched-out dark-red ulcer with swollen margins, causing pain and inflammation in the eye. More rarely, the cornea may become involved, with superficial punctate **keratitis** or a more serious stromal diskiform keratitis accompanied by plastic **iridocyclitis.** A late immune keratitis or recurrent VZV dendritic ulcerations may appear. **Iritis, retinitis, optic neuritis, ophthalmoplegia,** and **cataract** are infrequent.

2. **Therapy** includes the following:

a. **Acyclovir** 200 mg pills or suspension 20 mg/kg/day (not more than 800 mg) p.o. qid for 5 days or 30 mg/kg/day i.v. divided q8h for 7 days in immunocompromised patients.

b. **Good hygiene,** cool compresses, low illumination.

c. **Cycloplegics** for iritis or keratitis.

d. Vidarabine 3% **antiviral ointment** five times a day for 10 to 14 days for surface vesicles or ulcers and antibiotic bid prophylaxis.

e. **Cautious use of mild topical steroid** for nonulcerative interstitial or diskiform stromal keratitis. Dissemination of varicella in children from exogenous systemic steroids is a well-recognized hazard.

G. **Adenoviral** infections are frequent and classic causes of acute follicular conjunctivitis. Clinically, they are usually encountered as *epidemic keratoconjunctivitis (EKC),* usually associated with adenovirus types 8 and 19, and *pharyngoconjunctival fever (PCF),* usually associated with adenovirus type 3. After an incubation period of 5 to 12 days following droplet or fomite inoculation onto the conjunctival surface, symptoms of irritation and watery discharge are accompanied by hyperemia of the conjunctiva and follicle formation, often in association with preauricular adenopathy. Patients are *highly contagious for 10 to 12 days* starting one day before onset and should avoid close contact or sharing towels with others during this time (patients should take sick leave from work). Medical personnel examining or treating patients with this condition should be very vigilant about handwashing and cleansing of instruments.

1. **EKC** usually is *not* accompanied by systemic symptoms, and one eye is often involved prior to the other. The conjunctivitis runs a course of

7 to 14 days, at which time a superficial diffuse epithelial keratitis may develop and be superseded by slightly focal elevated epithelial lesions that stain with fluorescein. Focal subepithelial opacities may develop in weeks 2 to 3. There may be conjunctival hemorrhages or membrane formation, and marked lid swelling.

2. **PCF** is characterized by pharyngitis, fever, and follicular conjunctivitis. The highly contagious (10 to 12 days) condition is usually unilateral and self-limited over 5 to 14 days. In the early stages, the condition can be confused with herpes conjunctivitis, acute inclusion conjunctivitis, and acute hemorrhagic conjunctivitis. The keratitis is similar to EKC, but is usually bilateral and much milder.

3. **Treatment** is primarily supportive management, using astringent drops and cool compresses. Currently available antivirals have been ineffective in limiting the severity or course. Topical antibiotics prevent secondary bacterial infection. Some patients may be so immobilized by the symptoms that they will require mild topical steroids tid to qid, e.g., 1/8% prednisolone. Topical steroids will inhibit the appearance of subepithelial corneal infiltrates in EKC and PCF, but on discontinuation of the steroids infiltrates will recur. A few patients require a long and gradual tapering of the steroid dose because of symptom recurrence. With time, all infiltrates generally clear spontaneously.

H. **AIDS,** caused by HIV-1, causes a progressive, profound T-lymphocyte cellular immunodeficiency characterized by multiple opportunistic infections and malignancies. Kaposi sarcoma is due to human herpesvirus 8. Prior to current therapy, more than 60% of patients had ocular lesions, most chorioretinal. The virus has been isolated from the tear film and almost all ocular structures including cornea, vitreous, and chorioretinal tissues. Anterior ocular lesions include follicular conjunctivitis, Kaposi sarcoma of the conjunctiva (a deep purple-red soft tumor), a punctate or geographic ulcerative keratitis that may mimic herpes infection, and nongranulomatous iritis. These are HIV-1 induced and occur independently of any opportunistic infection. Opportunistic anterior infections include herpes simplex, herpes zoster, fungal amoebic, and bacterial ulcers. **Therapy** of AIDS is effective and now usually combines protease inhibitors with nucleoside reverse-transcriptase inhibitors (Chapter 9, sec. **VIII.A.5.**). Opportunistic infections are discussed in their respective sections by diagnosis.

I. **Molluscum contagiosum virus** is a large member of the pox group that causes epithelial tumor-like eruptions involving the skin and *chronic conjunctivitis.*

1. **Ophthalmic** interest centers around the lesions that affect the brow area, eyelids (particularly the eyelid margins), and, rarely, the conjunctiva. The skin lesion often starts as a discrete papule that eventually becomes multiple pale nodules up to 2 mm in size (larger in AIDS patients) with umbilicated centers from which a cheesy mass can be expressed. When one of the pearly umbilicated lesions affects the lid margin, a chronic follicular conjunctivitis and an epithelial keratitis can result that is thought to be the result of toxicity to products released by the lesion into the cul-desac. The keratitis is fine diffuse or focal epithelial that can, if chronic and untreated, lead to subepithelial infiltration and vascularization from the periphery that resembles a trachomatous pannus. The lid lesion(s) must be differentiated from other eyelid tumors, including sebaceous cyst, verruca, chalazia, keratoacanthoma, and small fibroma.

2. **Treatment** consists of complete eradication of the lesion. Following removal of the skin lesion, the conjunctivitis and keratitis rapidly clear. Cauterization and cryotherapy have been successful, but simple superficial excision or curettage is easily accomplished. HIV-positive patients are very prone to recurrence of multiple lesions.

J. **Ocular vaccinia** occurs following an inoculation to the eye. The vaccine is no longer in use but the virus is stored in the United States and Russia. There are pustular skin lesions that can extend to the adjacent conjunctiva or cornea to produce an acute ulcer or late diskiform opacity. In a previously vaccinated individual with a good level of immunity, little more than an acute focal purulent blepharoconjunctivitis can be seen; in the unvaccinated or weakly immune individual, a severe reaction may occur. **Treatment** is with *hyperimmune vaccinia immune globulin* 0.25 to 0.5 mL per kg body weight i.m., repeated in 48 hours if there is no improvement. Systemic *oral antivirals* or i.v. acyclovir should be effective. *Vidarabine* antiviral ointment and antibiotic qid, and cycloplegia are used for acute infection. Topical *steroids* bid to qid are used for diskiform keratitis if the epithelium is healed and the infection is resolved.

K. Other viral causes of interstitial keratitis (IK)
   1. An evanescent IK can accompany **mumps** but usually clears very rapidly.
   2. **Epstein-Barr virus** (mononucleosis) may cause a prolonged nebulous IK responsive to topical steroids but not to antivirals (see Chapter 9, sec. **VIII.A.6**).
   3. **Lymphogranuloma venereum** can produce a segmental and highly vascularized IK. Specific antiviral treatment is usually not effective, but control of the IK with atropine and topical steroids may be of benefit.

L. Spirochetal infections
   1. **Syphilis (*Treponema pallidum*; lues).** Ocular findings in lues include IK, conjunctivitis, episcleritis, scleritis, dacryoadenitis, Argyll Robertson pupil, uveitis, chorioretinitis, and optic neuritis. More than 90% of the cases of diffuse IK are **congenital,** starting with widespread, deep, infiltrative inflammation of the corneal stroma, and iritis. **Acquired** syphilis produces IK much less frequently. It is usually uniocular, whereas the congenital variant is most often bilateral. Even in congenital disease, the keratitis is usually not apparent until ages 10 to 20 years. Disease begins with endothelial and deep stroma associated with pain, circumcorneal injection lacrimation, photophobia, and blepharospasm that progresses to a diffuse corneal haze which often obscures iritis. The acute inflammatory edema resolves with the progressive vascular invasion from the periphery, leaving deep opacities and *ghost vessels* with hyaline excrescences on Descemet's membrane as secondary guttae. Hearing impairment and chorioretinal scarring (bone corpuscle or salt and pepper fundus) are often associated with the congenital variety of lues and IK. Neurosyphilis and cardiovascular syphilis are late forms of the systemic disease. Any patient with syphilis should be evaluated for AIDS and other sexually transmitted diseases (see Chapter 9, sec. **VIII.B.3.**). **Diagnosis** is confirmed with blood tests: fluorescent treponemal antibody-absorption test (FTA-ABS) or microhemagglutination-*Treponema pallidum* tests that never revert to negative (or may never become positive in concurrent HIV and syphilis). *Response to therapy* is followed with Venereal Disease Research Laboratory or rapid plasmin reagin blood tests because these will revert to negative (1:4) within 1 year of cure. HIV testing is indicated and lumbar puncture may be recommended by an infectious disease consultant.
      a. **Systemic treatment** of the newborn for **congenital syphilis** is indicated if the mother's serology (FTA-ABS) is positive or becomes positive during pregnancy, even if the infant remains seronegative. Benzathine penicillin 50,000 units per kg i.m. once or procaine penicillin 10,000 units per kg i.m. daily for 10 days is the therapy for such infants. Even this therapy may be insufficient for congenital ocular or neurosyphilis, and treatment of 50,000 units per kg benzathine penicillin weekly for 3 weeks may be required. Children or adults with acute syphilitic IK are usually treated with ampicillin, 1.5 g p.o., in combination with probenecid, 500 mg p.o. q6h, on an empty stomach, for 1 month. *Penicillin-allergic* patients may be treated effectively with doxycycline or, in children younger than 8 years, erythromycin 50 mg/kg/day p.o. in four divided doses for 2 weeks. Some strains are very *resistant* to erythromycin. A pediatric or infectious disease *consult* is recommended. Topical **steroids** such as 0.1% dexamethasone q2 to 4h and

cycloplegics (homatropine tid) are initiated and gradually tapered off as the disease responds. For severe IK, *subconjunctival* decadron 4 to 12 mg qd or 0.1 dexamethasone drops four to six times per day may be necessary as initial steroid therapy along with atropine cycloplegia.

   b. Treatment of adult early primary, secondary, or latent acquired syphilis (<1 year duration) is 2.4 million units of i.m. benzathine G penicillin once, or once weekly for 3 weeks if disease is **late (>1 year duration)**. For **neurosyphilis**, treatment is 3 to 4 million U aqueous penicillin i.v. q4h for 10 to 14 days. For *penicillin-allergic* patients, treatment is doxycycline 100 mg p.o. bid for 14 days (early) or 4 weeks (late) with nondairy-product meal, or tetracycline 500 mg on an empty stomach, p.o. qid for 4 weeks. Use neither for neurosyphilis. An internist or infectious disease *consult* should be obtained. Topical treatment with steroids and mydriatic cycloplegics is similar to that for congenital syphilis.

2. Lyme disease (erythema chronicum migrans), an infectious and immune-mediated inflammatory disease caused by the spirochete *Borrelia burgdorferi,* has numerous ocular, neuroophthalmic, and systemic manifestations. There are three defined stages of disease.

   a. Stage 1. Within 1 month of an infected deer tick bite, a characteristic macular *rash* of varying severity and often with a clear center usually appears at the area of the bite. There may be associated fever, chills, fatigue, and headache. A malar rash and *conjunctivitis* (11% incidence) may also occur.

   b. Stage 2. After several weeks to months, neurologic (meningitis, radiculoneuropathies, severe headache) and cardiac (atrioventricular block, myopericarditis) signs may begin. **Neuroophthalmic** findings include optic neuritis and perineuritis, papilledema, ischemic optic neuropathy, optic nerve atrophy, pseudotumor cerebri, diplopia secondary to third and sixth nerve palsies, Bell's palsy, and multiple sclerosis-like disease. Other **ocular manifestations** include retinal hemorrhages, exudative retinal detachments, iritis followed by panophthalmitis, and bilateral keratitis. The keratitis is characterized by multiple focal, nebular subepithelial opacities at all levels of the stroma, limbus to limbus, and may progress to corneal edema and neovascularization.

   c. Stage 3. Up to 2 years after the bite, a migratory oligoarthritis may develop initially without joint swelling, but later with effusions and degeneration. Extreme fatigue, lymphadenopathy, splenomegaly, sore throat, dry cough, testicular swelling, mild hepatitis, and nephritis are not uncommon. The ocular manifestations of Lyme disease may appear at any stage, but are more common in the later two stages and may occur despite "adequate" treatment. Most resolve spontaneously, waxing and waning.

   d. Diagnosis. Either the indirect fluorescent antibody method or the enzyme-linked immunosorbent assay is reliable; confirm with Western blot for *B. burgdorferi*. Lyme titers of 1:256 are diagnostic. In chronic Lyme disease, absence of antibodies against the spirochete does not exclude the disease; a specific T-cell blastogenic response to *B. burgdorferi* may make the diagnosis in seronegative patients. There is cerebrospinal fluid pleocytosis.

   e. Systemic treatment is still controversial, and any manifestation of the disease may recur and require treatment.

     (1) Definite neuroophthalmic, ocular, neurologic, or cardiac disease

       (a) Adults. Penicillin G i.v., 24 million units per day in four divided doses for 14 days, or ceftriaxone i.v., 2 g per day for 14 days.

       (b) Children. Penicillin G 250,000 units/kg/day in four divided doses for 14 days, or ceftriaxone 100 mg/kg/day in two divided doses i.m. or i.v. for 14 days.

(2) Nonspecific symptoms with positive Lyme titers
- **(a) Adults.** Doxycycline 100 mg p.o. bid, or tetracycline 500 mg p.o. qid; penicillin V or amoxicillin 500 mg qid; or azithromycin 500 mg p.o. qd for 3 to 4 weeks.
- **(b) Children.** Penicillin V potassium p.o. 50 mg/kg/day in four divided doses, amoxicillin 125 to 250 mg p.o. tid, or erythromycin 40 mg/kg/day in four divided doses, each regimen 3 to 4 weeks.

    f. Topical treatment is adjunctive to systemic therapy. Keratitis is responsive to 1% prednisolone qid with taper over several months and reinstitution as needed. Iritis may self-resolve and require only mydriatic–cycloplegic therapy (0.25% scopolamine bid) or be more severe, requiring addition of topical steroids four to six times per day with taper.

M. Mycobacteria

  1. Leprosy (Hansen's disease). The IK of leprosy *(Mycobacterium leprae)* is a deep infiltration, usually bilateral and extending from the periphery to the center of the cornea. The IK may be associated with a punctate epithelial keratitis, and, although corneal nerves are notably thickened and beaded, the interstitial vascularization is not prominent. The keratitis rarely occurs alone, but can occur with involvement of the ciliary body or a limbal leukoma. Nodular lepromas are frequently seen in the subconjunctival tissues and iritis is severe. The cornea can be greatly thickened, and the opacity usually does not clear. **Treatment.** Systemic sulfones (Dapsone) with topical steroid and atropine are needed to control disease. Tuberculoid (neurasthetic) leprosy is treated with dapsone 100 mg p.o. qd and 600 mg of rifampin monthly for 6 months. For lepromatous (granulomatous) leprosy, 50 mg of clofazimine is added to this regimen daily and 300 mg is given monthly. Such treatment should be carried out by a physician familiar with lepromatous disease.

  2. *M. fortuitum* and *M. chelonae*, the two most common causes of nontuberculous keratitis, result in indolent whitish infiltrates diagnosed by cultures and scrapings. **Therapy** is effective using topical clarithromycin 20 mg per mL, ciprofloxacin 0.3%, or amikacin 10 mg per mL with vancomycin 25 mg with gradual tapering over weeks.

  3. *M. tuberculosis* (see Chapter 9, sec. **VIII.B.2.**).

N. Fungal keratitis. Fungal infection of the eye poses a threat not only because of the damage that can be caused by the fungus, but also because of the limited number of approved antifungal agents available for treatment.

  1. Yeast fungi. *Candida* ulcers commonly occur in eyes with predisposing alterations in host defenses, including chronic use of corticosteroids, exposure keratitis, keratitis sicca, herpes simplex keratitis, and prior keratoplasty. *Candida* is a common offender in the northern and coastal regions of the United States, constituting 32% to 43% of keratomycoses. It is unwise and often not possible to determine the species of infecting organism by the clinical features, but the clinical appearance may suggest the infecting agent. *Candida* ulcers occasionally have distinct oval outlines with a plaque-like surface, or can produce a relatively indolent stromal infiltration with smaller satellite lesions.

  2. Filamentous fungi. *Fusarium, Cephalosporium,* and *Aspergillus* are the most common filamentous fungi in the United States, with *Fusarium* more common in the South and *Aspergillus* in the North, causing 45% to 61% of filamentous keratitis cases. These organisms usually infect normal eyes following mild abrasive corneal trauma, especially after injury from vegetable matter. The organisms are ubiquitous and can be isolated readily from soil, air, and organic waste. These organisms are particularly responsible for keratitis in the southern United States. The clinical appearance can be characteristic, with a gray or dirty-white dry, rough, textured surface that often has an elevated margin. There may be feathery extensions beneath epithelium into the adjacent stroma. Satellite lesions separated from the central infectious area may occur and correspond to microabscesses in the surrounding tissue. Occasionally, **ring abscesses** have been described. If the infection is deep, there can be endothelial plaque formation. Anterior chamber reaction and hypopyon can occur with large or deep infections. In **contact lens wearers,** filamentous fungi are more associated with cosmetic lens wear, and yeasts are more associated with therapeutic lenses.

3. **Diagnosis.** Scraping and inoculation of media should be performed (see sec. **III.C.,** above, and Table 5.3). It is important to scrape multiple sites in the ulcer crater, particularly at the margins, to enhance recovery of organisms. Because the organisms tend to be deep within the stroma, superficial keratectomy (corneal biopsy, see sec. **IV.B.3.b.,** above) may be necessary to obtain diagnostic material. Because the organism is often not seen on the scraping, it is important to inoculate each culture medium with multiple scrapings. Although Gram stain may identify some fungal forms, particularly the yeast forms of *Candida,* Giemsa stain is more likely to define the structure of filamentous fungi. Though not generally available, the Grocott modification of Gomori methenamine-silver stain often provides greater definition of fungal cytology. Sabouraud broth and agar and a blood agar plate kept at room temperature, as well as brain heart infusion broth, are essential. More specialized media (such as Nickerson media for identification of *Candida* organisms) may be used but are not essential.

4. **Treatment** is initially medical and potentially surgical because fungal infection can be rapidly destructive to the integrity of the eye. Hospital admission may be advisable. Lack of disease progression is the first sign of therapeutic response. Topical and systemic treatment usually lasts for several weeks (2 to 3 months).

   a. **Medical therapy** is limited by the number of approved **antifungal drugs** and by the poor penetration of the available agents. **Table 5.8** summarizes the most commonly used drugs, dosages, and indicated organisms. Prior to identification of the infectious agent, therapy should begin with as broad a spectrum as possible in highly suspect cases, e.g., no response to fortified antibiotics, clinical appearance, vegetable matter, injury, positive scrapings. The cornea should be cleaned of debris when needed to enhance drug penetration. Natamycin (Natacyn, pimaricin, Alcon corp.) 5% suspension or amphotericin B 0.075% to 0.3% is active against yeast and filamentous fungi. Cultures may take from 3 to 30 days to become positive. Substitution of a specific antifungal agent according to the clinical response or in vitro sensitivities may be indicated. When fungal elements are confirmed on direct smears, culture, or from histologic biopsy examination, therapy should be oriented toward the type of organism and extent of disease. **Filamentous** cases are usually responsive to the topical polyenes, natamycin, or amphotericin B, but refractory cases may be successfully treated with the addition of topical and subconjunctival miconazole. Ketoconazole p.o. is an effective adjunct therapy for patients who are unresponsive to purely topical medication. *Candida* or other yeasts usually respond to the **synergistic** combination of topical amphotericin B and oral flucytosine, or to topical and subconjunctival miconazole with or without adjunctive oral ketoconazole. Daily **epithelial débridement** by the physician (if the surface heals over) is useful in aiding drug penetration for at least the first several days of therapy. **Systemic amphotericin B** or fluconazole (Diflucan) is indicated if the infection spreads to sclera or perforation threatens or occurs (see Table 9.7). An infectious disease *consult* should be obtained because this drug can be quite toxic systemically.

   Cycloplegics such as atropine or scopolamine should be used liberally to prevent posterior synechiae and to help reduce uveal

TABLE 5.8. ANTIFUNGAL THERAPEUTIC REGIMEN USED IN FUNGAL KERATITIS[a,b]

Regimen	Drug Efficacious Against
Amphotericin B (Fungizone) Topical: 0.15% drop q1h Subconjunctival: 0.8–1.0 mg q48h for one to two doses (toxic) Systemic: Test dose 1 mg slow i.v. If tolerated, at 2–4 h start 0.25 mg/kg i.v. over 4–6 h/d. Work up to 0.5–1.5 mg/kg/d depending on fungus and tolerance. Hydrate well.	*Candida, Aspergillus, Cryptococcus, Coccidioides, Sporothrix, Blastomyces, Histoplasma, Paracoccidioides* mucormycosis
Fluconazole (Diflucan) 200 mg i.v./p.o. initial dose; 100 mg/d i.v./p.o. qd	*Candida, Cryptococcus, Coccidioides*
Flucytosine (5-FC, Ancobon) Topical: 10 mg/mL drop q1h; taper as above Oral: 50–150 mg/kg/d in four divided doses	*Candida, Aspergillus, Cryptococcus, Cladosporium*
Itraconazole (Sporanox) Oral: 200 mg qd to bid p.o. Topical: 1% drop q1h; taper as above	*Aspergillus, Cryptococcus, Histoplasmosis, Candida,* blastomycosis, paracoccidioidomycosis, sporotrichosis
Ketoconazole[c] (Nizoral) Oral: 200–400 mg/d p.o.	*Candida, Fusarium, Penicillium, Aspergillus, Alternaria, Rhodotorula, Histoplasma, Cladosporium, Coccidioides Paracoccidioides, Phialophora, Actinomyces*
Natamycin (pimaricin) Topical: 5% drop q1h; taper as above	See ketoconazole

i.v., intravenous; p.o., oral.
[a]See also Table 9.7.
[b]Only Pimaricin is approved by the U.S. Food and Drug Administration for ocular use.
[c]Oral absorption enhanced by taking with acidic beverage (e.g., orange juice, cola).

inflammation. Secondary glaucoma may require oral carbonic anhydrase inhibitors or hyperosmotic agents. During early therapy of a fungal ulcer, **corticosteroids** are **contraindicated** because of the documented enhancement of fungal growth. If there is evidence that an effective antifungal agent is being used and that the clinical infection is well under control, corticosteroids can be used cautiously late in the treatment to reduce stromal or anterior segment inflammation.
  b. **Surgical therapy** may be required not only for complications of the acute infectious processes, but also should medical management fail. Débridement and superficial keratectomy, although mostly of diagnostic benefit, may enhance the effectiveness of medical treatment. Conjunctival flaps have been advocated for nonhealing ulcers and are often effective, although fungal organisms have been found to persist under a conjunctival flap. Lamellar keratoplasty may be ineffective in treating fungal keratitis because of the inability to remove

completely the infectious agent. If the area of infection can be completely encompassed by a penetrating graft and if there has been inadequate response to medical treatment, the corneal graft may provide an effective cure. Lens extraction should be avoided if the posterior segment is not involved.

O. Nontrue fungi of the family Actinomycetaceae and Nocardiaceae. Two organisms that superficially resemble fungi but are related to the true bacteria cause disease in humans.

1. *Actinomyces* can infect the lacrimal system, particularly the canaliculi, producing a chronic conjunctivitis and canaliculitis. Rarely, a nodular keratitis may be produced. The Gram-positive, non-acid-fast, nonmotile filamentous organism microscopically shows branching filaments when granules expressed or curetted from the canaliculi are smeared. The organism grows on blood agar or in chopped meat infusion, usually anaerobically. **Treatment** of the canaliculitis usually requires surgical removal or expression of the granules, but the organism is sensitive to **penicillin** and **sulfa** drugs (see Appendix B). Irrigation of the expressed canaliculus with a penicillin solution is often effective.

2. *Nocardia asteroides* is a Gram-positive filamentous organism and may stain acid-fast. The organism grows aerobically very slowly on many simple media. It can produce a chronic corneal ulcer with a gray sloughing base and undermined overhanging edges. *Nocardia* can rarely produce endophthalmitis. **Sulfonamides** are the drugs of choice (see Appendix B).

P. Amoeba (*Acanthamoeba*). Corneal ulceration and keratitis due to *Acanthamoeba* species are rare in the United States, but must be considered in a nonhealing, culture-negative infection. Typically, it has been noted in patients who wore contact lenses (even disposables) or who had exposure to hot tubs, communal baths, or just plain lake or tap water.

1. **Diagnosis.** About 65% are initially diagnosed as herpetic keratitis, and 30% of patients are not definitely diagnosed for 4 to 7 months after onset. *Inordinate pain* is one of the cardinal signs. The lesions are often multicentric, but a ring-shaped lesion with stromal infiltrate is characteristic. The peripheral corneal nerves may be quite visible due to radial keratoneuritis. Amoeba can be cultured from scrapings or biopsy on confluent layers of coliform bacteria or in *Enterobacter* suspensions. *Calcofluor white stain* of scrapings is positive in 70% of cases. *Confocal microscopy* is highly suggestive but not definitively diagnostic; however, a positive corneal biopsy for microscopy and PCR testing for amoebic DNA are diagnostic.

2. **Therapy** is still controversial and unsatisfactory; many medical cures have now been reported, but none are FDA approved. Penetrating keratoplasty in combination with medical treatment may still be required. *Epithelial débridement* combined with topical treatment is highly therapeutic in early cases. The organism exists in the cornea in both trophozoite and encysted states, thus requiring extremely prolonged therapy. Currently used regimens are various combinations of 1% *propamidine* isethionate (Brolene), one drop followed 5 minutes later by one drop of *neomycin–polymyxin B–gramicidin* (Neosporin, AK-Spore) every hour, 18 hours per day, or dibromopropamidine (Brolene ointment) and neomycin–polymyxin B–bacitracin drops q2h for 1 week. Frequency is then tapered over several weeks to qid to qd over 1 year. *Polyhexamethylene biguanide* antiseptic (Bacquacil) 0.02% drops q1 to 2h has been successful in difficult cases and is often combined with other topical and p.o. therapy following the above-described time regimen along with *chlorhexidine* 0.006% q2h for 1 week with taper over weeks to qid. In more severe infections, ketoconazole 200 to 400 mg p.o. qd and 1% clotrimazole may be added to the above regimen. Oral itraconazole 150 mg p.o. every morning coupled with 0.1% miconazole q1h for 20 days with gradual tapering of both medications and discontinuation after just 2 months of therapy, has been reported as successful. **Topical steroids** will reduce

inflammation and pain, inhibit trophozoite conversion to cysts, thus keeping them susceptible to amebicides, but may also allow deeper penetration of organisms. Their role is still unestablished.

Q. Microsporidia are spore-forming, intracellular protozoa which are ubiquitous opportunistic pathogens and may cause multifocal epithelial and anterior stromal keratitis, particularly in HIV-positive patients and contact lens wearers. Diagnosis is by trichrome stain of corneal scrapings, and treatment is albendazole 400 mg p.o. bid with topical brolene and norfloxacin q2h for several weeks.

V. Noninfectious keratitis, keratoconjunctivitis, and keratopathies

A. Exposure keratopathy.
Any loss of the normal protective mechanisms of corneal sensation or lid blinking function can lead to exposure keratopathy.

1. **Causes** are Bell's palsy, Ramsay Hunt syndrome (herpes zoster), neurotrophic keratopathy, traumatic facial palsy, or exophthalmos and other causes of incomplete lid closure.

2. **Clinically,** there is corneal desiccation, most notable in the inferior interpalpebral area of the conjunctiva and cornea, which can lead to a frank epithelial defect and a noninfiltrated ulceration. Superinfection is a constant threat.

3. **Treatment.** In addition to the treatments described below, *lateral tarsorrhaphy* (closure of the lateral 25% to 33% palpebral fissure) is generally indicated in persistent epithelial defects or other ocular surface problems with neurotrophic ulcer, penetrating keratoplasty, postinfection, exposure keratopathy, dry eye syndromes, radiation keratopathy, entropion, some ocular cicatricial pemphigoid, and Stevens-Johnson syndrome.

   a. **Mild exposure.** Frequent instillation of artificial tears during the day and lubricant ointment at night with taping of the lid closed is usually sufficient. Frequent observation is needed.

   b. **Moderate exposure.** Application of a soft contact lens with frequent instillation of lubricant may suffice. Usually lid surgery (intermarginal lid adhesions, starting laterally) is required.

   c. **Severe exposure.** Marked exophthalmos of thyroid endocrine etiology requires urgent treatment with high-dose systemic steroids, e.g., prednisone, 80 to 100 mg per day for a few days, to control the acute infiltrative ophthalmopathy most commonly into the maxillary and ethmoid sinuses or orbital decompression (Ogura technique). Antibiotic prophylaxis and lubrication should be instituted.

B. Thygeson's superficial punctate keratitis.
The clinical entity of a coarse punctate ("snowflake") epithelial keratitis in an uninflamed eye is often *misdiagnosed* as adenovirus (which has a red eye). It runs a chronic course with exacerbations and remissions, is associated with foreign body sensation, photophobia, and tearing, and is usually bilateral but can be asymmetric. These circular to oval epithelial lesions usually occur centrally and are slightly elevated, with central fluorescein staining and a cluster of heterogeneous, granular gray dots. It usually self-resolves in 6 years or less.

1. **Treatment.** The lesions and associated symptoms usually respond quickly to topical corticosteroids, which may be tapered rapidly, but recurrence of the keratitis is common. One drop of prednisolone 0.12% weekly or even less frequently may keep a patient asymptomatic. It is not necessary to treat until all lesions are gone, but only to the point of comfort. Application of a TSCL will often relieve symptoms if the use of steroids is not possible or advisable. *Antiviral drugs* are *not* advised, because they may induce scarring beneath the lesions.

C. Filamentary keratopathy.
A variety of conditions can produce filamentary keratopathy, which is probably best considered as a form of aberrant epithelial healing. Consequently, any condition that leads to focal epithelial erosions may produce filamentary keratopathy.

1. The **following conditions** are probably most commonly associated with this entity.

a. **Keratitis sicca.** Filaments frequently occur in corneas that are subject to the epitheliopathy of keratitis sicca. These filaments can be distributed diffusely and are often associated with areas that stain with fluorescein on the corneal surface. Excess mucous production in this syndrome probably aggravates filament formation.

b. **Superior limbic keratoconjunctivitis.** This condition, initially described as mild inflammation and vascular injection of the superior conjunctiva associated with rose bengal staining of the superior bulbar conjunctiva, often is associated with filaments distributed over the superior portion of the cornea.

c. **Other causes** include: *prolonged patching* following cataract or other ocular surgery, *epitheliopathy* due to aerosol or *radiation* keratitis, *herpetic epithelial defects,* and *systemic disorders,* including diabetes, psoriasis, and ectodermal dysplasias.

2. **Treatment.** The specific etiology of the filamentary keratopathy should be identified and treated.

a. **Débridement.** If only a few filaments exist, they may be removed at their base with a pair of jeweler's forceps following topical corneal anesthesia.

b. **Medication.** In the dry eye or in the eye with unstable tear film, lubricants in the form of drops q2h or ointments q4h may be tried. Lid hygiene should be encouraged.

c. **Therapeutic contact lens.** If symptoms are severe or if medication has failed, application of a high-water-content (70%) TSCL (Permalens, Kontur) will provide relief and usually allow adequate epithelial healing without filament formation. Antibiotic drops bid, e.g., Polytrim, should be used for the first few weeks of wear.

d. **Lateral tarsorrhaphy (see sec. V.A.3., above).**

D. **Superior limbic keratoconjunctivitis** presents as bilateral ocular irritation with dilated conjunctival vessels over the superior bulbar conjunctiva. It is often associated with superior corneal filaments. Rose bengal reveals prominent staining in the superior bulbar conjunctiva. The superior conjunctival cells are often keratinized. No organisms have ever been associated conclusively with superior limbic keratoconjunctivitis, and the role of the tarsal conjunctiva in provoking the reaction is speculative. Superior limbic keratoconjunctivitis has been reported to occur with greater frequency in patients with hyperthyroidism.

1. **Treatment.** Topical lubricants and low-dose topical steroids may alleviate the symptoms, but usually do not completely reverse the conjunctival changes. Some success has been achieved with topical application of silver nitrate solution 1.0% to the involved area, but application may need to be repeated. Silver nitrate cautery sticks should **not** be used for this purpose because severe conjunctival burn and necrosis can occur. Various surgical procedures have been advised. Acceptable results can be achieved after application of faint diathermy in a checkerboard pattern across the superior bulbar conjunctiva. Recession or resection of a perilimbal strip of conjunctiva from the superior limbus is usually effective if other measures fail. Long-term wear of TSCLs may be required.

E. **Neuroparalytic keratitis**

1. **Bell's palsy.** Acute "idiopathic" palsy of the facial nerve (VIIth) may be *herpetic* in etiology and may result in paralysis of the orbicularis muscle and lagophthalmos, with incomplete closure of the lids and incomplete lubrication of the ocular surface, with resultant desiccation and epithelial breakdown. If Bell's phenomenon is weak or absent, frank ulceration of the corneal surface may occur. ***Emergency*** treatment is needed to prevent permanent paralysis. Prednisone, 40 mg p.o. bid for 10 to 14 days, coupled with acyclovir 400 mg qid p.o. for 14 to 21 days should be initiated on presentation.

2. **Herpes zoster ophthalmicus.** Involvement of the eye by herpes zoster ophthalmicus can result in severe corneal epithelial defect during the

acute episode, but also in diminished to absent corneal sensitivity because of ganglionic (Vth) damage in the recovery stage. Loss of the protective corneal innervation results in a surface that breaks down readily and is very prone to desiccation with minimum exposure. The predisposition of the eye to inflammation makes treatment with contact lenses or surgery more complex (see sec. **IV.E.**). **Ramsay Hunt syndrome** is Bell's palsy combined with VIIIth nerve zoster, with the latter causing tinnitus, vertigo, and permanent hearing loss.

3. **Status posttrigeminal section for tic douloureux.** Neurosurgical procedures to interrupt the sensory root of the trigeminal nerve (V) often result in corneal anesthesia. There may be desiccation and exposure, with subsequent epithelial breakdown.

4. **Postradiation keratopathy.** After radiotherapy to lesions of the head and neck, trophic changes can occur in the eye, with corneal epithelial breakdown.

5. **Syphilitic (luetic) neuropathy.** Hypesthesia of the corneal nerves from luetic involvement predisposes to epithelial breakdown.

6. **Neuroparalytic keratitis treatment**
   a. **Lubricants.** Specific treatment for zoster is indicated for acute Bell palsy. The mainstay of treatment of exposure keratopathy, particularly in the mild stages, is topical lubricants consisting of artificial tears (the more viscous bases being more effective) instilled q1 to 2h during the day, with lubricant ointment or antibiotic ointment applied at night. In many cases this treatment will be sufficient.
   b. **Mechanical.** Significant lid dysfunction or lagophthalmos needs to be treated. Bedtime ointment or taping the lid shut at night is often efficacious, and, although inconvenient, can be used intermittently during the day. Lateral tarsorrhaphy usually produces good results (see sec. **V.A.3.**, above). Side shields for glasses worn during the day are also effective.
   c. **Soft contact lens.** Application of a therapeutic, high-water-content soft contact lens (Permalens, Kontur) in conjunction with copious artificial tears can provide a reservoir to prevent desiccation. It must be remembered, however, that eyes with impaired sensation are at greater risk than those with normal sensation, and the patient requires close follow-up to detect any signs of neovascularization, infiltration, or anterior chamber reaction. Antibiotics such as trimethoprim–polymyxin B (Polytrim) should be instilled to minimize the chance of infection.
   d. **Thinning ulcers** are treated as in sec. **IV.D.2.**, above.

F. A **pterygium** is a fleshy triangular band of fibrovascular tissue with a broad base on the nasal or temporal epibulbar area, a blunt apex or head on the cornea, and a gray zone, or cap, which just precedes the apex. It is most common in the 20- to 30-year age group, in males, in tropical climates, and in people exposed to the elements and ultraviolet light. The episcleral portion usually develops rapidly over 2 to 3 months, but corneal growth takes many years. Signs and symptoms include congestion, photophobia, tearing, foreign body sensation, progressive astigmatism, diplopia, and restriction of extraocular movement. Often pterygia will spontaneously become inactive before any vision-threatening lesions occur. There is absence of periodic congestion, loss of punctate staining over the body, and shrinkage of the cap. Involution usually occurs, leaving a flat inconspicuous scar. Because of a strong tendency to *aggressive recurrence* after surgical excision, and the good chance for involution, great care must be taken to document progressive, vision-threatening, or disturbing corneal or episcleral growth with recorded sequential size measurements and, if possible, photography before any surgical therapy is performed. The key to inhibition of pterygium if surgery is performed is excision of the pterygium down to bare sclera leaving wide conjunctival (2 to 3 mm) margins and excising the corneal head. Conjunctival autografts cover the bared sclera and *mitomycin-C* 0.01% to

0.02% either as a single application at surgery or bid for 5 days will significantly inhibit recurrence. Because of increased *complications* with delayed epithelial healing and avascularity of sclera and cornea, mitomycin should be used to treat severe pterygia only and *avoided* in patients with Sjögren syndrome, or other dry eyes.

G. **Climatic keratopathy (actinic keratopathy)** is a slowly progressive degeneration caused by years of outdoor exposure in any climate. There are coalescent, elevated yellowish nodules and plaques in the lower half of the cornea. Treatment is avoidance of outdoor exposure and as in sec. **V.E.6.,** above.

H. **Marginal degenerations, peripheral ulcerative keratopathies (PUK)**

1. **Terrien marginal degeneration** is an uncommon, painless, nonulcerative thinning of the marginal cornea. Often bilateral, the condition predominantly affects males in the late teens or older. The process usually begins superiorly with opacification and progresses over many years with thinning and superficial vascularization and, in younger patients, may be inflammatory. Lipid deposits may be seen at the leading edge. Symptoms of mild irritation may occur and respond to lubricants or, in the inflammatory cases, to intermittent mild steroid qd to bid (0.1% fluoro-methalone, FML). **Pellucid marginal degeneration** is painless, bilateral thinning of the inferior corneal periphery and may have similar complications. The most bothersome problem can be progressive astigmatism with some diminution of vision. Spontaneous perforation is rare, but trauma can rupture the thin cornea. **Treatment** is nonspecific. Gas-permeable rigid contact lenses or piggyback hard and soft lenses are effective in correcting astigmatism in mild to moderate cases. Surgical reinforcement with peripheral crescentic lamellar keratoplasty, sometimes coupled with penetrating keratoplasty, often provides stable visual recovery.

2. **Furrow degeneration** is a thinning of the peripheral cornea occurring in older patients in the area of an arcus senilis. There is no ulceration or epithelial defect, no vascularization, and no tendency to perforate. **Treatment** is usually not necessary.

3. **Furrow degeneration or inflammatory ulceration associated with rheumatoid arthritis** may occur in marginal and central cornea and is seen with greater infiltration than furrow degeneration. Progressive melting to perforation is common if systemic disease is not controlled. NSAIDs and systemic steroids are only palliative. *Immunosuppressive agents* such methotrexate coupled with the drugs such as sulfasalazine, cyclophosphamide, etanercept, infliximab, or leflunomide appear to control the ocular inflammation and may prolong survival by controlling other vasculitis. Such therapy for rheumatoid or collagen–vascular disease should be undertaken in consultation with a rheumatologist (see Chapter 9, sec. **X.**). Local ocular therapy is lubrication, antibiotic ointment, soft contact lenses, and, if perforation threatens, tissue adhesive (Dermabond). Topical mild steroids are useful in sclerosing or acute stromal keratitis, but should be avoided in furrowing or keratolysis.

4. **Mooren's ulcer** is a severe inflammatory ulcerating disease of the marginal cornea running a **painful** and progressive course. The characteristic clinical picture is that of an overhanging advancing edge of an epithelial defect with vascularization of the ulcer base. The condition has been described in two forms, the first a more benign unilateral affliction of older males, and the second a bilateral ulceration of relentless progression in younger patients. Advancement of the inflammatory ulceration is both centrally and peripherally around the limbus and may extend into the sclera in severe cases. Scleral involvement, however, usually means there is another diagnosis, i.e., vasculitis, not Mooren's. Spontaneous perforation is uncommon but certainly can occur. Vascularization can advance to cover the cornea (autoconjunctival flap).

Treatment is often disappointing. Systemic interferon has been useful in hepatitis C-associated Mooren. Topical and systemic steroids are of some help, and immunosuppression with cyclosporin A or cytotoxic agents may be quite useful (see sec. **V.H.3.**, above, and Chapter 9, secs. **VI.A.,C.,** and **D.** for use and dosage of these drugs), as is early tissue adhesive for filling the bed of the ulcer (see sec. **IV.D.2.b.**). Conjunctival excision and recession with or without cryotherapy of the recessed edge has been reported to be successful in some cases, but the condition can recur. Soft contact lens therapy may benefit milder cases. Lamellar or full-thickness corneal grafts often melt or vascularize. Topical and systemic corticosteroids and systemic immunosuppression may be quite effective.

5. **Infectious agents associated with PUK** include ocular infection with the viruses herpes simplex, varicella-zoster, or HIV, and a variety of bacterial (especially *Staphylococcus*), fungal, and parasitic agents. Systemic infections include gonococcus, HIV, bacillary dysentery, tuberculosis, and syphilis.

6. **Noninfectious systemic vasculitic diseases** associated with **PUK** include Wegener granulomatosis, relapsing polychondritis, systemic lupus erythematosus, Sjögren syndrome, polyarteritis nodosa, malignancy, and giant-cell arteritis. Other *immune disorders* include progressive systemic sclerosis, graft versus host reactions, Behçet syndrome, sarcoid, and inflammatory bowel disease. ***Hematologic*** diseases include porphyria and leukemia, and ***dermatologic*** diseases are acne rosacea, psoriasis, cicatricial pemphigoid, and Stevens-Johnson syndrome. Many of these are discussed in this chapter, in Chapter 9, and in Tables 15.1, 15.2, and 15.9.

VI. Dry eyes (keratoconjunctivitis sicca)

A. **Etiologies.** One of the most common causes of chronic low-grade irritations of the eyes, particularly in the elderly population, is lacrimal aqueous and meibomian lipid layer insufficiency, causing dry eye. Although reflex tearing can decrease with advancing age, a variety of diseases can also diminish basal tear secretion. The height of the tear meniscus or marginal strip (less than 0.3 mm), the presence of rose bengal staining, particularly of the inner palpebral conjunctiva and inferior cornea, or a consistently diminished Schirmer strip test is of diagnostic importance. Corneal epithelial disease correlates with decreased aqueous tear production and delayed tear clearance, whereas meibomian gland dysfunction correlates just with delayed tear clearance. Desiccation causes cytokine release and subsequent *inflammatory* response with further tear layer disturbance. Loss of mucous secretion (tear spreading agent) results from a variety of inflammatory illnesses.

1. **Idiopathic.** Many patients with chronic low-grade keratoconjunctivitis sicca, usually of a mild degree, will demonstrate no systemic disease or other ocular disease to account for the lacrimal insufficiency. It is important to exclude ***drug-induced*** tear hyposecretion, which can occur with a variety of drugs, including phenothiazines, antihistamines, oral contraceptives (although estrogen alone is helpful), antihypertensives, antidepressants, antiulcer agents, anti-muscle spasmodics, nasal decongestants, and anticholinergics (Parkinson).

2. **Lupus erythematosus.** Both systemic and discoid lupus erythematosus can result in the complex of keratoconjunctivitis sicca and xerostomia due to infiltration of the lacrimal and salivary glands. Superficial punctate epitheliopathy and corneal erosions accompany the dry eye. Diagnostic features of importance are the butterfly rash of the cheek, nose, and lower lids. Treatment is systemic with NSAIDs, steroids, and cytotoxic agents (see Chapter 9, secs. **VI.A.,C.,** and **D.**). Local ocular therapy is lubrication.

3. **Ocular pemphigoid** (essential shrinkage of the conjunctiva, benign mucous membrane pemphigoid). Although chronic low-grade inflammation is a common feature of this disease, the more severe dry eye is encountered late in the disease, after significant scarring of the accessory lacrimal glands and ducts has occurred. Keratinization of the surface is further

aggravated by distortion of the lid anatomy and trichiasis. Dry eye and keratinization with scarring may be prevented with early systemic therapy. Immunosuppressives such as cyclophosphamide control ocular pemphigoid in 90% of cases, but often induce dangerous side effects. Dapsone 100 mg p.o. qd is the first line of treatment and often arrests the disease, but the drug may cause hemolytic anemia. An effective alternative is sulfasalazine 1 to 4 g per day p.o. This precursor of sulfapyridine is used to treat other autoimmune diseases and is a good alternative to Dapsone if there are unacceptable side effects. All treatment should be done in consultation with an oncologist (see Chapter 9, sec. **VI.D.**).

4. **Sjögren syndrome** (Gougerot-Sjögren syndrome) with keratoconjunctivitis sicca, xerostomia, and arthritis has been described as the prototype of this disease state. Seventy-five percent of the patients have associated rheumatoid arthritis. Approximately 15% of patients with rheumatoid arthritis will develop the sicca syndrome.

5. **Erythema multiforme (Stevens-Johnson syndrome).** The postinflammatory mucosal scarring that occurs as a result of an acute episode of erythema multiforme involving the eyes can result in chronic dry eye. Resolution of the acute mucosal necrosis leaves symblepharon and scarring of the accessory lacrimal glands and the ducts of the main lacrimal gland. Keratinization can occur. Immunosuppressive agents (see Chapter 9, sec. **VI.D.**) may be useful in therapy of chronic complications and cycloplegia, and mild topical steroids may be needed for chronic iritis. Lubrication is discussed in sec. **IV.B.** and acute disease is discussed in sec. **VII.G.**, below.

6. **Scleroderma (progressive systemic sclerosis)** may have associated keratoconjunctivitis sicca.

7. **Periarteritis nodosa.** Keratoconjunctivitis sicca occurs as a late development in some patients with inflammatory ocular involvement from periarteritis.

8. **Sarcoidosis.** In this chronic granulomatous disease, infiltration of the lacrimal gland can result in keratoconjunctivitis sicca and occurs with relative frequency in older patients afflicted with the disorder.

9. **Status postexcision of the lacrimal gland.** In most patients, excision of the lacrimal gland or obliteration of its ducts by removal of the palpebral portion will not cause keratoconjunctivitis sicca because the basal and mucosal secretors are preserved. In a small number of patients, however, a frank keratoconjunctivitis sicca will develop.

10. **Mikulicz syndrome** results from a variety of infiltrative diseases such as tuberculosis, leukemia, Hodgkin's disease, amyloid, or sarcoidosis. Characterized by symmetric enlargement of the lacrimal glands and salivary (parotid) glands, the condition can result in keratoconjunctivitis sicca.

11. **Other diseases associated with dry eyes are** diabetes mellitus (especially diabetic retinopathy), graft versus host, polymyositis, post-head and -neck radiation, HIV, hepatitis B and C, syphilis, tuberculosis, trachoma, and seventh nerve palsy.

B. **Treatment.** The following sequence of therapy is indicated (see Appendix A).

1. **Lid hygiene** to stabilize the tear film using warm, wet facecloth compresses 2 minutes, two to four times a day to the lids. Apply baby shampoo lather with the fingertips and clean and rinse the lash line qd after a compress.

2. **Tear replacement and stimulation.** *Hypotonic* solutions have been recommended and are helpful in milder cases or when alternated with the thicker tear drops. More *viscous* vehicles, such as methylcellulose, polyvinyl alcohol, or mucoadhesives, provide a longer contact time. The many different brands confirm the variable effectiveness of these solutions (see Appendix A for available agents). Oral pilocarpine (Salagen) 5 mg bid to tid, or cevimeline (Evoxac) *stimulate salivary and tear secretion* and relieve dry mouth and often dry eyes in these patients.

3. **Associated conditions.** Interference with the normal lubrication and cleansing function of the tears as well as the association of decreased lysozyme content place these patients at risk for chronic low-grade infections. Such infections of the eyelid margin can aggravate the underlying tear deficiency, and anterior (seborrhea, eczema, bacterial) or posterior (meibomitis) **blepharitis** should be treated with adequate lid hygiene, antiinflammatory, and/or antibiotic therapy. Discontinue any unnecessary topical medications that may be causing toxic medicamentosa.

4. **Punctal occlusion.** Temporary punctal occlusion (2 to 3 weeks) can be achieved by insertion of 0.2- to 0.6-mm collagen plugs (Eagle Vision, Lacrimedics). Reversible "permanent" occlusion of the puncta is achieved by insertion of 0.4- to 0.8-mm silicone plugs (Eagle, Oasis) at the slit-lamp. These may easily be removed later. Six months after placement, about 85% of patients are asymptomatic and about 75% use little to no lubricants. About 40% will lose a plug within the first 6 months, especially upper lid plugs. Electrocautery after local anesthesia produces permanent closure. Temporary occlusion may be used to predict those patients who would suffer from epiphora if permanent occlusion were performed.

5. **Therapeutic contact lens therapy (TSCL).** Hydrophilic *bandage lenses* often provide a tear reservoir if used in conjunction with copious artificial tears. These patients are prone to contact lens intolerance and superinfection and should be followed carefully. Forniceal scarring may dislodge the lenses. Newer lenses, the *gas-permeable scleral contact lenses,* have been very effective is otherwise contact-lens-intolerant eyes with extensive ocular surface disease. Indications include Stevens-Johnson disease, cicatricial pemphigoid, exposure keratitis, toxic epidermal necrolysis, herpetic trophic ulceration, congenital meibomian gland deficiency, superior limbal keratitis, Sjögren syndrome, and inflammatory corneal degeneration (see sec. **XI.,** below).

6. **Lateral tarsorrhaphy** will decrease tear evaporation.

7. **Other methods.** *Moist chambers* achieved by an occlusive plastic shield across the eye have helped in some cases. Close-fitting glasses with *side shields* often achieve the same effect. *Amniotic membrane* and cadaveric epithelial *stem-cell transplantation* has been used successfully with increasing numbers of patients with severe ocular surface disorders including severe dry eye, chemical burns, and neurotrophic ulcers. Future treatments include topical *androgens* to stabilize meibomian oil secretion, and topical *cyclosporin A* to suppress cytolytic T lymphocytes and other destructive inflammation.

VII. **Allergy and hypersensitivity** present in the eye as type IV delayed hypersensitivity, usually a contact dermatitis, or as type I reaction, an immediate hypersensitivity from allergen–immunoglobulin E (IgE) reaction on the mast cell surface triggering mast cell degranulation and release of inflammatory mediators, including histamine. The ocular histamine receptors are H1 (itching) and H2 (erythema). Other mast cell inflammatory mediators include prostaglandins and leukotrienes, which increase local blood flow, activate pain receptors, release serotonin, are pyogenic, enhance vascular permeability and dilation, and are white cell chemotactic.

A. **Seasonal and perennial allergic conjunctivitis** (SAC, PAC, respectively) cause the vast majority of allergic conjunctivitis and may be associated with hay fever. SAC symptoms are itchy, watery eyes, often with rhinitis or allergic pharyngitis. Eye signs are mild lid edema, fine papillary hypertrophy, bulbar conjunctival hyperemia, and, in some cases, chemosis. Corneal involvement is rare. Common inciting antigens are grass and tree pollens in the spring and ragweed pollen in the fall. PAC is less common and less severe, but tends to occur year-round because of the nonseasonal nature of the antigens, e.g., dust, animal dander, house mite feces, mold, and some foods. Chronic symptoms of itching, burning, and tearing in normal-appearing eyes often indicate PAC as opposed to SAC, which is seasonal and has more florid clinical findings. In severe atopic conjunctivitis, there may also be subepithelial fibrosis, symblepharon, corneal ulcers, and neovascularization. Conjunctival scrapings reveal eosinophils, and serum IgE is markedly elevated. Differentiation from acute viral infections can be made by lack of adenopathy, but differentiation from contact or toxic exposure often relies on the history and IgE levels. Atopy does not resolve spontaneously over time.

B. **Atopic eczema** may rarely cause keratoconjunctivitis. Acute exacerbations of atopic eczema with scaly dermatitis affecting especially the face, neck, popliteal, and antecubital areas can be associated with keratoconjunctivitis that is characterized by thickening and hyperemia of the conjunctiva with superficial opacification and vascularization of the cornea. Multiple other allergies, including hay fever, rhinitis, asthma, and urticaria, are often concurrently present. All may cause allergic keratoconjunctivitis. A higher occurrence of keratoconus (KC) than in the normal population has been reported with this condition.

C. **Vernal conjunctivitis.** This seasonally recurrent bilateral inflammation of the conjunctiva, producing itching, tearing, photophobia, and foreign body sensation, occurs in two forms.

1. The **palpebral** form is distinguished by cobblestone papillae on the tarsal conjunctiva and may be associated with shield ulcers of the superior cornea. These may require antibiotic prophylaxis and occasionally soft contact lens therapy in the form of a hydrophilic bandage lens.

2. The **limbal** form occurs with papillary hypertrophy on the limbal conjunctiva associated with white, chalky concretions known as Trantas dots near the limbus.

3. **Diagnosis.** One of the main diagnostic features is the conjunctival scraping showing prominent eosinophils, many of which will be fractured, releasing their granules. A seasonal predilection is for the spring and early summer as well as for the fall. In addition to the clinical appearance of the papillary changes, a thick, ropy mucous discharge is a hallmark of the disease. The condition usually occurs in young people and tends to run a course of from 4 to 10 years before remission.

D. **Treatment of ocular allergy.** (See Appendix A for categories and dosage.) For contact dermatitis, remove the offending allergen and apply topical steroid tid for 4 to 7 days. Allergen identity is often difficult to establish for conjunctivitis. Rapid-onset (15 minutes) palliative treatment with topical *decongestants–antihistamines* bid to qid is often effective, with decongestants vasoconstricting blood vessels to reduce redness and chemosis and the antihistamine blocking H1 receptors to reduce lid and conjunctival edema, hyperemia, itching, and tearing (Livostin, Emadine, Naphcon-A, Vasocon A, Opcon A, generic).

1. Topical *mast cell stabilizers* qid prevent mast cell degranulation and mediator release (Alomide, Crolom, Opticrom). Because these agents do not block histamine that has already been released, there is a 2- to 4-day delay in onset of effect (which may be addressed by also using an antihistamine drop for a few days). They are excellent long-term prophylaxis and may be started a few weeks ahead of an anticipated reaction such as SAC. H1 blockers are good when only antihistamine is needed or when combination with pure mast cell stabilizers (rather than a precombined drug) is desired (Emadine, Livostin).

2. The topical *antihistamine–mast cell stabilizer* olopatadine (Patanol) is used only bid to block H1 receptors immediately to relieve itching and also to stabilize mast cells to block further mediator release.

3. The topical *antihistamine–mast cell stabilizers–NSAID* agents combine the first two listed effects with nonsteroidal antiinflammatory properties and also have only bid dosing (Alocril, Alomast, Optivar, Zaditor). NSAIDs block prostaglandin and thus block another cause of itching. They are usually used qid during the acute episode (Acular, Voltaren), but signs of corneal toxicity must be monitored.

4. Patients with a moderate to severe disease or history of atopy, hay fever, eczema, or other systemic allergy often respond well to newer "soft" *topical steroids* bid to qid because of excellent surface-acting antiinflammatory properties and low tendency for elevating intraocular pressure (loteprednol as 0.2% Alrex or 0.5% Lotemax suspension). Stronger topical steroids such as 1% prednisolone or 0.1% dexamethasone (qid taper to bid in 1 week) may be needed for severe allergic disorders such as vernal kerato-conjunctivitis (VKC) or atopic kerato-conjunctivitis (AKC), especially if there are corneal complications. *New drugs* in the antiallergy pipeline include azelastine, cyclosporine, anti-IgE drugs, and leukotriene modifiers. Adding a *steroid nasal inhaler* (Beconase, Vancenase, Rhinocort) bid is often additive therapeutically. *Desensitization* should be reserved for more severe cases in which a specific allergen can be unequivocally identified.

5. *Oral antihistamines* should be added if there is moderate to severe lid edema or chemosis. Nonsedating forms are fexofenadine 60 mg bid (Allegra), loratadine 10 mg qd (Claritin), and cetirizine 5 to 10 mg qd (Zyrtec). These are safer than other oral antihistamines in terms of drug interaction with macrolides or ketoconazole.

E. **Giant papillary conjunctivitis** (see sec **XI.D.,** below, and Chapter 14).

F. **Phlyctenular keratoconjunctivitis.** This nodular inflammatory response of the conjunctiva or cornea appears to be an allergic reaction to an antigen. The clinical evolution of the phlyctenule is usually that of a small vesicle that forms a nodule that subsequently breaks down, with subsequent spontaneous healing. A local leash of vessels is common and may be most prominent when the phlyctenule moves onto the corneal surface. Formerly associated with tuberculosis in a debilitated patient, it is now most commonly secondary to staphylococcal blepharoconjunctivitis. Symptoms of irritation, tearing, and redness tend to be more severe when corneal involvement occurs. The condition must be distinguished from an inflamed pinguecula, small pterygium, or from limbal corneal involvement by acne rosacea or limbal herpes simplex keratitis.

1. **Treatment.** Doxycycline 100 mg or erythromycin 250 mg p.o. tid for 3 months coupled with prednisolone 1% or dexamethasone 0.1% qid usually provides long term remission. If photophobia is severe, cycloplegics will provide comfort. Epithelial breakdown should be treated with prophylactic antibiotics. Metronidazole 0.75% skin gel bid for 6 months for associated **rosacea** is therapeutically useful (see sec. **III.D.3.,** above).

G. **Ligneous conjunctivitis** is a rare, chronic disorder of the conjunctiva and other mucous membranes characterized by multiple inflamed (lymphocytes, plasma cells, and eosinophils) granulomatous lesions. Treatment with excision followed by steroids, cromolyn, fibrinolysin, and silver nitrate usually fails with rapid recurrence. Recent success using excision followed by topical cyclosporine 20 mg per mL q2 to 6h over several weeks, has been reported (not FDA approved). Prophylactic topical antibiotics should be used under this treatment.

H. **Erythema multiforme (Stevens-Johnson syndrome).** Usually occurring before the age of 30 years, this potentially fatal disease presents as a **cutaneous eruption** of sharply defined erythematous vesicular and bulbous patches scattered about the hands, forearms, face, and neck. This condition also affects the mucous membranes, resulting in severe stomatitis and conjunctivitis. It results from a hypersensitivity reaction to infections (herpes, mumps, Coxsackie virus, echovirus, mycoplasma, psittacosis, scarlet fever) or to drugs (sulfonamides, sulfones, penicillin, barbiturates). Ocular complications are common. The **conjunctivitis** usually occurs in one of three forms: (a) catarrhal—circumscribed raised patches of edema that may lead to frank bullae formation that resolves with disappearance of the eruption, (b) purulent—usually severe and associated with extreme chemosis and corneal involvement (epithelial keratitis, ulceration) or exudative iridocyclitis, or (c) pseudomembranous—most common and associated with extensive discharge and pseudomembrane formation with subsequent symblepharon and scarring. Optic neuritis may develop in either eye. Corneal involvement is most likely to occur with the pseudomembranous eye form and can result in frank ulceration and perforation. Iritis or panophthalmitis may occur. Severe keratoconjunctivitis sicca is a sequela. **Treatment** of acute systemic disease with high-dose systemic steroids is controversial and has no bearing on ocular prognosis. Ocular therapy in acute disease is topical antibiotic particularly for staphylococcal infection, which is common. Bacitracin, erythromycin, gentamicin, or tobramycin drops or ointment is given q4h to qid. Topical corticosteroids will help to control inflammation—1% prednisolone qid initially with monitoring for corneal ulceration with thinning, in which case they should be stopped or changed to less potent drugs such as lotoprednol. Long-term efficacy of steroids is still under debate. The fornices should be gently swept qd to bid with a glass rod after topical anesthetic to break fresh adhesions, along with daily lid hygiene. Late management is that of keratoconjunctivitis sicca which may be severe, and iritis (see sec. **VI.,** above, and Chapter 9). Immunosuppressives may be effective. Surgical **keratoprosthesis** may restore good vision in end-stage disease, although the incidence of postoperative infection is higher in this group and in cicatricial pemphigoid than in chemical burns or in noncicatrizing corneal disease.

I. **Rosacea (acne rosacea)** is primarily a disease of the sebaceous glands of the skin, predominantly involving the malar and nasal areas of the face. There can be a **chronic blepharoconjunctivitis** present in up to 30% of cases. Of those showing ocular involvement, approximately 7% will develop *corneal ulceration.*

1. **Facial eruption.** The rash is often present as a butterfly configuration across the malar area and consists of numerous small telangiectasia and often macular, slightly scaling lesions on an erythematous base. The chronic form with hyperplasia of sebaceous glands and periglandular fibrosis presents as rhinophyma, particularly in males. The patient often gives a history of prominent blushing and facial erythema, particularly after ingestion of alcohol or coffee.

2. **Ocular findings**
   a. **Blepharitis** is primarily *posterior* (meibomitis) and probably the most common manifestation of ocular rosacea. It is usually bilateral with staining of the tarsal conjunctiva, lid margin telangiectasia, and prominent plugging and inspissation of meibomian glands, which can be expressed on pressure to the lid margin. Staphylococcal superinfection may be present.
   b. **Conjunctivitis.** A low-grade conjunctivitis that fluctuates in severity is frequently associated with the blepharitis.
   c. **Keratitis** may present as marginal infiltrate with a fascicle of vessels from the limbus or as a frank ulceration that progressively advances across the cornea. Rarely do these ulcers perforate unless intensive steroids are used in treatment. Chronic scarring at the site of the ulcer usually results.
   d. **Cutaneous** and **ocular** lesions of rosacea need not coincide in severity. Skin lesions should be sought in any patient with chronic blepharitis or vascularized keratitis.

3. **Treatment** (see also secs. **III.D.3.,** above)
   a. **Local measures.** Lid hygiene should be emphasized with daily massage, hot compresses, and removal of crusts from the lid margins with baby shampoo-lathered fingertips or special lid-cleaning pads available in drugstores (Eye Scrub). Topical antibiotics such as bacitracin ointment HS may be used to control infection. Instability of the tear film or surface irregularities often necessitate use of lubricant qid.
   b. **Systemic antibiotic treatment.** The most effective treatment for the ocular manifestations of acne rosacea is systemic doxycycline or

minocycline 100 mg p.o. qd for 14 to 21 days, then 50 to 100 mg qd p.o. for *3–6 months* with meals (avoid milk products or minerals within 2 hours). Equally effective but less convenient is tetracycline 250 mg qd to bid times a day on an empty stomach for a period of 21 days and then tapered to qd dosage, to be maintained for 3 to 6 months. The effect of the doxycycline and tetracycline is apparently independent of its antibiotic effectiveness and may relate to an antiinflammatory effect and stabilization of meibomian lipid composition. An alternative drug is erythromycin 250 mg p.o. qid. The usual precautions with use of the tetracycline family should be observed, and it should not be used in women who are pregnant or breast-feeding. Relapse of the condition after discontinuation of tetracycline may occur.

  c. **Steroids.** The inflammatory and vascular aspects of the keratitis are extremely sensitive to low doses of topical steroid. Steroids must be used with caution, however, because there is a tendency for ulceration to perforate. It is probably best to limit steroid treatment to 0.12% prednisolone qd to bid.

J. **Cicatricial pemphigoid (ocular pemphigoid, benign mucous membrane pemphigoid)** is a relatively rare chronic inflammatory systemic disease of the mucous membranes (especially oral and eye) probably due to anti-basement membrane antibody reaction. In the eye, there is mucoid discharge, redness, and conjunctival subepithelial fibrosis with foreshortening of the fornices, symblepharon formation, entropion, trichiasis, and ultimately dry eye with corneal ulceration, neovascularization, and keratinization.

  Treatment is primarily systemic, immunosuppressive, and done with a physician familiar with the drugs used. The earlier the treatment is started, the better the outcome. Initial treatment for mild, nonprogressive early ocular disease is suppression with *steroids,* e.g., prednisone 40 to 60 mg p.o. qd, tapering to alternate-day therapy ranging from 2.5 to 60.0 mg per day. Steroids do not stop progressive pemphigoid but the *sulfone, dapsone,* is effective for mild to moderately progressive oral and ocular lesions. The starting dosage is 50 mg p.o. qd for 1 to 2 weeks, then, if tolerated, increased to 50 mg p.o. bid, but monitored for the expected side effect of hemolytic anemia. Dosage should be adjusted up and down as needed. Successful maintenance doses range from 50 to 150 mg p.o. qd for years. *Glucose-6-dehydrogenase-deficient patients* should *not* receive this drug or hemolysis will be severe. Rapidly progressive pemphigoid is usually responsive to combined *cyclophosphamide* 1 to 2 mg per kg p.o. qd, and *prednisone* 1 mg per kg p.o. qd for 1 month. If disease activity is still significant, cyclophosphamide is increased in 25-mg amounts monthly and prednisone tapered to 40 mg p.o. qd. Once disease is controlled, therapy is usually continued for 12 to 18 months total. *Lid hygiene,* topical *lubricants,* and *blepharitis therapy* should be maintained indefinitely. Oculoplastic surgery may be required for more advanced cases and *keratoprosthesis* with a valve shunt has been successful in restoring vision. Unfortunately, these advanced disease states do not respond well to systemic or topical treatment. **Drug-induced pemphigoid** has been seen with echothiophate, pilocarpine, idoxuridine, and epinephrine. Administration of the offending drug should be stopped.

VIII. **Dystrophies.** Corneal dystrophy describes primary, inherited, bilateral changes of the cornea that occur unaccompanied by systemic disease. Characteristic corneal changes are also encountered in certain inherited metabolic and skin disorders.

  A. **Meesman's epithelial dystrophy.** This dominantly inherited dystrophy presents in the fully developed form a corneal epithelium diffusely studded with minute fleck-like opacities of variable density and distribution that, on retroillumination with the slitlamp, appear to be minute collections of debris in an otherwise clear, spherical microvesicle. These spherical microcysts may elevate the corneal surface sufficiently to disturb the tear film. Superficial corneal scarring is rare. The epithelial changes have been demonstrated as early as 7 months of age and tend to increase with age. Although usually asymptomatic, some pedigrees have shown mild ocular discomfort and slight decrease in visual acuity to the 20/40 range. This condition must be differentiated from bilateral microcystic epithelial changes that may also be seen with corneal edema, with vernal conjunctivitis, or in association with disturbed tear function. Pathologically, the small round intraepithelial cysts appear to represent degenerated epithelial cells and contain periodic acid–Schiff (PAS)-positive cellular debris. Pathologic changes are usually confined to the epithelium. **Hereditary epithelial dystrophy** (Stocker-Holt, Schneider) occurs as a dominantly inherited dystrophy presenting with minute epithelial droplets that are transparent and have predilection for the center of the cornea. There can be fluorescein staining but pathologic changes are confined to the epithelium. This condition may be a variant of the Meesman corneal dystrophy. **Treatment** is usually not necessary, but first line would be *lubrication* with artificial tears and ointments. If the discomfort is severe, *TSCLs* with continued tear lubrication may be helpful. If visual impairment is unusually severe, *laser keratectomy* or *lamellar keratoplasty* may be indicated.

B. **Anterior membrane dystrophy.** There is an increasing tendency to label the epithelial basement membrane disorders as anterior membrane dystrophies.

1. **Cogan's microcystic epithelial dystrophy.** This epithelial disorder, with no obvious hereditary tendency, appears in females as bilateral, gray-white, round or comma-shaped deposits in the corneal epithelium ("putty marks"). Mild foreign body sensation is often a complaint, but visual acuity and corneal sensation are unaffected. Histologically, the deposits represent intraepithelial cysts containing cellular debris. PAS-positive nodular substance on the anterior surface of an irregular basement membrane is also seen.

2. **Fingerprint dystrophy.** Bilateral curvilinear lucent opacities (seen best on retroillumination at the slitlamp) at the level of Bowman's layer and variously described as "fingerprint" or "mare's tail" lines are the characteristic of this condition in which no consistent hereditary pattern is described.

3. **Map-dot-fingerprint dystrophy.** Polymorphic epithelial and anterior Bowman's layer microcystic opacities described as a map-dot pattern or a fingerprint-like wrinkling of the basement membrane (seen best by slit-lamp retroillumination) have been observed in bilateral distribution idiopathically or after fingernail or other corneal abrasions, and are often associated with recurrent epithelial erosions.

4. **Recurrent corneal erosion syndrome (RES).** Anterior membrane dystrophies may be accompanied by recurrent epithelial erosions. Often a fourth category of dystrophic recurrent erosion is described with similar epithelial changes but occurring in a dominantly inherited fashion. All are probably associated with an abnormality of basement membrane adhesion that accounts for the recurrent erosive episodes, causing eye discomfort and foreign body sensation (see Chapter 2, sec. **V.C.**). Trauma such as a fingernail or paper cut may also cause RES.

5. **Treatment** of *anterior membrane–epithelial disorders* is essentially treatment of recurrent erosion and includes patching with an antibiotic during the acute phase and an attempt at aborting recurrences by use of artificial tears several times daily and tear ointment nightly. For frequent or more severe erosions, a **TSCL** (Permalens) should be fitted and left in place for 3 to 6 months. Antibiotic drops bid and lubrication should be used if the epithelium is disrupted. Abnormalities of the lids, including chronic low-grade blepharomeibomitis, can aggravate the epithelial changes and predispose to recurrent erosion. Meticulous lid hygiene and *control of any blepharitis* are often necessary to prevent

repeated attacks of erosion. Recalcitrant cases should be treated with the metalloproteinase-9 inhibitors, doxycycline 50 mg p.o. bid for 2 to 3 months, and topical steroid tid for 3 to 4 weeks, with antibiotic cover. *Superficial débridement* or *anterior stromal puncture* is advocated in persistent cases. The puncture technique is done under topical anesthesia at the slitlamp. A 20- to 30-gauge bent needle tip is used to place 20 to 40 micropunctures directly over and surrounding the erosion. Depth is through epithelium to its underlying basement membrane with the purpose of creating microfibrotic adhesions that will hold the epithelium in place. The visual axis may be included because scarring is negligible. After treatment, antibiotic ointment is instilled and a 24-hour pressure patch applied. Lubricants are used regularly starting 1 day postoperatively. Occasionally, the erosion will recur in the same area or adjacent to it, requiring retreatment with anterior stromal puncture or, if due to local edema, treatment with ointment only. *Excimer laser* has been successful in resolving difficult cases.

C. **Reis-Bücklers dystrophy** is an autosomal-dominant condition of the cornea characterized by a network of ring-like opacities occurring at the level of Bowman's layer and protruding irregularly into the epithelium, with subsequent distortion of the anterior corneal surface. The disorder may present at about 5 years of age and shows a progressive course, with increasing frequency of attacks of recurrent erosions that usually result in a diffuse anterior scarring corresponding to a reduction in visual acuity and a decrease in corneal sensation. Histopathologic studies show widespread destruction of Bowman's layer, with replacement by irregular scar tissue interspersed with aggregates of microfilamentous material. Absence of hemidesmosomal attachments accounts for the faulty adherence of epithelium. Early **therapy** with lubrication and TSCL (Permalens) is effective, but in severe cases laser keratectomy or lamellar keratoplasty may be indicated.

D. The **anterior dystrophy** described by **Grayson and Wilbrandt** is similar to Reis-Bücklers dystrophy, with variable effects on vision and of corneal sensation.

E. **Vortex dystrophy** was the diagnosis once applied to the pigment lines occurring in a whorl-like fashion over the surface of the cornea and located in the area of Bowman's layer and adjacent stroma. This appears to be the same corneal lesion seen in Fabry's disease and is thought to be a manifestation of the asymptomatic carrier state of females with X-linked **Fabry's disease.** In general, it must be distinguished from the corneal deposits seen in *phenothiazine keratopathy, amiodarone, chloroquine, indomethacin, or tamoxifen toxicity*, and occasionally the pattern of *fingerprint lines*. Drug-induced vortex keratopathy is *not* an indication to stop the drug if it is needed. The condition is often reversible if the medication is stopped, however.

F. **Granular dystrophy (Groenouw type I)** is an autosomal-dominant dystrophy characterized by stromal opacities of dense, milky, granular-appearing deposits occurring in the axial portion of the cornea, most prominently in the anterior stroma. Intervening stroma is clear. The lesions may be manifest in the first decade of life, but visual acuity is usually not affected until late in the disease. The histochemical characteristics are listed in **Table 5.9.** The deposits are principally hyaline degeneration of *collagenous protein.* When visual acuity is notably impaired, penetrating keratoplasty is indicated.

G. **Macular dystrophy (Groenouw type II),** an autosomal- recessive dystrophy, appears as a diffuse clouding in the central cornea between the ages of 5 and 9 years. Gradual increase in the density of the opacity with development of gray-white nodular deposits of varying size within the corneal stroma is accompanied by progressive diminution of vision and episodic irritation and photophobia. The severe decrease in visual acuity often necessitates penetrating keratoplasty. Histologically and histochemically, the deposits in and

TABLE 5.9. HISTOLOGIC STAINING CHARACTERISTICS
OF STROMAL DYSTROPHIES

Dystrophy	Masson Trichrome	PAS[a]	Congo Red	Birefringence
Granular	Bright red	Negative	Negative	Negative
Macular	Negative	Pink	Negative	Negative
Lattice	Red	Pink-red	Red	Positive

[a]PAS, periodic acid–Schiff (reaction).

around the keratocytes appear as accumulation of *mucopolysaccharide* as a result of a local enzyme deficiency. *Monoclonal gammopathy* may cause deposits similar to macular dystrophy and should be considered (serum protein electrophoresis), because it may be a forerunner of multiple myeloma (Table 5.9).

H. **Lattice dystrophy (Biber-Haab-Dimmer)** is an autosomal-dominant dystrophy characterized by the appearance in the corneal stroma of relucent branching filaments interlacing and overlapping at different levels and forming an irregular latticework with dichotomous branching. Fine dots, flakes, and stellate opacities may appear between the filaments. Although appearing as early as 2 years of age, the occurrence of recurrent erosive episodes and progressive clouding of the central cornea is apparent by the age of 20 years and is associated with decreased visual acuity such that penetrating keratoplasty is often indicated when the patient is in the fourth decade of life. Histopathologically and histochemically, the stromal deposits appear as hyaline fusiform deposits of *amyloid*. **Avellino dystrophy** is dominantly inherited and shares features of lattice and granular dystrophy (Table 5.9).

I. **Fleck dystrophy (central speckled dystrophy)** is an autosomal-dominant condition involving all layers of the cornea with oval to round gray-white opacities. The lesions are well circumscribed and separated from each other by clear cornea. Corneal sensation and visual acuity are usually not affected. Treatment is usually not necessary.

J. **Central cloudy and parenchymatous dystrophy** is an apparently autosomal-dominant condition that involves particularly the deep stroma, but sometimes extends to the Bowman layer. The condition is quite variable and usually does not result in visual impairment. Treatment is usually not indicated.

K. **Schnyder's crystalline dystrophy,** an autosomal-dominant condition, is characterized by a round, ring-shaped, central corneal opacity consisting of white-to-yellow or polychromatic crystals in the stroma. Peripheral deposits separated from the limbus by a clear line also appear. The lesions may be apparent as early as 18 months and may progress, but usually are not destructive to visual acuity. Corneal sensation is usually normal. Pathologically, the needle-like crystals contain *cholesterol*. Occasionally, the visual acuity is decreased and laser keratectomy or penetrating keratoplasty is indicated. Some patients with this dystrophy exhibit elevated blood lipids, xanthelasma, and corneal arcus.

L. **Congenital hereditary endothelial dystrophy (CHED)** is characterized by diffuse milky or ground-glass opacification of the stroma associated with a thickening of the cornea up to four times normal. It has been described as both a dominantly and a recessively inherited disorder. Despite the gross stromal edema, the epithelium has only a mild roughening associated with fine microbullae. Visual acuity varies according to the degree of corneal clouding. Corneal sensation is normal and vascularization is rare. Histopathologically, there are *rare to absent endothelial cells* and an *overall increase in thickness of Descemet's membrane*, in contrast to Fuchs dystrophy. Nystagmus is common and congenital glaucoma must be ruled out. The **prognosis** for penetrating keratoplasty in these patients is *fair*. Examination of asymptomatic relatives of patients with congenital hereditary endothelial dystrophy may reveal clear vacuolar lesions with surrounding white haze and an irregular endothelial mosaic despite normal corneal thickness and visual acuity. The high risk of producing offspring with CHED makes examination of relatives important.

M. **Fuchs endothelial dystrophy** is seen most often in females in the fifth to sixth decades of life and can be transmitted in a dominant fashion. The endothelium has scattered guttae (Descemet "warts") progressing to a "beaten silver" appearance. There may be increasing stromal edema from endothelial dysfunction that culminates in epithelial edema, painful bullous keratopathy, and peripheral vascularization. Frequently, the condition is associated with cataractous changes in the lens nucleus, and a higher incidence than normal of chronic open-angle glaucoma and angle-closure glaucoma has been reported. Histopathologically, there is a paucity of endothelial cells which may be quantitated on *specular microscopy,* which provides a measure of disease status. Initial palliative **therapy** includes the use of hypertonic sodium chloride ointments at night and drops during the day. If painful bullous keratopathy ensues, a soft contact lens will often provide relief, although it rarely improves visual acuity. Penetrating keratoplasty is the mainstay of therapy for both visual rehabilitation and relief of pain.

N. **Posterior polymorphous dystrophy,** a dominantly inherited dystrophy of the endothelium and Descemet's membrane, presents clinically with a variable number of round, elliptical, or irregular lesions, often with vesicular appearance, bulging into the stroma or projecting into the anterior chamber. Although generally benign and nonprogressive, it can be associated with corneal edema, requiring penetrating keratoplasty for restoration of vision. Abnormal iris processes and peripheral anterior synechiae have been described. Histopathologically, a thickening of the posterior lamellae of Descemet's membrane and the presence of atypical cells on the posterior corneal surface suggestive of metaplasia to a fibroblastic cell suggest that it may represent a form of the anterior cleavage syndrome.

O. **Keratoconus (KC, ectatic corneal dystrophy)** is a disorder characterized by conical ectasia (bulging) of the paracentral cornea, with thinning and scarring resulting in a painless, progressive loss of vision resulting from an increasingly severe irregular myopic astigmatism. Corneal topography is useful in detecting early cases and following progression. **Subclinical KC** may be detected by doing keratography in upgaze and looking for inferior steepening. *These patients should not have refractive surgery.* Familial occurrence has been noted, although the majority of cases show no definitive inheritance pattern. There is often a history of eye rubbing. In the early stages, distortion of the retinoscopic reflex, keratoscopic figures, and keratometric mires are apparent. As the condition advances, vertical striae *(Vogt striae)* may be seen in the posterior stroma along with axial thinning and an increase in the axial corneal curvature. Reticular scarring of Bowman membrane can occur, the appearance of a *Fleischer ring* (epithelial iron deposits at the base of the cone), and bulging of the lower eyelid *(Munson sign)* on downgaze are often noted. Stromal corneal nerves tend to be more visible and fine fibrillary lines may be seen along the internal edge of the Fleischer ring. Occasionally, a break in the endothelium and Descemet's membrane results in gross stromal edema with bullous epitheliopathy *(corneal hydrops)* accompanied by pain and a rapid decrease in vision. **Treatment** is correction of the refractive error by spectacles or gas-permeable hard contact lenses or, in advanced cases, penetrating keratoplasty, with good prognosis for this condition. Corneal *hydrops* is self-resolving and managed conservatively with antibiotic ointments and moderate pressure patching. Patients *should not be dilated postoperatively* because permanent mydriasis may ensue even years later. Preoperative dilation should be done with mild mydriatics only, e.g., 2.5% phenylephrine. KC has been described in association with various **ocular anomalies** such as blue sclera, ectopia lentis, cataract, aniridia, retinitis pigmentosa, and optic atrophy. It is also associated with *systemic conditions,* Down syndrome, Ehlers-Danlos syndrome, Marfan syndrome, Addison's disease, neurofibromatosis, Apert anomaly, and allergic disease, including vernal conjunctivitis and atopic eczema. Association with chronic rubbing of the eyes and eyelids has been suggested.

IX. **Corneal edema.** Corneal deturgescence is achieved when pump function of the corneal endothelium balances the fluid-accumulating effect of intraocular hydrostatic pressure and corneal swelling pressure. Disturbance of this balance or disruption of the limiting membranes of the cornea (epithelium and endothelium) results in corneal edema. Stromal edema may minimally decrease visual acuity; epithelial edema, however, results in significant visual impairment and painful surface breakdown.

A. **Causes of corneal edema**
  1. **Elevated intraocular pressure (IOP)**
    a. **Acute angle-closure glaucoma** results in marked and often rapidly increased IOP. Corneal stroma thickness may not be increased despite prominent epithelial edema, but in some cases the pressure will aggravate prior endothelial dysfunction or produce temporary dysfunction resulting in stromal edema. Epithelial edema is a classic sign of acute glaucoma with resultant decreased vision. Although both epithelial and stromal edema usually resolve with control of the IOP, there occasionally can be residual stromal haze, which does not greatly affect vision.
    b. **Congenital glaucoma** can produce corneal haze that is usually most marked centrally, but that can involve the entire cornea. Edema involves stroma and epithelium. Normalization of the pressure may permit clearing of the cornea, although residual endothelial damage as manifested by horizontal *(Haab)* striae of Descemet's membrane may predispose to future corneal decompensation and edema late in life.
  2. **Trauma**
    a. **Birth trauma** (forceps injury) results in relucent double-contoured striae of Descemet's membrane that signal endothelial damage. The cornea is often clear during youth but can become edematous after an interval of several decades, with both stromal and epithelial edema.
    b. **Nonsurgical contusion injury** can cause focal endothelial dysfunction, with typical annular or diskiform areas of endothelial and stromal edema. Often transient and resolving over a few days, these focal areas of edema usually cause little long-term visual disability.
    c. **Penetration of a foreign body** into the anterior chamber can result in a retained foreign body in the inferior anterior chamber angle, with resultant focal (wedge-shaped) inferior corneal edema. Removal of the foreign body can be curative.
    d. **Surgical trauma** from cataract extraction, intraocular lens implantation, and prolonged or profuse anterior chamber irrigation can damage endothelial cells to produce corneal edema. Of the 31,532 corneal transplants done in the United States in 2000, the greatest numbers were for pseudophakic edema (20%). The edema can occur following vitrectomy or retinal detachment surgery and is more prone to occur in diabetics. Extensive extraocular muscle detachment procedures can also result in corneal decompensation if **anterior segment necrosis** occurs. Vitreous adherent to the cornea following cataract extraction may produce focal edema and stimulate metaplasia of the endothelium with resultant persistent edema.
  3. **Dystrophy. Endothelial dystrophies** such as Fuchs, CHED, and posterior polymorphous (see secs. **VIII.L.–O.**) may all cause edema. Although usually not considered as a cause of corneal edema, the **anterior membrane dystrophies** are characterized by corneal changes that can be accompanied by epithelial edema in very discrete distribution, especially

if recurrent breakdowns have occurred. An acute and painful cause of corneal edema occurs in some cases of **KC (acute hydrops).**

4. **Endothelial dysfunction secondary to inflammation. Uveitis or intraocular inflammation** can temporarily depress endothelial function to produce edema. Control of inflammation often restores endothelial integrity and reversal of edema. Herpetic uveitis is a common offender and should be suspected in patients with unilateral corneal edema and uveitis. **Focal keratitis** (bacterial, fungal, or viral) can provoke edema both by local inflammatory response and by compromising endothelial function. The infectious nature of the disease process is often suggested by the clinical features of focal infiltration of inflammatory cells that accompany the edema. **Corneal graft rejection** in patients who have undergone penetrating keratoplasty is a classic example of endothelial damage. The clinician should be alert to any inflammation or the earliest sign of edema in a corneal graft no matter how distant the surgery.

5. **Epithelial damage** resulting from *mechanical, chemical,* or *radiation* injury disrupts the barrier effect of the epithelium, allowing passage of fluid into the anterior corneal stroma. Metabolic disturbance of the cornea, such as hypoxia of contact lens overwear or toxic effects of medications and anesthetics, can also provoke intra- and intercellular epithelial edema.

B. **Treatment** is first to address the primary problem to restore the normal physiologic balance of corneal hydration. Should that be impossible, attempts should then be made to compensate for the fluid accumulation. Although visual acuity may be improved, the treatment often must strive for comfort and protection of the cornea.

1. **Lower IOP.** If IOP is pathologically elevated, attempts should be made medically or surgically to lower that pressure. In patients with borderline endothelial function and early corneal edema, reduction of the pressure from high-normal to low-normal levels will often relieve the edema.

2. **Control of inflammation** may improve corneal edema if dysfunction is the result of that inflammation. Topical steroids often are sufficient to achieve this.

3. **Hypertonic agents** such as sodium chloride 5% (drops or ointment), colloidal osmotic solutions, or anhydrous may provide sufficient dehydrating effect. Discomfort from such applied solutions can be significant, especially with glycerine, and limits their acceptance. Other mechanical measures for encouraging evaporation of tears, such as dehumidification of the environment, glycerine, or gentle dehydration with a hand-held hairdryer may be used with some success.

4. **Graft rejection (penetrating keratoplasty)** usually presents with slight red eye, blurred vision, endothelial keratic precipitates (lymphocytes), and sectoral or total graft edema. It requires emergency **therapy** with *topical steroids*, e.g., 0.1% dexamethasone q1h by day and q2h by night for several days, followed by taper down to qid by about 3 to 4 weeks and to qd for 2 to 3 months. Rejections with edema delimited by an endothelial lymphocyte (KP) line respond far better than total diffuse edema of the entire graft. If there is no response to therapy within 3 to 4 weeks, the graft has probably failed due to permanent endothelial damage and may need to be replaced. *Herpetic graft rejections* should be treated with steroids (see sec. **IV.D.,** above), plus *antiviral* acyclovir p.o. 400 mg bid for 12 to 18 months because of the high incidence of dendritic keratitis in the face of rejection. *Topical 2% cyclosporine*, a selective T-cell immunosuppressant under FDA review for approval for dry eye therapy, has been used successfully as prophylaxis against rejection in high-risk patients (several graft failures, heavy neovascularization, severe alkali burn, severe dry eye).

5. **For those cases of painful corneal edema** unresponsive to more conservative measures, **penetrating keratoplasty** offers the most effective

method of restoring vision. Obviously, the prognosis for successful keratoplasty depends on the etiology of the corneal edema, with inflammatory conditions being less sure than dystrophic causes.

6. If **visual rehabilitation is not essential,** several procedures may be used to ensure comfort and protection of the edematous cornea. Therapeutic **soft contact lens therapy** (Permalens, Kontur) will often ensure comfort (see sec. **XI.A.,** below). **Conjunctival flap** surgery after epithelial débridement gives relief and does not preclude subsequent keratoplasty. **Keratoprosthesis** also has been successful and restores vision, but should be reserved for those patients with severe disease or prior keratoplasty failures.

X. **Congenital anomalies of the cornea.** Congenital lesions of the cornea may be inherited as developmental defects or errors of metabolism, or may result from intrauterine infection or injury.

A. **Anomalies of size, shape, and contour**

1. **Megalocornea** is an enlargement of the cornea beyond 13 mm in diameter. The cornea is usually clear with normal vision, but there may be astigmatic refractive errors. The condition is usually not progressive and requires no treatment. The developmental condition must be distinguished, however, from corneal enlargement due to congenital glaucoma. The buphthalmic cornea often has central or peripheral clouding and Haab striae or Descemet tears. IOP is elevated in buphthalmos but normal in megalocornea.

2. **Microcornea** is a cornea with a diameter less than 11 mm. Occurring as a developmental defect, the cornea is often steeper than normal, producing myopia. Microcornea can occur as part of other congenital abnormalities, including rubella syndrome. If there is no corneal opacification, **treatment** is often not necessary except for correction of the refractive error.

3. **Cornea plana** is a rare flattening of the anterior contour of the cornea. The cornea may be small in addition to its markedly flattened shape and marked astigmatism.

4. **Keratoglobus** is a rare bilateral enlargement of the cornea in which it assumes a globular shape. Myopic and astigmatic refractive errors often occur.

B. **Congenital corneal opacities**

1. **Edema** can occur as a result of congenital hereditary endothelial dystrophy or congenital glaucoma. Edema can also occur with Descemet ruptures resulting from forceps injury or birth trauma.

2. **Congenital malformations.** A rather confusing array of congenital corneal opacities associated with abnormalities of the anterior chamber angle have been described as part of the **anterior chamber cleavage syndrome.** A recent classification helps to categorize the appearance of central or peripheral opacification with or without corneal–iris or corneal–lenticular touch (Fig. 5.2).

3. **Epibulbar and limbal dermoid tumors** also can occur as congenital lesions. Treatment for these congenital malformations can be difficult and usually requires penetrating keratoplasty or anterior segment reconstruction with or without lensectomy. Because the surgical technique can be difficult and graft rejection is not uncommon, it is probably best to perform surgery on the worse eye only. Developmental abnormalities of the posterior segment may be present and further interfere with visual function.

4. **Inborn errors of metabolism** (see Chapter 11). **Mucopolysaccharidoses** occurring as autosomal-recessive traits can present with corneal hazy opacification, particularly in the Hurler, Scheie, Morquio, and Maroteaux-Lamy syndromes. *Corneal opacification* can also be noted in cystinosis, mucolipidosis, gangliosidosis, Lowe syndrome, Riley-Day syndrome, and von Gierke's disease.

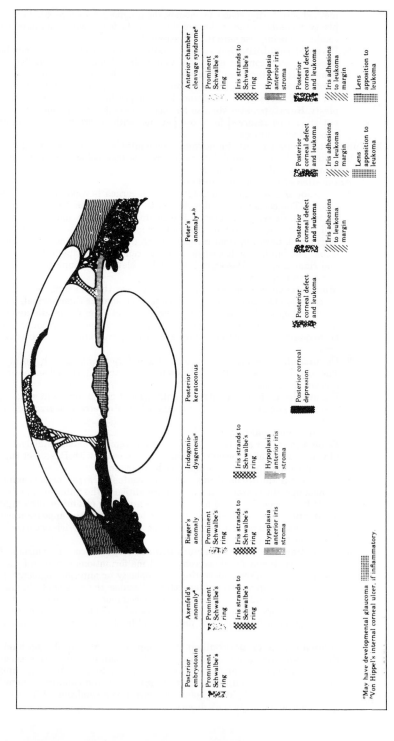

Posterior embryotoxin
Prominent Schwalbe's ring

Axenfeld's anomaly[a]
Prominent Schwalbe's ring
Iris strands to Schwalbe's ring

Rieger's anomaly
Prominent Schwalbe's ring
Iris strands to Schwalbe's ring
Hypoplasia anterior iris stroma

Iridogonio-dysgenesis[a]
Iris strands to Schwalbe's ring
Hypoplasia anterior iris stroma

Posterior keratoconus
Posterior corneal depression

Peter's anomaly[a,b]
Posterior corneal defect and leukoma
Iris adhesions to leukoma margin

Anterior chamber cleavage syndrome[a]
Prominent Schwalbe's ring
Iris strands to Schwalbe's ring
Hypoplasia anterior iris stroma
Posterior corneal defect and leukoma
Iris adhesions to leukoma margin
Lens apposition to leukoma

[a]May have developmental glaucoma
[b]Von Hippel's internal corneal ulcer, if inflammatory

5. **Chromosomal defects** can be associated with corneal opacification, especially with trisomy 21, trisomy 13 to 15, and trisomy 18 (see Chapter 11).

6. **Postinflammatory opacities** of the cornea can be present with the rubella syndrome, luetic IK, or congenital herpes simplex infection.

XI. **Therapeutic Soft Contact Lenses (TSCLs)** (see Chapter 14, sec. **VIII.** and Table 14.4).

A. **TSCL (bandage contact lens).** The hydrophilic soft contact lenses (*Permalens,* Coopervision; *Kontur,* Kontur Kontak Lens) offer a valuable method of treatment for a variety of corneal abnormalities. The Permalens has base curves from 7.7 to 9.0 and diameters 13.5 to 15 mm. The 14.5 mm *Plano T lens* (Bausch & Lomb) is most useful over tissue adhesive because of its greater thickness and low tendency to tear on the rough glue surface. The most frequent use for TSCLs is as a protective bandage for a diseased epithelial surface (epithelial defect, corneal edema), but the hydrophilic lens can also provide a reservoir for tears or medications and can be used for cosmetic or therapeutic occlusion. Antibiotic drops, e.g., Polytrim bid, are used where the epithelium is disturbed. *Ointments* are *not indicated* because they dislodge the lenses. ***Specific indications*** and ***precautions*** are as follows:

1. **Alkali burns.** After immediate removal of the offending chemical and appropriate irrigation, the ocular surface is often left deepithelialized or populated by a markedly abnormal epithelium. A TSCL applied to the alkali-burned eye when conjunctival edema has subsided will aid in the reepithelialization and provide protection to the fragile and easily dislodged epithelial layer. Encouragement of reepithelialization of the ocular surface is necessary to avoid the progressive ulceration that can occur in response to local collagenase production in the second to third week following the injury. Topical antibiotics are used to prevent infection.

2. **Bullous keratopathy.** Epithelial edema of aphakic bullous keratopathy or Fuchs dystrophy that does not respond to topical hyperosmotic agents can result in bullous epithelial lesions that are painful on breakdown. TSCLs can protect against recurrent epithelial breakdown and will provide comfort in many patients. Visual acuity is rarely improved but comfort is attained. Prolonged epithelial edema, particularly with the use of a large contact lens, can lead to vascularization that can interfere with future corneal surgery.

3. **Corneal perforations** Pinpoint perforations or flap lacerations that are otherwise in good apposition can often be splinted with a soft contact lens until wound healing occurs. Frank perforations that can be sealed with cyanoacrylate tissue adhesive are best managed by application of a TSCL to improve patient comfort and prevent the mechanical dislodgment of the adhesive by the action of the lids.

4. **Corneal transplants.** In cornea with diseased epithelium (chemical burns, herpes simplex keratitis), delay in epithelialization of the corneal donor or secondary breakdown of that epithelial layer frequently responds to soft contact lens treatment. Pinpoint leaks at the wound margin or slight anterior shifting of the wound edge that is not sufficient to require positioning of new sutures can often be splinted and sealed with

---

FIG. 5.2. Composite illustration of the anatomic findings in the anterior chamber cleavage syndrome. The stepladder table demonstrates the spectrum of anatomic combinations and terms by which they are commonly known. (Adapted from Waring GO III, Rodrigues M, Laibson PR. Anterior chamber cleavage syndrome: a stepladder classification. *Surv Ophthalmol* 1975;20:3.)

the use of a TSCL. TSCL therapy also provides comfort in those patients with epithelial defects.

5. **Dry eye syndrome.** Patients with lacrimal insufficiency that does not respond to replacement lubricants and lacrimal punctal occlusion may benefit from *preservative-free* artificial tear lubrication q1 to 2h plus a TSCL that provides a tear reservoir. These eyes may also be less tolerant of a TSCL, however. Topical antibiotic drops bid should be used as prophylaxis against infection. The **gas-permeable scleral contact lens** has been very effective in otherwise contact-lens intolerant eyes with extensive ocular surface disease (see sec. **VI.B.3.**, above).

6. **Epithelial erosions.** Epithelial defects occurring in a cornea prone to epithelial breakdown (diabetes mellitus, anterior membrane dystrophy, lattice corneal dystrophy) are effectively managed with a TSCL plus tear drop lubricants. Treatment is required for several weeks to months for complete reformation of the basement membrane adhesions.

7. **Filamentary keratitis.** This abnormality of the epithelial surface, probably the result of aberrant healing of multiple small erosions, usually responds well to TSCLs. Relief of the irritative symptoms and loss of the filaments is usually rapid. In a dry eye, the tear reservoir effect of the lens is also of some benefit.

8. **Irregular astigmatism.** Whereas a soft contact lens usually is not effective in relieving high degrees of astigmatism, a mildly irregular anterior corneal surface can be smoothed to better optical clarity with a TSCL, and any tendency to dellen formation can be minimized.

9. **KC.** TSCLs alone are inadequate to treat most cases of KC. It is possible, however, in patients who are intolerant of hard contact lenses, to provide a better surface for a hard contact lens by application of a soft contact lens. The "piggyback" technique can provide tolerance of an optically efficient lens system.

10. **Neuroparalytic keratopathy.** Patients with neurotrophic breakdown of the corneal epithelial surface (herpes zoster ophthalmicus, status posttrigeminal rhizotomy) often will have epitheliopathy and recurrent epithelial breakdown. These patients can be treated with a TSCL but great care is required, because the protective mechanisms of sensation are diminished and a greater incidence of intolerance with corneal infiltration and vascularization as well as superinfection is possible. If intolerance develops, partial tarsorrhaphy should be considered instead, adjunctively or prophylactically.

11. **Trichiasis.** Scarring of the lids or inturning of the lashes from any etiology will result in chronic irritation of the epithelium, which can be minimized by wearing TSCLs as a protective barrier. Posttraumatic or cicatricial entropion is especially well treated this way, particularly if lid surgery is difficult or inadvisable. Patients with benign mucous membrane pemphigoid are more difficult to fit because of the frequent shortening of the cul-de-sac. Extended-wear gas-permeable scleral lenses are more effective.

12. **Postherpetic or postinfectious (trophic) defects.** Following an infectious epithelial defect, when the primary infection has been adequately controlled, TSCLs are of great value in promoting reepithelialization. Control or several days of adequate drug therapy of the underlying infectious element is advisable before such lens insertion.

13. **Descemetocele.** In an eye that has sustained a thinning of the stroma to the point of descemetocele formation, a TSCL may be applied as reinforcement until such time as definitive therapy of tissue adhesive, lid adhesion, or keratoplasty may be done.

14. **Medications.** Although a TSCL can serve as a barrier to penetration of some medications, it is also possible by saturation of the lens to provide a higher and more uniform concentration of delivery to the anterior corneal surface. Instillation of drops into the eye with a soft contact

lens will also provide a mild reservoir effect. Epinephrine-containing compounds can become entrapped in the soft contact lens and oxidize to the adrenochrome pigments, producing a black tint to the lens. Fluorescein is a well-known stain that can be absorbed by the hydrophilic material, but wash out within a few hours. Collagen shields (Surgilens) are discussed in sec. **IV.B.6,** above.

B. **Care of the soft contact lens.** The flexibility of the soft contact lens sometimes poses problems on insertion and removal. The tendency of the lens to desiccate and deform its contour is also at times a problem. The lens should be kept hydrated at all times in a saline solution without preservatives. It should be cleaned and sterilized prior to insertion. Care should be taken not to apply any sharp object to the lens, because this may tear it. In many cases in which there are organic abnormalities of the cornea, it is advisable to use prophylactic antibiotic drops. Antiviral ointment will dislodge the lens.

C. **Complications of soft contact lens therapy** (see Chapter 14, sec. **VIII.** for cosmetic hard, gas-permeable, and daily- and extended-wear lenses).

1. **Tight lens syndrome** with a red, sore, tearing eye may occur weeks after placement. It has fairly sudden onset and is due to spontaneous tightening of the lens causing limbal compression and vascular engorgement. It resolves several hours after lens removal. A new, possibly larger, flatter lens, may be inserted at the time of removal or days later.

2. **Loss or damage to lens.** The flexibility of the lens and irregular contour of the diseased cornea can result in repeated loss of the lens. Tears or fractures in the lens can cause discomfort and irritation.

3. **Sterile infiltrates** are white and tend to appear peripherally, but can be paracentral or central, and are usually multiple and subepithelial. They disappear with removal of the lens. Pain, discharge, epithelial staining, and anterior chamber reaction are associated with an infectious etiology; their *absence* is associated with sterile infiltrates. Size of infiltrate is not a factor. Prophylactic quinolone drops qid for a few days until probable sterile infiltrate clears is advisable. Evaluation and therapy for infectious keratitis should be undertaken if there is any question about diagnosis.

4. **Infection.** The soft contact lens has been associated with the complication of infection. Although this is usually bacterial, fungal infection can also occur. It is therefore essential that the lens be periodically sterilized and that a prophylactic topical antibiotic be used if the epithelium is unhealthy. Frequent follow-up is essential (see sec. **IV.B., E.,** and **F.**).

5. **Anterior chamber reaction.** The inflammatory reaction that can be provoked by a contact lens can include flare and cell or frank hypopyon. This reaction is usually sterile and resolves after removal of the lens.

6. **Vascularization.** Peripheral vascularization can occur, particularly in a patient with chronic epithelial edema or postinfectious ulcer. The lens should be removed unless this will further compromise the cornea.

D. **Giant papillary conjunctivitis (GPC)** is a local allergy to antigen coating on soft or hard *contact lenses, ocular prostheses, and sutures*. Tear levels of IgE, IgG, and IgM are elevated and, as in vernal conjunctivitis which is clinically similar, the *mast cell* system is activated.

1. **Clinical findings** are decreased contact lens tolerance, itching, photophobia, mucous discharge, redness, punctate staining at the upper limbus, and giant papillae (>0.3 mm in diameter) on the upper tarsal conjunctiva.

2. **Treatment** includes:

a. Eliminate contact lens wear (or prosthesis or sutures) for several weeks until all inflammation and punctate staining are gone.

b. Start a mast cell stabilizer (such as lodoxamide, olopatadine, or cromolyn) qid and use for several weeks until GPC is resolved.

c. Once the eyes are quiet, fit new contact lenses, possibly of a material different from the original offending set. Instruct the patient in fastidious lens care and daily cleaning with nonpreserved solutions, and enzymatic lens treatment one to two times weekly. Use hydrogen peroxide or other cold disinfection daily, because heat may "cook" antigen on the lens surface.

E. Hard contact lenses are most effective in optically correcting high degrees of ametropia or corneal astigmatism as in KC or post-thinning distortion (see Chapter 14).

F. Microbiologic study of **contact lens-related keratitis** indicates that cosmetic contact lenses were worn in about 45% of cases, with extended-wear soft contact lens incidence 2.5 times that of daily-wear soft contact lenses and daily-wear hard lenses in only 3% of cases. Aphakic contact lenses were worn in about 32% of cases, with aphakic extended-wear soft contact lenses accounting for about 90% of this group. TSCLs were worn in about 25% of cases. Of organisms cultured, 52% were Gram-positive, 36% Gram-negative, 4% fungi, and 4% *Acanthamoeba. Pseudomonas* was highly associated with cosmetic soft lens use. Other studies on contact lens-related fungal keratitis indicate 4% incidence in cosmetic or aphakic hard or soft contact lenses and 27% incidence in therapeutic soft lenses. *Fusarium* and *Cephalosporium* predominated in cosmetic lenses and *Candida* predominated in therapeutic lenses. **Disposable** extended-wear soft contact lenses have also been associated with bacterial keratitis, even with proper lens care (70% *Pseudomonas,* 10% *Acanthamoeba,* 30% other bacteria).

G. Contact lens disinfection studies indicate that although available hard lens regimens and soft lens cold hydrogen peroxide or heat disinfection effectively eliminate *bacteria* from the lenses, bacterial contamination was found in the contact lens cases or solutions: 75% in chemical disinfection, 50% in peroxide disinfection, and 28% in heat procedure. *Acanthamoeba* was effectively eliminated from lenses by not less than 2-hour exposure to 3% hydrogen peroxide followed by enzyme catalyst. Also effective in eliminating the trophozoite and cysts from solutions and lens cases was 4-hour exposure to thimerosal 0.001% to 0.004% or benzalkonium chloride 0.005%, both with edetate or 1-hour exposure to chlorhexidine 0.005% with edetate. Other commercial preparations were not effective or effective only with prolonged exposure (12 to 24 hours). The safest and best proven method of *Acanthamoeba* disinfection is still **heat sterilization.** *HIV virus* and the *herpesviruses* are also all effectively killed by heat and the above-described disinfecting systems. Cold cleaning–disinfection effective against these viruses includes Boston cleaner and Boston conditioner for hard contact lenses and Pliagel, Miraflow, or Softmate for soft contact lenses.

XII. Radial keratotomy (see Chapter 6).

XIII. Sclera and episclera

A. Anatomy and physiology

1. **The sclera** constitutes five-sixths of the anterior tunic of the globe as an almost spherical segment 22 mm in diameter. It is continuous with the cornea at the limbus anteriorly and with the optic nerve posteriorly at the scleral fibers of the lamina cribrosa.

   a. **The thickness** of the sclera varies from a maximum of 1 mm near the optic nerve to 0.5 mm at the equator and 0.8 mm anteriorly. The thinnest portion (0.3 mm) is found just behind the insertions of the recti muscles.

   b. **The stroma** is composed of collagen bundles varying in size from 10 to 15 μm in thickness and 100 to 150 μm in length, interlacing in an irregular crisscross pattern roughly parallel to the surface of the globe. When compared to cornea, the scleral fibers have greater birefringence, absence of fixed spacing, and greater variation in fiber diameter. All of these anatomic features contribute to the opaque character of the sclera.

   c. The **avascular** sclera transmits blood vessels but retains scant supply for its own use, obtaining nutrition from the underlying choroid and the overlying episclera. The long posterior ciliary vessels course anteriorly in the horizontal meridian of the sclera, whereas six to seven oblique channels posteriorly transmit the vortex veins.

d. **Innervation** of the sclera is from the long and short posterior ciliary nerves and is especially prominent in the anterior portion where stimulation of the nerve endings by inflammation or distention can produce marked pain.

e. **The function of the sclera** is to provide a protective shell for the intraocular contents that will prevent distortion of the globe to maintain optical integrity, yet allow for variation in IOP. The viscoelastic ocular coat provides mobility without deformation by the attached muscles. Primarily supportive, the metabolic activity of the sclera is low and easily satisfied by the adjacent vascularity of episclera and choroid. The high hydration of the sclera contributes to the opaque nature of the tissue, which can become translucent if the water content is reduced to about 40%, as is seen clinically in scleral dellen. The collagenous nature of the sclera and its encasement by an episclera that acts much like a synovium have suggested the comparison of the eye to an exposed and modified ball-and-socket joint. This comparison has some merit because diseases that affect articular structures often can involve the scleral–episcleral coat.

2. **The episclera** provides much of the nutritional support of the sclera, which itself is permeable to water, glucose, and proteins. The episclera also serves as a synovial lining for the collagen and elastic sclera, and reacts vigorously to scleral inflammation. The fibroelastic episclera has a visceral layer closely opposed to the sclera and a parietal layer that fuses with the muscle sheath and the conjunctiva near the limbus. These two layers are connected and bridged by delicate connective tissue lamellae. The posterior episcleral plexus of **vessels** comes from the short posterior ciliary vessels. The anterior episcleral circulation is more complex, with communications among a conjunctival plexus, superficial episcleral plexus, and deep episcleral plexus that anastomose at the limbus with the superficial and deep intrascleral venous plexus. This interconnection of intrascleral and episcleral venous systems drains the anterior portion of the ciliary body. The conjunctival and episcleral vessels can be blanched with *1:1000 adrenalin or 2.5% phenylephrine*, whereas the deep vessels are little changed, thus providing a useful method of **differentiating superficial from deep** inflammatory congestion.

B. **Diseases of the sclera and episclera: inflammation.** The most important clinical afflictions of the sclera and episclera are inflammatory. Either condition may be associated with systemic disease (33% of episcleritis cases, >50% of scleritis cases). Although congenital, metabolic, degenerative, and neoplastic disease can also affect the sclera and episclera, the most common, diagnostically perplexing, and therapeutically difficult conditions are inflammatory.

1. **Classification**
   a. **Episcleritis**—simple and nodular.
   b. **Anterior scleritis**—diffuse, nodular, or necrotizing with or without inflammation (scleromalacia perforans).
   c. **Posterior scleritis**

2. **Clinical differentiation** of these types of inflammations is of diagnostic and therapeutic importance. Episcleritis is often a benign condition requiring modest treatment; scleritis, however, can signal destructive disease involving collagen tissues in general and can require potent therapy.

C. **Episcleritis** is a usually benign, uni- or bilateral inflammatory reaction localized to the superficial layers of Tenon capsule. In children there is almost always spontaneous regression in 7 to 10 days and rarely recurrence. In adults, 30% of cases are associated with an underlying connective tissue, inflammatory bowel disease, herpetic infection, gout, or various vasculitides. Systemic disease is rare in children.

1. **Simple episcleritis** (about 80% of cases). There is discomfort localized to the eye, accompanied by variable degrees of lacrimation and photophobia. Segmental or diffuse vascular engorgement and edema of the episclera are usually present, and, diagnostically, congestion of the superficial episcleral vessels disappears after administration of 1 drop of 2.5% *phenylephrine*. Women are more often affected than men, and the peak age incidence is the fourth decade.

2. **Nodular episcleritis** (about 20% of cases) is similar in its incidence and pattern but may run a more protracted course. The incidence of episcleritis is difficult to determine because many patients undoubtedly do not seek treatment. About three-fourths of the cases are simple and the remainder are nodular in character. About 30% of cases of nodular episcleritis can be associated with general medical problems: 5% occurring with collagen vascular disease (rheumatoid arthritis), 7% with prior herpes zoster ophthalmicus or herpes simplex, and 3% with gout or atopy. Extensive laboratory workup is not rewarding with most episcleritis cases, but clinical examination for evidence of rheumatoid arthritis, herpes zoster ophthalmicus, or gout can be supplemented by ***serologic tests for rheumatoid arthritis*** and serum ***uric acid***. Most cases of episcleritis resolve within 3 to 6 weeks without complication.

3. **Ocular complications** of episcleritis occur in approximately 15% of cases but are usually not severe or permanent. Elevation of the limbal area due to episcleral edema or nodule can result in corneal dellen. This local desiccation phenomenon may respond to patching, lubrication, or resolution of the limbal swelling. With significant inflammation, there can be superficial and midstromal infiltration and edema of the cornea that rarely provoke vascularization. IK, iritis (7%), and secondary glaucoma are uncommon.

4. **Treatment** is often not required, and symptoms can sometimes be relieved by topical decongestants. Symptomatic cases usually respond to modest topical steroid treatment (prednisolone 1% bid to tid) coupled with systemic NSAIDs, e.g., ibuprofen 400 mg p.o. tid, or naproxen 250 mg q12h with a meal over several weeks.

D. **Scleritis.** Inflammation of the sclera can result in severe destructive disease that causes pain and threatens vision. Occurring more commonly in females than in males, with a peak incidence in the fourth to sixth decades, the condition is bilateral in approximately 50% of cases. **Pain** can be severe and is often described as a deep boring ache. There is often associated photophobia and lacrimation as well as chronic systemic inflammatory disease.

1. **Anterior scleritis.** Ninety-five percent of cases of scleritis are in the anterior portion of the sclera. Superficial and deep episcleral vessels are congested and the deep ones remain so after 1 drop of 2.5% *phenylephrine*.

   a. **Diffuse anterior scleritis** occurs approximately 60% of the time, and **nodular anterior scleritis** approximately 25% of the time. **Necrotizing scleritis,** occurring 15% of the time, is usually more severe and is twice as frequent with inflammation as without. **Posterior scleritis** occurs in about 10% of cases. The specific pattern of scleritis is usually not distinctive enough to prove an etiology, although the clinical course and prognosis are often predictable on the basis of the pattern of inflammation. The necrotizing form is the most severe and unremitting. Only 8% of cases progress from one form of scleritis to another. *Ocular complications* occur in 50% of anterior scleritis cases and in about 90% of necrotizing or posterior scleritis cases.

   b. **Diseases** associated with the various types of scleritis vary; 45% of scleritis patients have a systemic disorder. These include rheumatoid arthritis, ankylosing spondylitis, Wegener granulomatosis, systemic lupus erythematosus, relapsing polychondritis, polyarteritis nodosa, herpes simplex or zoster, syphilis, psoriatic arthritis, Behçet's disease, temporal arteritis, Reiter syndrome, early HIV infection, sarcoidosis, thyroid disease, lymphoma, pancreatic carcinoma, multiple myeloma, primary biliary cirrhosis, and atopy. These diseases may be associated with any form of scleritis. Postoperative scleritis may occur without systemic disease.

(1) The **diffuse anterior** pattern can be associated with rheumatoid arthritis (24% of cases), prior herpes zoster ophthalmicus, and gout.

(2) The **nodular anterior** variety has been associated most frequently with prior episodes of herpes zoster ophthalmicus.

(3) The **necrotizing** variety is rare (3% of cases) but the most ominous, and can be associated with ocular or systemic complications in 60% of patients. Forty percent may show decreased visual acuity. Twenty-nine percent of patients with necrotizing scleritis may be dead within 5 years. The necrotizing variety must be distinguished on the basis of focal areas of avascular scleral dropout. In those cases of *necrotizing scleritis without inflammation* (**scleromalacia perforans**), most patients have long-standing rheumatoid arthritis involving multiple joints. More than half of the time the condition is bilateral in patients with rheumatoid arthritis. Clinically, large areas of avascular sclera may appear as a sequestrum with adjacent exposure of the uveal pigment through a markedly thin sclera. Anterior chamber reaction can occur with this type of scleritis and is an ominous sign. Perforation is not common but can occur.

2. **Posterior scleritis** is difficult to diagnose and often overlooked. One histopathologic series of enucleated eyes documented posterior involvement in 43% of eyes diagnosed with anterior scleritis. Certainly, posterior scleritis can occur alone but is then more difficult to diagnose. *Symptoms* of *deep, unremitting aching pain* unresponsive to topical or nonimmunosuppressive systemic therapy and, in some cases, decreased visual acuity suggest posterior scleritis. Physical *signs* suggesting posterior scleritis include occasional episcleral forniceal hyperemia, fundus changes (particularly exudative retinal detachment), annular choroidal folds or detachments, subretinal mass, patchy chorioretinal changes, vitritis optic nerve edema, or macular edema. Severe posterior inflammation can result in shallowing of the anterior chamber, proptosis, limited extraocular movement, and lower lid retraction. Posterior scleritis can be associated with rheumatoid arthritis or systemic vasculitis. **Ultrasound** or **computed tomography scan** will reveal diagnostic scleral thickening.

3. **Complications of scleritis**

   a. **Corneal changes** occur in approximately 37% of cases of anterior diffuse and nodular scleritis. There are four characteristic patterns of corneal involvement.

      (1) **Diffuse stromal:** midstromal opacities occurring with immune ring patterns and keratic precipitates.

      (2) **Sclerosing stromal keratitis:** edema and infiltration of the stroma with vascularization and scarring resulting in subsequent crystalline formation.

      (3) **Deep keratitis:** white, opaque sheets of infiltration at Descemet's membrane.

      (4) **Limbal guttering:** a limbal gutter progressing to ectasia and characterized by lipid deposits with or without vascularization.

   b. The **necrotizing** forms of scleritis can produce more significant corneal changes, occurring primarily in three forms.

      (1) **Acute stromal keratitis:** edema and dense white infiltration associated with ring infiltrates and keratic precipitates.

      (2) **Peripheral ulcerative keratitis (PUK):** marginal thinning with prominent inflammation indicative of a vasculitis that must be differentiated from Mooren's ulcer.

      (3) **Keratolysis:** diffuse areas of corneal infiltration that will suddenly thin by stromal melting to result in descemetocele surrounded by irregularly scarred and vascularized tissue. Without inflammation, this is scleromalacia perforans.

   c. Other ocular complications of scleritis include uveitis in approximately 35% of cases and scleral thinning in 27% of cases. There can also be both open-angle and narrow-angle glaucoma (13.5%), as well as cataract, retinal detachment, and optic neuritis.

4. Because of the high incidence of associated systemic or collagen disease, it is often wise to obtain ancillary **laboratory investigations** as a diagnostic routine.

   a. Hematology studies

      (1) Complete blood count and erythrocyte sedimentation rate.

      (2) Plasma protein and immunoglobulin level.

      (3) Antineutrophil cytoplasmic antibodies (ANCA). A negative ANCA posttreatment does not mean vasculitis is quiet. Nephritis may be ongoing. Obtain sedimentation rate and urinalysis.

      (4) Other immune profile tests as listed in Chapter 9.

      (5) Antinuclear and rheumatoid factors.

      (6) Serum uric acid.

      (7) Serologic tests for syphilis and HIV.

   b. X-rays of chest, hands and feet, lumbosacral spine.

   c. Fluorescein angiography, anterior or posterior segment, for evidence of vasculitis.

   d. B-scan ultrasound for posterior scleritis.

   e. Results of the tests need interpretation in light of the history, associated physical findings, and the pattern of positive results (see Chapter 9, sec. **V.**).

5. Treatment of noninfectious scleritis

   a. Medical therapy is the first line of defense. About 30% of scleritis patients require oral NSAIDs, >30% require oral corticosteroids, and >25% require immunosuppressive drugs.

      (1) Although **topical steroids** frequently increase comfort and occasionally maintain a remission, the topical preparations may not be sufficient to induce a remission and will exacerbate keratolysis.

      (2) In addition to topical steroids, **oral NSAIDs** are also effective. Such treatment, e.g., indomethacin 25 mg qid to 50 mg tid for 7 to 12 weeks may suppress the inflammation in diffuse and nodular varieties, but is not often effective for the necrotizing form. Naproxen 375 to 500 mg q12h, or diflunisal 500 mg q12h have also proved effective in nonnecrotizing scleritis. Cyclooxygenase-2 inhibitors (celecoxib [Celebrex] 100 mg bid, rofecoxib [Vioxx] 12.5 to 25 mg qd) are also effective.

      (3) For unresponsive cases or scleromalacia perforans, **initial treatment** is *systemic steroids* in a dosage of 80 to 120 mg prednisolone per day for the first week with tapering. Median duration of therapy is about 30 weeks in patients responding to prednisone alone. Topical steroids may be used to sustain a remission. Subconjunctival steroids are to be discouraged because the scleral thinning per se and sustained local suppression of wound healing by subconjunctival route can be hazardous.

      (4) Severe unremitting, unresponsive, or necrotizing **cases require treatment** with *immunosuppressive drugs*. Methotrexate 2.5 to 15 mg p.o. every week, cyclosporine 3 to 5 mg/kg/day, azathioprine 1 to 2 mg per kg p.o. qd, or cyclophosphamide, starting at 100 mg p.o. qd and increasing the dosage to 150 to 200 mg p.o. qd over 2 weeks are often effective regimens. Patients should be warned of the potential serious side effects (see Chapter 9, sec. **VI.D.**). Immunosuppressive agents are effectively coupled

with other antirheumatoid drugs such as sulfasalzine, cyclophosphamide, chlorambucil, etanercept, infliximab, or leflunomide to control the ocular inflammation, and may prolong survival by controlling other vasculitis. *An internist or other physician familiar with the use of these drugs should be consulted before and during the course of treatment.*

(5) If fluorescein angiography reveals a vasculitis or blood tests indicate immune complex disease, both life-threatening processes, and/or the presence of a progressive destructive ocular lesion, inflamed or not inflamed, cyclophosphamide 100 mg p.o. qd or less, with prednisolone 15 mg p.o. qd, may control the process. If there is little response, pulsed i.v. methylprednisolone over 1 to 2 hours should be given with 500 mg of cyclophosphamide i.v. over several hours and washed through with i.v. 5% dextrose with water or saline over 24 hours to decrease the incidence of hemorrhagic cystitis. This pulsed therapy is not without hazard and may be repeated if necessary under desperate circumstances to save not only vision but life itself. Once the disease process is under control using systemic therapy, *mild topical steroids* should be used qd to tid to maintain suppression and systemic treatment should be stopped. *Subconjunctival steroids* should *never* be given, because scleral or keratolysis may result.

(6) **Adverse effects.** It is important to recognize the potential serious adverse reactions to systemically administered antiinflammatory agents. The serious adverse effects of steroid therapy with adrenal suppression can be avoided with short-term therapy, but gastrointestinal disturbance, aggravation of hyperglycemia, fluid retention, and acute psychoses may occur. Long-term systemic or local steroid therapy obviously can produce cataracts and elevate IOP. Immunosuppressives may cause severe bone marrow suppression, gastrointestinal toxicity, and serious infection (see Chapter 9, sec. **VI.D.**).

b. **Surgical treatment**

(1) **Extreme scleral thinning** or **perforation** requires reinforcement. Whatever material is used must be covered with conjunctiva to maintain its integrity. Donor sclera or cornea may be used, but usually swells with edema and softens. Fascia lata or periosteum is somewhat more resistant to the melting process. All grafts should be completely covered by sliding conjunctiva or donor conjunctiva from the same or opposite eye should be used.

(2) **Extreme corneal marginal ulceration** or keratolysis may require corneal grafting, usually as a lamellar patch graft in addition to systemic therapy.

(3) **Treatment of infectious scleritis** involves aggressive, specific systemic and topical antibiotics and, if needed, conjunctival recession and local cryotherapy. *M. tuberculosis* is treated with amikacin 10 mg per mL drops q1h, and oral rifampin and isoniazid. Taper drops over 2 to 4 weeks and oral medication in 1 year (see sec. **IV.B.,** above, for other treatment).

6. KERATOREFRACTIVE SURGERY*

Dimitri T. Azar

Refractive surgical techniques have evolved rapidly over the past three decades, emerging as safer and more reliable means of treating myopia, hyperopia, and astigmatism, thus reducing the need for corrective lenses. Surgical techniques for the correction of presbyopia are under development, but have not yet been refined for widespread application. Technological advances, especially in the realm of laser surgery, continue to improve precision, accuracy, and patient satisfaction. Although a wide range of refractive procedures exists, we will discuss the following refractive procedures: (a) radial keratotomy (RK), (b) excimer laser photorefractive keratectomy (PRK) with the (c) laser-assisted in situ keratomileusis (LASIK), (d) laser-assisted subepithelial keratomileusis (LASEK), (e) laser thermokeratoplasty (LTK), (f) intra-corneal ring segments (ICRS), and (g) phakic intraocular lenses (IOLs).

Because of the permanent nature of refractive surgery, one of its most important aspects is adequate patient selection and counseling. Many potential refractive surgery candidates have great expectations. A patient may not be a good candidate because of unrealistic expectations, or because of inadequate knowledge about the risks and benefits, or alternatives of the procedure.

Spectacles and contact lenses are reasonable alternatives to refractive surgical procedures. Not only is the accuracy of these forms of optical correction greater than that of refractive surgery, but also they are totally reversible. Although operating on a normal eye to reduce the dependence on glasses or contact lenses may seem aggressive, most patients are delighted after successful refractive surgery. To achieve uniform satisfaction with newer refractive surgical procedures, they must be validated continuously through controlled and well-designed scientific investigations to ensure better predictability and reproducibility.

I. **History of keratorefractive surgery.** The phenomenon of corneal flattening after injury with a consequent change in the refractive power of the eye was first recognized in the late 19th century. RK to correct myopia was introduced in Japan in the 1940s using anterior and posterior corneal incisions. This approach fell into disfavor 10 to 20 years later when resulting endothelial cell injury led to irreversible corneal edema and bullous keratopathy. Russian investigators improved the procedure in the 1970s by using only anterior incisions. Since its introduction to the United States in 1978, RK underwent continual refinement, but long-term studies showed significant instability and progressive hyperopic shifts that led to virtual abandonment of this surgical procedure in the late 1990s.

The excimer laser is named for the "excited dimers" of halogen gases used to generate photons of energy in the ultraviolet end of the electromagnetic spectrum. Initial excimer laser experiments with plastics revealed a high degree of ablative precision without thermal damage to surrounding areas. Early excimer laser techniques mimicking the surgical blade incisions of RK have been superseded by PRK to perform large-area central ablation for refractive correction. U.S. Food and Drug Administration (FDA) trials of PRK for myopia established its efficacy for the correction of myopia, astigmatism, and hyperopia. Subsequent FDA approvals included the LASIK and LTK techniques. Several other refractive procedures are pending approval.

II. **Patient selection and evaluation.** Meticulous patient selection and evaluation are essential to ensure that medical and surgical requirements are met and that patient expectations match what is realistically offered by surgery.

*Updated from Talamo JH, Kornstein HS. Keratorefractive surgery. In: Pavan-Langston D. *Manual of ocular diagnosis and therapy*, 4th ed. Boston: Little, Brown, 1996:123–129.

TABLE 6.1. MAJOR CONTRAINDICATIONS TO KERATOREFRACTIVE SURGERY

Absolute	Relative
Refractive instability	Blepharitis
Unrealistic expectations	Dry eye
Age less than 21 years	Chronic eye rubbing
Keratoconus	Other ocular surface disease
Contact lens warpage	Diabetes mellitus
Chronic steroid and antimetabolite use; immunosuppression	Glaucoma
Glaucoma	
Herpes simplex keratitis (active disease)	
Connective tissue disease	

A. **Motivation** for refractive surgery revolves around the desire to have reduced dependence on spectacles or contact lenses. This motivation may be based on occupational requirements, cosmetic or recreational needs, contact lens intolerance, or feelings of threatened safety. Patients must understand that refractive surgical procedures rarely eliminate the need for optical aids.

B. **Contraindications.** Any uncontrolled ocular surface disease including blepharitis and dry eye, or poorly controlled glaucoma, should preclude surgery. Patients who are immunosuppressed, taking chronic steroids or antimetabolites, or suffering from connective tissue or other systemic diseases may have altered wound healing ability that can compromise the accuracy of intended corrections. Additional contraindications include refractive instability over time and corneal ectasias such as keratoconus (KC) or contact lens-induced warpage, which may yield erratic results postoperatively (Table 6.1).

C. **Physical examination** including manifest refraction and slitlamp biomicroscopy of the anterior segment is performed to exclude underlying disease. To avoid overcorrection of myopia, refraction is repeated after cycloplegia.

   1. **Myopic refraction.** The myopic eye brings a pencil of parallel rays of light into focus at a point anterior to the retina in the vitreous. Manifest and cycloplegic refractions aim to determine the location of the far point located between infinity and the anterior surface of the cornea. Rays that diverge from this point are brought to focus on the retina without the aid of accommodation. For the full correction of myopia, a distance corrective lens placed in front of the eye with its secondary focal point coincident with the far point corrects the refractive error. The newly created optical system allows parallel rays that come from infinity to diverge as if they originated from the far point of the eye, and thus focus on the retina. In refractive surgical procedures for myopia, the refractive power of the cornea or the crystalline lens is reduced so that parallel rays from infinity focus on the retina.

   2. **Hyperopic refraction.** The hyperopic eye brings a pencil of parallel rays of light into focus at a point behind the retina. Accommodation of the eye may produce enough additional plus power to allow the light rays to focus on the retina. Cycloplegic refraction is aimed to determine the location of the far point of a hyperopic eye, which is behind the eye. A corrective lens placed in front of the eye with its secondary focal point coincident with the far point will converge parallel rays from infinity toward the far point of the eye, and hence could focus on the retina without the aid of accommodation. In the prepresbyopic age group, low to moderate hyperopia is less visually significant than myopia. Older hyperopes or patients with high degrees of hyperopia that exceed their accommodative reserve require optical correction for clear distance vision. They can benefit from refractive surgical procedures in which the corneal curvature is steepened

or the power of the crystalline lens is increased to converge rays of light that emanate from distant objects onto the retina without the aid of accommodation.

3. **Astigmatism.** Astigmatism is caused by a toric cornea or, less often, by astigmatic effects of the crystalline lens. Manifest refraction will allow classification of the astigmatism as simple or compound, according to whether one or both meridians, respectively, are focused outside the retina. If one meridian focuses in front of the retina and the other meridian focuses behind it (mixed astigmatism), it is important to confirm the manifest refraction by performing cycloplegic refractions to eliminate accommodation during testing.

Binocular spectacle correction of oblique astigmatism tilts each eye's view and may distort the perceived three-dimensional image. When astigmatism is corrected at the corneal plane, such as with contact lenses or keratorefractive surgery, full correction reduces meridional magnification and eliminates the optical distortion.

D. **Cycloplegic refraction.** A cycloplegic refraction is an essential part of the evaluation of a refractive surgery candidate, however, the pupil dilates and spherical aberrations are produced. The rays of light reaching the periphery of a spherical cornea and lens are bent more than the central rays. The asphericity of the cornea and lens where they flatten toward the periphery may be insufficient to counteract these spherical aberrations associated with cycloplegia. The benefit of relaxing the accommodative tone is especially important in young individuals. It may be useful to measure the cycloplegic refraction through a 3- to 4-mm aperture to account only for the accommodative tone; in this way the effects of the peripheral cornea and the lens on the refraction are negated.

E. **Pupil size and centration of refractive procedures.** Most keratorefractive procedures are centered around the pupil under mesopic or scotopic conditions. The pupil diameter might reach 6 to 8 mm under decreased light conditions. The optical zone in a keratorefractive procedure is defined as the area of the central cornea that bears the refractive change caused by the surgery. As the pupil dilates beyond the edge of the optical zone, the rays of light are refracted differently in the midperipheral and the central cornea. This may result in edge glare and halos around objects, especially at night (or in cases of decentration of the optical zone). Some patients with particularly large pupils may have a mismatch between pupil size and optical zone diameter, and should be warned about possible postoperative symptomatic optical distortions especially under mesopic conditions.

The active reorientation of the photoreceptors toward the center of the pupil plus the possibility of edge glare if the entrance extends beyond the optic zone of the keratorefractive procedure favor the centration of refractive procedures on the pupil uninfluenced by miotics, because the center of the pupil may move in the nasal direction with miosis, which produces temporal edge glare when the pupil dilates after surgery.

F. **Presbyopia.** Presbyopia is an important aspect in relation to informed consent of keratorefractive patients. Patients over 40 years old who consider refractive surgery for myopia must appreciate the extent to which they exchange dependence on distance spectacles for dependence on near-vision spectacles. Surgically corrected presbyopic myopes will need reading glasses as they age, whereas before surgery they could remove their spectacles to read.

G. **Screening tests. Pachymetry** readings are important to rule out abnormally thin corneas at greater risk for perforation. Keratometry readings should be obtained, but are limited in their ability to uncover early, barely noticeable irregularities. Computerized videokeratography has become a more useful adjunct that provides high-resolution topographic analysis of the cornea. This is especially helpful for discovering subtle abnormal patterns in corneal steepness, often seen in KC, contact lens warpage, and other causes of irregular astigmatism (Fig. 6.1).

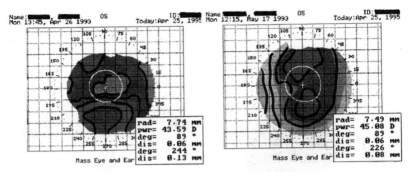

FIG. 6.1. Reversible contact lens-induced warpage. The topographic analyses show inferior corneal steepening *(left)* that resolved 3 weeks after discontinuing contact lens use *(right),* returning the cornea to "bow tie" regular astigmatism. (Adapted from Gangadhar D, Talamo J. The use of computerized videokeratography in keratorefractive surgery. *Semin Ophthalmol* 1994;9:82.)

H. Informed consent. Patients must be aware of the risks and benefits of the intended procedure, the range of potential complications, and side effects **(Table 6.2),** and the variability of individual response. Patients should fully comprehend that they may still need spectacles or contact lenses to achieve best-corrected vision after surgery. Patients who are becoming presbyopic may require near-vision correction. Future contact lens use may be difficult because of alterations in corneal shape. Presbyopic patients should be prepared for possible glare, "starbursts" around lights, and diurnal fluctuations in vision; these phenomena are usually transient, but in rare cases persist for many months or longer postoperatively.

After RK, 1% to 3% of patients may lose one or more Snellen lines of best-corrected vision. Patients considering incisional keratotomy should be warned that a gradual hyperopic shift over time may occur in up to 40% of all cases. Patients should be forewarned of the greater propensity for corneal rupture from blunt ocular trauma following RK.

Excimer PRK and LASIK patients should be counseled regarding the small but real possibilities of delayed regression of effect, disabling corneal haze, and the steroid-induced side effects of cataracts and glaucoma if prolonged use of such medication is required. Serious complications that are rare but can occur after either RK or PRK procedure include infectious keratitis, endophthalmitis, and corneal scarring. Diffuse lamellar Keratitis (DLK) and flap folds and wrinkles may occur after LASIK.

TABLE 6.2. COMPLICATIONS AND SIDE EFFECTS OF KERATOREFRACTIVE SURGERY*

Haloes/glare/"starbursts" around lights	Corneal haze (PRK)
Instability, Ectasia (LASIK)	Corneal scarring
Hyperopic shift (RK)	Perforation (RK)
Diurnal fluctuation (RK)	Flap wrinkles (LASIK)
Regression (PRK)	Steroid-induced glaucoma (PRK)
Irregular astigmatism	Infectious keratitis; DLK (LASIK)
Poor contact lens fit	Endophthalmitis

*Partial list.
RK, radial keratotomy; PRK, photorefractive keratectomy; LASIK, laser in situ keratomileusis; DLK, diffuse lamellar keratitis.

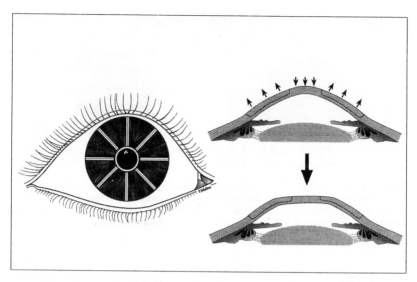

FIG. 6.2. The mechanism of action of radial keratotomy. Paracentral weakening results in midperipheral corneal steepening and central corneal flattening. Corneal ectasia may also occur after LASIK surgery.

III. RK

A. Mechanism. RK refers to the placement of deep paracentral and peripheral incisions in the cornea, producing central flattening and thus reducing central corneal refractive power and myopia. The most accepted theory holds that normal intraocular pressure (IOP) pushes out the peripheral cornea weakened by the incisions, leaving a relatively flatter center. Incisions are ideally 80% to 90% of corneal depth. Deeper incisions give greater flattening effect, but should not extend to Descemet's membrane to avoid the danger of mechanical instability and perforation. Incisions that approach the pupil center produce greater corneal flattening, but any incision breaching a 3-mm optical zone diameter runs a higher risk of producing disabling glare and irregular astigmatism (Fig. 6.2).

B. Technique. Several surgical approaches have been developed. The incision direction may be frontcutting, backcutting, or combined.

1. **Frontcutting** involves centripetally directed incisions from the limbus to the optical zone. This approach achieves greater and more uniform incision depth; hence the potential for increased correction. The drawbacks include higher risks of microperforation and violation of the central clear zone.

2. **Backcutting** moves in the opposite, centrifugal direction from the optical zone to the limbus. This places the optical zone at less risk, but produces slightly shallower incisions with a smaller range of correction.

3. **A combined (or two-pass method)** first makes a centrifugal cut and then deepens it by returning along the same groove toward the optical zone. This provides deeper incisions and a greater correction range while also minimizing the chance of central clear zone invasion. In general, no more than eight radial cuts with a 3.0-mm central clear zone and two enhancements are recommended. This lessens the chance of hyperopic overcorrection, which is difficult to reverse.

The degree of myopia and age are significant factors (older patients respond more to a given incision than do younger patients). IOP, gender, corneal thickness, curvature, topography or diameter, and scleral rigidity are less important factors influencing outcomes.

C. **Results.** The National Eye Institute-sponsored Prospective Evaluation of Radial Keratotomy (PERK) Study began gathering data in 1980 on 427 patients (793 eyes) who underwent a standardized eight-cut RK with 4.0-, 3.5-, and 3.0-mm optical zones for low, moderate, and high myopes, respectively. The surgical nomogram did not adjust for patient age or astigmatism. There were few subsequent enhancements (12%). The 10-year follow-up results showed an uncorrected visual acuity of 20/40 or better in 85% of all operated eyes, including 92% of low myopes (−1.50 to −3.12 D), 86% of moderate myopes (−3.25 to −4.37 D), and 77% of high myopes (−4.50 to −8.87 D). Overall, 70% of patients stated they no longer required corrective lenses for distance vision. Three percent of eyes lost two or three lines of spectacle-corrected vision, with the poorest corrected vision no worse than 20/30; 98% of eyes were correctable to 20/20 or better. Forty-three percent of eyes had a +1.00 D or greater shift toward a more hyperopic refraction over the 10-year period.

IV. Astigmatic keratotomy (AK)

A. **Mechanism.** AK constitutes the placement of transverse or arcuate incisions perpendicular to the steepest corneal meridian to correct astigmatism (Fig. 6.3). The incised meridian flattens while the meridian 90 degrees away steepens by nearly the same amount. Incisions are ideally between 5 and 7 mm from the pupil center. As with RK, deeper, longer, and more centrally located incisions give greater effect, but increase the risk of irregular astigmatism, microperforation, and overcorrection. Irregular astigmatism refers to corneal astigmatism that cannot be corrected by spherocylindrical lenses and requires application of a rigid contact lens to elicit best-corrected visual acuity; irregular astigmatism is generally not amenable to correction by AK. Examples of irregular astigmatism also include KC and contact lens warpage.

B. **Technique**

1. **Transverse incisions** (T-cuts) are usually done in pairs along the steepest meridian and extend for 3.0 mm. Sometimes a second pair is added to the same meridian for greater effect. Because the incisions are tangent to a given optical zone size, the center of the incision is more remote from the central cornea and incremental flattening power decreases accordingly as the incision is lengthened. The amount of correction per incision increases when combined with RK.

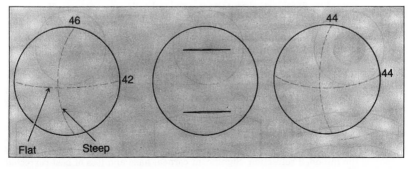

FIG. 6.3. Astigmatic keratotomy. Paired transverse incisions flatten the steepest meridian and produce the opposite affect 90 degrees away. (Adapted from Talamo J, Steinert R. Keratorefractive surgery. In: Albert D, Jakobiec F, eds. *Principles and practice of ophthalmology,* Vol. 1. Philadelphia: WB Saunders, 1994.)

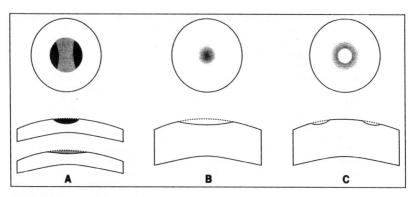

FIG. 6.4. Excimer laser photorefractive keratectomy directly alters the central cornea, flattening to correct astigmatism *(left),* myopia *(center),* or steepening to treat hyperopia *(right).*

2. **Arcuate incisions** remain at a constant distance from the pupil center at any length and may be more effective than T-cuts at a given optical zone size. Longer incisions give more flattening up to a maximum length of 90 degrees.

3. **Nomograms** exist to adjust surgery for patient age and the amount of astigmatism. As with RK, response to an incision has a positive correlation with age. Some surgeons correct preoperative astigmatism simultaneously with RK, whereas others prefer to manage astigmatism in a staged fashion after correcting the myopia.

V. **Excimer laser PRK**

A. **Mechanism.** Whereas RK incisions avoid the central cornea, PRK directly removes layers of tissue in this area to resculpt the anterior refractive surface of the eye (Fig. 6.4). Ultraviolet photons break molecular bonds, precisely ablating Bowman membrane and the anterior corneal stroma while causing minimal residual thermal damage. This central area, or ablation zone, altered by PRK, produces corneal flattening over the visual axis, thus reducing myopia. The surgeon achieves the intended change in dioptric power by varying the diameter and depth of the ablation zone. Deeper ablations lead to greater corneal flattening, but may increase the risk of subepithelial haze caused by fibroblastic keratocytes and local collagen synthesis. Postoperative topical steroids are routinely prescribed for 1 to 3 months to limit haze and refractive regression through inhibition of normal wound healing. By changing the pattern of surface ablation, hyperopia and astigmatism can be corrected as well, but to date in a less predictable fashion.

B. **Technique.** Treatment of myopia can involve a single ablation or multiple ablations of different diameters, with multizone ablations often performed for higher degrees of nearsightedness. Although larger ablation zone sizes are desirable because they minimize the chance of optical side effects, the depth of the ablation zone varies with the square of the diameter.

C. **Results.** In FDA Phase III trials for PRK in low myopia (-1 to -6 D), 88% to 92% of patients had uncorrected vision of 20/40 or better at 1 year, with 50% to 60% better than or equal to 20/20, and 70% to 80% within 1.0 D of the intended refraction. Significant corneal haze and loss of best-corrected vision were uncommon complications. Excimer laser PRK for higher levels of myopia and for hyperopia is somewhat less predictable. LASIK has virtually replaced PRK for the treatment of hyperopia and higher degrees of myopia.

VI. **Excimer laser phototherapeutic keratectomy (PTK).** PTK diminishes corneal opacities and irregularities by recontouring the anterior surface of the cornea. Patients with disabling corneal scars may benefit from PTK, thus avoiding more complicated procedures such as lamellar or penetrating keratoplasty.

VII. LASIK combines lamellar dissection with the microkeratome and a refractive ablation in the bed with the excimer laser. The exponential growth of LASIK refractive correction makes it the most commonly performed refractive surgery throughout the world today (Fig. 6.5).

LASIK is similar to PRK in that an excimer or ultraviolet laser is applied to the cornea to modify its radius of curvature. The difference is that in PRK the laser is applied directly to Bowman's layer, whereas in LASIK the laser is applied to the midstroma after a flap has been lifted from the cornea. In contrast to PRK, no visually significant haze follows LASIK, but when the flap is too thin or is ablated accidentally with the laser, haze may occur, suggesting that a critical amount of unablated flap keratocytes is needed to inhibit haze formation after routine LASIK. An additional factor to take into account after LASIK is the biomechanical response of the corneal lamellae after creation of the flap; there seems to be peripheral steepening and central flattening of the cornea.

The disadvantages of LASIK include microkeratome malfunction and flap malpositions. Optical aberrations are more frequent for higher degrees of myopia and hyperopia. Postoperative LASIK patients frequently have disturbed *tear function* for 1 or more months and should be managed with artificial tears and ointments to prevent surface damage.

VIII. LASEK. By cleaving the epithelial sheet at the basement membrane with dilute alcohol, applying the laser as in conventional PRK, and repositioning the epithelium afterwards, there is some decrease in pain, quicker visual rehabilitation, and less haze than after a classic PRK.

IX. Thermokeratoplasty shrinks the peripheral and paracentral stromal collagen to produce a peripheral flattening and a central steepening of the cornea to treat hyperopia. Solid-state infrared lasers, such as the holmium:yttrium, aluminum, and garnet (Ho:YAG) laser, have been used in a peripheral intrastromal radial pattern (laser thermokeratoplasty) to treat hyperopia of 2.50 D and less. However, the long-term effects and refractive stability of Ho:YAG laser thermokeratoplasty are unknown. The use of a handheld radiofrequency probe to shrink the peripheral collagen has also been employed.

X. ICRS

ICRS are placed in the peripheral cornea and act by compressing the peripheral cornea and changing the radius of curvature of the central cornea. The second mechanism takes advantage of the fact that the arc of the cornea (the distance from limbus to limbus) remains constant at all times, so when the anterior surface is lifted focally over the ring, a compensatory flattening of the central cornea occurs. ICRS are threaded into a peripheral midstromal tunnel. A potential advantage of intracorneal segments over other refractive surgical techniques is reversibility. The main drawback is the limited range of correction (up to -3 D in myopia and up to $+2$ D in hyperopia).

XI. Refractive lensectomy

The extraction of the clear lens in the correction of high myopia, originally performed in 1890, was later abandoned because of an unacceptable high rate of complications. With more recent operative techniques, such as phacoemulsification, and better IOLs, there has been renewed interest in managing high refractive errors by clear lens extraction. The procedure seems more useful in high hyperopes than in high myopes because of the lower incidence of complications in the hyperopes. One drawback is the loss of accommodation. The use of accommodating or multifocal IOLs could obviate this problem.

XII. Phakic intraocular lenses

The iris-claw lens originally devised by Worst for the correction of aphakia was later modified by Fechner et al. to correct high myopia in phakic patients. It is enclaved in the midperipheral, less mobile iris and presently requires a 6.0 mm incision for its insertion. The *angle-supported* phakic IOL was introduced by Baikoff and Joly for the correction of myopia and has gone through several modifications. Long-term follow-up has reported progressive pupil ovalization

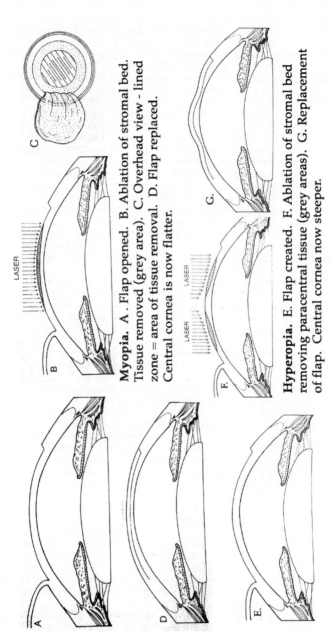

Myopia. A. Flap opened. B. Ablation of stromal bed. Tissue removed (grey area). C. Overhead view – lined zone = area of tissue removal. D. Flap replaced. Central cornea is now flatter.

Hyperopia. E. Flap created. F. Ablation of stromal bed removing paracentral tissue (grey areas). G. Replacement of flap. Central cornea now steeper.

FIG. 6.5. Excimer laser in situ keratomileusis (LASIK) for correction of myopia and hyperopia. (Adapted from Doane J, Slade S, Talamo J, et al. Lamellar refractive surgery. In: Albert D, Jakobiec F, eds. *Principles and practice of ophthalmology*, 2nd ed. Philadelphia: WB Saunders, 2000.)

with an older model. The *posterior chamber* phakic IOL was introduced by Fyodorov et al. in 1990. It must accommodate to the space between the posterior iris and the crystalline lens. If it vaults too much, pigment dispersion and even papillary block glaucoma could result. If it lies against the anterior surface of the crystalline lens, cataract could result. Long-term follow-up is needed for all types of phakic IOLs regarding endothelial cell loss, glaucoma, iris abnormalities, cataract formation, and ease of explantation to determine the exact role of this form of optical correction.

XIII. **Ciliary muscle–zonular complex surgery.** Recent attempts have been made to treat presbyopia based on the alternate theory of its pathogenesis: relaxation of the equatorial zonules. These zonules have been made taut by either scleral expansion or infrared laser application. Further studies are needed to evaluate the safety and effectiveness of these presbyopia treatments. An alternative to offset the problems of presbyopia is making the nondominant eye myopic (monovision).

XIV. **The future.** The future of keratorefractive surgery will likely include a wide array of new procedures. A refractive procedure that is predictable, stable, safe, and titratable, but also uses large optical zones and preserves or eventually treats presbyopia may not be far away. In the meantime, refractive surgeons have to choose the procedure among the large number of possible techniques that best fits the need of the patients. For patients left with small amounts of residual myopia, treatment with other procedures may become a viable option. For high myopia, *LASIK may be complemented by ICRS* to reduce the chance of postoperative ectasia. In this procedure, a microkeratome is used to mobilize a partial-thickness anterior corneal flap attached at one edge after an ICRS tunnel. The stromal wound bed is then ablated with the excimer laser to achieve the desired refractive effect. The corneal flap is then replaced after insertion of the ICRS segments. Although PRK, LASIK, and LASEK are likely to continue as the procedures of choice for most patients in the short term, the future holds great promise for newer, more sophisticated refractive surgical techniques.

XV. **Wavefront deformation.** The principles of wavefront deformation measurements, adapted from astronomical optics, will undoubtedly be incorporated in most future refractive surgical procedures. In a perfect optical system, all of the refracted rays are focused on a single plane (wavefront). Optical aberrations induce deformations on this plane and represent the optical performance of the entire visual system, not only the anterior surface of the cornea as in most corneal topography machines. In addition to correcting second-order optical aberrations (sphere and astigmatism), higher-order aberrations (spherical aberration and coma, i.e., irregular astigmatism) can be treated. With the use of advanced lasers and wavefront deformation measuring devices, the correction of these distortions of the human eye will continue to gain widespread use.

7. THE CRYSTALLINE LENS AND CATARACT*

Dimitri T. Azar

I. **Basic anatomy, physiology, and biochemistry.** The crystalline lens is a biconvex avascular structure suspended by thin filamentous zonules attached to the ciliary processes between the iris anteriorly and the vitreous humor posteriorly. The lens is the lesser of the two refractive diopteric elements in the eye accounting for approximately 18 D in the unaccommodated state, increasing with accommodation. It is an encapsulated multicellular organ surrounded by a basal lamina, the lens capsule, with an anterior layer of cuboidal epithelium covering concentric layers of fibers **(Fig. 7.1).** The lens capsule is rich with type IV collagen. The anterior lens capsule is thicker than the posterior capsule and contains another matrix protein, laminin. The epithelial cells contain nuclei, mitochondria, endoplasmic reticulum, and other cytoplasmic organelles; metabolic activity is both aerobic and anaerobic. At the equator, epithelial cells undergo mitotic division and differentiate into lens fibers. With aging and differentiation, all cells are gradually incorporated into the lens by anterior and posterior elongation to form the fiber cells of the lens. Cellular organelles are lost during differentiation. The lens sutures are formed by interdigitation of the anterior and posterior tips of the spindle-shaped fibers. Additional branches are added to sutures as the lens ages. No cells are lost from the lens. Newly laid fibers crowd and compact previous fibers; thus the oldest (embryonic and fetal) layers are the most central. The outermost fibers constituting the lens cortex are the most recently formed fibers. In lens fibers aerobic metabolic activity is absent.

The nucleus, the innermost part of the lens, contains the oldest cells, and metabolic activity in this region is virtually nonexistent. Metabolic activity supports active transport of amino acids and cations across the epithelium as well as protein synthesis in the fibers. Cations move actively across the anterior epithelium, but passively across the posterior lens capsule—a so-called pump–leak system. The maintenance of homeostasis is essential to lens clarity. Physiologic stresses may disrupt this homeostasis and lead to cataract formation, or opacification of the lens.

II. **Optics.** The lens and cornea form an optical system that focuses light from a distant object on the retina (emmetropia), anterior to the retina (myopia), or posterior to the retina (hyperopia). Myopic and hyperopic refractive errors are corrected with spectacle or contact lenses. The lens has a higher refractive index than its surroundings, resulting from the high concentration of α-, β-, and δ-crystallins in the lens fiber cytoplasm. The ability of the lens to change the refractive power of the eye and focus near objects is called ocular accommodation. The most commonly accepted mechanism of accommodation is that ciliary muscle contraction relaxes zonular tension on the lens and allows the intrinsic elasticity of the lens capsule to increase the central convexity of the anterior lens. This change reduces the focal length of the lens and moves the point of clear vision closer to the eye. When accommodation is relaxed, the equatorial edge of the lens moves toward the sclera (see Chapter 9, sec. **I.B.,** and Chapter 14, sec. **V.B.).** The accommodative response resulting from the same amount of ciliary muscle contraction, or accommodative effort, may vary depending on the age of the patient. It may be expressed as the diopteric change of lens power (amplitude of accommodation) or as the distance between the far point and the near point of the eye (range of accommodation).

*Updated from Gregory JK, Talamo JH. The crystalline lens and cataract. In: Pavan-Langston D. *Manual of ocular diagnosis and therapy,* 4th ed. Boston: Little, Brown, 1996:131–154; Pavan-Langston D. The crystalline lens and cataract. In: Pavan-Langston D. *Manual of ocular diagnosis and therapy,* 3rd ed. Boston: Little, Brown, 1991:125–148.

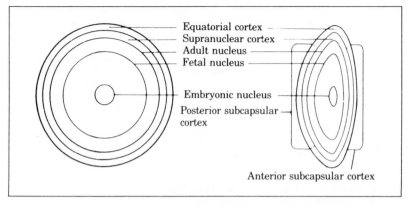

FIG. 7.1. Anatomic layers of the crystalline lens. Between the fetal and adult nuclei lie the lamellae of the infantile and adolescent nuclei.

Infants possess great powers of accommodation; with age, this power decreases. By about age 40 years, a substantial amount of accommodative power has been lost and reading glasses are needed for clear near vision. This is known as presbyopia, which is one of the earliest age-related lenticular changes. The amplitude of accommodation is helpful to calculate the power of the add used in bifocal spectacles to correct presbyopia.

In addition to presbyopia, ultrastructural deterioration and various biochemical changes of the crystalline lens take place with aging. The lens nucleus also becomes increasingly yellow with age (nuclear sclerosis), and in some cataracts the nuclear color may be brown or black. Nuclear sclerosis per se is not associated with loss of clarity. Often it is associated with an increase in the refractive index of the lens and a myopic shift in refraction, known as lenticular myopia. A change in color perception may result from the superimposition of a yellow filter between the retina and the incident light.

III. **Age-related changes.** Age-related cataracts are a major cause of visual impairment in older adults. When the transparency of the crystalline lens decreases enough to disturb vision, a clinically significant cataract exists. Such a decrease is usually the result of scattering of light rays or absorption in the axial part of the lens; similar changes in the peripheral parts of the lens may exist without loss of vision. Although these changes in the periphery are strictly cataractous in nature, surgical intervention is rarely warranted in the absence of visual symptoms.

A cataract is characterized by the zones of the lens involved in the opacity: anterior and posterior subcapsular, anterior and posterior cortical, equatorial cortical, supranuclear, and nuclear. In certain congenital cataracts, the nuclear zone is further subdivided into adult, adolescent, infantile, fetal, and embryonic zones (Fig. 7.1). There is a gradual transition but no distinct morphological differentiation between the layers of a cataract. The distinctions between these regions relate primarily to potential differences in their behavior and appearance during surgical procedures.

A. **Epidemiology of cataracts.** Ninety-five percent of individuals older than 65 years of age have some degree of lens opacity; many have cataracts sufficiently dense to warrant cataract extraction. The Beaver Dam Eye Study reported that 38.8% of men and 45.9% of women older than 74 years had visually significant cataracts. It is estimated that more than 1 million cataract extractions are performed each year in the United States alone. Cataract accounts for more than 15 million cases of treatable blindness in the world;

extraction often leads to complete visual rehabilitation. The Baltimore Eye Survey showed that untreated cataract was the source of blindness in 27% of African-Americans and 13% of whites.

B. Optics of cataracts. Visual disturbances resulting from a cataractous lens are secondary to fluctuation in the index of refraction creating light scattering and/or a loss of transparency. In cortical, supranuclear, and subcapsular cataracts, protein-deficient fluid collects between fibers. The index of refraction of this fluid is much less than that of fiber cytoplasm, and light scattering occurs at this interface. Light scattering also occurs from large protein aggregates linked to the cell membrane by disulfide bonds. This may cause monocular diplopia. Progressive yellowing of the lens in nuclear sclerotic cataracts causes poor hue discrimination, particularly at the blue end of the visible spectrum. The myopic shift associated with nuclear cataracts may transiently enable presbyopic patients to read without spectacles, a condition referred to as "second sight."

IV. Evaluation and management of cataracts

A. Symptoms of cataract formation

1. Decreased vision. Cataracts cause painless progressive decrease in vision. Clinically significant cataracts cause a decrease in distance or near visual acuity. Posterior subcapsular cataracts of even mild degree can reduce visual acuity substantially. Nuclear sclerotic cataracts cause image blur at distance but not at near. Image blur occurs when the lens loses its ability to differentiate (resolve) separate and distinct object points. When this occurs, near visual tasks, such as reading and sewing, become more difficult. Many older patients may tolerate considerable reductions in distance acuity if their night driving is minimal, but they may not be as tolerant of a blur that interferes with their indoor activities.

2. Glare. One of the symptomatic manifestations of light scattering is glare. When a patient looks at a point source of light, the diffusion of bright white and colored light around it drastically reduces visual acuity. The effect is akin to looking at automobile headlights at night through a dirty windshield. Posterior subcapsular opacification is responsible for much of the glare.

3. Distortion. Cataracts may make straight edges appear wavy or curved. They may even lead to image duplication (monocular diplopia). If a patient complains of double vision, it is essential to determine if the diplopia is binocular or monocular. If monocular, the examiner is usually dealing with corneal, lenticular, or macular disease.

4. Altered color perception. The yellowing of the lens nucleus steadily increases with age. Artists with significant nuclear sclerosis may render objects more brown or more yellow than they actually are.

5. Unilateral cataract. A cataract may occur in only one eye or may mature more rapidly in one eye than in the other. Unless the patient is in the habit of checking the acuity of each eye, he or she may not be aware of the presence of a dense cataract in one eye. It is not uncommon for a patient to claim that the vision in the cataractous eye was lost precipitously. Because cataracts rarely mature precipitously, it is more likely that the slowly evolving lens opacity was unrecognized until the patient happened to test his or her monocular acuity.

6. Behavioral changes

a. Children with congenital, traumatic, or metabolic cataracts may not verbalize their visual handicap. Behavioral changes indicative of a loss of acuity or binocular vision may alert the parents or teachers to the presence of a visual problem. Inability to see the blackboard or read with one eye may be one such symptom; loss of accurate depth perception, e.g., the inability to catch or hit a ball or to pour water from a pitcher into a glass, may be another.

b. Prepresbyopic adults. Difficulty with night driving is frequently an early sign of **cataract.**

   c. **Presbyopic adults.** Frequently, maturation of nuclear cataracts is associated with the return of clear near vision as the result of increasing myopia secondary to the higher refractive power of the rounder, harder nuclear sclerotic lens. Reading glasses or bifocals are no longer needed. This change is called "second sight." Unfortunately, the improvement in near vision is only temporary as the nuclear zone becomes more opaque.

B. **Signs of cataract formation**
   1. **Reduced visual acuity.** Although it is not part of the usual general physical examination, the measurement of visual acuity will alert the examiner to the presence of cataract as well as other ocular disorders. The examiner should always inquire about monocular acuity when conducting a review of systems.
   2. **Lenticular opacification.** Examination of the red reflex with the direct ophthalmoscope set on $+5$ (black) D at approximately 20 cm from the patient frequently will reveal a black lens opacity against the reddish-orange hue of the reflex. This is an extremely sensitive method of detecting cataractous change. If on upgaze the opacity appears to move down, the opacity is in the posterior half of the lens; if the opacity moves up with upgaze, it is located in the anterior half of the lens or in the cornea.
   3. **Leukokoria.** The white pupil is seen in mature cataracts; in certain immature cataracts, whitish patches are seen in the pupillary zone, the result of foci of light scattering, located in the anterior subcapsular or cortical zone.

C. **Diagnostic tests and spectacle correction for cataract**
   1. **Uncorrected and spectacle-corrected Snellen visual acuity.** Distant and near acuity with and without the appropriate glasses should be tested. Some patients with cataracts complain of poor visual function despite good Snellen visual acuity. Snellen charts measure high-contrast visual acuity. Cataracts can cause decreased appreciation of contrast, leading to subjective visual dysfunction. Snellen visual acuity in a brightly lit room versus a dark room may be substantially worse secondary to glare.
   2. **Non-Snellen acuity.** Tests of contrast sensitivity may be used to objectively document subjective decrease in contrast, although they have yet to be widely standardized for this purpose. Cataracts, especially posterior subcapsular and cortical, may cause debilitating glare. Several readily available instruments can document the effect of glare on visual acuity, e.g., **brightness acuity testing.** Confrontation visual fields and Goldmann and automated visual field testing may be valuable to evaluate the degree of preoperative visual field loss. **Potential acuity meter** testing can be helpful in evaluating the lenticular contribution to visual loss. Similarly, **laser interferometry** is predictive of final visual acuity in moderately dense cataracts.
   3. **Flashlight examination of lens and pupil.** The direct and consensual pupillary responses are not affected by lens opacities if a bright light is used; if a dim flashlight is used, the responses may be less pronounced when illuminating the eye in the presence of a dense cataract. A flashlight may also render anterior lens opacities more visible to the examiner if pupil size is not reduced excessively.
   4. **Direct ophthalmoscopy.** With the pupil dilated, nuclear cataracts often appear as a lens within a lens when viewed against the red reflex with a $+5$ to $+10$ D lens.
   5. **Slitlamp biomicroscopy** allows the most detailed examination of the anterior part of the eye. The extent, density, type, and location of the cataract can be easily determined. Slitlamp examination is also helpful in determining the position of the lens and the integrity of the zonular fibers. Excessive distance between the lens and the pupillary margin may indicate lens subluxation. Slitlamp biomicroscopy may have limitations, especially in detecting oil droplet cataracts, which may be easier to detect using the direct ophthalmoscope through the 10 D lens.

6. **Refraction and retinoscopy.** Myopia induced by the early stages of nuclear cataract formation can be detected by routine refraction. Patients may be well corrected for years with a stronger myopic distance lens and reading add. Retinoscopy will reveal the abnormal reflexes associated with lenticonus, a condition in which the anterior or posterior surface of the lens (or both) is excessively convex or conical.

7. **Fundus evaluation.** Both the direct and indirect ophthalmoscope can be used to evaluate the anatomic integrity of the posterior segment. Dilated fundus examination is necessary to evaluate the macula, optic nerves, vitreous, retinal vessels, and retinal periphery. Attention to macular degeneration, diabetic retinopathy, macular edema, retinal ischemia, vitreoretinal traction, neovascularization, optic nerve pallor, extensive cupping, and posterior capsular ruptures is important because these conditions may limit visual rehabilitation after cataract surgery.

8. **A-scan and B-scan ultrasonography** are techniques for measuring the thickness and location of a cataract. A-scan ultrasound techniques to measure the eye's axial length paired with keratometric measurement of corneal curvature allow precise calculation of appropriate intraocular lens (IOL) power, thus minimizing postoperative spherical refractive error. B-scan techniques are particularly useful in evaluating partial or total dislocation of the lens, and also provide a means of detecting abnormalities in the posterior half of the eye in the presence of a very dense cataract that precludes direct visualization. Some secondary cataracts form in response to posterior segment tumors or inflammation, thereby necessitating ultrasonography to ascertain the anatomic state of the eye behind the lens (see Chapter 1, sec. **III.H.**).

V. **Abnormalities of the lens**
   A. **Ectopia lentis (dislocated lens)** (see Chapter 11, secs. **VII.E.** and **F.,** and Chapter 15).
      1. **Homocystinuria.** This autosomal-recessive condition is associated with a deficiency of cystathionine beta-synthetase, an enzyme responsible for condensing homocystine and serine to cystathionine. Bilateral lens dislocation occurs in this disease; if the lens dislocates into the anterior chamber, acute pupillary block glaucoma may develop. Cataractous changes are unusual. Systemic manifestations include malar flush, mental retardation, osteoporosis, pectus excavatum, decreased joint mobility, and eczema. Abnormal physical findings are usually apparent by age 10, but may be delayed until the third decade. Surgical removal of dislocated lenses is fraught with complications, including vitreous loss, iris prolapse, and retinal detachment. **General anesthesia is to be avoided,** if possible, because of the increased risk of vascular thrombosis.
      2. **Marfan syndrome.** Inheritance of this disorder is autosomal dominant. In contrast to homocystinuria, in which lens dislocation is usually inferior, in Marfan syndrome dislocation is superior and only occasionally into the anterior chamber. Surgical extraction of these lenses is complicated by many of the same problems encountered in homocystinuria. The systemic manifestations of this disease include a tall and thin body habitus, scoliosis, arachnodactyly, elastic skin, hyperextensible joints, aortic insufficiency, and aortic aneurysm. Abnormalities in the expression of fibrillin have been found in some patients with Marfan syndrome. The diagnosis is usually established by the physical examination and the characteristic patient habitus.
      3. **Weill-Marchesani syndrome** is inherited as an autosomal-dominant or -recessive trait. Patients are short with broad hands and fingers. There may be joint stiffness, prominence, and decreased mobility. Carpal tunnel syndrome may result from fibrous tissue hyperplasia. Lenses are small, spherical, and frequently dislocate anteriorly, precipitating acute glaucoma. Patients are easily distinguished from those with Marfan syndrome or homocystinuria by their characteristic body habitus.

4. **Other heritable conditions with ectopia lentis:** hyperlysinemia, Crouzon syndrome, oxycephaly, Sprengel deformity, sulfite oxidase deficiency, Sturge-Weber syndrome, Ehlers-Danlos syndrome, dwarfism, polydactyly, and mandibulofacial dysostosis.

5. **Traumatic dislocation.** During ocular injuries, particularly blunt ocular trauma, expansion and compression of the globe equator can lead to lens dislocation or subluxation. The direction of dislocation could be vertical, horizontal, anterior (into the chamber) or posterior (into the vitreous). Very often this condition is associated with traumatic mydriasis, vitreous prolapse, rosette-shaped cataract formation, blood in the anterior chamber (hyphema), and glaucoma.

B. **Congenital cataracts** (see Chapter 11, sec. **VI., XVI.,** and Chapter 15)

1. **Galactosemia** is the result of an autosomal-recessive inborn error of galactose metabolism, a deficiency of galactose-1-phosphate uridyltransferase, the enzyme that converts galactose-1-phosphate to uridine diphosphogalactose. In the presence of milk sugar (lactose), this deficiency leads to the accumulation of galactose-1-phosphate and galactose. Galactose is converted by the enzyme aldose reductase to the sugar alcohol, galactitol. The accumulation of this sugar alcohol within lens cells creates a hypertonic intracellular milieu that is neutralized by the influx of water. The entry of water leads to swelling, membrane disruption, and opacification of the lens. Cataracts are not apparent at birth, but usually develop within the first few months of life. A central nuclear opacity resembling a drop of oil appears within the lens. This opacity may progress to opacification of the fetal nucleus. The disease is manifest in **patients fed milk products** that contain the disaccharide lactose (glucose plus galactose). Mental retardation, growth inhibition, and hepatic dysfunction commonly ensue if the disease goes untreated. The diagnosis can be made by an assay for uridyltransferase in peripheral red cells.

2. **Galactokinase deficiency.** The enzyme galactokinase converts galactose to galactose-1-phosphate. In this autosomal-recessive disorder; lack of this enzyme leads to the accumulation of galactose, which is then converted to galactitol. The same osmotic events as in galactosemia occur and lead to cataract formation. Systemic manifestations of galactosemia are absent, however. Except for cataracts, these patients usually enjoy normal health. Treatment is dietary restriction of galactose-containing foods. Patients who are heterozygous for this genetic defect are also at increased risk of cataract formation during the first year of life.

3. **Hypoglycemia.** Neonatal hypoglycemia occurs in approximately 20% of newborns. The incidence is significantly increased in premature infants. Blood sugars of 20 mg per dL or less may cause repeated episodes of somnolence, diaphoresis, unconsciousness, and convulsions. Repeated hypoglycemic episodes may lead to a characteristic lamellar cataract in which layers of cortical opacity are separated from a deeper zonular cataract by clear cortex. The cataract does not usually appear until the child is at least 2 to 3 years old; in many patients, no visual disability is encountered. Experimental evidence suggests that this cataract may be the result of an inactivation of type II hexokinase. Treatment of this condition is aimed at the restoration and maintenance of normal glucose levels in the blood.

4. **Lowe syndrome (oculocerebral renal syndrome).** Bilateral nuclear cataracts and microphakia are always found in this X-linked recessive disorder. Aspiration of these cataracts is associated with a poor prognosis for full visual recovery. Other ocular abnormalities include glaucoma and malformation of the anterior chamber angle and iris. Most striking is the **blue sclera,** a manifestation of scleral thinning. Frequently, there is associated mental retardation, failure to thrive, absence of eyebrows, and vitamin D-resistant rickets. Vomiting, glucosuria, proteinuria, renal caliculi, and convulsions are not unusual. The exact biochemical defect is unknown. Female genetic carriers have punctate cortical opacities.

5. **Myotonic dystrophy** is inherited as an autosomal-dominant trait and is the result of a defect in the gene encoding myotonin protein kinase; the defective gene contains increased repeats of a trinucleotide sequence. Early cataracts are characteristic and consist of fine, scattered, dust-like opacities in the cortex and subcapsular region. Multicolored (especially red and green) refractile bodies are scattered among these finer dust-like opacities; this finding is commonly referred to as a "christmas tree" cataract. Later in the disease, a granular, posterior subcapsular cataract develops. Cataract extraction usually is performed in adulthood, and the visual prognosis is good if there is no serious posterior segment abnormality such as optic atrophy or retinal degeneration. Associated systemic findings include dystrophic changes in muscles, including impaired contraction and relaxation, gonadal atrophy, and frontal baldness.

6. **Rubella cataract** results from fetal infection with rubella virus before the ninth week of gestation. This virus is known to inhibit mitosis and cell division in many fetal tissues. Involvement of the lens vesicle at the time of elongation of the posterior epithelial cells leads to abnormal lens development. The cataract has a characteristic morphology: slightly eccentric, dense, white core opacity and lesser opacification of the surrounding cortex. The anterior suture may be visible. Other ocular manifestations of this disease are microphthalmos, pigmentary retinopathy, and iritis. Because of the involvement of dilator fibers, pupillary dilation is frequently incomplete. Early referral to an ophthalmologist will optimize chances for successful cataract extraction. Surgery is frequently difficult because of poor pupillary dilation, shallow anterior chamber depth, and the small size of the eye. The newest techniques, however, with phacoemulsification and other forms of cataract aspiration, give this procedure a better prognosis. Rubella prevention, through vaccination, probably offers the safest and most effective method of reducing the incidence of this disease.

7. **Other congenital abnormalities** in which cataracts are found include Werner syndrome, congenital ichthyosis, Rothmund-Thomson syndrome, Fabry's disease, incontinentia pigmenti, Refsum's disease, gyrate atrophy of the choroid and retina, Stickler syndrome, neurofibromatosis type II, cerebrotendinous xanthomatosis, Wilson's disease, Niemann-Pick disease Type A, mannosidosis, mucolipidosis I, and Hallermann-Streiff-François syndrome (see Chapter 10, sec. **IX–XII.**).

C. **Age-related cataracts.** The term *senile* was previously used to describe cataracts in older adults with no specificity with regard to morphology or etiology. However, with the emergence of surgical procedures specifically suited to certain forms of cataracts, it has become more important to specify the degree of nuclear sclerosis, which often correlates with hardness, when distinguishing one form of cataract from another. Typically, cataracts are now described by their cortical, nuclear, and subcapsular components.

D. **Metabolic cataract**

1. **Diabetic cataract**

   a. **Osmotic cataract.** In the pre-insulin era, the acute onset of a mature cataract in an untreated or brittle diabetic was not uncommon. Because blood sugar control is now relatively easy with insulin, this form of acute osmotic cataract is extremely rare. It is possible to precipitate this cataract, however, by abruptly lowering a markedly elevated blood sugar with insulin. The intracellular hypertonicity, which results from the accumulation of sorbitol and glucose, remains after the serum osmolarity decreases precipitously with the blood sugar. A rapid influx of water leads to acute swelling and opacification of the lens.

   b. **Poorly controlled diabetics** frequently experience changes in their refractive status. Increasing blood sugar is associated with myopic change; decreasing blood sugar is associated with hyperopic change. These changes are most noticeable during periods of poor control. Restoration of control eliminates these refractive error fluctuations.

   c. **The reversible appearance and disappearance of a posterior subcapsular cataract** have been documented in adult diabetics. These are believed to be a somewhat lesser response to the same osmotic stress that opacifies the entire lens of the uncontrolled juvenile diabetic.
   d. **Incidence.** Cataract extraction is done more frequently and at an earlier age in adult diabetics when compared to the general population. It is not clear whether this is because of the increased incidence and more rapid maturation of cataract in diabetics, or whether it is a manifestation of the increased detection of cataracts in a population already under medical supervision. Abundant experimental evidence suggests that diabetes is a significant cataractogenic stress that, added to other age-related stresses, may lead to earlier maturation of cataracts. The development of aldose reductase inhibitors to block the conversion of glucose to sorbitol may provide a means of eliminating this cataractogenic stress. The morphology of the adult diabetic cataract is indistinguishable from that of the nondiabetic senile cataract.
 2. **Hypocalcemic (tetanic cataract).** The morphology of the cataract associated with hypocalcemia varies with the age at which hypocalcemia occurs. In the infant, depression of serum calcium produces a zonular cataract with a thin, opacified lamella deep in the infantile cortex. In the adult, acquired or surgical hypoparathyroidism is associated with punctate, red, green, and highly refractile opacities occurring in the subcapsular area. In **pseudohypoparathyroidism,** lamellar opacities are found in the nucleus of the lens. Ocular involvement may include papilledema, diplopia, photophobia, and strabismus. It is believed that calcium is necessary to maintain membrane integrity and that calcium deficiency leads to membrane disruption and increased permeability.
 3. **Aminoaciduria** (see secs. **V.A.** and **B.,** above; Chapter 10, sec. **VII.**).
 4. **Wilson's disease** is an autosomal-recessive disorder of copper metabolism. Ocular involvement includes the Kayser-Fleischer ring of golden peripheral discoloration of Descemet's membrane and the formation of a characteristic sunflower cataract. The latter is due to the deposition of cuprous oxide in the anterior lens capsule and subcapsular cortex in a stellate pattern. Sunflower cataracts, however, do not generally induce significant reductions in visual acuity.
 5. **Galactosemia** (see Chapter 10, sec. **VII.** and **V.B.,** above)
 6. **Myotonic dystrophy** (see sec. **V.B.5.,** above)
E. **Drug-induced cataracts**
 1. **Corticosteroids.** The use of topical, inhaled, and systemic corticosteroids is associated with the appearance of axial posterior subcapsular cataracts. These cataracts frequently assume a discoid morphology and, by virtue of their axial position near the nodal point of the eye, cause significant visual disability. The higher the dose of corticosteroid and the longer the course of treatment, the more likely the patient is to develop cataract. By reducing the dose and duration of treatment, the cataractogenic process can be slowed or stopped. All patients with diseases requiring prolonged corticosteroid therapy should be periodically evaluated by an ophthalmologist.
 2. **Miotics (anticholinesterase drugs including echothiophate, diisopropyl fluorophosphate, and demecarium bromide)** are used to treat glaucoma and some forms of strabismus in children. Prolonged use is associated with the appearance of anterior subcapsular vacuoles and granular opacities. Removal of the drug reduces the risk of progression and may even be associated with reversal of cataract.
F. **Traumatic cataract.**
 1. **Contusion cataract.** Lens opacification may occur in response to blunt and penetrating trauma.
 2. **Infrared radiation** (glassblower and glassworker cataract). Prolonged exposure (over several years) to infrared radiation leads to exfoliation of

the anterior lens capsule. In contrast to the pseudoexfoliation seen in elderly patients, in true exfoliation large pieces of the lens capsule flake off and may curl back on themselves in the pupillary zone of the lens. Although this is not a true cataract, prolonged exposure may lead to the appearance of a discoid posterior subcapsular opacity with many highly refractile spots. This cataract is rarely seen currently, but was common in the 19th century.

3. **X-ray radiation.** Ionizing radiation can produce a characteristic posterior subcapsular opacity. The degree of cataract formation is a function of the radiation dose. As little as 300 to 400 rad as a single dose may lead to cataract formation. These opacities do not necessarily progress. With higher doses, the cataract may progress to involve the entire posterior subcapsular zone, and rare cases may involve the entire lens. There is usually a latent period between the exposure and the onset of cataract that may be as brief as 6 months (after intensive exposures such as atomic bomb injury) or as long as several years. Neutron and alpha beams produce the greatest ionization and pose the greatest risk of cataract formation. Gamma and x-rays are the most frequently used forms of radiation in medicine; therefore, these forms are most frequently associated with cataract formation. Appropriate shielding of the lens is necessary when tumors around the eye are being treated.

4. **Microwave radiation.** Although it is possible to produce cataracts in animals exposed to high doses of microwave radiation, microwave exposure in humans has not been associated with cataract formation. Surveys of armed services personnel exposed to microwave radiation at radar installations have not revealed an increased incidence of cataracts. This remains, however, a potential cataractogenic factor.

5. **Ultraviolet (UV) radiation.** Exposure to UV radiation has been linked to human cataracts in many studies. This radiation is divided into three wavelength bands: UV-A (400 to 320 nm), UV-B (320 to 290 nm), and UV-C (290 to 100 nm). UV-A induces suntanning, UV-B induces blistering and skin cancer, and UV-C does not normally reach the earth's surface. Depletion of the ozone layer, however, is allowing more UV-B and potentially UV-C to penetrate our atmosphere. The cornea absorbs some of the UV-B (snow blindness is UV-B keratitis), but all wavelengths longer than 300 nm are transmitted into the eye. Although the lens tends, in turn, to transmit UV-A, it absorbs almost all intraocular UV-B, the wavelength shown experimentally and clinically to be most damaging to the lens, particularly in formation of cortical and nuclear cataracts. Only the retina is susceptible to damaging effects from visible light. Ocular exposure to UV-B may be reduced by 50% by just wearing a hat with a brim, 95% by wearing ordinary glasses with glass lenses, and 100% by using a UV coating or UV screener incorporated into spectacle lenses. UV screeners may protect against cataract formation.

The ability of the natural lens to absorb UV light may have a protective effect on the retina. UV irradiation may cause macular degeneration in patients whose natural lenses have been removed because of cataracts. Because of this, manufacturers of IOLs incorporate filters that block transmission of wavelengths below 400 nm. All polymethylmethacrylate (PMMA) and many silicone IOLs now contain UV filters. Similar filters are being used in spectacles. The patient benefits from both the filtered spectacles and the implants by experiencing less glare in bright light and perhaps greater macular longevity. Darkly tinted glasses block transmission of visible light but an incorporated UV block or coating must be present to offer full UV protection.

6. **Electrical cataract.** Electrocution injury can be associated with cataract formation. The cataracts may involve both the anterior and the posterior subcapsular and cortical regions and are usually more extensive on the side with the greater electrical burn. The morphology of these cataracts

varies, but may include punctate dust-like vacuoles as well as linear and cortical spokes. Nuclear opacification is unusual.

7. **Copper (chalcosis) and iron (siderosis) cataracts.** Intraocular foreign bodies containing copper and iron may lead to cataract formation. Both intraocular copper and iron may lead to significant loss of vision.

   a. **Copper** is extremely toxic to the eye and produces a sunflower cataract with small yellowish-brown dots in the subcapsular cortex within the pupillary zone. The petals of the sunflower may extend toward the equator.

   b. **Intraocular iron** may produce a brownish subcapsular opacity without characteristic morphology. Intralenticular iron may produce a mature cataract. The brown color may involve other parts of the eye such as the iris or the cornea.

8. **Syn- and cocataractogenic factors.** Many investigators have advocated the concept of cataractogenesis as the result of multiple subthreshold cataractogenic stresses. Each stress acting alone is insufficient to cause cataract; however, when these stresses act in concert, a cataract may form. It is possible that age is one of these cataractogenic stresses, and that the superimposition of other toxic stresses on an aging lens may accelerate the rate of cataract formation. Conversely, the elimination of one or more subcataractogenic stresses may delay or entirely prevent cataract formation.

G. **Other forms of secondary cataract**

1. **Cataract secondary to ocular inflammation.** Chronic keratitis, iritis, and posterior uveitis may all lead to cataract formation. The exact mechanism of lens opacification is poorly understood, but treatment of this cataract is addressed primarily to the control of the ocular inflammation while minimizing the dose of corticosteroid used to treat the inflammation.

2. **Neoplasia.** Anterior and posterior segment tumors such as ocular melanoma and retinoblastoma may lead to cataract formation. Metastatic tumors involving the choroid or anterior segment may also cause cataract.

H. **Miscellaneous lenticular abnormalities**

1. **Pseudoexfoliation.**

   Pseudoexfoliation is the deposition of a dandruff-like material on the anterior lens capsule, posterior iris, and ciliary processes, and is associated with a form of open-angle glaucoma. The material does not derive from the lens capsule and is therefore called pseudoexfoliation. It is of visual significance because severe **glaucoma** and **weak lens capsule zonules** frequently coexist, which may make ciliary sulcus placement of a posterior chamber lens implant advisable at the time of cataract surgery despite a successful extracapsular procedure.

2. **Lens-induced inflammation.** A hypermature cataract may leak lens protein into the anterior chamber. These proteins may act as antigens and induce antigen–antibody formation, complement fixation, and inflammation. Although topical steroid therapy will temporarily suppress the inflammation, a permanent cure of this condition is obtained only by cataract extraction.

3. **Lens-induced glaucoma.** In a similar manner, the leakage of lens protein into the anterior chamber may elicit a macrophage response. Macrophages engorged with lens protein and/or free high-molecular-weight lens proteins obstruct the trabecular meshwork outflow tract, and aqueous humor produced within the eye cannot exit freely. An acute glaucoma called **phacolytic glaucoma** may arise. Treatment is by immediate cataract extraction.

4. **Pupillary block glaucoma.** As a mature lens swells and becomes hypermature, the disintegration of protein molecules into smaller molecules results in intralenticular hypertonicity, and swelling may obstruct the flow of aqueous humor around the iridolenticular interface. This leads to iris bombé and an acute form of **angle-closure glaucoma.** Peripheral iridectomy is inadequate treatment. The lens must be extracted to relieve

the pupillary block. In other forms of pupillary block glaucoma in which an intumescent lens is not involved, peripheral iridectomy is sufficient treatment.

VI. Medical treatment of cataract

A. Dietary factors. Epidemiologic studies have recently indicated that patients with diets high in the antioxidant carotenoid alpha carotene had a notably lower incidence of nuclear cataract, those high in the carotenoid lycopene were lowest in cortical cataract, and those high in the carotenoids lutein and possibly zeaxanthin were lowest in posterior subcapsular cataract. Vitamins C and E had no notable effect.

B. Mydriatics. The patient with a small axial cataract may occasionally benefit from pupillary dilation (mydriasis); this allows the clear, paraxial lens to participate in light transmission, image formation, and focusing, eliminating the glare and blur caused by these small central cataracts. Phenylephrine 2.5%, one drop bid in the affected eye, may clarify vision. In the hypertensive patient, the use of a short-acting, mydriatic-cycloplegic drug such as tropicamide 1% or cyclopentolate 1% will exacerbate hypertension.

C. Diabetes

1. **Age-related cataracts,** as stated earlier, are widely believed to occur more frequently and mature more rapidly in diabetics. Just as careful control of blood sugar levels can minimize the troublesome changes in refractive error that occur in patients with poorly controlled diabetes, some mild cataracts can be reversed through diabetic control. Advanced cataracts are not benefited by better control of diabetes.

2. **Aldose reductase inhibitors** have been used successfully in animals to prevent "sugar cataract" (diabetic and galactosemic) formation; such drugs may be beneficial in human diabetics. Blocking the conversion of glucose to sorbitol by aldose reductase might delay or prevent the adverse osmotic stress resulting from the intracellular accumulation of sorbitol, a sugar alcohol.

D. Removing cataractogenic agents. Irradiation (infrared and x-ray radiation) as well as **drugs** (corticosteroids, phenothiazines, cholinesterase inhibitors, and others) can cause cataracts. Conversely, their removal may delay or prevent further progression of the cataract. Any drug or agent with known cataractogenic properties should be used as briefly, at as low a dose as possible, or both. Ophthalmologic evaluation before and during treatment can alert the physician to signs of cataract formation.

VII. Surgical treatment of cataract

A. Timing of surgery

1. **Visual considerations.** The mere presence of a cataract is insufficient reason for its removal: It is important to establish the patient's specific visual needs before undertaking surgery. If the cataract is uniocular, surgery may be delayed until the cataract is mature, as long as visual function in the fellow eye is sufficient for the patient's needs and the patient does not need stereoscopic vision. If bilateral cataracts are present, extraction of the cataract from the eye with the worse visual acuity may be done when the patient regards the visual handicap as a significant deterrent to the maintenance of his or her usual lifestyle.

B. Preoperative evaluation and considerations

1. **The preoperative ophthalmologic evaluation** should include a complete examination to rule out comorbid conditions, such as longstanding amblyopia, pseudoexfoliation, retinal tears or holes, macular lesions, or optic nerve abnormalities that may affect the visual or surgical outcome. An accurate refraction of both eyes, measurement of corneal refractive power with a keratometer, and measurement of axial length with an A-scan ultrasound are all necessary to calculate the appropriate IOL power. Some surgeons measure macular acuity using devices that project either Snellen letters or gratings onto the macula through a relatively clear part of the lens (potential acuity meter). These measurements give the surgeon and patient an indication of the visual acuity that can be obtained

postoperatively, but they are not foolproof. These tests tend to underestimate postoperative visual acuity in some situations, while overestimating visual acuity in some macular diseases.

2. **Preoperative medical evaluation.** Each patient should be evaluated by an internist or general practitioner before surgery for any conditions that may affect the patient's surgical or postsurgical course. The necessary testing depends on the patient's age and prior medical history.

3. **Preparation for surgery** should include a full explanation of the potential risks and benefits of proposed surgery and anesthesia, as well as the technique for administering eye drops and ointments and other postoperative care. Any blepharitis, dacryocystitis, or other ocular surface disease should be treated and resolved before proceeding with intraocular surgery.

4. **Both outpatient and inpatient** surgical facilities are used for cataract surgery, with the latter reserved for patients at risk for medical complications. Well-designed, certified outpatient surgical facilities offer the patient the briefest possible surgical experience and reduce to a minimum the disruption of the patient's normal living routine. Such facilities offer the surgeon an opportunity to deliver state-of-the-art surgical care in an efficient outpatient environment at minimal cost.

C. **Preoperative medications**

1. **Mydriasis.** For planned extracapsular cataract extraction (ECCE) and phacoemulsification, it is crucial that the pupil be widely dilated throughout most of the procedure. This is most often achieved with a preoperative combination of an adrenergic agent (such as phenylephrine), an anticholinergic agent (such as cyclopentolate or tropicamide), and a cyclooxygenase inhibitor (such as flurbiprofen). The cyclooxygenase inhibitor is believed to contribute to maintaining and preventing formation of intraoperative mydriasis. Intraoperative mydriasis may also be maintained with the use of dilute epinephrine in the irrigating solution.

2. **Anesthesia options.** Cataract extraction may be performed under local, topical, or general anesthesia. Local anesthesia minimizes the risk of wound rupture, a complication frequently associated with coughing during extubation and postoperative nausea and vomiting. The use of 1:1 mixed 2% to 4% xylocaine and 0.75% bupivacaine in facial and peribulbar or retrobulbar blocks achieves rapid anesthesia, akinesia, and postoperative analgesia for several hours. Care to avoid intravascular injections of anesthetic is essential, because refractory cardiopulmonary arrest may result from an inadvertent intravenous or intraarterial injection. Many patients express dread of the facial and retrobulbar injections; proper preoperative sedation and good rapport with the surgeon make them quite tolerable.

   Topical anesthesia, in conjunction with intravenous sedation and clear corneal incisions, has been used with increasing frequency in very cooperative patients and does not carry the risks of local anesthesia. This is becoming the most commonly used approach for managing uncomplicated soft cataracts. It permits very early postoperative use of the eye, because there is no lid ptosis, diplopia, or amaurosis. Although topical anesthesia for cataract surgery is a relatively new approach, it will be some time before safety comparable to retro- or peribulbar techniques can be demonstrated in patients with dense nuclei. Patients who are extremely apprehensive, deaf, mentally retarded, unstable, or cannot communicate well with the surgeon are discouraged from having topical anesthesia.

3. **Intraocular pressure (IOP) lowering.** Preoperative IOP reduction can prevent such operative complications as vitreous loss, expulsive choroidal hemorrhage, and shallowing of the anterior chamber. This can be accomplished by mechanical pressure (digital massage or Honan balloon) or osmotic means (intravenous mannitol).

4. **Preoperative prepping–antibiosis** is designed to prevent postoperative endophthalmitis, a condition that is devastating but rare. Many surgeons prescribe a topical antibiotic such as tobramycin preoperatively to eradicate conjunctival bacterial flora. Most surgeons prepare the lids and facial

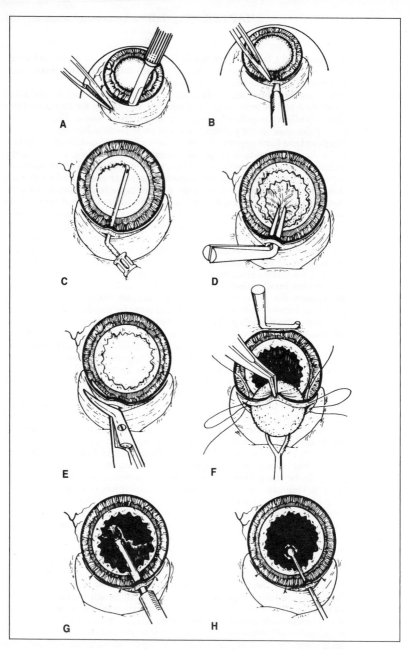

FIG. 7.2. Planned extracapsular cataract extraction by irrigation–aspiration technique. **A:** Posterior limbal groove, 10 to 11 mm, 2/3 scleral depth. **B:** 3.5-mm entry into anterior chamber, viscoelastic substance in anterior chamber. **C:** 360-degree round cystotome opening of anterior capsule. **D:** Removal of anterior capsule. **E:** Corneal scissors angled at 45 degrees extend wound to 10 mm. **F:** 10-0 nylon sutures 7 mm apart displaced from wound and nucleus expressed by gentle pressure at 6 o'clock (muscle hook) and 12 o'clock (lens loop). Assistant lifts cornea and rotates and "teases" nucleus out with 19-gauge needle. **G:** Irrigate anterior chamber, tie sutures, and place third suture at 12 o'clock before irrigation–aspiration of residual lens. **H:** Polishing posterior capsule. (Adapted from Hersh P. *Ophthalmic surgical procedures.* Boston: Little, Brown, 1988:91–93.)

skin with 10% povidone–iodine. Many surgeons will also place one drop of 5% povidone–iodine into the conjunctival cul-de-sac.

D. Surgical techniques

1. **Intracapsular cataract extraction (ICCE).** Removal of the entire lens (with capsule intact) is performed with a forceps or cryoprobe. Usually the supporting zonules are dissolved with the enzyme alpha-chymotrypsin. This procedure was the most widely used surgical technique of cataract extraction for nearly 60 years, but has been almost entirely replaced by extracapsular and phacoemulsification techniques.

2. **ECCE (Fig. 7.2).** This technique is designed to remove the opaque portions of the lens without disturbing the integrity of the posterior capsule and anterior vitreous face. Compared to ICCE, there is a significantly lower incidence of postoperative cystoid macular edema (CME) and retinal detachment, improved prognosis of subsequent glaucoma filtering surgery or corneal transplantation, reduced incidence of vitreocorneal touch and bullous keratopathy, and reduced secondary rubeosis in diabetics. In ECCE, the anterior capsule is opened widely, the nucleus expressed through a 9- to 10-mm incision, and the residual equatorial cortex aspirated, using either automated irrigation–aspiration machines or manual handheld devices. The posterior capsule may be polished, but is otherwise undisturbed, and serves as the resting site for posterior chamber lens implants. Some posterior capsules may opacify within a few months or years of surgery. These are easily opened on an outpatient basis using the infrared neodymium:yttrium, aluminum, and garnet (Nd:YAG) laser mounted on a slitlamp delivery system (see sec. **VII.E.9.,** below).

3. **Phacoemulsification (Fig. 7.3)**

   a. **Technique**

      (1) **Wounds.** Numerous wound configurations have been developed for use with phacoemulsification. In one popular technique, a partial-thickness scleral groove long enough to accommodate the width of the IOL is made perpendicular to the sclera, 2 mm posterior and tangential to the limbus. A 2.8- to 3-mm scleral tunnel is then fashioned, with entry into the anterior chamber occurring in clear cornea. The length of the anterior chamber entry wound is initially kept just long enough for the diameter of the phacoemulsification probe and is extended after phacoemulsification to accommodate the IOL. This type of wound has a triplanar configuration and is usually self-sealing. Another method involves making the entire stepped wound through clear cornea. With any wound configuration, one or two paracenteses are made 90 degrees from the primary

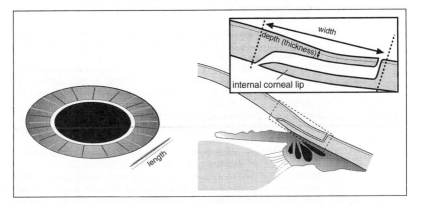

FIG. 7.3. Scleral tunnel wound construction (front and side views).

wound and a viscoelastic substance is injected into the anterior chamber before entry through the primary wound. This paracentesis provides entry for a second instrument useful for handling the nucleus during phacoemulsification.

(2) **Capsulotomy versus capsulorrhexis.** Most surgeons performing phacoemulsification now use the capsulorrhexis technique to create a small opening in the anterior capsule. This involves making a smooth, continuous, circular tear in the anterior capsule. The "beer can" capsulotomy technique is used exclusively with ECCE, making multiple small tears in the anterior capsule that are joined just before the removal of the capsulotomy flap. Capsulorrhexis produces a small opening in the anterior capsule that is less likely to tear than the beer can capsulotomy, possibly producing a loss of capsular support for the IOL. The small opening also allows "in-the-bag" placement of IOLs with much greater certainty.

(3) **Lens removal.** After hydrodissection and hydrodelineation (injection of balanced salt solution into the lens to delineate its structures and provide for easier nucleus rotation), removal of the lens nucleus is accomplished with the phacoemulsification probe. The nucleus is emulsified by a titanium needle vibrating at ultrasonic frequencies (28 to 68 kHz) and aspirated by the probe that also passes irrigating fluid into the eye through a concentric soft or rigid sleeve. Many different techniques are used to accomplish phacoemulsification. The "chip and flip" technique involves using the probe to sculpt the nucleus into a bowl, the superior pole of which is then flipped anteriorly so that the probe can work from below it. Phacoemulsification can be carried out in the anterior chamber as well with the nucleus being prolapsed there after capsulorrhexis. Most surgeons use the "divide and conquer" supranuclear phaco, or the "chopping" method.

The former method, in which a cross is fashioned in the nucleus with the phacoemulsification probe, produces four fragments that are then manually split and phacoemulsified separately. Supranuclear phaco requires a large capsulorrhexis opening and elevation of the nucleus above the anterior capsular rim for emulsification. The chopping technique can be used after deep nuclear sculpting to create a vertical trough. A second instrument designed for chopping is inserted through the paracentesis and the nucleus is cracked. The phaco tip is used for stabilization and the phaco chop instrument is inserted below the anterior capsule to be embedded in the periphery of the epinucleus, creating a free wedge that is easier to emulsify with the phaco tip. The size of the nuclear wedges can vary depending on the nuclear consistency; hard nuclei require smaller wedges than softer nuclei.

(4) **Irrigation–aspiration.** After phacoemulsification of the nucleus, removal of the soft cortex is accomplished with an automatic or manual irrigator–aspirator.

(5) **IOL placement.** After removal of the cortex, viscoelastic material is injected to expand the capsular bag and deepen the anterior chamber. The wound is extended, if needed, to accommodate the IOL, but this may not be necessary when using a foldable IOL. The lens is placed between the posterior capsule and the remaining anterior capsule if possible, because this in-the-bag placement results in a more stable IOL.

(6) **Wound closure.** After insertion of the IOL, scleral tunnels sometimes may need to be closed with a single horizontal suture that helps reduce the astigmatism associated with radial sutures. Failure to use sutures to close large cataract wounds may be associated with an increased risk of endophthalmitis, but this has not

been conclusively demonstrated. For small self-sealing phacoemulsification wounds, sutures are needed only when the security of the wound is not ascertained.

b. Benefits. Although there is no significant difference in the final visual acuity outcome among patients with 3.5-, 7.0-, and 10-mm incisions, there are a number of advantages of phacoemulsification over ECCE: earlier visual recovery, earlier return to usual activities, decreased astigmatism, greater wound stability, decreased risk of wound rupture, and the use of a safer, closed fluidics system during surgery that minimizes IOP fluctuations, and perhaps the chance of debilitating expulsive choroidal hemorrhage.

c. Risks. The difficulty of phacoemulsifying hard brunescent cataracts has deterred ophthalmic surgeons from offering phacoemulsification to patients with this type of cataract. Despite new titanium needle designs (thin-walled, oval, 15-, 30-, and 45-degree tip angles) and more powerful sonicators, which facilitate emulsification of brunescent nuclei, many surgeons believe that excessive energy release may limit its safety. Emulsification of the nucleus in the posterior chamber (behind the iris plane) has reduced the risk of damage to the corneal endothelium and, in certain patients, has reduced the importance of corneal endothelial dystrophy as a contraindication to phacoemulsification. In inexperienced hands, however, there may be an increased risk of posterior capsular rupture compared to ECCE. With the advent of synthetic hyaluronic acid and chondroitin sulfate (viscoelastic substances), topical nonsteroidal antiinflammatory drugs (NSAIDs) (e.g., flurbiprofen), and iris retractor hooks, it has become possible in many cases to deal with shallow chambers and poorly dilated pupils—two additional conditions that dissuaded surgeons from considering this operation. Because the number of contraindications to phacoemulsification has decreased dramatically over the past few years as the result of improved instrumentation and techniques, phacoemulsification has become by far the preferred method of cataract extraction for most ophthalmologists.

4. Pars plana lensectomy and phacofragmentation. Cataracts frequently obscure vitreous pathology. To deal surgically with such pathology, the cataract may have to be removed. This may be accomplished with an ultrasonic needle introduced via an anterior approach or through the sclera and pars plana. The emulsified lens is aspirated through the same needle; irrigation fluid enters the eye through a separate portal. Pars plana techniques are not used for cataract extraction alone, because the posterior capsule cannot be preserved.

E. IOLs (intraocular lens implants). In the last 20 years, the replacement of a cataractous crystalline lens with a clear lens of PMMA has become an integral part of almost every cataract procedure. Of these lenses, the vast majority are the posterior chamber type (PC IOL). Although the vast majority of IOLs used to be made of PMMA, silicone and acrylic lenses now account for the majority of the IOL market. Iris-fixation and iridocapsular IOLs are no longer used because of a higher complication rate. The number of implants today largely reflects new cases of visually significant cataracts. The rapid increase in IOL implants and their popularity is a function of many factors such as increasing acceptance by physicians and patients, a growing appreciation of the improved visual rehabilitation and quality of vision compared to aphakia corrected by spectacles or the lesser convenience of contact lenses, the lowered postoperative complication rate of CME and retinal detachment with the extracapsular techniques, improved instrumentation, better lens design, and the advent of viscoelastic substances.

1. Anterior chamber intraocular lenses (AC IOLs) are relatively easy to insert after ICCE or ECCE, and most are easy to remove if so indicated **(Fig. 7.4A, B).** The first AC IOLs to gain acceptance were either rigid, vaulted, four-footed lenses, or rigid, closed-loop lenses, some of

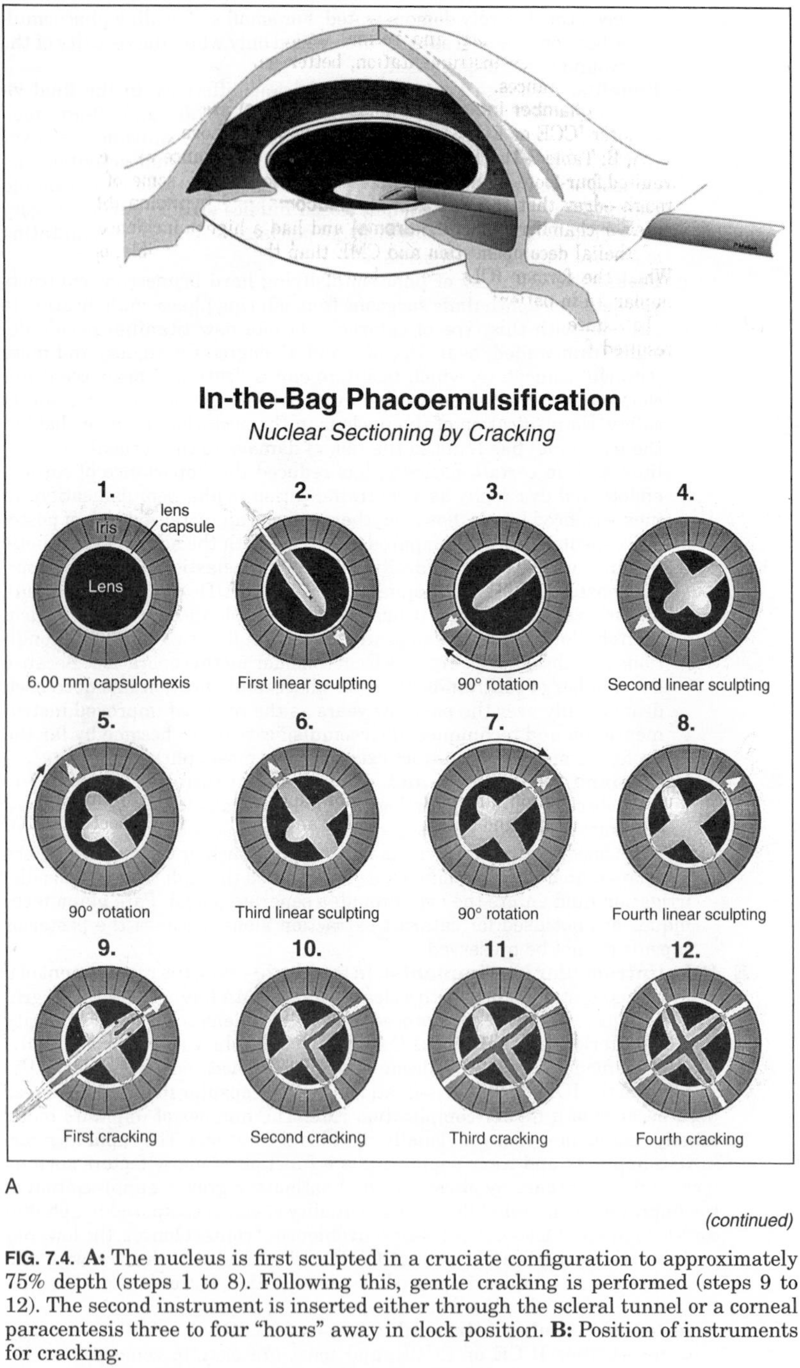

In-the-Bag Phacoemulsification

Nuclear Sectioning by Cracking

1. 6.00 mm capsulorhexis

2. First linear sculpting

3. 90° rotation

4. Second linear sculpting

5. 90° rotation

6. Third linear sculpting

7. 90° rotation

8. Fourth linear sculpting

9. First cracking

10. Second cracking

11. Third cracking

12. Fourth cracking

A

(continued)

FIG. 7.4. A: The nucleus is first sculpted in a cruciate configuration to approximately 75% depth (steps 1 to 8). Following this, gentle cracking is performed (steps 9 to 12). The second instrument is inserted either through the scleral tunnel or a corneal paracentesis three to four "hours" away in clock position. **B:** Position of instruments for cracking.

FIG. 7.4. *(continued)*

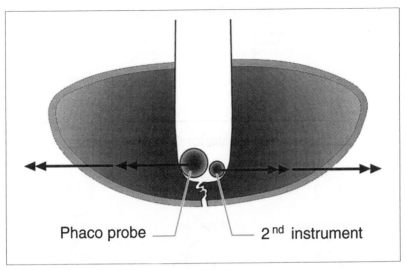

Phaco probe ——| |—— 2nd instrument

B

which had rough edges that induced **uveitis, glaucoma,** and **hyphema** (blood in the anterior chamber) **(UGH syndrome)** and had a higher incidence of corneal endothelial decompensation and CME than the newer flexible, open lenses. Although the former IOLs are no longer available, large numbers are still implanted in patients with well-functioning eyes.

To reduce postoperative complications and to avoid sizing problems that resulted from rigid, oversized lenses eroding into and painfully inflaming intraocular structures, or too-small lenses "propellering" in the AC, manufacturers developed AC IOLs with flexible supporting loops that rest gently against the angle structures (Fig. 7.5 A, B). It has been shown that all closed-loop and open broad-loop AC IOLs have varying angle contact during flexion of the globe. This results in chronic irritation, secondary angle synechiae, endothelial cell loss, CME, or all of these. Current evidence indicates that the optimal AC IOLs are the three- and four-footed flexible open design (Kelman style) that maintain a small but constant area of angle contact with external ocular pressure. In general, visual results are excellent, complications are low, and surgical outcomes may be comparable to those obtained with PC IOLs. Even with flexible loops, an occasional patient may have ocular tenderness upon touching the eye postoperatively. This may be an indication for removal of the IOL only if symptoms do not abate when the patient stops rubbing the eye.

2. **Secondary IOLs.** For those patients who did not have an IOL implanted at the time of primary cataract extraction, a **secondary IOL** may be put in at a later date, thus avoiding the need for contact lenses or aphakic spectacle correction. Preoperative evaluation for suitability should include specular microscopy (endothelial cell count should be greater than 1,200 mm^2), no active intraocular inflammation, an intact posterior capsule (for PC IOLs), and a sufficiently intact iris and anterior chamber angle for the AC IOL feet to rest on with stability.

3. **Rigid PC IOLs** are by far the IOLs most commonly inserted after ECCE with the posterior capsule relatively intact (a small defect may still allow use of a PC IOL in many cases) **(Fig. 7.5)**. The loops fit either within the capsular bag of the lens or in the ciliary sulcus, a ridge just anterior to

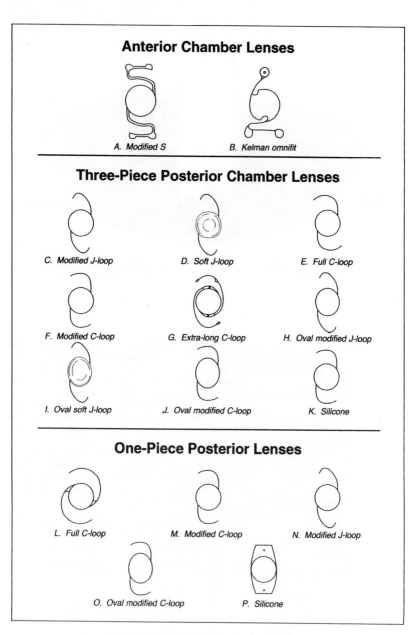

FIG. 7.5. Common intraocular lens styles.

the ciliary processes. The loops prevent the lens from moving by becoming enmeshed in a fibrous cuff. The optic rests against the posterior capsule. In certain patients with insufficient capsular support, iris or scleral fixation with 10-0 Prolene sutures may be utilized. The advantages of this technique over AC IOLs have not yet been conclusively demonstrated.

    a. Design modifications. The first PC IOLs had simple J-loop Prolene haptics and PMMA optics all in one plane. Since then, modifications in designs in Fig. 7.5 include (a) a gentler J-curve or broadening of the haptic all the way to a C-curve to increase the fixation contact, with sizes ranging from 10 to 14 mm, (b) anterior angulation of the loops to minimize iris capture, (c) reduction or elimination of fixation holes that might cause glare in an inordinately large pupil, (d) variable optic sizes from 5.0 to 7.0 mm, (e) variable haptic-to-haptic diameters to allow for in-the-bag or sulcus fixation, (f) incorporation of UV chromophores to screen out harmful UV-B rays, (g) use of PMMA for both haptic and optic construction to reduce potential inflammatory reaction to Prolene degradable haptics, (h) use of single-piece construction, (i) biconvex optics to decrease posterior capsule hazing, (j) laser ridges, and (k1) introduction of multifocal and soft foldable IOLs (see secs. **VII.E.5.** and **6.,** below).

    All of the above are generally aimed at various levels of IOL improvement, but each lens design must be selected on the basis of its suitability for a given patient, and not all modifications invariably achieve the desired end point.

    b. Disadvantage. Although the reduced incidence of cystoid macular edema and retinal detachment following ECCE with PC IOL implantation is well documented, the technical difficulty of removing a PC IOL remains a major potential disadvantage of this type of implant. Fortunately, the need for explantation of PC IOLs has been far less than for all other styles of implants, and it is the hope of all ophthalmologists that this risk will remain a potential one.

4. Complications of AC and PC IOLs are rare, often self-resolving or resolved with medical therapy, and usually occur in fewer than 1% or 2% of patients. In order of approximate decreasing frequency, the most common complications are macular edema, secondary glaucoma, hyphema, iritis, corneal edema, pupillary block, retinal detachment, vitritis, endophthalmitis, and cyclitic membrane.

5. Foldable PC IOLs made of hydrogel or silicone are now the most commonly used lens after phacoemulsification surgery.

    a. Advantages of such lenses are (a) insertion through a small incision (3 to 4 mm); (b) good to excellent tolerance and flexibility; (c) hydrophilic properties that reduce endothelial damage through low interfacial energy; (d) autoclavability; (e) reduced astigmatism and faster rehabilitation due to smaller incisions; and (f) a thicker lens (silicone), which fills and distends the posterior capsular bag more fully, possibly decreasing the incidence of capsular haze (however, see sec. **VII.E.9.,** below).

    b. The disadvantages of the current generation of foldable PC IOLs occasionally reported are (a) a tendency to decenter, particularly after YAG posterior capsulotomy; (b) imperfect surface finishing, especially with silicone lenses (possible potential for UGH syndrome); (c) severe iris chafing; (d) weak tensile strength with lens tears and increased susceptibility to damage; (e) groove marks from insertion instruments; (f) tissue damage when lens is released from folding instrument; (g) visual acuity possibly decreased; (h) suboptimal insertion instruments and difficulty inserting lens without tissue damage; (i) pitting during YAG capsulotomy; (j) lack of UV filters in some models; and (k) unknown long-term effects on ocular tissues.

6. Multifocal PC IOLs. These lenses focus both near and far objects, placing images on the macula simultaneously. The brain decides which image to concentrate on via selective vision. Success is determined by whether the patient can distinguish between the two objects. For "best-case patients" in a U.S. Food and Drug Administration (FDA) study, 82% had near vision of J-1 to J-3 with distance correction only. A variety of styles are undergoing clinical trials. Thousands of multifocal lenses have been implanted worldwide, but adequate follow-up is needed to produce reliable safety and efficacy data.

7. **Contraindications to IOL implantation** include active, uncontrollable uveitis (see sec. **VII.G.,** below) or proliferative diabetic retinopathy, glaucoma with progressive visual field loss (although with PC IOLs this may be a relative contraindication), and youth. The lower limit of age at which it is safe to implant a lens is not known. Ophthalmologists in some centers are implanting lenses in children, and they are doing so according to carefully designed and monitored research protocols. Most centers regard 18 years of age as the limit below which patients may be too young for IOL implantation. There is considerable difference of opinion regarding this lower limit; some surgeons believe it to be too low, others too high. Other contraindications include aniridia and a history of IOL intolerance in a fellow eye, unless judged the result of suboptimal lens style or intraoperative complication. Over the years, the list of contraindications has decreased in size as surgical techniques and implant quality have improved.

8. **Results of IOL implantation** have been generally excellent, with final visual acuity of 20/40 or better in greater than 90% of AC and PC IOLs. PC IOLs may give slightly better results regardless of age by currently available studies (94% versus 90%). There is evidence, however, that ECCE surgery coupled with an AC IOL or suture-fixated PC IOL may give equally good results and should be considered in certain patients, e.g., pseudoexfoliation with weak zonules.

9. **YAG capsulotomy.** In patients over 65 years of age, the posterior capsule usually remains clear behind the optic. In younger patients, and in some older patients, the capsule often opacifies and must be opened. Before the advent of the YAG laser, the posterior capsulotomy with a PC IOL in place was a formidable surgical challenge. The YAG laser has simplified this procedure, however, and in fact has prompted lens manufacturers to place small ridges on the posterior surfaces of the optic to keep the capsule away from the surface of the optic and avoid inadvertent damage to the optic when the laser light is used to cut the posterior capsule. The laser ridge is probably not essential to successful lens design. If the lens dislocates sideways during normal postoperative fibrosis, however, otherwise-clear vision may be blocked by the ridge. It is possible to fracture or pit the optic with the YAG laser beam, but fortunately these small imperfections are usually insignificant. Photodisruptive powers used range from 0.6 mJ for thin capsules to 4.0 mJ for dense fibrous bands (usually posttraumatic).

F. **Postoperative care**

1. **Wound healing** occurs slowly over a 4- to 8-week period, but small refractive changes from further healing of the incision occur up to 9 months postoperatively. As corneal anesthesia decreases, contact lenses can be fitted if the patient did not receive an IOL. Nonabsorbable radial sutures may be cut or removed if protruding or inducing astigmatism usually between 6 and 8 weeks from ECCE wounds, and as early as 3 to 4 weeks from scleral tunnel wounds used for phacoemulsification; some are not removed. Topical corticosteroids used to control postoperative inflammation may retard healing slightly, but patients with sedentary jobs are often back to work in 3 to 5 days.

2. **Postoperative medications.** Patients undergoing general or local anesthesia often receive a subconjunctival injection of an antibiotic such as cefazolin (100 mg) and a steroid such as methylprednisolone (50 mg). A topical antibiotic ointment is instilled at the end of the procedure after topical anesthesia. If elevated pressure is anticipated, an oral carbonic

anhydrase inhibitor such as sustained-release acetazolamide 500 mg may be given immediately postoperatively, administered at bedtime, or both. A common postoperative regimen also includes antibiotic–steroid combinations initially qid and tapered over 3 to 4 weeks.

3. **Dressings.** An eye patch is used for only a few days postoperatively if topical anesthesia is not performed; a protective shield is worn for a few weeks at night to avoid injury to the eye during sleep.

4. **Activities and limitations.** Because of the advances in wound construction and suture materials, postoperative wound strength is sufficient to allow resumption of quiet daily activities with little risk of wound rupture. It is still prudent, however, to avoid contact sports, vigorous exertion, excessive bending from the waist, and heavy lifting for approximately 3 weeks after phacoemulsification and 6 weeks after ECCE.

5. **General medical considerations.** Constipation, coughing, and wheezing should be avoided. Any stressful diagnostic procedure, such as sigmoidoscopy, barium enema, pulmonary function studies, and exercise tolerance tests, should be delayed if possible for 3 to 6 weeks. Anticoagulant therapy can be resumed 1 or 2 days postoperatively if no bleeding is observed. Most topical medications used postoperatively (topical steroid drops and antibiotics) have minimal and easily recognizable systemic side effects. Carbonic anhydrase inhibitors used to treat postoperative glaucoma may lead to potassium depletion, depression, and cardiac arrhythmias. The control of diabetes mellitus is usually easily reestablished, but sometimes ocular and nonocular (headache, nausea, and vomiting) complications of cataract surgery may interfere with this.

G. **Cataract surgery in uveitis patients.** Posterior subcapsular cataracts are common complications of uveitis, particularly those with cyclitis. It is possible, however, to control the uveitis and place an **IOL** successfully in many of these patients through judicious use of perioperative antiinflammatory therapy.

Inflammation should be suppressed to 0 to 2 leukocytes per 0.2-mm-high slit beam in the aqueous or anterior vitreous for at least 3 months preoperatively. This may be done through the use of topical, periocular injected, and systemic corticosteroids, NSAIDs, and, where indicated, immunosuppressive agents. For the few days before surgery, patients may be treated with 1 mg/kg/day of oral prednisone with breakfast, diflunisal 500 mg p.o. bid, and topical 1% prednisolone or 0.1% dexamethasone qid along with continuation of any immunosuppressive therapy on which the patient may have been placed. If an IOL is to be placed, a posterior chamber IOL in the capsular bag is recommended to minimize uveal tissue contact. IOLs coated with heparin, a hydrophilic substance, have been shown to be less inflammatory in animals and may cause less inflammation in human uveitic patients. At the end of the surgical procedure, 80 mg of subconjunctival methylprednisolone is injected as well as an antibiotic such as 100 mg of cefazolin. Postoperatively, topical 1% prednisolone or 0.1% dexamethasone is used four to eight times daily, depending on the anterior chamber inflammation. Systemic prednisone is tapered and discontinued after the inflammation has cleared (unless the patient is maintained on this drug for systemic disease). Diflunisal is continued for 2 months postoperatively along with an immunosuppressive indicated for the primary disease.

H. **CME therapy.** A leading cause of visual loss after cataract extraction, occurring in about 3% to 5%, is aphakic or pseudophakic CME. Although the majority of affected eyes will ultimately regain good vision, CME prolongs the postoperative recovery period and causes concern for physician and patient alike.

1. **Etiology.** CME is a nonspecific response, which may result from a variety of ocular conditions, leading to a disruption of the blood–ocular barrier as well as clinical and histologic evidence of inflammation, particularly following cataract surgery. These factors include excessive or prolonged postoperative uveal inflammation, intraoperative vitreous loss, ICCE, and

ECCE with primary capsulotomy. Prostaglandins are unsaturated fatty acid derivatives formed from arachidonic acid. Their effects on the eye include disruption of the blood–ocular barriers, dilation of iris vessels, miosis, and alteration of the IOP. Prostaglandins are found in increased concentrations in the aqueous during cataract extraction and are hypothesized to be an etiologic factor in the development of postoperative CME.

2. **Aphakic CME** frequently undergoes transient periods of relapse and recovery and, although not entirely benign, is generally considered self-limited regardless of treatment regimen.

3. **Pseudophakic CME** is more persistent and often requires therapeutic intervention, although the natural history of this process is that in the absence of obvious anatomic precipitations (vitreous touch, IOL capture, etc.), most cases usually resolve within 6 months.

4. **Medical therapy** of CME is still a controversial topic, because there are few well-controlled studies. Corticosteroids (topical, periocular, or oral) have been used to treat CME even though there have been no prospective randomized trials demonstrating efficacy. Two prospective randomized trials have demonstrated improvement in visual acuity in chronic CME patients treated with ketorolac, one drop qid (Acular), an NSAID. (NSAIDs block production of prostaglandins.) One regimen that has been successful in numerous patients is flurbiprofen 0.03% (Ocufen), one drop to the affected eye q2h for 1 week followed by one drop q4h for 2 weeks. If improved, patients are then continued on flurbiprofen three to six times daily for 1 to 3 months, then bid for 8 to 12 months or for at least 2 months after fluorescein angiogram has shown resolution of CME. Systemic NSAIDs, e.g., naproxen 250 mg or indomethacin 25 mg p.o. tid, may also have a role in cases refractory to topical therapy. No prospective study has compared corticosteroids with NSAIDs in the treatment of CME. In addition, acetazolamide 250 mg p.o. qd and hyperbaric oxygen have both been shown to increase visual acuity in small uncontrolled studies of patients with aphakic or pseudophakic chronic CME.

I. **Optical correction of aphakia**

1. **Temporary cataract glasses** are dispensed to patients who have not received an IOL immediately postoperatively if the vision in the unoperated eye is poor. Although vision with these glasses is not perfectly clear, acuity is usually sufficiently good that patients accept them. Aphakic spectacles contain thick convex lenses; unavoidable optical aberrations with these lenses are (a) 30% to 35% magnification of objects in the field of view; (b) a dramatic restriction of the width of the visual field; (c) a circular zone around the central field in which the patient sees nothing; and (d) the annoying "jack-in-the-box" phenomenon, an apt term describing the manner in which objects in the blind circular paracentral field suddenly pop into view. If the patient's unoperated eye has good vision, usually he or she will reluctantly wear temporary or permanent cataract glasses for ambulation and driving because of these optical problems. It is not possible to use an aphakic lens over only the operated eye, because this would lead to intolerable diplopia based on image size discrepancy. It would also lead to tilting of the glasses, because the weight of the cataract lens is greater than the phakic lens. To many patients, monocular aphakia is a visual handicap far greater than the blurred but otherwise normal vision before cataract surgery. It is therefore advisable to defer cataract extraction of a unilateral cataract unless the patient has a mature lens, a lens-induced complication, or a willingness to use contact lenses or IOLs.

2. **Contact lenses** (soft, hard, gas permeable). Without going into the specific advantages and disadvantages of each form of contact lens, it is important to understand that contact lenses offer many advantages to the postoperative cataract patient who did not receive an IOL. Image magnification is usually less than 7% and does not lead to image size diplopia. Binocular fusion is possible, so depth perception is normal. Visual field

size is unrestricted, and none of the other optical disadvantages of apha-kic spectacles is present. Contact lenses may be more difficult to insert and remove, however, and the rate of contact lens failure increases with age. **Continuous-wear lenses** are available as hard, semisoft, and soft lenses. They may be worn continuously, being removed for cleaning only every 6 months in the ideally fitted patient. It is difficult, however, to pre-dict the likelihood of a successful fit. The success rate decreases with in-creasing age, climate (patients in dry, dusty areas do poorly), and intercur-rent illness (e.g., keratitis sicca, arthritis, senility, seborrheic blepharitis). Approximately 70% of all patients are successful with continuous-wear aphakic lenses (see Chapter 5, sec. **XI.,** and Chapter 14, sec. **VIII.**).

3. **IOLs,** which are placed in almost all patients who undergo cataract ex-traction, spare patients the challenge of wearing contact lenses and the op-tical aberrations associated with aphakic spectacles. Image magnification is usually less than 3% and visual field size is unrestricted. It is necessary, however, to measure corneal curvature and axial length of the eye accu-rately to select an IOL based on A-scan ultrasound calculations that will yield a refractive error postoperatively that is similar to the unoperated eye. It is not advisable to insert an "average" IOL, because many patients will have significant inequality of refractive errors postoperatively. Sev-eral techniques have been described to suture PC IOLs to the sclera in aphakic patients. This approach may offer several advantages over using AC IOLs, but the learning curve may be steep. The use of 10-0 Prolene sutures and modified IOLs with islets in the haptics has facilitated the surgical technique.

8. RETINA AND VITREOUS

Peter Reed Pavan and Deborah Pavan-Langston

I. **Normal anatomy and physiology** (see frontispiece)

A. **The retina** is the innermost layer of the eye and is derived from neuroecto-derm. It is composed of two layers: the outer **retinal pigment epithelium (RPE)** and the inner **neural retina,** with a potential space between the two layers. The RPE, a single layer of hexagonal cells, is continuous with the pigment epithelium of the pars plana and ciliary body at the **ora serrata.** The inner sensory retina is a delicate sheet of transparent tissue varying in thickness from 0.4 mm near the optic nerve to approximately 0.15 mm anteriorly at the ora serrata. The center of the **macula** contains the thin sloping **fovea** that lies 3 mm temporal to the temporal margin of the optic nerve. The macula is close to the insertion of the inferior oblique muscle and is made almost entirely of cones. It is the site of detailed fine central vision (20/20 normal). Visual acuity decreases rapidly in the paramacular areas and is only 20/400 at a distance of 2 or 3 mm from the fovea. The ora serrata is located 6 mm posterior to the corneoscleral limbus nasally and 7 mm temporally. The scleral insertions of the medial rectus and the lateral rectus serve as landmarks for the location of the ora serrata nasally and temporally.

Nutritional support for the sensory retina comes largely from the Müller cell, which spans almost the entire thickness of the retina. The inner two-thirds of the retina is nourished by the retinal vessels to the level of the outer plexiform layer. The outer one-third consists of the outer part of the outer plexiform layer, the photoreceptors and the RPE is nourished by the choriocapillaris of the choroid.

B. **Histology.** The retina consists of ten parts. Proceeding from the outside in, they are

   1. RPE.
   2. Photoreceptor cells (rods and cones).
   3. External limiting membrane.
   4. Outer nuclear layer.
   5. Outer plexiform layer.
   6. Inner nuclear layer.
   7. Inner plexiform layer.
   8. Ganglion cell layer.
   9. Nerve fiber layer.
   10. Inner limiting membrane.

C. **Physiology.** The neuronal component of the retina consists of rods and cones that transduce light signals into electric impulses, which are amplified and integrated through circuitry involving bipolar, horizontal, amacrine, and ganglion cells, and transmitted through the nerve fiber layer to the optic nerve.

D. **Vitreous.** The vitreous body, which makes up the largest volume of the eye, provides support for the delicate inner structures of the eye. It is limited by the lens anteriorly and by the ciliary body, pars plana, and retina posteriorly. The vitreous is a clear jelly-like substance consisting of a delicate framework of **collagen** interspersed with a hydrophilic mucopolysaccharide, **hyaluronic acid.** Delicate collagen fibrils attach the vitreous to the internal limiting membrane of the retina, the attachment being strongest around the ora serrata and at the optic disk and fovea.

II. **Tests of retinal function** (see Chapter 1, secs. **II.A., C., I.,** and **III.D., F.,** and **G.;** Chapter 13, sec. **I.A.**)

A. **Visual function** is classified under the terms *light sense, form sense,* and *color sense.* Scientifically, these characteristics of incident light striking the eye are analyzed in terms of spatial, luminous, spectral, and temporal functions.

1. **Visual acuity.** In clinical practice, form sense is assessed by use of tests such as the Snellen chart test (see Chapter 1, sec. **II.A.**). This test is primarily of macular function. It is subjective and depends on patient cooperation. Objective tests are of value in assessing visual acuity of infants, mentally disturbed patients, and malingerers. The amplitude of the visual evoked response (VER) or the optokinetic nystagmus response can be correlated with visual acuity. Thus, it is estimated that the visual acuity at birth is approximately 20/600 and improves by the age of 5 months to 20/60 and to adult levels by the age of 2 years.

2. **Visual fields.** Light sense is assessed by visual field examination, which reflects any damage to the visual pathway from the retina to the visual cortex. The conventional method of testing the visual field is called **kinetic perimetry** and consists of moving a target to identify points of equal retinal sensitivity. The normal visual field extends at least 90 degrees on the temporal side, 70 degrees nasally and inferiorly, and 60 degrees superiorly. **Static perimetry** involves the determination of the differential light threshold in chosen areas of the retina. This method is more sensitive and reproducible than kinetic perimetry (see Chapter 1, sec. **II.I;** Chapter 13, sec. **I.A.–F.**).

3. **Color vision.** The retinal cones mediate color vision. Many abnormalities of visual function are characterized by defects in color vision. The simplest and best-known method of testing color vision is by the use of *Ishihara* pseudoisochromatic plates. The Ishihara plates can only identify defects in red-green discrimination, whereas the American Optical *Hardy-Rand-Ritter* plates are useful in detecting red-green and blue-yellow defects. The Farnsworth-Munsell *100-hue* test and anomaloscopes are more sophisticated devices used in clinical research on color vision testing (see Chapter 1, sec. **II.C.**).

4. **Dark adaptation.** This test depends on the increase in visual sensitivity occurring in the eye when it goes from the light-adapted state to the dark-adapted state. The Goldmann-Weekers machine is used to plot the dark-adaptation curve. The eye to be tested is exposed to a bright light for 10 minutes and then all lights are extinguished. At intervals of 30 seconds, a measurement of light threshold is made in one area of the visual field by presenting a gradually increasing light stimulus until it is barely visible to the patient. The graph of decreasing retinal threshold against time shows an initial steep slope denoting cone adaptation and a subsequent gradual slope due to rod adaptation. Depression of the dark-adaptation curve occurs in conditions affecting the outer retina and RPE, such as retinitis pigmentosa.

5. **Fluorescein angiography** is the study of retinal and choroidal vasculature using fluorescein (see Chapter 1, sec. **III.D.**).

   a. **Technique.** Fluorescence is a physical property of certain substances that, on exposure to light of short wavelength, emit light of longer wavelength in a characteristic spectral range. Sodium fluorescein, a yellow-red substance, absorbs light between 485 and 500 nm in aqueous solution and exhibits a maximum emission between 525 and 530 nm. A 5-mL bolus of dye is rapidly injected via the antecubital vein, and rapid retinal photographs are taken with a fundus camera containing an excitatory filter with maximum transmission between 485 and 500 nm and a barrier filter peaking close to the maximum of the fluorescein emission curve (between 525 and 530 nm). The value of fluorescein angiography is based on the fact that fluorescein dye does not penetrate healthy RPE and normal retinal capillaries because of the tight endothelial junction present in the latter. Fluorescein does leak freely from the normal choriocapillaris. Under optimum conditions, the smallest retinal capillaries (5 to 10 μm in diameter) can be seen with this technique, a feat impossible by ophthalmoscopy or by color photography.

b. **Use in retinal and choroidal disease.** Fluorescein angiography is of particular value in elucidating small vessel disease such as diabetic retinopathy, outlining clearly such changes as microaneurysms, shunt vessels, and sites of early neovascularization. Vascular abnormalities within the retina commonly leak fluorescein because of damage to the endothelium. New vessels, both those anterior to the retina and those arising from the choroid under the retina, characteristically leak fluorescein because of the absence of tight endothelial junctions. Angiography provides a valuable means of identifying such vessels in macular degeneration, diabetes, sickle cell disease, and retinal vein obstruction. It also provides a means of assessing the efficacy of treatment, particularly photocoagulation, in eliminating these vessels and in sealing leaks from vascular abnormalities within the retina, as in clinically significant diabetic macular edema.

c. **Use in RPE and optic nerve evaluation.** Although angiography does not provide any clue regarding the function of RPE, it anatomically delineates the true extent of RPE atrophy in diseases affecting RPE, such as rubella, retinitis pigmentosa, and age-related macular degeneration. Angiography is also helpful in distinguishing early papilledema, in which both the superficial and deep vascular networks become dilated and leak fluorescein, from "full" disks or disks with buried drusen. Papillitis shows many of the fluorescein characteristics of early papilledema. In optic atrophy, a loss of vessels occurs in both the superficial and the deep networks.

6. **Electrophysiology.** There are three major electrophysiologic tests used in the investigation of the visual system (see also Chapter 1, secs. **III.F.** and **G.**).

a. **Electrooculography (EOG)** measures slow changes in the standing potential of the retina caused by the interaction of the RPE with the photoreceptors. Electrodes are attached to the skin over the orbital margin opposite the medial and lateral canthi, and the potential difference between the electrodes is amplified and recorded, after both light and dark adaptation as the patient is asked to look back and forth at targets to the right and left. The maximum height of the potential in light divided by the minimum height of the potential in dark gives the **Arden** ratio, which is normally 1.85 or greater. Its principal diagnostic usefulness is in distinguishing Best vitelliform degeneration (in which the ratio is abnormal but the electroretinography [ERG] is normal) from other macular diseases such as Stargardt's disease or pattern dystrophies.

b. **ERG** reflects the chain of graded electric responses from each layer of the retina. The human response, for clinically useful purposes, is a biphasic wave, an early negative a wave, generated by the rods and cones, followed by a larger positive b wave, generated in the Müller and the bipolar cell layer. The recording is done with a corneal contact lens electrode and a reference electrode on the forehead. Cone responses predominate under photoptic testing conditions when a bright flash stimulates the retina. Rod responses predominate in a scoptic environment when a dim flash is used. A bright flash under scotopic conditions elicits a combined response. In addition, the ERG can distinguish the differences in response between the rods and cones to flickering flash; only the cones respond at 30 Hz because they have a much higher temporal resolution than the rods. The ERG is very useful in evaluating early retinal function loss before ophthalmoscopic changes are evident. The ERG is normal in diseases involving only the ganglion cells and the higher visual pathway, such as optic atrophy.

c. **Visual evoked response (VER).** The VER is the response of the electroencephalogram recorded at the occipital pole and is a macula-dominated response, due to the disproportionately large projection of the macular retina in the occipital cortex. The VER can be recorded using an intense flash stimulation or a pattern stimulation. The VER is the only clinically objective technique available to assess the functional state of the visual system beyond the retinal ganglion cells. The flash VER can assess **retinocortical function in infants and demented or aphasic patients,** and it can distinguish patients with psychological blindness from those who have an organic basis for poor vision.

III. **Retinal vascular disease**

A. **Retinal vascular anomalies** cause loss of visual function primarily through incompetence of the endothelial lining of the anomalous vessels, permitting escape of exudate and, less often, blood into the retinal tissues and the subretinal space. The serous component of the exudate is resorbed, leaving behind clinically visible bright yellow deposits with sharp borders called *hard exudates,* often in the macular area. The presence of such deposits in the absence of leakage in the posterior pole on fluorescein angiography should lead to a search of the peripheral retina for a vascular anomaly. Effective methods of treatment of these lesions include *photocoagulation* and *cryotherapy,* with repeated freezing and slow thawing. More severe cases may require vitrectomy (hemorrhage), endolaser, and retinal reattachment. Photocoagulation can be effective even after serous detachment of the retina has occurred. Once the lesion is destroyed, the subretinal fluid will absorb. Retinal vascular anomalies may be classified as follows.

1. **Retinal telangiectasia or Coats's disease.** The basic lesion in Coats's disease is a congenital anomaly of the vasculature of the retina, manifested ophthalmoscopically as telangiectasias. There is a marked male predominance (85%), and more rapid progression in children under 4 years of age, simulating retinoblastoma. Fluorescein angiography shows an abnormally coarse net of dilated capillaries, often with irregular aneurysmal dilations, which leak fluorescein. The telangiectasis may involve superficial or deep retinal vessels and can be associated with hemorrhages and hard exudates. Even advanced cases may regress spontaneously. Retinal telangiectasia is usually unilateral. Patients with loss of central vision from subretinal or intraretinal exudation are ideal candidates for photocoagulation. There is a high incidence of recurrence after treatment; therefore, these patients should be followed indefinitely.

2. **Retinal angiomatosis or von Hippel-Lindau disease.** The basic lesion in the phakomatosis, von Hippel-Lindau disease, is a vascular hamartoma consisting of capillaries with proliferating endothelial cells, a feeding artery, and draining veins. This disease is bilateral in 50% of patients. It can occur spontaneously or be dominantly inherited. Partly through abnormal hemodynamics and partly through hypertrophy and hyperplasia of the constituent elements, these lesions may enlarge over a period of time. However peripheral the lesion may be, abnormal permeability can result in changes at the macular region, including development of hard exudates, retinal edema, and serous detachment. Repeated photocoagulation of the tumor will usually eliminate the exudation. Long-term follow-up is needed to detect new lesions. Treatment of angiomas on or near the temporal margin of the optic nerve head is difficult without destroying central vision. Appropriate systemic evaluation is necessary to detect associated central nervous system vascular abnormalities (hemangioblastomas), renal cell carcinoma, and pheochromocytoma (see Chapter 11, sec. **VIII.** for other phakomatoses).

3. **Retinal cavernous hemangioma** may arise in the retina or optic nerve head. The lesion is composed of clusters of saccular aneurysms filled with dark venous blood. Fluorescein angiography shows that these lesions do

not leak and that they have a sluggish blood flow. Dermal vascular lesions and intracranial lesions may be associated with this condition. Photocoagulation may be used when spontaneous hemorrhage occurs.

4. **Arteriovenous (AV) malformations,** a rare condition, have been called "racemose" or "cirsoid" angioma. There is a direct communication between the artery and vein with no intervening capillary bed. The retinal vessels appear dilated and tortuous. Smaller caliber malformations are well compensated, stationary, and usually do not require any treatment. Large-caliber AV malformations can have a breakdown of the blood–retinal barrier with development of macular edema. Photocoagulation may be of benefit in these cases. Severe cases of widespread AV malformations, often with face, orbit, and intracranial associations, are not amenable to therapy because of widespread retinal disorganization (i.e., **Wyburn-Mason syndrome**).

5. **Retinal macroaneurysms** occur in the retinal arteries of arteriosclerotic and often hypertensive elderly patients. The aneurysms appear as outpouchings of the arteriolar wall which leak on fluorescein angiography. They can bleed into the vitreal, retinal, subretinal, or subretinal pigment epithelial spaces. The blood will often resorb, and there will be no further hemorrhaging. The artery beyond the aneurysm may become sclerosed and occluded. If macular edema or exudate formation is present, gentle photocoagulation of the aneurysm without occluding the associated arteriole may help.

B. **Vascular retinopathies**
1. **Mechanisms of visual loss.** These diseases reduce vision through either **abnormal vascular permeability** or **retinal ischemia.** The former decreases vision principally through exudation of fluid into the macula. Clinically, exudation is seen as thickening of the retina, cystic changes in the retina, and/or as hard exudates. On fluorescein angiography, the leakage can be diffuse or specific, such as that coming from a microaneurysm.

Retinal ischemia is seen as capillary dropout on fluorescein angiography. Capillary dropout may correlate with areas of retinal whitening about one-quarter of a disk diameter in size. Because of their fuzzy or ill-defined edges, these lesions are sometimes called soft exudates. This feature plus their bright white appearance has also earned them the eponym **cotton-wool spots (CWSs).** A CWS results when there is interruption of axoplasmic flow in the nerve fiber layer. In ischemic retinal disease, this interruption is caused by a nerve fiber layer infarct secondary to closure of a precapillary arteriole. CWSs are seen in *diabetic retinopathy, hypertension, anemia, leukemias, collagen vascular diseases, dysproteinemias, endocarditis, preretinal macular fibrosis, and acquired immunodeficiency syndrome (AIDS).* Retinal ischemia may also correlate with widespread retinal whitening as seen in acute central retinal artery occlusion. More commonly, however, there is no retinal whitening in areas of capillary dropout, which can only be detected on fluorescein angiography.

Ischemia can cause visual loss in a variety of ways. Ischemic areas can contribute to leakage in the macula. The perifoveal capillary network may be partially or totally destroyed. **Vascular endothelial growth factor (VEGF)** released by partially ischemic tissue may induce the proliferation of new vessels on the disk or surface of the retina. These new vessels become tightly bound to the posterior vitreous. They leak fluid into it. This fluid induces contraction of the vitreous gel resulting in traction on the new vessels, which can then bleed into the vitreous cavity. Depending on the size of the hemorrhage, only a few floaters might be seen or there can be a sudden and severe decrease in vision. The blood components can cause further contraction of the vitreous and further bleeding, setting up a vicious cycle of recurrent hemorrhaging. In addition to, or instead of, inducing vitreous hemorrhaging, the traction can lead to pulling and detachment of the retina under and around the new vessels *(traction retinal detachment)*. If the fovea is involved, vision will decrease. Retinal ischemia may also induce new vessel formation on the iris and trabecular meshwork blocking Schlemm's canal, leading to severe pressure elevations *(neovascular glaucoma)*. In diabetic retinopathy, posterior proliferative changes predominate with vitreous hemorrhaging and traction retinal detachments, whereas in central retinal vein occlusion, neovascular glaucoma is more common. In artery occlusions, total ischemia with destruction of the perifoveal capillary network is the mechanism of visual loss. New vessel formation either anteriorly or posteriorly is rare, presumably because little VEGF is produced by totally ischemic tissue.

2. **Management** of the vascular retinopathies consists of treatment of the underlying medical condition. Depending on the underlying cause, *laser photocoagulation* has been shown in controlled clinical trials to be of visual benefit in treating the exudation of fluid into the macula and the retinal complications of the partial ischemia by reducing or eliminating new vessel growth. Pars plana vitrectomy is useful in managing vitreous hemorrhages and traction retinal detachments.

3. **Hypertensive retinopathy.** The retinal changes in hypertension are essentially the same as in the retinopathies seen in the collagen diseases and are secondary to local ischemia. At least 50 million Americans suffer from hypertension, with its effects on the arteries of the heart, brain, kidneys, and the retina.

   a. **Pathology.** Essential hypertension is associated with thickening of the arteriolar wall caused by hypertrophy of muscle fibers in the media. There is no intima in ocular arterioles. Sustained elevations of blood pressure cause necrosis of vascular smooth muscle and seepage of plasma into the unsupported wall through a damaged endothelium. Angiography at this stage will demonstrate a focal leak of fluorescein. Progressive plasma insudation into the vessel wall with further muscle necrosis results in secondary occlusion and the typical picture of advanced **fibrinoid necrosis.**

   b. **Clinical findings**

      (1) **Retinal.** In its milder forms, hypertension causes increased arteriolar light reflexes called copper and silver wiring. Thickening of the common adventitial sheath compresses venules where they pass under the arterioles and causes **arteriovenous (AV) nicking.** In its extreme form, this compression can cause a **branch retinal vein occlusion (BRVO)** (see sec. **III.B.4.a.,** below). With higher levels of blood pressure, intraretinal hemorrhages (typically flame shaped, indicating they are in the nerve fiber layer), CWSs, and/or retinal edema are seen. **Malignant hypertension** is characterized by papilledema, and with time, a macular star figure.

      (2) **Choroidal.** Young patients with acute, severe elevations in blood pressure from pheochromocytoma, preeclampsia, eclampsia, or accelerated hypertension can develop **hypertensive choroidopathy.** Pale or reddish areas of RPE (Elschnig spots) indicate poor choroidal perfusion. Focal serous or large exudative retinal detachments occur in more severe disease.

   c. **Prognosis.** Serious impairment of vision does not usually occur as a direct result of the hypertensive process unless there is local arteriolar or venous occlusion. Patients with hemorrhages, CWSs, and edema without papilledema have a mean life expectancy of 27.6 months. With papilledema, life expectancy is 10.5 months.

4. **Venous retinopathy.** Retinal vein occlusion can manifest itself as a **central retinal vein occlusion** (CRVO), in which the site of occlusion

is behind the cribriform plate, or as a **branch retinal vein occlusion (BRVO),** in which the occlusion is anterior to the cribriform plate. Obstruction of outflow occurs in retinal vein occlusion, resulting in an increase of intravascular pressure and stagnation of flow. The increase in intravascular pressure is responsible for the **edema, abnormal leakage, and hemorrhage** leading to the formation of **collaterals** over several weeks. Stagnation of flow is manifest by delayed perfusion, leading to ischemia of endothelial cells and the surrounding retina, resulting in capillary nonperfusion and **CWSs.** The development of large areas of capillary closure stimulates the growth of new vessels. In BRVO, these new vessels are usually at the junction of the normal and ischemic retina. They can lead to vitreous hemorrhage. In CRVO, the new vessels are usually on the iris and trabecular meshwork and cause neovascular glaucoma.

a. **BRVO**

(1) The **site of occlusion** in BRVO is usually at AV crossings. Thickening of the arteriolar wall within the common adventitial sheath around the two vessels compresses the venule and induces thrombosis. When a BRVO is not at an AV crossing, vasculitis should be suspected.

(2) **Conditions predisposing** to BRVO are systemic arterial **hypertension,** cardiovascular disease, increased body mass index at age 20 years, and glaucoma. The superotemporal quadrant is affected more than 60% of the time. The clinical picture consists of superficial and deep intraretinal hemorrhages with a variable number of CWSs indicating areas of focal retinal infarction. Subhyaloid and vitreous hemorrhages occur rarely.

(3) The **natural history** of BRVO varies from complete resolution with no long-term visual difficulties to severe visual loss. Patients presenting acutely should be followed for at least 3 months to allow for the development of collaterals and spontaneous improvement. In general, about 55% of patients retain vision of 20/40 or more after 1 year. In those who do not, the most common causes are **macular edema** and **preretinal neovascularization.** Macular edema occurs in 57% of cases with temporal branch occlusion. The Branch Vein Occlusion Study showed that **photocoagulation** was effective treatment of macular edema in patients who had had a BRVO for at least 3 months, acuity 20/40 or worse, and an intact perifoveal capillary network. This same study showed that panretinal photocoagulation in the distribution of the occluded vein significantly lessened the chance of a vitreous hemorrhage in eyes that developed retinal or disk neovascularization. For macular disease, a light grid pattern of 100- to 200-μm spots is given to areas of leakage identified by fluorescein in the macular region extending no closer to the fovea than the edge of the foveal avascular zone and not extending peripheral to the major vascular arcade. Areas of dense intraretinal hemorrhage are avoided. There is no effective treatment for visual loss secondary to macular ischemia.

b. **CRVO**

(1) **Clinical course.** CRVO presents a wide spectrum of clinical appearances. The variations depend on the severity of obstruction of venous outflow. In the mildest cases, minimum dilation of veins and hemorrhages are present with little macular edema and little decrease in vision. In the severe cases, vision may deteriorate to hand motions, with extensive deep and superficial hemorrhages with stagnant blood columns in grossly dilated veins and numerous CWSs throughout the fundus. Mild to severe disk edema may be present. As in BRVO, the principal vascular response in CRVO

consists of dilation of retinal capillaries, abnormal vascular permeability, and retinal capillary closure. *Macular edema* is often present in the *nonischemic* CRVO with dilated, leaking capillaries. *Ischemic* CRVO is characterized by widespread capillary closure as demonstrated on fluorescein angiography. Serious neovascular complications are common, leading to *rubeosis iridis and neovascular glaucoma.* If it is going to occur, rubeosis iridis and/or neovascularization of the angle is usually visible within 6 months of the occlusion. The incidence of the latter complication depends upon the amount of retinal ischemia. In eyes with less than 10 disk areas of nonperfusion, less than 10% will develop rubeosis or angle neovascularization. In eyes with more than 80 disk areas of nonperfusion, approximately 50% will have rubeosis or angle neovascularization on follow-up.

(2) **Diseases predisposing to CRVO** include cardiovascular disease, systemic hypertension, diabetes, and open-angle glaucoma. Increased physical activity lowers the chance of a CRVO as does the use of estrogen in postmenopausal women.

(3) **Differential diagnosis.** There are four conditions from which CRVO must be differentiated.

(a) **Venous stasis retinopathy or retinopathy of carotid occlusive disease** has been described in patients with internal carotid stenosis or occlusion. Unlike CRVO, venous stasis retinopathy is characterized by the presence of only mild hemorrhages, arterial dilation, and the absence of disk hyperemia. The hemorrhages are typically in the midperiphery and appear as large (greater than or equal to one disk diameter), round blots.

(b) **Hypertension** often coexists with CRVO. Severe hypertensive retinopathy, however, is usually bilateral and often symmetric with superficial hemorrhages and a macular star of hard exudates present. Retinal hemorrhages do not extend to the periphery as in CRVO. Severe macular edema and visual loss are rare in hypertensive retinopathy.

(c) **Hyperviscosity syndromes** such as macroglobulinemia, leukemias, polycythemias, and some hyperlipemias show a clinical picture similar to CRVO. These conditions are usually bilateral with few hemorrhages and little macular edema.

(d) **Diabetic retinopathy** is usually bilateral. Beading and reduplication of the vein is rare in CRVO.

(4) **Treatment.** Underlying medical conditions such as hypertension, elevated blood sugar, or congestive heart failure should be corrected. Increased intraocular pressure (IOP) in either the involved or uninvolved eye should be corrected. Focal photocoagulation for macular edema does not improve acuity. A careful *undilated* slitlamp examination and gonioscopy should be done every month for 6 months. If neovascularization is detected, give panretinal photocoagulation promptly to prevent neovascular glaucoma. Eyes presenting with good vision (>20/40) have a fair chance of retaining good vision. Eyes with poor vision are more likely to have widespread ischemia, are not likely to recover their vision, and have an increased incidence of rubeosis and angle neovascularization.

5. **Diabetic retinopathy** is the leading cause of new cases of blindness in the United States in patients between the ages of 20 and 74. In the developing Western countries, at least 12% of all blindness is due to diabetes. In the United States, a diabetic patient has more than a 20-fold chance of becoming blind compared to a nondiabetic counterpart.
a. **Risk factors.** The duration of insulin-dependent diabetes is the main

factor in the appearance of diabetic retinopathy. When diabetes is diagnosed before age 30 years, the risk of developing retinopathy is about 2% per year. After 7 years and 25 years, 50% and 90% of diabetic patients, respectively, will have some form of retinopathy. After 25 to 50 years of diabetes, 26% will have the proliferative form. Puberty and pregnancy both stimulate development of retinopathy. The 10-year rate of vision loss to less than 20/40 bilaterally is about 10% in juvenile diabetics, 38% in adult-onset, insulin-dependent disease, and 24% in adult-onset, non-insulin-dependent diabetes. The Diabetes Control and Complications Trial (DCCT) showed that intensive insulin treatment to *control blood sugar levels tightly* decreased the risk of developing severe nonproliferative or proliferative retinopathy and reduced the need for laser surgery by about 50%.

b. Types of diabetes

   (1) Type I (juvenile onset) diabetes cases are autoimmune (pancreatic destruction) and have a high risk for developing severe proliferative retinopathy.

   (2) Type II (adult onset) cases have normal to high insulin production but insulin-resistant receptor cells. There are more type II patients with blinding sequelae because of the greater number of type II diabetic patients.

c. Medical evaluation. Every diabetic patient deserves the benefit of a comprehensive evaluation, with careful attention paid to determine the presence of symptoms of diabetic retinopathy such as decreased vision, distortion of vision, loss of color vision, and the presence of floaters. The duration of diabetes and the method of control of diabetes should be assessed. The presence of associated systemic disease should be noted. Hypertension is present in 20% of insulin-dependent diabetics and in 58% of non-insulin-dependent diabetics. Optimal medical control is key to minimizing ocular and systemic complications.

d. Clinical appearance. Diabetic retinopathy is classified into four groups.

   (1) Background retinopathy (nonproliferative retinopathy). The diabetic lesions of background retinopathy are dilated veins, intraretinal hemorrhages, microaneurysms, hard exudates, edema, and CWSs. Dot-blot hemorrhages, retinal edema, and hard exudates result from increased vascular permeability. Microaneurysms cluster around areas of capillary nonperfusion.

   (2) Preproliferative diabetic retinopathy represents the most severe stage of background retinopathy (nonproliferative retinopathy). Preproliferative retinopathy is categorized by the presence of many intraretinal hemorrhages and microaneurysms, intraretinal microvascular abnormalities (dilated vessels within the retina), and venous beading. There is widespread capillary closure. Approximately 10% to 50% of patients with preproliferative retinopathy develop proliferative retinopathy within a year.

   (3) Proliferative diabetic retinopathy occurs in 5% of patients with diabetic retinopathy. In the proliferative stage, vascular abnormalities appear on the surface of the retina or within the vitreous cavity, starting postequatorially. Visual loss can be severe. New blood vessels grow on the surface of the retina and the optic nerve and are usually attached to the posterior hyaloid surface of the vitreous body. In the cicatricial stage, contraction of the vitreous body causes traction on the retinal neovascularization, resulting in vitreous hemorrhage and/or traction retinal detachment.

   (4) Diabetic maculopathy may result from increased vascular permeability with or without intraretinal lipoprotein deposits (hard exudates), or, less commonly, from ischemia due to closure of foveal capillaries. Diabetic maculopathy may be seen in any phase of retinopathy except for very early background disease.

e. **Pathology.** Histology of eyes with diabetic retinopathy shows loss of intramural pericytes and extensive capillary closure in trypsin-digest flat preparations of the retina. The blood–retinal barrier is compromised mainly by defects in the junctions between abnormal vascular endothelial cells. The most widely accepted working hypothesis for the pathogenesis of proliferative retinopathies such as diabetes, retinopathy of prematurity (ROP), and CRVO is that retina rendered ischemic by widespread capillary closure elaborates ***VEGF,*** which stimulates retinal neovascularization and/or rubeosis of the iris.

f. **Management.** Diabetic eyes should be inspected for rubeosis with a slitlamp before the pupil is dilated because fine vessels on the iris are almost impossible to see once mydriasis is induced. Gonioscopy is necessary if new vessels are seen on the surface of the iris with the slitlamp. To properly inspect the retina, wide pupillary dilation is needed. Diabetic retinas are best examined using a binocular viewing system which provides moderate magnification such as a slitlamp at 10× in conjunction with a 90-D lens to allow the detection of retinal thickening and tractional retinal detachments with stereoscopic vision. It is important to have the patient look in various fields of gaze so the more peripheral retina to the equator can be inspected, because approximately 27% of retinal abnormalities are found outside the central 45-degree area. Indirect ophthalmoscopy provides a view of the retina at, and anterior to, the equator. Color photography is used to document the progress or regression of retinopathy following treatment. Fluorescein angiography defines areas of leakage and ischemia, and confirms the presence of neovascularization of the retina or disk.

(1) **Three major clinical trials** have been carried out by the National Eye Institute to determine the retinal history of nonproliferative and proliferative diabetic retinopathy, as well as guidelines for treatment.

(a) The **Diabetic Retinopathy Study (DRS)** showed that scatter argon laser photocoagulation (panretinal photocoagulation [PRP]) reduced the incidence of severe visual loss (vision less than or equal to 5/200) by half or more in eyes with **neovascularization** on the disk or within one disk diameter of the disk. A similar reduction in the rate of severe visual loss was obtained in eyes with neovascularization elsewhere associated with vitreous hemorrhage.

(b) The **Early Treatment Diabetic Retinopathy Study** showed that eyes with *clinically significant macular edema* benefited from focal argon laser to discrete areas of leakage and grid photocoagulation to areas of nonperfusion or diffuse leakage. Moderate visual loss was defined as a doubling of the visual angle; e.g., going from 20/20 to 20/40. Laser treatment reduced the risk of such visual loss by 50% or more, increased the chance of improved vision, and had only minor visual field effect. Focal photocoagulation for vision-threatening macular edema should be given before scatter photocoagulation (PRP) for approaching high-risk proliferative retinopathy. Aspirin had no clinical effect. Observation only was indicated for eyes with mild to moderate nonproliferative retinopathy.

(c) The **Diabetic Retinopathy Vitrectomy Study** showed that type I diabetic patients with recent, severe **vitreous hemorrhage** associated with vision equal to or less than 5/200 undergoing early vitrectomy (within 6 months) had a notably better chance of attaining 20/40 or better vision than those whose vitrectomy was deferred a year. Type II or mixed diabetic patients did not benefit from early vitrectomy for severe vitreous hemorrhage. Patients with severe proliferative retinopathy with vision equal to or greater than 10/200 had a better chance of attaining 20/40 or better vision if they had early vitrectomy than those managed with conventional therapy.

(2) **Follow-up and management guidelines for diabetic retinopathy, as recommended by the American Academy of Ophthalmology**

    (a) Normal or rare microaneurysms: annual examination, good diabetic control.

    (b) Mild nonproliferative diabetic retinopathy (NPDR) (few hemorrhages and microaneurysms in one field or several fields, but no macular edema or exudates): examination every 9 months, good diabetic control.

    (c) Moderate NPDR (hemorrhages and/or exudates in all fields, intraretinal microvascular abnormalities [IRMAs] or CWSs): examination every 6 months, good diabetic control.

    (d) Severe NPDR (one or more of the following: severe number of retinal hemorrhages and microaneurysms, moderate IRMAs, venous beading): examination every 4 months.

    (e) Macular edema at any time: examination every 3 to 4 months, focal laser if clinically significant edema develops.

(3) Clinically significant **macular edema** includes any of the following features:

    (a) Thickening of the retina at or within 500 μm of the center of the macula.

    (b) Hard exudates at or within 500 μm of the center of the macula.

    (c) Zones of retinal thickening one disk area or larger, any part of which is within one disk diameter of the center of the macula.

        Appropriate argon laser photocoagulation reduces the risk of visual loss substantially.

(4) **Non-high-risk proliferative diabetic retinopathy** occurs when there are any new vessels but the eye does not yet have **high-risk characteristics (HRC)** as defined by the DRS. These eyes should be followed every 2 to 3 months. In patients with bilateral non-high-risk proliferative retinopathy, PRP should be considered in one eye.

(5) **Proliferative retinopathy with HRC.** Panretinal laser photocoagulation is the treatment of choice for this stage, which is characterized by one or more of the following.

    (a) Neovascularization on or within one disk diameter of the disk greater than one-fourth to one-third of the disk area.

    (b) Vitreous or preretinal hemorrhage associated with less extensive neovascularization of the disk (NVD) or neovascularization elsewhere (NVE) one-half disk area or more in size.

(6) **Laser applications.** The risk of severe visual loss in patients with HRC is substantially reduced by means of **panretinal laser photocoagulation** done with the argon green laser. If nuclear sclerotic cataract or vitreous hemorrhage is present, there is less wavelength absorption with yellow or red lasers, such as the Krypton. The goal is to achieve regression of existing vessels and inhibition of new vessel growth. Treatment is commonly done in two to four stages separated by 1 or more weeks. Typically, 400 to 600 burns of 500-μm diameter are placed in the retinal periphery in one session. They come to within 500 μm of the disk on

the nasal side. To preserve central vision, none are placed within two disk diameters of the center of the macula. To preserve peripheral field, burns are placed one to one-half burn width apart. The duration of each burn is 0.1 to 0.2 seconds and the power is adjusted to achieve definite retinal whitening. Flat new vessels away from the disk receive confluent burns. Areas of significant fibrosis, traction retinal detachment, and vitreous or preretinal hemorrhage are avoided. If proliferative diabetic retinopathy continues to be active despite panretinal laser photocoagulation in all quadrants, additional laser spots may be added between, or anterior to, the old laser scars. *Panretinal cryoablation* is useful in selected patients. If a blinding vitreous hemorrhage occurs despite these measures or before laser can be given, pars plana vitrectomy should be performed within 6 months in type I diabetics. Intraoperative laser photocoagulation is often performed when these patients undergo pars plana vitrectomy. If B-scan ultrasonography suggests an underlying traction retinal detachment of the macula, vitrectomy should be done in all patients. Of course, when a recent traction *macular detachment* or a combination traction and rhegmatogenous *retinal detachment* is present even when there is no vitreous hemorrhage, vitreous surgery is indicated.

PRP is not necessary in phakic eyes if there is peripupillary rubeosis but no abnormal new vessels on the trabecular meshwork. Such eyes should be followed every 3 months. If there are new vessels in the angle, the eye is aphakic, or the eye is pseudophakic with a broken posterior capsule, prompt PRP is needed to prevent neovascular glaucoma even when proliferative diabetic retinopathy with HRC is absent.

Focal macular laser therapy for clinically significant macular edema commonly uses 100- to 200-μm spot sizes and 0.1-second duration. The goal is to change the color of leaking microaneurysms through direct treatment; grid treatment is given to areas of diffuse leakage and ischemia. Leaks within 500 μm of the center of the macula are usually not treated with the laser unless previous treatment has failed, vision is less than 20/40, and treatment will not damage the perifoveal capillary network on the edge of the foveal avascular zone.

6. **Sickle cell retinopathy.** The mutant hemoglobins S and C are alleles of hemoglobin and cause sickle trait (HbAS), sickle cell disease (HbSS), and hemoglobin SC disease in 8%, 0.2%, and 0.2% of patients, respectively; most patients affected by these alleles are African-American. Sickle cell thalassemia (S Thal), in which beta polypeptide chain synthesis is severely depressed as well as defective, is rare (0.03%). The initial event in the retinopathy is intravascular sickling, hemostasis, and thrombosis. Any hemoglobinopathy may cause nonproliferative or proliferative retinopathy, but severe proliferative disease is more common in HbSC and S Thal than HbSS, which causes more systemic complications. The incidence of significant visual loss is about 4%.

   a. **Diagnosis** is by positive sickle test and hemoglobin electrophoresis, which is the only way to distinguish homozygous from heterozygous disease.

   b. **Nonproliferative sickle retinopathy** is characterized by salmon patch hemorrhages occurring after peripheral retinal arteriolar occlusion; refractile spots, which are resorbed hemorrhages leaving hemosiderin deposition; and black sunburst lesions, which are areas of RPE hypertrophy and hyperplasia with posthemorrhage hemosiderin. Central retinal artery occlusion (CRAO) may also occur with or without retinopathy.

    c. **The five progressive stages** of proliferative sickle cell retinopathy are

    (1) Peripheral arteriolar occlusion due to intravascular sickling.

    (2) Peripheral arteriovenous anastomosis.

    (3) Sea fan (retinal arterial) neovascularization, which is most frequent at about the equatorial plane superotemporally. Fluorescein angiography is valuable for detecting early sea fans.

    (4) Vitreous hemorrhage.

    (5) Retinal detachment, which usually begins in areas affected by fibrovascular proliferation and local vitreous traction.

    d. **Treatment.** Application of low-energy scatter argon laser photocoagulation to the involved ischemic areas induces regression in neovascular fronds. Application of high-energy laser photocoagulation to close fronds is **not recommended** because of the high incidence of complications such as hemorrhaging, choroidal ischemia, and neovascularization with vitreal extension and retinal detachment. Peripheral **cryotherapy,** causing mild retinal whitening of the nonperfused areas, is an alternative mode of therapy. Pars plana vitrectomy is useful in treating patients with vitreous hemorrhage. Special precautions should be taken if retinal detachment surgery is undertaken, because these eyes are prone to develop **anterior segment ischemia.** These measures include nasal oxygen, omission of vasoconstrictors such as epinephrine from local anesthetics, and avoidance of elevated IOP at all times. Sparing use of cryotherapy is preferable to extensive applications. Diathermy should be avoided. Muscles should not be detached. Subretinal fluid is drained where technically possible. A segmental scleral buckle is preferable to one with an encircling band. The rate of anterior segment ischemia is greatly reduced if vitrectomy is done in combination with, or instead of, a scleral buckle. This allows complete control of the IOP so the pressure spikes associated with conventional buckling are avoided and intraocular sickling is prevented. Epinephrine is omitted from the intraocular irrigating solutions. With vitrectomy, the partial exchange transfusions used in the past are usually not necessary.

7. **Retinopathy of prematurity (ROP)** (see Chapter 11, sec. **XIV.**)
8. **Ischemic retinopathies**

    a. **Cotton wool spots (CWSs)** are seen in the early stages of ischemic retinopathies and are local infarcts of the inner retina. They fade over 2 to 3 months.

    b. **Systemic etiology** should be searched for in any patients with CWSs. Although diabetes, AIDS, and hypertension are the most frequent associated disorders, CWSs also occur in collagen vascular diseases such as dermatomyositis, systemic lupus erythematosus, polyarteritis nodosa, and giant-cell arteritis. Other conditions where CWSs are found include cardiac valvular disease, radiation retinopathy, carotid occlusive disease, pulseless disease, syphilis, leukemia, trauma, metastatic carcinoma, intravenous drug abuse, sarcoid, ulcerative colitis, hemoglobinopathies, and partial retinal artery obstruction. With severe ischemia, development of optic disk and retinal neovascularization occurs.

    c. **Treatment.** In addition to treating the underlying systemic condition, photocoagulation may be used when the ischemic condition is well established, the guidelines being the same as in the management of proliferative diabetic retinopathy. To rule out *lupus erythematosus vasculitis,* lupus anticoagulant, an acquired serum immune globulin, should be considered in all patients with collagen vascular diseases, retinal artery occlusion, ischemic optic neuropathy, or transient visual loss or diplopia. It is important to recognize lupus anticoagulant in young and middle-aged patients not otherwise at high risk for stroke. Lupus anticoagulant and other vascular occlusive disease (see Chapter 9, sec. **V.B., C.**) may be screened for using anticardiolipin antibodies.

9. **Retinal arterial occlusion**

   a. The **branch retinal arterial occlusion (BRAO)** may take hours or days to become **clinically apparent** as an edematous, whitish retinal infarction in the distribution of the affected vessel. Ultimately, the vessel recanalizes, resolving the edema but leaving a permanent visual field defect in the area of damaged retina.

   b. **Central retinal artery occlusion (CRAO)** results in *infarction* of the inner two-thirds of the retina, reflex constriction of the whole retinal arterial tree, and stasis in all retinal vessels. CRAO may be preceded by *transient ischemic attacks* of visual blurring or blackout in embolic or inflammatory vasculitic disease, e.g., temporal arteritis. As in BRAO, bright cholesterol emboli (Hollenhorst plaques) from carotid atheromata may lodge at branch arterial bifurcations. The central infarct is ischemic; therefore, unlike retinal vein occlusion, hemorrhage is minimal. The retina at the posterior pole becomes milky white and swollen, and the choroid is seen through the fovea as a **cherry-red spot.** Usually the patient has painless loss of vision to 20/400 (unless the patient retains central vision via a cilioretinal artery supplying the papillomacular nerve fibers: 15% to 30% of patients). Vision with no light perception suggests choroidal ischemia due to **ophthalmic artery occlusion** in addition to the CRAO. Commonly, circulation is reestablished and the acute retina whitening resolves within a few weeks to months. The only clue that an eye without vision has had an old CRAO may be the loss of the B-wave with preservation of the A-wave on the ERG.

   c. **Histology.** The retinal cells undergo necrosis, disintegrate, and are phagocytosed by macrophages. These macrophages appear foamy because of the high lipid content of the retina. In time the edema and necrotic tissue are resorbed, leaving a thin retina with loss of bipolar cells, ganglion cells, and nerve fibers. Gliosis is minimal because glial cells are destroyed along with the nerve cells. Extensive hyalinization of the retinal vessels is seen in late stages.

   d. **Etiology.** The most common cause of retinal arterial occlusion is *embolization* of the retinal vascular tree due to emboli arising from the major arteries supplying the head or from the left side of the heart. The emboli may be fatty material from *atheromas,* calcium deposits from diseased heart valves, septic and nonseptic fibrin, and platelet thrombi. In the absence of visible emboli, other causes include *giant-cell (temporal) arteritis, collagen vascular diseases, oral contraceptives,* and increased orbital pressure in conditions such as *retrobulbar hemorrhage* and *endocrine exophthalmos.* Rare causes include *sickle cell disease* and *syphilis.*

   e. **Treatment.** Retinal arterial occlusion is an ophthalmic emergency, and prompt treatment is essential. Completely anoxic retina in animal models causes irreversible damage in about 90 minutes. However, because clinical occlusions may be partial, the following suggestions should be carried out immediately for anyone presenting within 24 hours of visual loss due to a CRAO. Specific precipitating events should be corrected; e.g., orbital decompression for acute retrobulbar hemorrhage or ocular hypotension for acute glaucoma. Nonspecific methods to increase blood flow and dislodge emboli include digital massage, 500 mg intravenous (i.v.) acetazolamide and 100 mg i.v. methylprednisolone (for possible arteritis). A 95% oxygen–5% carbon dioxide mixture has been recommended in the past to dilate retinal vessels. However, after initially dilating vessels, this mixture induces a severe acidosis. The acidosis, in turn, will cause vasoconstriction and may induce cardiac arrest. Consequently, any gas containing 5% carbon dioxide should be used very cautiously or, better yet, not at all. Additional measures include paracentesis of aqueous humor to decrease IOP acutely. A sedimentation rate should be drawn to detect possible temporal arteritis. Improvement can be determined by visual acuity and visual field testing, and by ophthalmoscopic examination. Patients with **transient blurring of vision (amaurosis fugax)** should have a thorough evaluation of the carotid artery. Amaurosis fugax demands urgent attention because it is a warning sign of an impending stroke. If carotid occlusive disease results in **ophthalmic artery occlusion,** general ocular ischemia may result in retinal neovascularization, rubeosis iridis, cells and flare, iris necrosis, and cataract. PRP appears effective in reducing the neovascular components and their sequelae [see sec. **III.B.5.f.(6), above**].

10. **Retinal vasculitis** is a complex group of conditions in which there is evidence of retinal vascular disease along with signs of inflammation such as cells in the aqueous or vitreous. Fluorescein angiography shows staining of the vessel walls with leakage, macular edema, and all the other signs associated with ischemic response of the retina. Retinal vasculitis is seen in a number of conditions such as **temporal arteritis, Behçet syndrome, lupus erythematosus, polyarteritis, inflammatory bowel disease (Crohn), multiple sclerosis, sarcoidosis, syphilis, pars-planitis, masquerade syndrome, toxoplasmosis,** and **viral retinitis. Eales's disease** is idiopathic retinal vasculitis and is responsible for idiopathic vitreous hemorrhage, especially in young males. The etiology of Eales's disease is obscure. Photocoagulation is of benefit if an ischemic response has been established with retinal and disk neovascularization.

11. **AIDS** (see Chapter 9, sec. **VIII.A.5.**)

IV. **Degenerative diseases of the macula.** Macular degenerations form the most common cause of patients being reported to the Registry of the Blind. Their treatment presents a formidable clinical challenge. Fluorescein angiography and photocoagulation in selected cases represent major advances in the classification and therapy of these conditions. The basic pathology in these conditions appears to be confined to the choriocapillaris, Bruch membrane, and the RPE. The sensory retina is affected secondarily, in contrast to retinal vascular disease, in which the sensory retina is affected primarily. The choroid and the RPE may be affected by inflammation or degeneration that can be the result of a variety of factors, such as vascular, metabolic, or toxic influences. The response of the macula can be either a serous (or hemorrhagic) detachment of the retina or a primary atrophic or degenerative response.

A. **Serous detachment of the macula**

1. **Central serous choroidopathy (CSC)**

a. **Clinical characteristics.** CSC, formerly called *central serous retinopathy,* usually occurs in young adult males and has an unknown etiology. The usual symptoms are decreased visual acuity, distortion, generalized darkening of the visual field, increased hypermetropia, and a decreased recovery from glare. Patients can be symptomatic even if their vision is 20/20. Ophthalmoscopy shows shallow detachment of the sensory macular retina, although the detachment may occur anywhere in the posterior pole. Fluorescein angiography demonstrates one or more points of progressive hyperfluorescence, demonstrating the site of origin of leakage through the RPE into the subretinal space. The leaking point may lie anywhere within the serous detachment and may or may not be associated with pigmentary changes seen clinically in the RPE.

b. **Differential diagnosis.** Serous detachment of the macula can occur in association with a **congenital pit of the optic disk** or **choroidal neovascular membrane.**

c. **Treatment.** The disease usually lasts 1 to 6 months and 80% to 90% of the patients recover good visual acuity, although mild metamorphopsia, color vision defects, and faint scotoma may persist.

The condition is not inflammatory in nature, and *systemic steroids are not indicated.* The duration of the disease, the initial visual acuity, the age of the patient, and laser treatment to the point of fluorescein leakage do not appear to have any effect on the final visual outcome. Almost all patients show some disturbance of the RPE, even after complete visual recovery. Duration of the disease for longer than 4 to 6 months, detectable morphologic changes in the retina (such as cystic edema and lipid deposition on the outer retinal surface), recurrence in eyes with previous CSC, and the need for prompt return of visual acuity are frequently accepted as indications for laser treatment to the point(s) of fluorescein leakage.

2. **Age-related macular degeneration (AMD;** formerly called *senile macular degeneration)* is the chief cause of vision loss in patients over 50 years old in the United States. This condition has both a *dry* and a *wet* form.

   a. **Dry AMD. Drusen** are the hallmark of **dry AMD.** They are commonly associated with RPE pigment mottling and geographic atrophy of the RPE and underlying choriocapillaris. Histologically, drusen are composed of basal laminar deposits and basal linear deposits. The basal laminar deposits are long-spacing collagen between the plasma membrane and the basement membrane of the RPE. Basal linear deposits accumulate in the inner part of Bruch membrane. They consist of electron-dense granules and phospholipid vesicles. Clinically, drusen appear as yellow deposits deep to the retina. Their size is variable. Larger drusen are serous elevations of the RPE and inner part of Bruch membrane. Drusen are often associated with RPE clumping and atrophy. Areas of complete loss of the RPE with sharp borders are called geographic atrophy. In these areas, the choriocapillaris is missing and the larger choroidal vessels stand out against the pallor of the underlying sclera. As long as the center of the macula is not involved with geographic atrophy, visual loss is usually mild in dry AMD.

   b. **Treatment** of **dry AMD** is symptomatic with stronger near adds and low-vision aids as required. Recently, The Age-Related Eye Disease Study (AREDS) published that patients with dry AMD who take *high-dose vitamins and zinc* have a reduced risk of developing visual loss from advanced or wet AMD (23% versus 29% in placebo-treated patients). To be considered for this therapy, patients should have at least one drusen >125 μm in diameter or noncentral geographic atrophy. If drusen are <125 μm in diameter, they must be >63 μm in diameter and cover an area >360-μm-diameter circle if soft indistinct drusen are present or an area >656-μm-diameter circle if soft indistinct drusen are absent. Patients with advanced AMD or vision loss due to AMD in one eye should be treated. The *doses of vitamins and minerals* were as follows: vitamin C 500 mg, vitamin E 400 IU, beta-carotene 15 mg, zinc 80 mg as zinc oxide, copper 2 mg as cupric oxide (copper should be taken with zinc because high-dose zinc is associated with copper deficiency). This represents about 5 times the usual intake of vitamin C from diet alone, 13 times the recommended daily allowance (RDA) for vitamin E, and 5 times the RDA for zinc oxide. Smokers and former smokers should probably not take beta-carotene because other studies have shown an increased incidence of lung cancer in smokers who take this supplement. In addition, *smoking is the one risk factor* consistently associated with any form of AMD.

   Patients with dry AMD should also be tested with Amsler grids. If they notice distortion of the lines on the grid, they should contact their eye care professional immediately.

   AMD is predominantly a disease of white persons, with an ill-defined inheritance pattern. When drusen are found in younger (<50 years old) individuals, they are sometimes called dominant or familial drusen, but the inheritance pattern is rarely proven. Some patients have cuticular or basal laminar drusen. Here the drusen are myriad, especially on fluorescein angiography, and tend to be smaller. These eyes are prone to develop a central, subretinal, yellowish, soft-edged, deposit about three-fourths of the disk diameter in size, or a so-called vitelliform lesion. It is surprising that vision often remains reasonably good (greater than or equal to 20/80). Drusen must also be differentiated from pattern dystrophies (see secs. **VI.B.5.** and **6.,** below). These patients have central yellowish deposits, sometimes in specific shapes such as a butterfly. These patients have a better prognosis than patients with AMD and usually retain good vision in at least one eye.

c. **Wet AMD.** Eyes with drusen or geographic atrophy which meet the AREDS criteria for treatment with vitamins and zinc (see sec. **IV.A.2.a.,** above) are at increased risk of developing the **wet type of AMD.** In this condition, the retina and RPE are detached from the underlying structures by serous fluid, and the subpigment epithelial space is occupied by blood vessels derived from the choroid, the so-called **choroidal neovascular membrane (CNV).** The CNV may cause subretinal and subpigment epithelial hemorrhages. The subsequent organization of these hemorrhages and/or the normal maturation of the CNV gives rise to a typical subretinal fibrovascular **diskiform scar,** most often located in the macular region. In contrast to dry AMD, eyes with wet AMD usually lose central vision fairly rapidly. The serous fluid leakage from the CNV detaches the RPE and/or the neurosensory retina, causing images to distort **(metamorphopsia).** The neurosensory detachment is often visible on careful binocular stereoscopic examination of the macula. Other signs of CNV on clinical exam include cystic changes in the central macula **(cystoid macular edema),** hard exudates, bright red subretinal blood, and dark gray subretinal pigment epithelial blood. Left untreated, the lesion will eventually develop into a white-appearing fibrous scar often associated with an extensive RPE atrophy and an overlying neurosensory detachment.

d. **Treatment of wet AMD** consists of obliteration of the CNV by **photocoagulation** as reported by the Macular Photocoagulation Study or treatment with **photodynamic therapy (PDT).**

(1) **Types of CNV.** CNV is identified and delineated by **fluorescein angiography.** CNV is divided into two types, classic and occult, by its appearance during this test. During the initial transit of dye, classic CNV displays early hyperfluorescence, which progressively increases in size and intensity. In some instances a lacy meshwork or a bicycle-wheel pattern of CNV can be identified before there is a progressive leakage of dye from the abnormal new vessels into the subretinal space, which obscures these details. Occult CNV does not fluoresce during the early phases of the fluorescein angiogram. Only late pooling of dye in the subretinal space is seen. Eyes with classic CNV lose vision faster than eyes with occult CNV.

(2) **Photocoagulation.** Because CNV and its complications may be responsible for up to 90% of severe visual loss (visual acuity of 20/200 or less) in AMD, and because AMD is responsible for 14% of all new cases of blindness in the United States in persons over the age of 65 years, in 1979 the National Eye Institute initiated a series of collaborative clinical trials of laser photocoagulation in the treatment of CNV. These studies demonstrated that laser photocoagulation is effective in reducing the risk of visual loss from extrafoveal choroidal neovascular membranes (CNM) (between 0 and 2,500 μm from the focal center). Treatment, which should be done as soon as possible after identification of the CNV by fluorescein angiography, consists of high-energy, contiguous **laser burns** over and adjacent to the CNV. After the initial treatment, patients

should be followed at close intervals with repeat fluorescein angiography because of a high risk of recurrence, and, if necessary, re-treated if residual or recurrent CNV is still present.

A wide variety of laser wavelengths are available to treat CNV. Blue wavelengths such as that found in unfiltered blue-green argon light should be avoided when working close (within 200 μm) to the center of the macula because these wavelengths are absorbed by the macular xanthophyll. If blue light is used, burns placed near the center spread into the center due to this absorption, causing unnecessary vision loss. Green lasers are now very popular because they are not absorbed by the macular xanthophyll; because green light is well absorbed by hemoglobin, making it a good choice to treat leaking microaneurysms in diabetic retinopathy; and because this wavelength is easily generated by diode lasers, which are compact, relatively inexpensive, mobile, and easy to maintain.

Thermal lasers burn the retina overlying the CNV, leaving a permanent blind spot. Partial treatment of CNV is not advised because it often results in accelerated growth of, or bleeding from, the residual, untreated portion. Hence, if CNV extends under the center of the macula, treatment results in an instantaneous, profound, and permanent visual loss. The Macular Photocoagulation Study showed that despite this loss, many patients were better off with such treatment because they would have even worse vision after 1 to 2 years if the CNV were left untreated. Nevertheless, this was an obviously less-than-ideal situation. Because many CNVs extend under the center of the macula, there was a great need to develop a way to treat subfoveal CNV without destroying either the overlying retina or underlying RPE–choriocapillaris complex that nourishes it.

(3) **Photodynamic therapy (PDT) or ocular photodynamic therapy (OPT).** In response to this need, OPT was approved by the U.S. Food and Drug Administration (FDA) for treatment of subfoveal CNV in AMD in the spring of 2000. A light-activated dye **(Verteporfin)** is infused intravenously over 10 minutes. This drug preferentially attaches to lipoproteins, which are concentrated in the actively proliferation capillaries of the CNV. Fifteen minutes after the start of the infusion, the CNV is illuminated with laser light, the wavelength of which (689 nanometers) photoactivates the Verteporfin. The time of exposure is 83 seconds at an intensity of 600 mW/cm^2 for a total dose of 50 J/cm^2. This amount of laser irradiation does not cause a thermal burn. The photoactivated Verteporfin converts normal oxygen to a highly energized form called "singlet oxygen." The singlet oxygen damages the endothelial cells of the CNV, causing their death and occlusion of the neovascular lesion.

The initial trials of Verteporfin OPT showed it was effective for primarily classic (greater than or equal to 50%) *subfoveal CNV in AMD.* Approximately 60% of Verteporfin-treated eyes lost less than 15 letters compared to only 30% of placebo-treated patients. It did not seem to work for minimally classic (less than 50% but greater than 0%) CNV. Lesions commonly recurred and the protocol called for repeat treatment at 3-month intervals if there was leakage on fluorescein angiography. An average of 3.4 and 2.2 Verteporfin treatments were given in the first and second years, respectively.

Subsequent publications have shown that Verteporfin OPT is effective in 100% occult subfoveal CNV secondary to AMD except in eyes with both large lesions (greater than 4 MPS [Macular Photocoagulation Study] disk diameters) and good acuity

(20/50 or better). Prospective, controlled trials have also shown eyes with subfoveal CNV secondary to pathologic myopia benefit from Verteporfin treatment. An open-label, uncontrolled trial showed improvement in acuity in treated eyes in patients with CNV secondary to the ocular histoplasmosis syndrome.

   e. **Other causes of CNV** include any disease that disrupts Bruch membrane, or CNV can occur without apparent cause (idiopathic). Some of the more common conditions associated with CNV are

   (1) **Ocular histoplasmosis syndrome** (see Chapter 9, sec. **VIII.D.**).

   (2) **High myopia.**

   (3) **Angioid streaks** are dark lines radiating from the region of the disk and represent breaks in Bruch membrane. Angioid streaks occur bilaterally and may superficially resemble retinal vessels in their appearance and course. They are associated with *pseudoxanthoma elasticum, Paget's disease of the bone* (osteitis deformans), *sickle cell disease, and Ehlers-Danlos syndrome.*

   (4) **Traumatic choroidal rupture.**

   (5) **Drusen of the optic nerve.**

   (6) **Retinal dystrophies** such as Best's vitelliform dystrophy.

B. **Pigment epithelial detachments (PED)** are classified as serous or fibrovascular. Serous PEDs are dome-shaped elevations of the RPE with sharp borders that fill early and uniformly with dye on fluorescein angiography. They are seen in CSC and in AMD. In CSC the prognosis for resolution and preservation of vision is good. In AMD, vision is usually fair until signs of associated CNV appear, such as subretinal pigment epithelial or subretinal blood, hard exudates, or irregular filling on fluorescein angiography. Fibrovascular PEDs are seen in AMD. They appear as a variable elevation or thickening of the RPE, which fills with dye irregularly and slowly during fluorescein angiography. The borders may be ill defined. These lesions are a form of occult CNV.

   No treatment is necessary for serous PED in CSC. Thermal laser ablation of extrafoveal serous PEDs and extrafoveal, well-defined, fibrovascular PEDs in AMD should be considered. Treatment of subfoveal serous PEDs in AMD can be delayed until signs of CNV develop. Then these lesions and subfoveal fibrovascular PEDs in AMD should receive Verteporfin OPT if the lesion meets the published criteria for treatment.

C. **Cystoid macular edema (CME)** is intraretinal edema with numerous cystoid spaces and is usually due to abnormal perifoveal retinal capillary permeability, although leakage can come from beneath the retina as in CNV. Vitritis and disk edema may be associated.

   1. **Numerous conditions are associated with CME,** including diabetic retinopathy, anterior or posterior uveitis, retinal vein occlusion (central or branch), retinitis pigmentosa, and ocular surgery (cataract [Irvine-Gass syndrome], keratoplasty, glaucoma procedures, scleral buckle, photocoagulation, and cryopexy). Intraocular lens implantation at extracapsular cataract surgery does not increase the risk of CME. CME usually occurs 6 to 10 weeks postoperatively and 75% of uncomplicated cases resolve spontaneously within 6 months. Surgical complications such as undue inflammation, vitreous loss, or iris prolapse increase the risk of CME and permanent vision impairment.

   2. **Medical treatment** includes topical, periocular, and systemic steroids, especially for established CME, but the recurrence rate is high when treatment is stopped, thus the condition often requires long-term, low-dose topical steroids and occasionally a periocular drug. Antiprostaglandin nonsteroidal antiinflammatory drugs such as topical ketorolac (Acular) or indomethacin 25 mg bid to qid orally (p.o.) are also useful over several weeks to months (see Chapter 9, sec. **VII.D.**). The carbonic anhydrase inhibitor, acetazolamide p.o. 500 mg per day, is effective in some cases and may be added for several weeks to any of the above

medications. Indomethacin p.o. 25 mg per day reduces the incidence of CME recurrence.

3. **Surgical treatment** has been shown to be effective in cases where there is vitreous entrapment in the inner aspect of a corneoscleral incision. Removal of the entrapped vitreous via pars plana vitrectomy will frequently eliminate the CME. Yttrium, aluminum, and garnet (YAG) laser lysis of such vitreous adhesions has not been shown to be effective in a controlled trial.

D. **Toxic maculopathies.** Certain drugs have a toxic effect on the macula by producing degeneration of RPE and loss of vision. It is important to detect these changes at an early stage, by either fluorescein angiography or electrophysiologic diagnostic tests (see Chapter 16).

1. **Chloroquine.** This aminoquinoline along with hydroxychloroquine is used in the long-term treatment of rheumatoid arthritis and lupus erythematosus. A total dose of 100 to 300 g or more of chloroquine leads to a toxic effect on the macula characterized by a horizontally oval area of RPE atrophy, giving rise to a bull's-eye appearance of the macula. Hydroxychloroquine is tolerated in large cumulative doses (1,000 to nearly 5,000 g) as long as the daily dose does not exceed 400 mg per day or 6.5 mg per kg body weight per day. **Bull's-eye maculopathy** can be detected at its earliest stages by *fluorescein angiography*. The earliest functional changes are a relative or absolute scotoma to red, red-green defect on the Ishihara color test, an abnormal EOG, and elevation of threshold on static perimetry.

2. **Thioridazine** also has toxic effects on the RPE. Patients receiving high doses (>1 g per day) may develop pigmentary retinopathy with central or ring scotomas and diminished photopic and scotopic responses of the ERG.

3. **Chlorpromazine,** when taken in large doses (>2 g per day for a year) may cause mild pigmentary changes of the retina with no significant functional deficits.

E. **Hereditary macular dystrophies.** A number of genetically transmitted conditions such as Stargardt's disease, Best vitelliform dystrophy, and cone dystrophy show a marked similarity in appearance to the toxic maculopathies (see sec. **VI.B.,** below).

F. **Vitreoretinal macular diseases.** Disturbances at the vitreoretinal interface are common causes of reduced central vision in elderly patients.

1. **Idiopathic preretinal macular fibrosis.** These patients, who present themselves with blurry vision and metamorphopsia (distorted vision), show a glinting reflex, traction lines (retinal striae), occasional CWS, and mild, gray preretinal fibrosis in the macula. These characteristics may arise spontaneously or may be related to vitreous detachment, or they may be secondary to local vascular or inflammatory changes. Preretinal macular membranes may also arise after photocoagulation or after retinal detachment surgery. Pars plana vitrectomy with peeling of the epimacular membrane is done if there is significant visual loss due to epimacular membranes.

2. **Senile macular holes.** Idiopathic macular hole is a common cause of reduced central vision in otherwise healthy patients, usually women, in the sixth and seventh decades. Full-thickness holes must be differentiated from "lamellar" holes, cysts, and pseudoholes in idiopathic preretinal macular fibrosis. If a full-thickness hole is present, the patient will commonly state there is a complete break in the middle of a thin line of light shone on the center of the macula (positive **Watzke-Allen sign**). Small cuffs of subretinal fluid often surround these holes, and they are commonly associated with CME and epiretinal membranes. Ten percent to 20% of patients will develop a hole in their second eye. These holes rarely give rise to extensive retinal detachment. The cause of this condition is abnormal vitreoretinal adhesion and traction to the center of the

macula. Vitrectomy with gas fluid exchange followed by face-down positioning can close a large number of holes and improve acuity. Peeling the posterior hyaloid, epiretinal membranes, or the internal limiting membrane increases the chance of hole closure.

V. **Retinal inflammatory diseases.** A variety of diseases cause inflammation primarily of the sensory retina, the RPE, or both the choroid and the retina. These diseases cause loss of central vision either by direct involvement of the macula or from secondary retinal edema or detachment from a paramacular lesion. Cells in the vitreous are always present.

A. **Infectious chorioretinitis.** A variety of **bacterial** and **fungal** agents can be carried to the retina and/or choroid as septic emboli. If the agent can be identified by cultures of blood, aqueous humor, or vitreous, and appropriate therapy instituted immediately, many of these eyes can be saved with maintenance of varying degrees of visual function. Intravitreal antimicrobials and/or **pars plana vitrectomy** may be used to supplement systemic therapy in selected cases (see Chapter 9, secs. **VIII.** and **XII.**).

CMV **retinitis** is commonly seen in AIDS patients with CD4 counts of less than 50. CMV retinitis must be differentiated from **progressive outer retinal necrosis (PORN)** and **toxoplasmosis.** CMV is associated with more intravitreal hemorrhage and less vitritis than toxoplasmosis. Like CMV, PORN has minimal vitritis. However, the retina lesions in PORN have less hemorrhage than CMV. In the early stages, they appear as large, deep, ovoid areas of retinal whitening with minimal involvement of the overlying retinal vessels. The cause is usually varicella-zoster virus. In immunocompetent individuals, the same virus causes **acute retinal necrosis** and **bilateral acute retinal necrosis.** Here there is marked vitritis and arteritis. Toxoplasmosis also occurs spontaneously in immunologically competent individuals. In this setting, acute retinal whitening is usually seen next to an old, pigmented toxoplasmosis scar, and there is an overlying focal vitritis. Syphilis should not be forgotten as a cause of retinitis in immunocompetent or immunocompromised patients. Therapy is available for all of these conditions (see Chapter 9, sec. **VIII.**).

B. **Infectious disease of the RPE.** Certain viral diseases appear to primarily involve the RPE.

1. **Rubella retinitis.** Children born of mothers who contracted rubella in the first trimester of pregnancy show a high incidence of salt-and-pepper mottling of the RPE. Multiple other ocular and other organ involvement may be present. In the absence of other ocular problems, such as cataracts or glaucoma, these children may have normal visual function. Fluorescein angiography shows mottled hyperfluorescence due to extensive and irregular loss of pigment.

2. **Acute posterior multifocal placoid pigment epitheliopathy (APMPPE),** appears to involve the RPE, particularly in the macular region, causing visual loss with subsequent spontaneous resolution and residual pigmentation. The affected patients are young (average age 25 years) and often have a history of viral illness preceding the onset of visual symptoms, although a specific agent has not been identified. Bilateral involvement is present. One or more flat, gray-white, subretinal lesions are present in the posterior pole. These lesions block out background choroidal fluorescence during the early stages, but stain in the late stages of fluorescein angiography. Healed, quiescent APMPPE may show extensive pigmentary changes and appear similar to atrophic macular degenerations or widespread retinal dystrophies. Unlike the latter conditions, patients with APMPPE retain good visual acuity and good electrophysiologic function (see Chapter 9, sec. **X.C.**).

C. **Retinochoroiditis** (see sec. **V.A.,** above; Chapter 9; and Chapter 11, sec. **II.**). Focal or diffuse retinitis or choroiditis may be associated with a number of conditions such as peripheral uveitis, sarcoidosis, and rare diseases such as Bechet syndrome and subacute sclerosing panencephalitis.

VI. **Retinal dystrophies** are genetically transmitted diseases of the retina that lead to premature cell changes and cell death (see Chapter 11, sec. **XIX.A.**). These conditions must be differentiated from congenital stationary retinal disorders such as stationary night blindness or achromatopsia (autosomal recessive [AR]). Electrophysiologic tests are important in diagnosing these disorders, especially in young children, the main tests being **ERG** and **EOG.** An abnormality of the RPE photoreceptor complex plays a primary role in these diseases, with probable secondary abnormality of the choriocapillaris. In three conditions—retinitis pigmentosa, choroideremia, and sex-linked retinoschisis—the female carrier may show ocular signs. In most instances, the female carrier is asymptomatic and has normal test findings. Although a metabolic abnormality—hyperornithinemia—has been shown to be associated with gyrate atrophy of the choroid and retina, most retinal dystrophies do not appear to have any systemic or metabolic associations. DNA probes have identified the genetic defect in dominant retinitis pigmentosa and choroideremia.

A. **Primary retinal dystrophies**
   1. **Retinitis pigmentosa** is the most common retinal dystrophy. The most common symptom is *night blindness.* Ophthalmoscopy demonstrates attenuation of the retinal vessels, retinal pigmentary changes consisting of bone-corpuscular clumping of pigment clustering around retinal vessels in the midperiphery of the fundus, and waxy pallor of the optic disk. The visual fields show annular scotomas. The EOG and scotopic ERG are primarily affected; the photopic ERG is relatively spared. The AR and X-linked forms are, in general, more severe than the autosomal-dominant (AD) form. Treatment with 15,000 units of vitamin A, palmitate form, slows the progression of the disease.
   2. **Differential diagnosis of retinitis pigmentosa.** A number of diseases and syndromes are associated with retinitis pigmentosa (see Chapter 11).
      a. **Acanthocytosis (Bassen-Kornzweig syndrome)** is an AR disorder characterized by crenated red cells, serum abetalipoproteinemia, and spinocerebellar degeneration. In its early stages the pigmentary retinopathy can be reversed by large doses of vitamin A.
      b. **Alström syndrome** is a rare AR disease whose clinical features include profound childhood blindness, obesity, diabetes mellitus, and neurosensory deafness. Chronic renal disease is seen in later stages.
      c. **Bardet-Biedl syndrome** is an AR disorder characterized by polydactyly, obesity, mental retardation, and hypogonadism.
      d. **Cockayne syndrome** is a rare, autosomally inherited condition. Afflicted patients have a prematurely senile appearance, mental retardation, deafness, peripheral neuropathy, and photosensitive dermatitis.
      e. **Friedreich syndrome** is a recessively inherited spinocerebellar ataxia with deafness and mental deficiency.
      f. **Kearns-Sayre syndrome.** The symptoms of this disease, which begins in childhood, include progressive external ophthalmoplegia and cardiac conduction defects. Early recognition and the use of a cardiac pacemaker may avert a fatal cardiac arrest.
      g. **Leber congenital amaurosis** is an autosomal recessively inherited disease and is associated with profound visual loss at birth or in the first year of life. The ERG is nondetectable and provides an important means of differentiating retinal disease from "cortical blindness."
      h. **Mucopolysaccharidosis.** There are two types of mucopolysaccharidoses associated with pigmentary retinopathy. In **Hunter syndrome** (type II) the clinical features are gargoylism, mental retardation, hepatosplenomegaly, and early death. **Sanfilippo syndrome** (type III) is characterized by mental retardation, seizures, and deafness (see Chapter 11, sec. **VII.**).
      i. **Refsum's disease** is a recessively inherited condition characterized by peripheral neuropathy, deafness, and cerebellar ataxia. There is an increase of *phytanic acid* in the blood. Early dietary control

consisting of withholding phytol, a precursor of phytanic acid, may retard neurologic and retinal changes.
  j. **Syphilis.** Both acquired and congenital syphilis show extensive signs of pigmentary retinopathy.
  k. **Usher's syndrome** is an autosomal recessively inherited condition responsible for 3% to 6% of severe childhood deafness and 50% of deafness–blindness. Both the cochlear and vestibular systems are involved.
  l. **Pseudoretinitis pigmentosa.** Certain retinal degenerations and inflammations may culminate in a clinical and electrophysiologic picture similar to that seen in retinitis pigmentosa. This condition is encountered with detachment of the retina and following injury, especially concussive ocular injuries occurring early in life.

B. **Primary macular dystrophies.** Most macular dystrophies show ophthalmoscopic and retinal functional changes outside the macular area; however, their early manifestations are first seen in the macular area. All have varying degrees of central scotoma.
  1. **Vitelliform dystrophy (Best's disease)** is an AD disorder that begins in childhood and is characterized by an egg-yolk-like lesion in the macular region bilaterally. It is compatible with near-normal visual acuity. The EOG is specifically afflicted; the ERG is normal. The yolk-like material eventually absorbs, resulting in extensive pigmentary degeneration of the macula and a decrease in acuity.
  2. **Stargardt's disease.** This well-known macular dystrophy occurs between the ages of 6 and 20 years and is inherited as an AR condition. Unlike vitelliform dystrophy, Stargardt's disease begins with rapid loss of vision with minimal ophthalmoscopic changes. Subsequently, the macula shows pigmentary disturbance. Many yellowish flecks surround this central area of beaten bronze atrophy. Central vision typically decreases to the 20/200 range, but the visual fields remain intact. The ERG is normal. On fluorescein angiography, there may be a dark choroid due to blockage of choroidal fluorescence by lipofuscin-like pigment in the RPE. *Fundus flavimaculatus* is reserved for cases without macular involvement, whereas Stargardt's disease denotes atrophic macular dystrophy with fundus flavimaculatus.
  3. **Progressive cone or cone–rod dystrophy** is an AD disease starting in the first to third decades and characterized by decreased central vision, severe photophobia, and severe color vision loss. There may be bull's-eye maculopathy with a ring-like depigmentation around the center or the macula and optic disk pallor. Fluorescein angiography shows window defects and/or diffuse transmission defects in the posterior pole. Photopic ERG is very abnormal and scotopic ERG is near normal. The EOG is very useful in following disease progress. The end stage has the same appearance as retinitis pigmentosa.
  4. **Familial drusen** has its onset in the second to fourth decades and probably represents early AMD. Inheritance pattern is usually uncertain. There are no symptoms unless macular degeneration begins. The fundi have round yellow-white deposits of the posterior pole to midperiphery (drusen) that often coalesce. RPE detachment and CNV may develop, requiring laser photocoagulation. On fluorescein angiography, drusen may block then stain and the RPE is mottled. ERG is normal; EOG is abnormal.
  5. **Foveomacular vitelliform dystrophy, adult type,** has its onset in the fourth to sixth decades and resembles Best's disease clinically except there is only a slight decrease in vision. The ERG and EOG are normal, and color vision slightly defective (tritan).
  6. **Butterfly pigment dystrophy of the fovea** is an AD disease with onset in the second to fifth decades and causes only a slight decrease in

vision. It is one of the pattern dystrophies. The central macula has a butterfly-shaped reticular pattern, and there may be pigment stippling in the peripheral retina. Fluorescein angiography shows a reticular hyperfluorescence. The ERG and color vision are normal, and the EOG is abnormal.

7. **Central areolar dystrophy (choroidal sclerosis)** is an AD disease with onset in the third to fifth decades that causes a slowly progressive decreased central vision. Early, there is mild foveal granularity. Later, RPE disruption as well as geographic atrophy of the RPE and choriocapillaris appears. Fluorescein angiography shows transmission defects early; later, there is late staining of edges of areas of geographic atrophy. The photopic ERG is abnormal and the scotopic ERG and EOG are essentially normal. Vision correlates with the degree and location of the pigmentary changes seen clinically, and color vision defect parallels vision loss.

C. **Primary choroidal dystrophies** (see Chapter 9, sec. **XV.**). The best-known disorders in this group are the sex-linked choroideremia, the AR gyrate atrophy of the choroid and retina, and the AD central areolar choroidal dystrophy.

D. **Primary vitreoretinal dystrophies** primarily affect the superficial retina and the vitreous body, and include juvenile retinoschisis, Goldmann-Favre dystrophy, Wagner's disease, and clefting syndromes with palatoschisis and maxillary hypoplasia (see Chapter 11, sec. **XIX.C.**). These clefting syndromes are closely related to the **Pierre Robin syndrome** of glossoptosis, micrognathia, and cleft palate. **Retinal detachment** is frequently associated with clefting syndromes.

VII. **Retinal detachment.** In retinal detachment, fluid collects in the potential space between the sensory retina and the RPE that remains attached to Bruch membrane. Fluid may accumulate by three major mechanisms. It may escape from the vitreous cavity into the subretinal space through a **retinal hole or tear** (break) in the retina. In this instance, it is called a **rhegmatogenous retinal detachment.** Extravasation from the choroid or the retina may result in retinal detachment in the absence of a tear or traction, the so-called **exudative retinal detachment.** Exudative detachments differ from rhegmatogenous detachments in that they do NOT extend to the ora serrata and shift with changes in head position; i.e., the subretinal fluid migrates quickly to the most dependent portion of the retina. They are also not associated with retinal breaks. Lastly, the retina can be detached from its normal position by contraction of adherent vitreous or fibrous bands, resulting in a **traction retinal detachment.**

A. **Rhegmatogenous retinal detachment** occurs more commonly in patients over the age of 45 years, males, and myopes. Rarely do patients present with bilateral detachments.

1. **Pathogenesis, signs, and symptoms.** Rhegmatogenous retinal detachments usually occur in one of two ways. Rarely, they will result from the slow accumulation of fluid through a round hole or break in the peripheral retina. The patient's only symptoms will be loss of side vision (frequently spontaneously described as a "curtain" by the patient) or loss of central vision when the macula becomes involved. More commonly, retinal detachment results from the relatively rapid flow of fluid through an acute tear created by an acute **posterior vitreous detachment (PVD).** The posterior vitreous is normally surrounded by a pseudomembrane, the posterior hyaloid. As the eye ages, pockets of liquefaction form in the vitreous in a process called **syneresis.** At some point in many people's lives (about one-third by autopsy studies), fluid flows from one of these pockets of liquefaction through a hole in the posterior hyaloid separating it from the back of the eye and creating the so-called **PVD.** This typically happens very quickly, over minutes to hours. Frequently fibrous tissue on the disk adheres to the posterior hyaloid as it separates and condensations form in the collapsed vitreous gel. These opacities throw shadows on the retina, and the patient complains of new **floaters.** The detached

posterior hyaloid cannot separate from the peripheral retina, and in some patients it exerts intermittent traction on the peripheral retina, creating the sensation of bright, peripheral, split-second, light flashes (**photopsia**). In most patients, a retinal tear will not occur, the floaters become less noticeable, and the photopsia wanes. However, if the traction on the peripheral retina is great enough, a tear will occur. Fluid from the vitreous cavity can then flow through this tear, creating a rhegmatogenous retinal detachment. The patient will complain of a **curtain** coming over his or her vision, which corresponds to the area of the detachment.

Ophthalmoscopy shows that the retina has lost its pink color and appears gray and opaque. If the collection of subretinal fluid is large, the retina shows a ballooning detachment with numerous folds. Binocular indirect ophthalmoscopy with scleral depression is valuable in locating the retinal breaks to repair the retinal detachment. Surgical reattachment should be performed as soon as possible as the macula undergoes cystic changes, with progressive degeneration of rods and cones, because the photoreceptors are separated from the choriocapillaris, their normal source of nourishment.

2. **Differential diagnosis** of rhegmatogenous retinal detachment includes **senile retinoschisis.** This condition results from a splitting of the retina in older patients, particularly in the inferotemporal periphery. It appears as smooth, dome-shaped elevation unlike rhegmatogenous detachment, which is usually irregular in its contour. Other contrasting features with rhegmatogenous detachment include frequent bilateralism and lack of associated pigmentary changes in the RPE. It produces an absolute field defect, whereas rhegmatogenous retinal detachment has a relative field defect. Thermal laser burns and cryopexy cause a visible white lesion on the outer wall of a schisis cavity, whereas no whitening is seen under a full-thickness retinal detachment because there are no retinal elements to turn white.

3. The following conditions **predispose** to retinal detachment:

   a. **Lattice degeneration** of the retina is characterized by ovoid patches of retinal thinning with overlying vitreous liquefaction and abnormal vitreoretinal adhesions on their borders. These patches are usually concentric with the ora serrata and in the periphery. Sometimes crisscrossing white lines that represent atrophy retinal vessels are seen within these lesions; hence, the term "lattice" degeneration. Pigmentary changes and round hole formation within the lesions are common. Small cuffs of subretinal fluid may form around the holes, but usually do not need treatment unless they extend beyond the borders of the lattice degeneration. Vitreous traction can cause large horseshoe breaks at the posterior margin of lattice degeneration when an acute PVD occurs. Lattice degeneration is present in 6% to 10% of patients and in about one-fifth to one-third of eyes with rhegmatogenous retinal detachment. However, the risk of developing retinal detachment in eyes with lattice degeneration is only 1%. Hence, prophylactic treatment with laser or cryopexy in asymptomatic eyes is usually not indicated.

   b. **Cystic retinal tufts** appear as small elevations in the peripheral retina. They are associated with chronic traction on the retina by vitreous strands. Frequently, there is underlying hyperpigmentation of the RPE. When an acute PVD occurs, tears can occur at these tufts due to the abnormal vitreoretinal adhesions. About 5% to 10% of all rhegmatogenous detachments are associated with a cystic retinal tuft. Nevertheless, prophylactic treatment of asymptomatic lesions is usually not indicated because less than 0.3% of the 5% of eyes with this lesion will go on to have a retinal detachment.

   c. **Zonular traction tuft** is similar to a cystic retinal tuft but it is due to the insertion of a lens zonule into the peripheral retina.

d. **Outer layer breaks in senile retinoschisis.** There are often breaks in the thin inner layer of schisis. If outer layer breaks occur, fluid can then flow from the vitreous cavity through the inner layer breaks and then under the retina through the outer layer breaks. Outer layer breaks are usually large and round with thickened edges. They are easily treated with laser around their edges to prevent fluid flow under the retina, although in most instances they can be safely observed without therapy. The risk of a retinal detachment from double-layer holes in retinoschisis is about 1.4%.

e. **Dialysis** or disinsertion of the retina from its attachment to the ora serrata can occur spontaneously or as a result of trauma. Most dialyses occur in the inferotemporal retina, although superonasal dialyses can be seen after ocular contusion. A **giant retinal break** is when the tear extends 90 degrees or more along the circumference of the globe. It is often due to a traumatic dialysis.

4. **Common peripheral conditions which do not predispose to retinal detachment are**

   a. **Peripheral cystoid degeneration** is generally found in eyes after age 20 years. These microcysts are considered to be a normal aging change and are located from the ora serrata extending backward into the retina.

   b. **Peripheral chorioretinal degeneration, also called paving stone degeneration and cobblestone degeneration.** These lesions develop after age 40 years. They are usually located inferiorly near the ora serrata and are bilateral. They appear as areas of complete RPE absence showing a few large choroidal vessels against bare sclera; they have sharp borders.

5. **Treatment.** Rhegmatogenous retinal detachment is treated with **pneumatic retinopexy, scleral buckling, or vitrectomy.** All retinal breaks are localized and a chorioretinal adhesion is initiated around the break with diathermy, laser, or the cryoprobe. In pneumatic retinopexy, a gas bubble is injected into the vitreous cavity, and the patient is positioned so the gas pushes the retina around the retinal break against the outside of the eye until the chorioretinal adhesion forms in 1 to 2 weeks. The subretinal fluid is resorbed by the RPE. In scleral buckling, the subretinal fluid is drained surgically, and the sclera overlying the retinal break is indented or buckled inward by sewing material to the outside of the eye. The buckled sclera pushes the choroid against the retina around the break, sealing the hole and allowing the chorioretinal adhesion to form. In vitrectomy, the vitreous pulling on the break is severed, and gas is used to then push the retina around the break against the choroid.

B. **Secondary retinal detachments** can occur with systemic or retinovascular diseases, or as a response to inflammation of the retina or choroid.

   1. **These conditions** include

      a. Severe hypertension, especially toxemia of pregnancy.

      b. Chronic glomerulonephritis.

      c. Retinal venous occlusive disease.

      d. Retinal angiomatosis.

      e. Papilledema.

      f. Postoperative inflammation.

      g. Primary or metastatic choroidal tumor.

      h. Vogt-Koyanagi-Harada syndrome.

      i. Retinal vasculitis.

   2. **The differential diagnosis** includes **choroidal detachments.** Choroidal detachments have a solid, smooth, dome-shaped appearance. Their color is the orange-red of the normal fundus. They are common after intraocular surgery complicated by hypotony or inflammation.

   3. **Treatment** is directed toward correcting the underlying condition. Secondary retinal detachments are not amenable to standard scleral

buckling surgery. Systemic steroids are effective in Vogt-Koyanagi-Harada disease.

C. **Traction retinal detachments** are due to contraction of the vitreous after abnormal vitreoretinal adhesions have formed. They are most often seen in proliferative diabetic retinopathy where the posterior hyaloid develops abnormal attachment to areas of new vessel formation on the surface of the retina. The leakage of fluid and blood from these new vessels and the vascular abnormalities within the retina stimulate the vitreous to contract. The vitreous then pulls on areas of adhesion to the retina, lifting the retina off. New membranes can form on the surface of the retina in rhegmatogenous retinal detachment and can contract. This condition is called **proliferative vitreoretinopathy (PVR)**. The retina will not reattach because these membranes hold the retinal breaks away from the back of the eye. Other stimulants to membrane formation, contraction, and traction retinal detachments include **intraocular foreign body, perforating ocular injury,** and **vitreous loss** after cataract surgery. **Pars plana vitrectomy** with vitreous membrane cutting and pealing often reattaches the retina.

VIII. **Retinal malignancy** (see Chapter 11, sec. **XIII.A.**)

IX. **Vitreous.** The vitreous undergoes significant physical and biochemical changes with **aging.** The most striking changes are liquefaction **(syneresis)** and **PVD** (see sec. **VII.A.1.,** above). Complications of PVD include retinal break and vitreous hemorrhage from tearing either superficial retina vessels or from the creation of a full-thickness retina break through the vascular retina. Syneresis and PVD occur an average of 20 years earlier in myopes than in emmetropes. Aphakic eyes have a much higher prevalence of PVD. Forward movement of the vitreous may be a reason for the higher prevalence of retinal detachment in aphakic eyes and also for development of **pupillary block glaucoma** and **malignant glaucoma.**

A. **Developmental abnormalities** (see Chapter 11, sec. **XI.F.**). Persistent hyperplastic primary vitreous (PHPV) and the various vitreoretinal dystrophies belong to this group. Eyes with PHPV, which are microphthalmic, develop cataract, pupillary block, and secondary glaucoma. Early intervention with a vitrectomy instrument to remove the cataract and retrolental tissue, either via the anterior or pars plana approach, is advisable. Visual results are naturally poor because of the associated amblyopia.

B. **Vitreous opacities**

1. **Blood.** Vitreous hemorrhage usually comes from the retina and may be preretinal or diffusely dispersed in the vitreous cavity. Massive hemorrhages may reduce vision severely. The blood in a long-standing vitreous hemorrhage often becomes converted to a white opaque mass resembling an inflammatory exudate, endophthalmitis, or an intraocular tumor. A detailed history along with a complete ocular examination combined with **ultrasonography** usually establishes the diagnosis. The components of blood such as platelets and leukocytes probably contribute to the development of pathologic vitreous membranes.

   Vitreous hemorrhage and membrane formation are seen in a number of ocular conditions. *Diabetic retinopathy* is the most important cause, followed by *retinal tear.* Other conditions include PVD, retinal vein occlusion, sickle cell retinopathy, congenital retinal vascular anomalies, trauma, diskiform macular lesions, choroidal malignant melanoma, and subarachnoid hemorrhage.

2. **Asteroid hyalosis,** also known as **Benson's disease,** is characterized by minute white or yellow solid bodies suspended in an essentially normal vitreous. This condition probably represents a dystrophy with fairly weak penetrance. Calcium soaps of palmitate and stearate are present in these vitreous deposits.

3. **Cholesterolosis bulbi (synchysis scintillans)** is typified by freely floating, highly refractile crystals in liquefied vitreous and is seen in eyes with severe intraocular disease.

4. Other conditions. Vitreous opacification can be seen in **primary amyloidosis** and **reticulum cell sarcoma.** In **retinoblastoma,** tumor cells may be seen freely floating in the vitreous.

C. **Inflammation.** The response of the vitreous is characterized by liquefaction, opacification, and shrinkage whenever it is exposed to inflammatory insult. The vitreous is an excellent culture medium for the growth of bacteria, leading to **endophthalmitis.** The presence of white blood cells results in the laying down of fibrous connective tissue and varying degrees of capillary proliferation. Organization of these membranes may lead to a **cyclitic membrane,** formed by the cells from the ciliary body and the adjacent retina and located along the plane of the anterior hyaloid surface. Cyclitic membranes often lead to total retinal detachment. In addition to bacteria and fungi, vitreous abscesses with intense eosinophilia may be seen with **parasitic infections,** such as *Taenia,* microfilaria, and nematode infections due to *Toxocara canis* and *Toxocara cati* (see Chapter 11, sec. **III.B.**).

D. **Vitrectomy** is the most significant advance in the surgical management of vitreous disease. The technique is used to clear vitreous opacities and relieve or prevent vitreoretinal traction. Vitrectomy through the pars plana approach is the best-established procedure. A variety of vitrectomy units are currently available. All instruments perform vitreous cutting and aspiration, the procedure being performed under microscopic control with the aid of fiberoptic illumination. The following are indications for pars plana vitrectomy:

1. Nonresolving vitreous opacities (e.g., diabetic hemorrhage).
2. Certain retinal detachments:
   a. Traction detachments involving the macula
   b. Giant retinal tears
   c. Rhegmatogenous detachment with vitreous hemorrhage or PVR
3. Macular diseases:
   a. Preretinal macular fibrosis
   b. Macular hole
   c. Aphakic or pseudophakic CME with vitreous entrapped in corneoscleral incision
   d. Subinternal limiting membrane hemorrhage in the macula.
4. Trauma:
   a. Penetrating injuries of the posterior segment with vitreous loss and vitreous hemorrhage
   b. Double-penetrating injuries involving the posterior segment
   c. Selected magnetic and nonmagnetic intraocular foreign bodies.
5. Vitreous biopsy (amyloidosis, reticulum cell sarcoma).
6. Anterior segment reconstruction (pupillary membranectomy).
7. Vitreous complications in the anterior segment:
   a. Vitreous "touch" with corneal edema
   b. Aphakic pupillary block glaucoma
   c. Malignant glaucoma.
8. Secondary open-angle glaucoma:
   a. Hemolytic glaucoma
   b. Phacolytic glaucoma.
9. Endophthalmitis if initial vision is only light perception.
10. Severe proliferative diabetic retinopathy.

X. **Trauma** (see Chapter 2; Chapter 9, sec. **XVII.**). Ocular injuries often cause vitreoretinal and choroidal changes. Vitreoretinal trauma can be considered under the following headings.

A. **Contusion injuries** are caused either by a direct blow applied to the eye or from indirect force, as in head injuries or explosions. The force distorts the globe and alters pressure relationships in the retinal and uveal vessels. The following are the sequelae of contusion.

1. **Commotio retinae** appears as widespread deep retinal whitening with scattered hemorrhages following blunt injury to the globe. Damage to

the outer segments of the rods and cones has been proposed as a mechanism. If the center of the macula is involved, vision is initially decreased. Vision usually recovers as the whitening resolves over several days to weeks, unless there are secondary pigmentary changes. No treatment is indicated.

2. **Purtscher retinopathy,** also known as traumatic retinal angiopathy, occurs after crushing injuries of the head, chest, or long bones. The condition is usually bilateral. The characteristic appearance is of multiple patches of superficial whitening and hemorrhages surrounding the optic disk. The whitening and hemorrhages disappear, but there may be some loss of vision. A similar picture can occur in acute pancreatitis, lupus erythematosus, and amniotic fluid embolization. The condition appears to be due to acute capillary ischemia.

3. **Macular holes** may occur following blunt trauma.

4. **Choroidal ruptures** are common following blunt trauma. They appear as curvilinear white lines at the level of the RPE concave toward the disk. Acutely, they are often associated with subretinal hemorrhages. Days to years later, CNV may grow from their edges.

5. **Retinal tears** or dialysis of the retina along with retinal detachment occurs after trauma. There is a high incidence of retinal dialysis after blunt trauma. This is a major cause of retinal detachments in children and young adults. Retinal dialysis appears to occur at the time of ocular contusion. If it is not recognized initially, it may go undetected until a symptomatic retinal detachment develops. Patients who have had blunt trauma should be examined periodically, especially if vitreous hemorrhage obscures part of the retinal periphery.

6. **Retinal hemorrhages.** The effects of retinal hemorrhages vary considerably according to their sizes and locations. Small retinal hemorrhages absorb completely without any significant visual defects. Hemorrhages trapped under the internal limiting membrane over the macula may induce epiretinal membrane formation and macular pucker.

7. **Nonclearing vitreous hemorrhages** may cause **erythroclastic or ghost cell glaucoma** or they may organize, causing traction retinal detachment.

8. **Occult rupture** should be suspected in any eye with **hypotony** following blunt trauma. It commonly occurs just posterior to a muscle insertion. Careful exploration of the globe and closure of the rupture are indicated.

B. **Perforating injuries** of the posterior segment associated with vitreous loss and vitreous hemorrhage should be considered for vitrectomy to prevent retinal detachment from PVR secondary to fibrovascular ingrowth. Similar considerations apply to eyes that have suffered a double perforating injury. Provided there is no retinal detachment, the surgery may be delayed for 2 to 3 weeks following the initial trauma to allow resorption of choroidals and formation of a PVD, thus simplifying the procedure.

Endophthalmitis is always a risk in perforating injuries. Intravitreal injection of broad-spectrum antibiotics such as 1 mg of vancomycin and 2.2 mg of ceftazidime at the time of initial repair lessens this risk considerably. If intravitreal antibiotics cannot be given for technical reasons, the patient should receive 5 days of high-dose i.v. vancomycin and ceftazidime.

C. **Intraocular foreign bodies.** A computerized axial tomography scan should always be done to rule out an intraocular foreign body in any perforating injury. Hammering steel on steel often sends up small chips from the hammerhead at high speed. These can enter the eye causing not much more than a foreign body sensation and a very small self-sealing entrance wound, which can be overlooked. Although most of these high-velocity steel foreign bodies are sterile, all foreign bodies must be assumed to be contaminated and prophylactic antibiotic therapy as for any perforating injury must be instituted. Depending on the velocity, shape, and mass of the object, it may come to rest anywhere in the eye or pass through the eye, causing a double perforating injury. In the latter case, the entry wound should be closed but attempted closure of the more posterior wound can result in loss of intraocular contents and so should be avoided in most instances. Steel chips from hammerheads not uncommonly come to rest on the retina. Acute whitening rapidly develops around the touch site. After the removal of the foreign body, it is not necessary to treat the touch site with laser unless there is a frank retinal tear. It will scar to the choroid. If there is a double perforation or vitreous hemorrhage associated with vitreous loss, appropriately timed vitrectomy should be done as prophylaxis against retinal detachment from PVR secondary to fibrovascular ingrowth.

Intraocular foreign bodies may be divided into two types, based on the ocular reaction they elicit (see Chapter 2, sec. **VII.**).

1. **Inert substances** such as gold, silver, glass, and plastics cause no specific reaction in the eye based on their composition. Apart from traumatic infection and hemorrhage, these substances can cause slow liquefaction and opacification of the vitreous and fibroglial proliferation in the posterior segment, leading to retinal detachment from PVR. If they are loose inside the vitreous cavity, they can also cause retinal detachment by shredding the retina as they bounce off it with everyday eye movements.

2. **Irritant metals.** Iron and copper have serious effects on the eye (see Chapter 2, sec. **VII.**).

   a. **Iron foreign bodies. Siderosis** is the complication of intraocular iron foreign bodies. The degree depends on the size, number of ferrous particles, and location in the eye. Retained iron, especially soft iron, undergoes electrolytic decomposition, combines with tissue cells, and causes eventual cell death. Siderosis affecting the retina results in diminution and ultimate extinction of the ERG. Iron can be demonstrated in tissues by **Perls stain,** a specific histochemical test. Late effects of siderosis include **heterochromia,** cataract, and secondary glaucoma. **Treatment** consists of removal of the foreign body either by a magnet or with intraocular foreign body forceps usually in combination with vitrectomy. High-grade steel alloys are poorly magnetic and cannot be removed by a magnet.

   b. **Copper foreign bodies** cause profuse suppuration in the eye. Copper is oxidized as readily as iron. Intraocular foreign bodies with less than 85% of copper cause **chalcosis,** signs of which include a greenish-blue peripheral ring in Descemet's membrane in the cornea, a greenish-red iridescent sunflower cataract, and retinal atrophy. **Management** consists of pars plana vitrectomy and removal of the foreign body using vitreous forceps.

D. **Radiant energy.** Ocular lesions can be produced by radiant energy of almost any wavelength. Vitreoretinal pathology is seen in the following conditions.

   1. **Solar retinopathy (foveomacular retinitis)** refers to a specific foveolar lesion occurring in patients who gaze directly at a solar eclipse, sunbathers, and people gazing at the sun while under the influence of a hallucinogenic agent. Soon after exposure, these patients complain of metamorphopsia and a central scotoma. Vision is reduced to between 20/40 and 20/200, but almost complete recovery is seen over the ensuing months. During the period immediately after the exposure, a small gray zone develops around the foveolar area, resulting from photochemical injury to the sensory retina and the RPE. This zone is slowly replaced by a sharply circumscribed lamellar hole.

   2. **Radiation retinopathy** describes alterations in the retinal vasculature in patients several months or years after receiving brachytherapy or heavy particle irradiation (e.g., proton beam) for intraocular tumor (e.g., malignant melanoma) or roentgen radiation to the skull and orbital region. An ischemic ocular response may be established as is seen

in diabetic retinopathy. Macular function may be affected with decrease in central vision. Photocoagulation may be of value in controlling these complications.

3. **Retinal phototoxicity.** Wavelengths between 400 and 1,400 nm are transmitted by the mammalian ocular media to the retina, causing mechanical, thermal, and photochemical damage. Melanin granules in the RPE play a key role in mediating all three types of damage. Absorption of energy by the RPE and choroid causes elevation of temperature above the ambient temperature present in the neural retina, with thermal denaturation of sensitive macromolecules such as proteins. Photochemical damage results from extended exposure of the retina by shorter wavelengths in the visible spectrum (450 to 550 nm). The lens absorbs wavelengths below 450 nm, with the result that fewer photons in the blue and near-ultraviolet region reach the retina.

The physician, especially the ophthalmologist, should be aware of retinal irradiance levels for all ophthalmologic instruments such as ophthalmoscopes, intraocular fiberoptic light sources, surgical microscopes, and overhead surgical lamps. Infrared radiation should preferably be filtered from these sources because it causes actinic damage and does not contribute to visibility. Aging or diseased retinas may be more susceptible to actinic damage, compared to normal retinas.

XI. **Lasers** have been a major therapeutic modality in the management of the retinochoroidal and vitreal disorders. Lasers have been variously used to perform **photocoagulation, photodisruption, photovaporization,** and **photoradiation.**

A. **Photocoagulation** is the most commonly used modality. The incident light energy is absorbed and converted into heat by the pigment in the target tissues such as RPE. The threshold temperature rise for retinal photocoagulation is approximately $10°C$. Excessive temperature increase can cause vaporization and hemorrhage in target tissues. The wavelength of the incident light contributes to the efficiency of the photocoagulation process.

B. **Photocoagulation is used to** (a) apply confluent burns under flat neovascularization not on the disk; (b) seal focal intraretinal leakage points; (c) perform grid therapy to areas of diffuse leakage and ischemia within the macula; (d) scatter PRP in the periphery to reduce angiogenic factor production by the oxygen-deprived retina; (e) focally treat RPE abnormalities such as central serous choroidopathy; (f) obliterate extra and parafoveal choroidal neovascularization; and (g) produce chorioretinal adhesions as in scleral buckling surgery.

C. **Photodynamic laser therapy** [see sec. **IV.A.2.c.(3),** above]

D. **Laser types** (see Chapter 10, sec. **VI.**).

1. The blue-green and green **argon** lasers have been a major advance in the treatment of major blinding conditions such as diabetic retinopathy, AMD, severe open-angle glaucoma, and angle-closure glaucoma. The blue-green laser has both blue (488 nm) and green (614 nm) wavelengths. The advantage of the argon laser is that it is well absorbed by hemoglobin and also by melanin in the RPE. The delivery system is precise with a wide range of possible power densities, thereby affording a large coagulation range. The argon laser is minimally absorbed by the ocular media. It can be delivered through fiberoptic systems so that laser photocoagulation can be done intraoperatively, such as during vitreous surgery for diabetic traction detachments and hemorrhages. Its major disadvantage is that the blue-green argon laser cannot be applied close to the fovea because of the absorption of the laser energy by the xanthophyll pigment in the macula. Because the green laser is well absorbed by melanin and hemoglobin, but not xanthophyll, it has replaced the blue-green laser for treating retinal vascular abnormalities and CNVs.

2. The **krypton** laser with the red wavelength (657 nm) is an excellent alternative when CNV is present in the parafoveolar area, because this

wavelength is minimally absorbed by the macular xanthophyll. The red krypton laser is less absorbed by nuclear sclerosis and vitreous hemorrhage than green wavelengths; hence, it is useful in patients with these conditions. It can also prove useful when trying to penetrate intraretinal blood.

3. **Tunable dye lasers,** with intermediate wavelengths between green and red, are used for photocoagulation in the macular region. These lasers are expensive to produce and maintain.

4. **Dye yellow lasers** are well absorbed by hemoglobin and have low xanthophyll absorption, making them useful in treating retinal and subretinal lesions.

5. **Diode lasers** are currently available for retinal photocoagulation at a variety of wavelengths. They are inexpensive to produce, small, and easy to maintain. Because no studies have shown any advantage to any wavelength over green in the treatment of retinal diseases, green diode is now the laser of choice for general retina work.

6. The short-pulse **neodymium (Nd):YAG** laser is an example of a **photodisruptor.** This laser delivers a very high-power density in the pico-to nanosecond range (10^{-12} to 10^{-9} seconds), thereby ionizing tissue in a small volume of space at the laser beam focus, creating a **"plasma."** The clinical Nd:YAG laser delivers energy in the near infrared (1064 nm) and is coupled with a helium–neon laser to provide a visible, red focusing beam that identifies the focal point of the invisible Nd:YAG laser beam. This modality is primarily used to disrupt relatively transparent targets in the anterior segment, such as lens capsular membranes and anterior vitreous bands.

7. **Excimer lasers** are currently being used to alter the refractive power of the cornea (see Chapter 6).

8. The **xenon arc** was invented before true lasers. It emits polychromatic white light (400 to 1,600 nm) and can produce intense burns if great tissue damage is desired, but it cannot be well focused for vascular disease therapy. Currently, this device is rarely used.

9. UVEAL TRACT: IRIS, CILIARY BODY, AND CHOROID

Deborah Pavan-Langston and Victor L. Perez

I. **Normal anatomy and physiology.** The middle vascular layer of the eye, the uveal tract, is composed of three portions: **iris, ciliary body,** and **choroid.** The primary function of this tract is to supply nourishment to the ocular structures (see frontispiece).

A. **The iris** is the anterior extension of the ciliary body dividing the aqueous compartments into anterior and posterior chambers. The anterior surface of the iris consists of loosely structured stromal tissue of mesodermal origin lined posteriorly by a pigmented layer that extends from the pupillary margin of the iris back to the ciliary body. The pupil is the central iris aperture that changes in size to control the amount of light entering the eye. The pupillary sphincter muscle is supplied by the parasympathetic fibers of cranial nerve III, and the dilator pupillary muscle is supplied by the sympathetic nervous system (see Chapter 13, sec. **III.**).

B. **The ciliary body** is the posterior extension of the iris and contains the ciliary muscle, which functions in accommodation. The epithelium extending posteriorly from the iris becomes two distinct layers. The outer pigmented epithelial layer is continuous posteriorly with the retinal pigment epithelium (RPE). The inner nonpigmented epithelial layer of the ciliary body produces aqueous humor and extends posteriorly to become the sensory retina.

1. **The aqueous humor** from the ciliary body epithelium contributes to the maintenance of intraocular pressure (IOP) and supports the metabolism of the avascular lens and cornea. The composition of aqueous is approximately that of blood plasma with nearly all protein removed. Once secreted, the aqueous concentration is modified by water and chloride in the posterior chamber and by accumulation of lactic acid from the lens. The aqueous also contains proteins and peptides that regulate immune responses in the eye. The pressure of the eye depends on the rate of secretion of aqueous humor, which is approximately 1.0 to 2.0 μL per minute, and on the ease with which the aqueous passes through the trabecular meshwork to the canal of Schlemm and then into the aqueous veins.

2. **Accommodation,** or focusing of the lens, is a function of both the inner radial muscle lying posterior to the iris root and the outer longitudinal muscle running between scleral spur and choroid. Between these muscles run the oblique muscles of the ciliary body. Contraction of the round muscle shortens the diameter between the ciliary processes, allowing relaxation of tension on the lens capsule. The lens, by virtue of its own elasticity, tends to assume a more spherical shape, thus increasing its refractive power to focus on an object closer to the eye. Contraction of the longitudinal and oblique muscles has a similar effect. Conversely, relaxation of these three muscle bundles increases tension on the zonular fibers, thereby increasing tension on the elastic lens capsule to flatten the lens, causing the eye to become focused on a more distant object.

C. **The choroid** makes up the major portion of the uveal tract. It runs between retina and sclera from the ora serrata to the optic nerve. This vascular layer supplies nutrition to the external half of the retina and is composed primarily of an inner layer of capillaries known as *choriocapillaris* and externally by succeeding larger collecting veins (medium vessels—Sattler layer; outer large vessels—Haller layer). The choroid is thickest posteriorly (0.25 mm) and thin near the ora serrata (0.1 mm). The anterior uveal tract is fed primarily by long posterior ciliary arteries; the posterior uveal tract is fed primarily by short ciliary arteries, although there is free anastomosis between vessels. Bruch membrane is part of the choroid and lies between the choriocapillaris and the retinal rods and cones. Uveal melanocytes are scattered throughout the choroid, and their numbers account for variation in degree of choroidal pigmentation. The nerve supply to the choroid is from both short posterior and long anterior ciliary nerves.

II. Uveitis

A. Definition. *Uveitis* is a general term referring to inflammation of the uveal tract. It may be divided into iritis, cyclitis (ciliary body inflammation), iridocyclitis, and choroiditis, according to specific areas of the uveal tract involved. Although the term *uveitis* refers primarily to inflammation of this vascular structure, adjacent structures such as retina, vitreous, sclera, and cornea are also frequently involved secondarily in the inflammatory process.

B. Incidence. In a population of 100,000 people, over a period of 1 year, 15 individuals will develop uveitis. Uveitis afflicts 2.3 million people in the United States, with 45,000 cases reported each year. Uveitis is responsible for 10% of all blindness. Among patients with ocular inflammation, about 75% will have anterior uveitis (iritis, iridocyclitis), 8% intermediate uveitis (pars-planitis), and 17% posterior or panuveitis.

C. Demography

1. **Age.** Uveitis can affect patients of any age. Patients most commonly afflicted are 20 to 50 years of age. In the young, juvenile rheumatoid arthritis (JRA), congenital toxoplasmosis, toxocariasis, and intermediate uveitis are found. In the adult, sarcoidosis, Behçet syndrome, intermediate uveitis, toxoplasmosis, and heterochromic uveitis are seen. There is a marked decrease in incidence in individuals more than 70 years of age. In the elderly patient, the most common forms of uveitis are toxoplasmosis, herpes zoster, aphakic uveitis, and masquerade syndromes.

2. **Sex.** Forms of uveitis more common in men are sympathetic ophthalmia, due to a greater incidence of penetrating injury, sexually transmitted diseases, and acute anterior nongranulomatous uveitis secondary to systemic ankylosing spondylitis and Reiter syndrome. In women there is a greater incidence of chronic anterior uveitis of unknown etiology, toxoplasmosis, pauciarticular JRA, and the multifocal white dot syndromes.

3. **Race.** In the United States, toxoplasmosis and histoplasmosis are less common in African-Americans than in whites. Sarcoid is more common in African-Americans, and Behçet disease is more common in Japanese (not Americans of Japanese extraction).

4. **Geographic location.** Sympathetic ophthalmia is almost unheard of in the Southwest Pacific. Histoplasmosis is found almost exclusively in the Midwestern United States. Sarcoidosis is most common in Sweden and the South Atlantic and Gulf regions of the United States. Leprosy is found almost entirely in the subtropics. Onchocerciasis is found in tropical Africa and Central America; Behçet syndrome is found in the Mediterranean and Japan. Vogt-Koyanagi-Harada (VKH) syndrome is several hundred times more common in Japan than in the United States.

5. **Social factors.** Fungal endophthalmitis and acquired immunodeficiency syndrome (AIDS) are seen more frequently in intravenous drug users, and AIDS and syphilitic ocular disease are seen more frequently in promiscuous heterosexuals, homosexual males, and their sexual contacts. Nearly 30% of AIDS patients suffer cytomegaloviral chorioretinitis.

6. **Immunologic factors.** The histocompatibility leukocyte antigen (HLA) system in humans influences immunologic homeostatic functions and cellular and humoral immune responses, as well as coding for histocompatibility antigens on cell surfaces. The uveitis syndromes for which there is a strong HLA–disease association may be due to inherited genetic factors that control the expression of HLA antigens, immune responses, and possibly responses to endogenous inflammatory mediators (see sec. **V.C.5.**, below).

III. Signs and symptoms of uveitis may be unilateral or bilateral, isolated attacks or repeated episodes, and acute or chronic. Autoimmune disease tends to

be bilateral, whereas unilateral disease is often infectious or of unknown origin. Table 9.1 lists signs or symptoms of diagnostic significance in uveitis. Infectious and noninfectious uveitides may also be ruled out on the basis of location alone. Table 9.2 lists potential anatomic locations of several uveitis types.

A. **Granulomatous versus nongranulomatous uveitis.** Although morphologic description is still of some value, the rigid division of uveitis into these two categories has become largely anachronistic. By the original definition, *nongranulomatous uveitis* was typically acute or chronic, located in the iris and ciliary body, and characterized by a cellular infiltrate of lymphocytes and plasma cells that tended to form hypopyon and fine precipitates on the corneal endothelium known as **keratic precipitates (KPs).** The etiology was thought to be noninfectious, such as in Fuchs heterochromic uveitis. *Granulomatous uveitis* was thought to be chronic and to involve any portion of the uveal tract, but with a predilection for the posterior area. It was typically characterized by nodular collections of epithelioid cells and giant cells surrounded by lymphocytes. The KPs were larger than those seen in nongranulomatous disease, greasy in appearance (mutton fat), and composed primarily of epithelioid cells and pigment. The etiology was thought to be infectious and due to such organisms as tuberculosis (TBC), toxoplasmosis, and spirochetes; however, granulomatous uveitis was also seen in noninfectious disease such as sarcoidosis and sympathetic ophthalmia. It is now known that *transitional forms* of uveitis are not uncommon, and that the basic pathology lies somewhere between the rigidly defined granulomatous and nongranulomatous uveitides. Nonetheless, the classification is often useful in orienting the physician toward workup and therapy.

B. **Anterior uveitis** clinical findings vary between the acute and chronic form. In acute nongranulomatous uveitis, there is an acute onset of ocular pain (a few days) with hyperemia, photophobia, and blurred vision, lasting 2 to 6 weeks. There is perilimbal flush caused by dilation of the radial vessels and frequently fine white KPs on the posterior corneal, inferiorly in a vertical or base-down pyramidal distribution. KPs can also be found in the trabecular meshwork. The pupil is miotic, and cells and flare are found in the anterior chamber with or without fibrin exudation. Posterior synechia formation between iris and lens may be present, but **iris nodules** (pupillary Koeppe and anterior iris Busacca) and vitreous haze are typically absent. However, in severe iritis, spillover cells may be present in the anterior vitreous. The disease course is acute and the prognosis relatively good, although recurrence is not uncommon. More than 50% of cases are associated with HLA-B27 or HLA-B8. Chronic anterior uveitis is often insidious in onset and lasts longer than 3 months. Chronic iridocyclitis may be either nongranulomatous or granulomatous in character and usually is not associated with much hyperemia. In fact, in several forms the eyes may be white (JRA, white iritis in young girls, and Fuchs heterochromic iridocyclitis). Old KPs, iris stromal atrophy, posterior synechiae, and cataract formation are common findings. Diagnoses associated with chronic iridocyclitis are sarcoidosis, TBC, and Fuchs heterochromic iridocyclitis.

C. **Intermediate uveitis (pars-planitis)** is usually bilateral, with patients presenting with signs and symptoms of blurred vision (macular edema), floaters, and little or no pain, or both, photophobia, or anterior segment inflammation. Active inflammatory cells in the vitreous are white, round, and with equal distribution in the formed and liquid vitreous. Old vitreous cells are small, irregular, pigmented, and confined to the formed vitreous. The ora serrata is the site of vitritis and exudates that may progress to "snowbank" appearance, especially inferiorly. Progression of vitreous gel damage can result in membrane formation, with retinal traction and detachment. *Multiple sclerosis* and *sarcoid* are often associated. Twenty percent of children with uveitis have pars-planitis.

D. **Posterior uveitis.** In disease limited entirely to the posterior segment of the eye, the onset may be acute, but is often more insidious with little or no pain, minimum photophobia and blurring of vision (unless the macular

TABLE 9.1. SIGNS AND SYMPTOMS OF POSSIBLE DIAGNOSTIC SIGNIFICANCE IN UVEITIS

Sign or Symptom	Possible Clinical Diseases
Alopecia	VKH, psoriasis, lupus, syphilis
Arthritis	Behçet, colitis, JRA, rheumatoid arthritis, Reiter, psoriasis, Lyme, *Brucella,* syphilis, Whipple disease, RP, lupus, sarcoid
Cerebrospinal fluid pleocytosis	APMPPE, Behçet, sarcoid, VKH
Cough, shortness of breath	Sarcoid, tuberculosis, malignancy, Churg-Strauss syndrome, Wegener granulomatosis, systemic toxocara
Diarrhea	Crohn, ulcerative colitis, AIDS, *Giardia,* amoeba, Whipple disease
Erythema nodosum	Behçet, sarcoid, APMPPE, tuberculosis
Epididymitis	Polyarteritis nodosa, Behçet
Genital ulcers	Behçet, Reiter, syphilis
Headaches	Sarcoid, VKH, cryptococcus (AIDS), leptospirosis, tuberculosis, Lyme, VZV, CNS lymphoma, Whipple disease, systemic vasculitides, APMPPE
"Healthy"	Pars planitis, HSV, ocular histoplasmosis, toxoplasmosis, toxocara, Fuchs heterochromia, birdshot retinochoroidopathy, sympathetic ophthalmia, serpiginous chorioretinitis
Hematuria	Lupus, polyarteritis nodosa, Wegener
Immunosuppression	CMV, HSV, VZV, AIDS, fungal (especially, *Candida*), parasitic (pneumocystitis, *Toxoplasma*), chorioretinitis, other opportunistic infections
Lymphoid swelling	AIDS, sarcoid, malignancy, tuberculosis
Neurosensory deafness	Sarcoid, VKH, Lyme, syphilis
Oral ulcers	Behçet's, colitis, Crohn, Reiter, HSV
Paresthesia, weakness	Behçet's, multiple sclerosis, leprosy sarcoid, malignancy, polyarteritis nodosa
Psychosis	VKH
Salivary or lacrimal gland swelling	Sarcoid
Sacroiliitis	Ankylosing spondylitis, colitis, Reiter
Saddle nose	Syphilis, Wegener, RP
Sinusitis	Sarcoid, Wegener, RP, Whipple, Churg-Strauss syndrome
Skin nodules	Onchocerciasis, sarcoid, Behçet, leprosy
Skin rash	Behçet, HSV, psoriasis, RNA viral exanthem (mumps, measles, rubella), sarcoid, syphilis, VZV, systemic vasculitides
Systemic vasculitis	Behçet, RP, sarcoid, Cogan, arthritis, Lyme, syphilis, malignancy, primary vasculitides
Tracheal, nasal, or ear lobe pain	RP
Vitiligo, poliosis	VKH, sympathetic uveitis, APMPPE

AIDS, acquired immunodeficiency syndrome; APMPPE, acute posterior multifocal placoid pigment epitheliopathy; CMV, cytomegalovirus; CNS, central nervous system; HSV, herpes simplex virus; JRA, juvenile rheumatoid arthritis; RP, relapsing polychondritis; VKH, Vogt-Koyanagi-Harada syndrome; VZV, varicella-zoster virus.
(Adapted from Nussenblatt R, Palestine A. *Uveitis: Fundamentals and clinical practice.* Chicago: Mosby-Year Book, 1988:58; Opremcak EM. *Uveitis: A clinical manual for ocular inflammation.* New York: Springer-Verlag, 1995:38; and Jones NP. *Uveitis: An illustrated manual.* Butterworth-Heinemann, Oxford, 1998:38–40.)

TABLE 9.2. ANATOMIC LOCATIONS POTENTIALLY INVOLVED IN MAJOR TYPES OF INFECTIOUS AND NONINFECTIOUS UVEITIS

Anterior Only	Both Segments	Posterior Only
Infectious		
AIDS	AIDS	AIDS
Herpes simplex	Brucellosis	ARN
Herpes zoster	Coxsackie virus	Aspergillosis
Syphilis	EBV	Candidiasis
Tuberculosis	Herpes simplex	Cryptococcosis
Herpes zoster	Cysticercosis	
Rubella	CMV	
Rubeola	Histoplasmosis	
Syphilis	Lyme disease	
Toxoplasmosis	Nocardiosis	
Tuberculosis	Onchoceriasis	
Syphilis		
Toxocariasis		
Toxoplasmosis		
Tuberculosis		
Noninfectious		
Ankylosing spondylitis	APMPPE	APMPPE
Behçet disease	Behçet disease	Behçet disease
Heterochromic iridocyclitis	Inflammatory bowel disease	Birdshot choroidopathy
Idiopathic	Relapsing polychondritis	Eale disease
Reiter disease	Sarcoidosis	Geographic choroiditis
Sarcoidosis	Sympathetic ophthalmia	Harada disease
Lupus	Masquarade	
VKH syndrome	MEWDS	
Wegener granulomatosis	Polarteritis nodosa	
Sarcoidosis		
Serpiginous choroiditis		
VKH syndrome		

Intermediate

Infectious	*Noninfectious*
Lyme disease	JRA
Syphilis	Lens-induced uveitis
Tuberculosis	Multiple sclerosis
	Pars plantis
	Sarcoidosis

AIDS, acquired immunodeficiency syndrome; APMPPE, acute multifocal placoid pigment epitheliopathy; ARN, acute retinal necrosis; CMV, cytomegalovirus; EBV, Epstein-Barr virus; JRA, juvenile rheumatoid arthritis; MEWDS, multiple evanescent white dot syndrome; VKH, Vogt-Koyanagi-Harada syndrome.

area is involved), and no perilimbal flush. Inflammation of the posterior segment can affect the sensory retina, retinal vasculature, the retinal pigmented epithelium, the choroid, and optic nerve. Retinitis is associated with yellowish-white thickening, with secondary hemorrhages and focal ischemia. Inflammation of the retinal vessels usually is segmental, seen as a perivascular whitish cuff or sheathing. Choroidal lesions may be diffuse, but tend to be focal patchy yellow-white areas of infiltrate with overlying vitritis. Because of the anatomic relationship between choroid and retina, a retinitis is also usually present, and resolution of the process results in a chorioretinal scar with a corresponding visual field scotoma. If the macula is not involved, central visual acuity may return to normal. Examples of diseases involving predominantly the choroid are sympathetic ophthalmia and VKH (often with exudative retinal detachment). Optic nerve pathology in uveitis can be due to direct inflammation, ischemia secondary to vasculitis, glaucoma, or papilledema caused by involvement of the central nervous system.

Toxoplasmosis is a necrotizing retinitis with secondary inflammation in the choroid, as are the viral infections cytomegalovirus (CMV), herpes simplex, herpes zoster, rubella, and rubeola. Behçet's disease, however, is a retinitis with retinal vasculitis and only rarely has choroidal involvement. It is not, then, truly a uveitis, although it is almost always included in this ocular disease category.

E. **Panuveitis** may involve the entire uveal tract in any inflammatory type. Onset may be acute or insidious and the course variable, depending on etiology. The KPs, if present, tend to be large and greasy (mutton fat), and the pupils small and occasionally scarred down to the lens by posterior synechiae. In the anterior chamber, cells and flare are sometimes present, but not to the extent commonly seen with acute anterior uveitis. Iris nodules and vitreous haze are occasionally present. The course tends to be chronic, with a fair to poor prognosis, and recurrence occasionally is seen despite an apparent cure.

IV. **Differential diagnosis of uveitis.** It is first necessary to determine whether a lesion is an inflammation, a tumor, a vascular process, or a degeneration. Although flare and cells in the anterior chamber are a hallmark of uveitis, they themselves are not diagnostic. Necrotic or metastatic tumors may produce an inflammatory response. Vitreous cellular debris may result from degenerative conditions such as retinitis pigmentosa or retinal detachment. Study of cells from the aqueous or vitreous or both may be diagnostic (see Chapter 1, sec. III.L.).

A. **Conjunctivitis** is an inflammatory condition of the mucous membrane overlying the sclera. Hyperemia is usually diffuse or may be confined to just the lateral and medial angles, but is not primarily confined to the perilimbal area as in iritis. In conjunctivitis, vision is generally not blurred and pupillary responses are normal. A watery or purulent discharge may be present. There is no notable photophobia or deep pain. Moderate irritation and itching may also be present.

B. **Anterior scleritis,** while not a disease of the retinal vasculature, may have a sufficiently intense inflammatory reaction to induce an anterior or intermediate uveitis in about 40% of patients (see Chapter 5, sec. **XIII.D.**). **Posterior scleritis** is also not a uveitis but may cause ocular pain, boggy conjunctiva, vitritis, and chorioretinal edema. Ultrasound will reveal the posterior scleral inflammatory process, indicating the need for systemic steroid therapy.

C. In **acute angle-closure glaucoma** the vision is markedly reduced, and pain may be so severe that the patient presents with nausea and vomiting. Attention may be incorrectly misdirected to the gastrointestinal tract and the red eye ignored as the source of this disturbance.

The pupil is fixed in middilation at about 4 to 5 mm and nonreactive. The cornea is diffusely hazy. Occasionally, it may be difficult to differentiate angle-closure glaucoma from glaucoma secondary to uveitis. Gonioscopy of an eye with angle closure will reveal obstruction of the trabecular meshwork by iris, whereas an eye with acute glaucoma secondary to uveitis will have a normal open angle unless there has been extensive peripheral anterior synechia formation to the posterior cornea. In this latter case the scarring will be self-evident (see Chapter 10, sec. **IX.**).

D. **Retinoblastoma** is seen in young children and is characterized by pseudohypopyon with nodules in the iris as well as free-floating cells in the aqueous humor. The fundus should be carefully searched for retinal lesions. An x-ray of the globe revealing calcification scattered throughout the retinoblastic tumor is helpful in differentiating the disorder. **Anterior chamber aspiration** should be performed only if there is serious doubt concerning diagnosis (see Chapter 1, sec. **III.L.**; Chapter 11, sec. **XIII.**).

E. **Juvenile xanthogranuloma of the iris (nevoxanthoendothelioma)** is characteristically associated with recurrent hyphema (blood in the anterior chamber), elevated IOP, and yellowish, poorly defined tumors. Therapy varies and includes local systemic corticosteroids, local irradiation, and excision. This disease is most commonly seen in the first year of life, but it may occur in adults. The physician should look for yellow tumors in the skin.

F. **Malignant lymphoma (large cell lymphoma)** such as lymphatic leukemia involving the anterior chamber is diagnosed primarily by the absence of KPs and by cell type on aqueous aspiration. This differs from **central nervous system (CNS)** lymphoma, which presents as malignant masquerade syndrome (see sec. **IV.L.**, below).

G. **Neurofibromas** of the iris appear as brownish pinhead-sized tumors level with the iris stroma or projected in a mushroom from the stroma. They may be congenital or develop after birth, puberty, pregnancy, or menopause. Pigmentation may appear and disappear spontaneously.

H. **Pigment "cells"** in the anterior chamber may be confused with iritis. The anterior chamber should be graded for flare and cells before dilating drops, especially phenylephrine hydrochloride, are used, because the process of dilation may release cells into the aqueous that are actually benign pigment granules. This is most common in patients over the age of 40 years and in myopes. These cells are one-tenth the size of white cells and brownish in color. This benign pigment dust may also appear on the back of the cornea and is finer in appearance and more diffuse than that seen with leukocytic KPs.

I. **Pseudoexfoliation of the lens** presents as blue, white, or gray dandruff-like flecks on the pupillary margins, anterior surface of the lens, trabecular meshwork in the angle, lens zonules, or ciliary body. Diagnosis is confirmed by the presence of a dandruff ring, the central edge of which is lifted and curled, on the anterior lens capsule.

J. **Primary familial amyloidosis** may present as globules that are slightly larger than inflammatory cells suspended in the anterior vitreous or as dense veil-like opacities of wavy contour resembling glass wool. Protein electrophoresis and biopsy are indicated.

K. **Reactive lymphoid hyperplasia** frequently presents as an iridocyclitis. This condition may also simulate malignant melanoma. These pseudotumors respond to topical or systemic corticosteroid.

L. **Masquerade syndrome** (non-Hodgkin lymphoma of the CNS or systemic) involving the eye frequently presents as a uveitis. Occasionally, the diagnosis may be made by aqueous or vitreous tap, with the better yield being from vitrectomy. Malignancy should be suspected in individuals over 40 years of age, particularly those with neurologic manifestations.

V. **Diagnostic tests in uveitis.** The three stages of diagnosis are (a) integrate information, (b) name the uveitis, and (c) order indicated tests. After a careful history, review of systems and physical examination (Table 9.1), **name** the uveitis, e.g., a nongranulomatous iridocyclitis with band keratopathy in both eyes of a 4-year-old girl with arthritis in one knee. These characteristics suggest JRA, thus the main test would be an antinuclear antibody (ANA), which is positive in 80% of patients with iridocyclitis in JRA. However, not all uveitides require an extensive workup. Laboratory testing is performed in cases of recurrent, chronic, or refractory to treatment episodes of ocular inflammation. Cases of intermediate and posterior involvement should also be evaluated with the appropriate laboratory tests. Any patient with uveitis associated with systemic symptoms or signs of a systemic disorder needs to undergo diagnostic testing. Tests that should be considered are as follows (Table 9.3):

A. **Skin testing** is a frequently used useful diagnostic tool, although the risks of severe local reaction or reactivation of quiescent ocular lesions, e.g, macular histoplasmosis, must be borne in mind.

TABLE 9.3. DIAGNOSTIC AIDS FOR UVEITIS BY ANATOMIC CLASSIFICATION

Anterior Uveitis	Intermediate Uveitis	Posterior Uveitis
Anergy skin tests	Anergy skin tests	Anergy skin tests
ACE	ACE	ACE
ANA	ANA	ANA
Anterior chamber paracentesis	Brain CT scan	Antiviral antibodies
Antiviral antibodies	CBC	Brain CT scan
CBC	Chest x-ray	Cardiolipin antibodies
Chest x-ray study	Conjunctival biopsy	CBC
Conjunctival biopsy	Complement (3, 4, CH50)	Chest x-ray
Complement (3, 4, CH50)	CRP	Chorioretinal biopsy
CRP	ESR	Complement
ESR	FTA-ABS	CRP
FTA-ABS	Fluorescein angiography	Doppler ultrasound
Gallium scan	Gallium scan	Echography
Hand x-ray studies	Echography	ERG/EOM
HLA typing (HLA-B27)	Laser interferometry	ESR
Immune complexes (Raji, C1q)	Liver function tests	Fluorescein angiography
Lacrimal gland biopsy	Lyme titers	FTA-ABS
Laser interferometry	Lumbar puncture	Gallium scan
PPD	MRI brain scan	HIV testing
RF	PPD	HLA typing (HLA-A29)
Sacroiliac x-rays	Stool evaluation	Immune complexes
Skin snips	Toxocara titers	Laser interferometry
Stool evaluation	Vitreal biopsy	Liver function tests
Lyme titers		
Lumbar puncture		
MRI brain scan		
PPD		
Stool evaluation		
Toxocara titers		
Toxoplasmosis titers		
Visual evoked responses		
Vitreal biopsy		

ACE, angiotensin converting enzyme; ANA, antinuclear antibodies; CBC, complete blood count; CRP, C-reactive protein; CT, computed tomography; EOM, electrooculogram; ERG, electroretinogram; ESR, erythrocyte sedimentation rate; FTA-ABS, fluorescent treponemal antibody absorption; HIV, human immunodeficiency virus; HLA, human leucocyte antigen; MRI, magnetic resonance imaging; PPD, purified protein derivative; RF, rheumatoid factor.
(Adapted from Nussenblatt R, Palestine A. *Uveitis: Fundamentals and clinical practice.* Chicago: Mosby-Year Book, 1988:58. Opremcak EM. *Uveitis: A clinical manual for ocular inflammation,* New York: Springer-Verlag, 1995:38, and Foster CS, Vitale A. *Diagnosis and treatment of Uveitis.* Philadelphia: WB Saunders, 2002:94–95.)

1. The **tuberculin** and **histoplasmin** tests are among the most important skin tests in uveitis. Even a very small area of reactive induration may be significant. The intermediate-strength purified protein derivative (PPD) should be used routinely (0.1 mL of 5 tuberculin units [TU]). A positive test is regarded as an indication of tuberculous disease unless the patient was vaccinated with bacille Calmette-Guérin previously. A positive PPD does not, however, rule out other etiologic factors, because it may be a coincidental finding. A negative response should be confirmed by performing a PPD using a 250-TU dose.
2. **Anergy panel** or hyporeactivity to skin testing may be of diagnostic value, because it is a phenomenon seen in sarcoidosis, lepromatous

leprosy, pars-planitis, and possibly herpes zoster or other immunocompromised patients. Subcutaneous injections of a panel of common antigens such as *Candida* and mumps are performed.

3. **Older skin tests.** The **Kveim test** for sarcoid is essentially obsolete. The **Behçetin** skin test for pathergy is rarely used currently; it appears to be effective primarily in Behçet's disease patients from the Middle East, but not in the United States.

4. **Systemic steroids** taken every other day will not suppress skin test reactions. If, however, a patient is taking corticosteroids daily, the physician must not require much of a reaction for a positive response; the response may be drug suppressed altogether or, rarely, anergy may be reversed by these drugs. Systemic **cyclosporine** may also suppress a positive skin test.

B. **Blood tests** used in diagnosis of uveitis are numerous; the shotgun approach is rarely rewarding and is very expensive. The tests should, therefore, be based on a high index of suspicion based on clinical findings and review of systems. Some of these are obvious in their objective, e.g., Venereal Disease Research Laboratory (VDRL) or fluorescent treponemal antibody (FTA) test for syphilis. Others warrant the following discussion, and all are listed in Table 9.3. The laboratory workup can be divided into three broad categories: (a) hematology/chemistry, (b) special chemistry, and (c) immunological tests.

1. **Hematology–chemistry**

   a. A **complete blood count** (CBC) with differential showing eosinophilia indicates parasitic infestation or some systemic vasculitis (Wegener granulomatosis and Churg-Strauss syndrome).

   b. **Elevated erythrocyte sedimentation rate** (ESR) is a nonspecific indication of systemic disease that may or may not be related to the ocular disease. Elevation of ESR represents an elevation of acute-phase reactant proteins and supports a more widespread systemic inflammatory process. Other more representative test for the evaluation of acute-phase reactant products include C-reactive protein.

   c. A **urine analysis** is performed to determine the presence of hematuria or proteinuria in cases where a vasculitic disorder is suspected.

   d. **Electrolytes** and **liver function tests** are indicated when damage to the kidney or liver occur, and in patients who will be undergoing systemic treatment of the uveitis with chemosuppression

   e. **Serum globulin** and **calcium** are elevated in sarcoidosis, as is **urine calcium.**

2. **Special chemistry**

   a. **Angiotensin converting enzyme** is often routinely drawn in cases of suspected sarcoid, yet it is not specific for this disease. Normal values in children are not known, and the diagnostic value is not established in the absence of other signs of sarcoid.

   b. **FTA-antibody absorption** (FTA-ABS) and **VDRL** are the tests for syphilis. This condition can present in different forms of uveitis, and should always be considered in the differential diagnosis and must be ruled out. The FTA-ABS test is the most sensitive test for syphilis. It becomes positive at the beginning of the disease and always remains positive. A VDRL test can be performed on patients with active or resolving infection. It is used to monitor efficacy of treatment.

   c. **Antibody titers against other infectious organisms.** A *Toxoplasma* fluorescent antibody or hemagglutination titer is considered positive at any level, even 1:1. Other available serological tests for infectious organisms include Lyme immunoglobulin IgG/IgM, *Rickettsia typhi* IgG/IgM, *Toxocara* IgG/IgM, and catscratch disease. Antiviral titers (herpes simplex virus [HSV], varicella-zoster virus [VZV], CMV, Epstein-Barr virus [EBV], and others listed in Table 9.3) are, with the exception of human immunodeficiency virus (HIV) titers (AIDS), meaningful only when drawn as acute and convalescent sera about 1 month apart and demonstrating at least a two-to-fourfold increase in titer. A single "positive" test for virus does not indicate whether a viral infection took place recently. Elevated IgM indicates recent infection, whereas detectable IgG represents previous exposure. These tests should be ordered only if indicated by pertinent positive data obtained in the history, review of systems, and physical exam.

3. **Immunological tests**
   a. **HLA** testing is of significance when positive in a patient exhibiting signs of disease compatible with the appropriate known HLA immunogenetic test. HLA tests associated with specific ocular inflammatory states include
      (1) Acute anterior uveitis: HLA-B27, HLA-B8.
      (2) Ankylosing spondylitis: HLA-B27, HLA-B7.
      (3) Behçet's disease: HLA-B51.
      (4) Birdshot retinopathy: HLA-A29.
      (5) Multiple sclerosis, uveitis and optic neuritis: DR2.
      (6) Ocular pemphigoid: HLA-B12, DQw7.
      (7) Presumed ocular histoplasmosis: HLA-B7, DR2.
      (8) Reiter syndrome: HLA-B27.
      (9) Rheumatoid arthritis: HLA-DR4.
      (10) Sympathetic ophthalmia: HLA-A11, DR4, Dw53.
      (11) VKH disease: DR4, Dw53, DQw3.

   HLA typing is now considered an important diagnostic test in determining the etiology of certain uveitides. The HLA system is the main human leukocyte isoantigen system. Human leukocyte antigens are present on most nucleated cells and comprise the major histocompatibility systems in humans. In practice, the blood lymphocyte is tested by cytotoxicity methods by incubation with antiserum complement. The genetic loci belonging to the system are designated by the loci A, B, C, and D. These alleles are designated by numbers. In practice, it is seen that HLA-B27 is commonly associated with iridocyclitis in ankylosing spondylitis. A patient with a positive HLA-B27 has a 35% chance of developing acute iritis, compared with a 7% chance for those with a negative HLA-B27. Patients with VKH syndrome have an increased frequency of positive HLA-BW22J, a unique Japanese antigen. HLA-B7 appears to predispose a patient to the development of histoplasmic maculopathy. This testing is generally done in university hospital centers.

   b. Autoantibody production in connective tissue disorders can be evaluated by testing for **ANAs, rheumatoid factor (RF),** and other antiextracted nuclear antigens such as **anti-double-stranded DNA** and **anti-Ro/anti La** (Sjögren syndrome). The presence of these antibodies is suggestive of an active autoimmune disorder; however, to make a specific diagnosis, a clinical correlation is needed.
   c. **Anticardiolipin antibodies** should be drawn in cases of retinal vascular occlusive disease, especially suspected lupus with vasculitis (see Chapter 8, sec. **III.B.10.**).
   d. **Antineutrophil cytoplasmic antibodies** (ANCAs) for diagnosis of vasculitic disease such as Kawasaki, polyarteritis nodosa, and Wegener granulomatosis (p-ANCA is for polyarteritis nodosa, c-ANCA is for Wegener). Efficacy of cyclophosphamide or trimethoprim–sulfisoxasole DS tablets daily can be monitored using sequential ANCA titers.
   e. **Circulating immune complexes** present in ocular inflammatory disease may be a secondary or protective reaction rather than a destructive primary cause of disease. A positive ANA is of diagnostic significance in JRA and lupus erythematosus. Tests that are used to detect circulating immune complexes include **C1q binding assay** (IgM complexes) and **Raji cell assay** (IgG complexes).
   f. **Complement.** Low levels of complement factors in serum will occur in infectious or autoimmune disorders where complement consumption is

active. This can be determined by testing for CH_{50} **total complement** (50% total hemolyzing dose of complement), **C3, C4,** and **properdin factor B** serum levels.

    g. Cytokines (**interleukin-1 [IL-1], IL-2, IL-2R, IL-6, IL-10, IL-12, and tumor necrosis factor [TNF]**) are soluble proteins made by cells of the immune system (T cells, B cells, and macrophages) during an immune response. The detection of these cytokines and soluble receptors in the serum of patients with uveitis is another marker that can be used to assess active immunological activity.

    h. The **lymphocyte transformation test** may demonstrate T-cell or cellular hypersensitivity to many antigens in the laboratory. These highly specialized tests may or may not aid in diagnosis and are still being refined.

C. Radiographic and other imaging analyses of diagnostic significance are
1. **Chest x-ray** for sarcoid, TBC, or malignancy.
2. **Gallium scans** of the lungs, salivary, or lacrimal glands for sarcoidosis.
3. **Computed tomography (CT) scans** of the chest and mediastinum can be more sensitive for sarcoidosis.
4. **Sinus films (plain x-ray and CT scan)** for orbital inflammatory disease are important in diagnosing diseases affecting the orbit and periocular tissue.
5. **Sacroiliac and spinal x-rays** for evidence of ankylosing spondylitis.
6. **Hand, wrist, foot, and knee x-rays** for arthritic changes of rheumatoid disease or Reiter syndrome.
7. **Magnetic resonance imaging (MRI) scan and magnetic resonance angiography** for early demyelinating lesions of multiple sclerosis, vasculitis of lupus, or other vasculitides with CNS manifestations.
8. **Doppler ultrasonography** for enhanced images of poorly visualized lesions of retina, choroid, and sclera.

D. Fluorescein angiography may be of use in diagnosis and clinical follow-up of chorioretinitis secondary to toxoplasmosis, toxocariasis, and histoplasmosis, and as an invaluable aid in following the clinical course of the many changes seen in a variety of uveitis patients.
1. The most common **fluorescein angiographic changes** found in uveitis include
    a. Cystoid macular edema.
    b. Disk leakage.
    c. Late staining of the retinal vasculature.
    d. RPE disturbances.
    e. Retinal capillary dropout, ischemia, and neovascularization.
    f. Subretinal neovascular membranes.
2. **Visual acuity impairment** is correlated directly with increased macular thickening, but not with late-phase leakage as determined by angiography.
3. **Indocyanine green (ICG) angiography** for choroidal lesion evaluation.

E. Echography (ultrasound) is extremely useful in evaluating **anterior and posterior disease,** particularly when the **view is obscured.** Methods include anterior immersion technique and ultrasound biomicroscopy, and posterior A- and B-scans (see Chapter 1, sec. **III.I.**). This test is helpful in the evaluation of
1. **Vitreal disorders:** hemorrhage versus inflammation, pars-planitis, retained lens fragments.
2. **Optic disk edema** and **cupping.**
3. **Macular disease:** edema, exudative detachments.
4. **Choroidal thickening:** uveal effusion, scleritis, Harada's disease, sympathetic ophthalmia, and hypotony.
5. **Masquerade syndromes:** lymphoma, diffuse melanoma, and benign lymphoid hyperplasia.

F. **Other ophthalmic tests** of use in uveitis are as follows:
   1. The **electroretinogram** (**ERG;** local retinal damage) and the **electrooculogram** (**EOG;** RPE status assessed by corneal retinal potentials) will indicate the extent of widespread damage to the eye, but are not diagnostically specific (see Chapter 1, sec. **III.G.**).
   2. **Laser interferometry** is a useful predictor of which patients will do well with immunosuppressive therapy. Visual acuity measured by laser interferometry is often better than that measured by standard eye charts. The difference probably indicates potentially reversible macular disease. Thus, if a patient reads two lines better with laser testing than on the eye chart, one may predict about a two-line potential improvement with therapy with better than 80% accuracy.
G. **Ocular tissue sampling** can be extremely valuable in the diagnosis of a systemic disorder in patients with uveitis.
   1. **Conjunctival biopsy** is useful in sarcoidosis only if there is an obvious lesion. Even if shown to be a granulomatous reaction, it may be hard to prove that it is not an old chalazion. In vasculitides and other immune-mediated processes, histological evaluation and immunofluorescence staining of the conjunctiva specimen can help to identify the presence of immune complex deposition, and identification of inflammatory cells and vasculitis.
   2. **Anterior chamber aspiration.** Cytology examination and antibody titers of the aqueous humor through a paracentesis may be of diagnostic assistance (see Chapter 1, sec. **III.L.**).
      a. **Cytology** may vary depending on etiology. A small drop of **aqueous** is placed on a slide from the aspirating needle, fixed in absolute methanol for 10 minutes, and allowed to air-dry. The slide is stained with Giemsa solution for 1 hour and then rinsed with 95% ethanol and allowed to dry. Acute uveitis involving binding of complement to immune complexes (Behçet syndrome) may have an abundance of neutrophils. Lens-induced uveitis produces many macrophages as well as some neutrophils. In parasitic infections numerous eosinophils are present. Bacterial uveitis may reveal both organisms and multiple neutrophils. Gram staining should be performed on another single-drop slide preparation of aqueous to confirm the type of bacteria seen.
      b. **Local production of antibody** resulting in higher intraocular than serum titers may be indicative of an active intraocular lesion such as toxoplasmosis, HSV, or VZV. A normal antibody coefficient is 1.0. A range of 2 to 7 is suggestive, and over 8 is diagnostic. These tests are done only in major medical centers.
   3. **Diagnostic pars plana vitrectomy** can be extremely helpful in making the diagnosis of masquerade syndromes in patients with posterior uveitis and vitritis.
      a. **Cytology** of vitreous fluid can be used to identify atypical or malignant cells in patients with intraocular lymphoma. The absence of malignant cells and the presence of inflammatory lymphocytes can be diagnostic of an inflammatory uveitis.
      b. **Flow cytometry analysis** can be performed in vitreous cells from vitreous samples. Using fluorescent antibodies to cell surface markers, flow cytometry can identify a specific population of cells expressing such marker. Expression of kappa and lambda variable chains in B cells is representative of a monoclonal expansion typical of lymphoma. Flow cytometry can be used to identify kappa and lambda expression and confirm a diagnosis of intraocular lymphoma.
      c. **Polymerase chain reaction (PCR)** allows the detection of a small number of DNA fragments by exponential replication. By using specific DNA probes for certain microorganisms, PCR can locate the DNA fragment in the sample and allow its identification. This technique is

extremely sensitive and is used more frequently to diagnose microbiological infections. PCR has been used in the diagnosis of intraocular infections caused by herpesviruses, *Mycobacterium tuberculosis*, *Toxocara gondii*, and CMV.

  d. Cytokines can also be measured in vitreous fluid. As in serum, they are representative of intraocular inflammatory disease. The presence of IL-10 (B-cell cytokine) can be suggestive of intraocular lymphoma.

H. Ancillary tests

  1. Stool samples are of diagnostic value if parasitic disease is the suspected etiologic agent.

  2. Lumbar puncture for cerebrospinal fluid cytology is indicated in cases of suspected VKH syndrome or intraocular neoplasm.

  3. Skin snips are biopsy specimens used in making a diagnosis of onchocerciasis and vasculitic diseases. The snip should be taken from one or two of the skin nodules or purpuric lesions.

VI. Nonspecific treatment of uveitis. The main goal of the treatment in patients with intraocular inflammation is to down-modulate immune responses. Because the etiology of noninfectious uveitis is often unknown or no specific treatment is available despite specific diagnosis, nonspecific measures are frequently employed. These measures include *topical and systemic corticosteroids, mydriatic–cycloplegics, nonsteroidal antiinflammatory agents (NSAIDs), immunosuppressive drugs, and photocoagulation.* The chronic use of topical or systemic steroid in the treatment of uveitis must be avoided, in order to prevent the devastating ocular and systemic side effects. If intraocular inflammation cannot be controlled without the use of corticosteroids, then a stepladder approach should be strategized, beginning with NSAIDs, followed by immunosuppressive drugs as necessary.

A. Corticosteroids are very effective, not too difficult to administer, not too expensive, and therefore are the most common agents used. These drugs reduce inflammation by (a) reduction of leukocytic and plasma exudation, (b) maintenance of cellular membrane integrity with inhibition of tissue swelling, (c) inhibition of lysozyme release from granulocytes and inhibition of phagocytosis, (d) increased stabilization of intracellular lysosomal membranes, and (e) suppression of circulating lymphocytes. Corticosteroids should be used with caution in uveitis secondary to an infectious process, particularly that of HSV, bacterial etiology, TBC, and toxoplasmosis, and they should never be used with fungus. The relative drug potency, the aqueous penetration, and relative ocular antiinflammatory effect are listed in Table 9.4. Corticosteroid can be administered locally or systemically.

  1. Local administration of corticosteroids can be very effective in the treatment of uveitis. Their action in suppressing inflammation in the eye is rapid and can spare the use of systemic medications.

  a. Topical corticosteroid administration. For an anterior iridocyclitis, the frequency of corticosteroid drops is dependent on the severity

TABLE 9.4. RELATIVE POTENCY OF SYSTEMIC CORTICOSTEROIDS AND AQUEOUS PENETRATION OF TOPICAL PREPARATIONS

Drug	Systemic Relative Potency	Peak Aqueous Concentration (ng/mL)	Relative Antiinflammatory Effect
Prednisolone acetate 1%	4	670	26
Dexamethasone alcohol 0.1%	25	31	7
Prednisolone sodium phosphate 0.5%	4	26	1
Betamethasone sodium phosphate 0.1%	25	8	2

of the reaction and varies from one drop q2 to 4h around the clock for the first few days. If the uveitis is posterior to the lens iris diaphragm, drops or ointments will not be adequate. Titration should be slow over many days to weeks and generally reduced by 50% at each step as the disease improves. The starting point is dependent on the severity of the reaction. In general, the presence of a fibrinous hypopyon uveitis would indicate high-dose therapy starting at q1 to 2h; the presence of a mild to moderate cell and flare reaction would indicate therapy starting at a level of strong corticosteroids six to eight times daily with taper within several days to the weaker steroid preparations over several weeks to months at qid, tid, bid, qd, qod, etc. dosages, depending on the clinical response. The strongest ophthalmic corticosteroid drop preparations are dexamethasone phosphate 0.1%, dexamethasone alcohol 0.1%, prednisolone acetate 1.0%, and prednisolone phosphate 1.0%. However, lipophilic preparations, such as prednisolone acetate, will achieve higher intraocular concentrations due to their effective penetration through the corneal epithelium (Table 9.4). Of lesser strength and of great use in tapering or treating less severe anterior segment inflammation are fluorometholone 0.1%. A new family of topical steroids has been developed, the members of which have a higher affinity for steroid receptors on inflammatory cells, providing antiinflammatory activity with fewer tendencies to cause an increase in IOP. **Rimexolone (Vexol 1%)** and **loteprednol etabonate (Lotemax 1%, Alrex 0.2%)** have been used successfully in the treatment of postsurgical inflammation after cataract surgery and in certain types of uveitis. Their role in the resolution of severe cases of intraocular inflammation remains to be investigated.

b. **Periocular injection.** Periocular injections are indicated to supplement systemic therapy in severe iritis, pars-planitis, and macular edema in patients who cannot be trusted to take their medications, during eye surgery in an eye with uveitis, and when topical and systemic steroids are not sufficiently effective. Children must be placed under general anesthesia and **never maintained on injected steroid without monitoring by a pediatrician** for adrenal suppression and other adverse side effects. Because of the danger of intraocular injection, only an ophthalmologist should give such medication.

Although **depot** medication remains in the periocular tissues for 6 weeks, its major effect is during the first week. (Depot methylprednisolone [Depomedrol], 40 to 80 mg subconjunctiva, subtenon, or retrobulbar, is commonly used.) These injections are ordinarily given once every 2 weeks four to five times in patients who have had no IOP increase with topical or previous short-acting local steroid injections. Some patients may require such an injection only once every 6 months. **Soluble, short-acting** steroids may be used for acute cases, in patients who have to take injections every week, or in patients in whom the physician is concerned about an increase in IOP from corticosteroids. **Aqueous** methylprednisolone 40 to 80 mg, triamcinolone 40 mg, or decadron 4 to 24 mg per mL may be given daily, every other day, or as needed to control inflammation.

The **injection** is most safely made above the temporal subtenon area over the pars plana, over the peripheral retina, or back near the macular region, depending on the disease target. Topical anesthetics are necessary, but mixing injectable anesthetic with steroid increases volume and initial pain. Injection through the lower lid into the orbit floor can also be effectively performed. Preinjection oral analgesics can be given for the lingering discomfort. Such injections may be used at the end of an intraocular surgical procedure, in unilateral uveitis, in cystoid macular edema (CME), and in children. All are situations in which systemic effects of steroids are minimized, yet good therapeutic doses are delivered to the target site.

2. **Systemic corticosteroids.** These are of use in noninfectious intractable anterior uveitis not responding satisfactorily to topical drops alone and for posterior uveitis or panuveitis where the deeper uveal structures can be reached only by systemic administration of drug or by periocular injection (see sec. **VI.A.1,2.**). With the exception of concurrent systemic disease that demands systemic therapy or severe vision-threatening disease, children should be treated only with topical and/or periocular injections, because immunosuppressive agents have lifelong effects on growth and development. **Systemic steroids, including periocular injection, should never be used in children without consultation with or the concomitant care of a pediatrician.** Table 9.4 lists the relative dose potencies of commonly used corticosteroids.

   a. **Daily therapy** for marked inflammatory activity, in which an immediate high dosage is necessary over a period of several days for maintenance of the integrity of critical visual structures such as the macula or optic nerve, is necessary for at least 7 days. Patients with panuveitis will require dosage of at least 60 to 100 mg of prednisone (1 mg per kg), whereas patients with intermediate uveitis or bilateral macular edema commonly are treated with 40 to 50 mg per day. Once the inflammation is controlled, the daily dose is reduced by 10 mg per day until 25 mg per day is reached. A slower tapering schedule is then performed, by reducing the dose 5 mg per day every month down to 15 mg per day, followed by 2.5 mg every month down to 5 mg per day, and 1 mg monthly to finalize the tapering schedule. It is important to monitor the patient for any signs suggestive of a flare-up. If a flare-up occurs, a substantial increase in the dosage should be prescribed (50% to 100%). Patients resistant to corticosteroid tapering should be considered for steroid-sparing therapy prior to the development of steroid therapy complications.

   b. **Intravenous methylprednisolone** can be used in cases of Behçet syndrome, VKH syndrome, severe scleritis, and other sight-threatening uveitides. The effects are rapid and dramatic, but are also of brief duration. This form of treatment allows a fast control of the inflammatory process, and is supplemented with oral steroids and if necessary, other forms of immunosuppression. Methylprednisolone is administered in dosages from 500 mg to 1 g. Pulse therapy can be used by repeating the dose at intervals of 24 hours, with a maximum of three doses. The intravenous infusion is done slowly during 1 to 2 hours with proper monitoring of the patient's vital signs and clinical status.

3. **Complications of corticosteroid therapy**

   a. **Topical therapy.** Potential side effects of topical therapy include temporary partial lid ptosis, pupillary mydriasis of 0.6 to 2.0 mm, increased IOP in approximately 30% of patients treated for 3 weeks or more, posterior subcapsular cataract formation that will not progress if corticosteroids are discontinued, bacterial or fungal superinfection secondary to suppression of cellular defense systems, and decreased wound healing.

   b. **Systemic and repeated periocular therapy.** Complications of systemic or repeated periocular therapy are all of those described above, plus extraocular muscle fibrosis (periocular injection), Cushing syndrome, peptic ulcers, systemic hypertension, sodium retention, hyperglycemia in diabetics, psychosis, failure of growth, amenorrhea, aseptic joint necrosis, osteoporosis, myopathy, fluid retention, and Addison's disease.

B. **Mydriatic–cycloplegics** are used to give comfort by relieving iris sphincter and ciliary muscle spasm and to prevent scarring between the pupillary border and anterior lens capsule (posterior synechiae). Atropine, the strongest mydriatic–cycloplegic, is used in strengths of 1%. It should be reserved for moderately severe to severe anterior uveitis and should be used one to two times daily. As uveitis lessens, the atropine dosage may be reduced or the patient placed on homatropine 5% at bedtime. For mild to moderate anterior uveitis, homatropine 5% qd to bid will suffice to move the pupil. Bedtime use is beneficial only in milder cases, because the pupil is mobilized primarily during sleep and iatrogenic presbyopia is not present during the day. Eyes with pupils that fail to dilate on atropine should have the lids taped shut between applications to increase the effect of the atropine. Phenylephrine 2.5% bid to tid (in the absence of significant cardiovascular disease) and cocaine 4% drops q30min tid are also useful in mobilizing the otherwise scarred-down pupil. Atropine may also complicate or precipitate urinary retention in patients with prostatism. Scopolamine 0.25% has almost the same cycloplegic strength as atropine and may be substituted in patients with urinary retention problems. Scopolamine itself, however, in very frequent doses may also aggravate this condition. **Cyclopentolate may aggravate iritis** because of its neutrophilic chemotactic effect; however, this has not been proven true in clinical experience.

C. **NSAIDs.** Oral NSAIDs appear to act by blocking local mediators of the inflammatory response such as the polypeptides of the kinin system, lysosomal enzymes, lymphokines, and prostaglandins. The prostaglandins are one of the many chemical mediators involved in the pathogenesis of uveitis; they are synthesized by the enzyme prostaglandin synthetase and found in all tissues of the eye. Prostaglandins cause a marked increase in protein content of the aqueous humor and mild smooth muscle contraction (pupillary miosis). Certain prostaglandins lower IOP, and others (E_1 and E_2) may increase it. The increased permeability of the ciliary epithelium may be a critical factor in inducing increased IOP secondary to prostaglandin release. All should be **taken with meals.**

1. **Indications.** There is no evidence that any NSAID is effective when used as the **primary agent** in therapy of intraocular inflammation, but they are often **steroid-sparing** agents. They are, however, useful in long-term therapy of **recurrent anterior uveitis, rheumatoid scleritis,** or **macular edema** initially controlled by steroid therapy. Diflunisal (Dolobid) 250 to 500 mg p.o. bid, diclotenac (voltaren 50 mg p.o. bid), naproxen (Naprosyn) 250 or 375 mg p.o. bid, or indomethacin (Indocin SR) 75 mg p.o. qd to bid, may allow a patient to reduce or even discontinue steroid therapy without reactivation of disease. Rofecoxib (Vioxx) 25 mg p.o. qd and celecoxib (Celebrex) 100 to 200 mg p.o. bid are in a new class of NSAID that selectively inhibits cyclooxygenase-2 and reduces prostaglandin synthesis (COX-2 inhibitor) and are better tolerated, causing less gastrointestinal discomfort. Their efficacy in the treatment of uveitis and CME is still under investigation.

2. **Salicylates** are effective in reducing inflammatory response and protein increase in the anterior chamber after keratocentesis. Aspirin must be used in the range of 4 to 5 g or more per day to be effective, and may be given in several divided doses.

3. **Toxicity** includes gastric mucosal ulceration and liver and renal damage. Urine, stool, and blood monitoring should be done every few months. COX-2 inhibitors should be avoided in patients with liver disease and when used, liver function tests should be performed.

4. **Topical NSAIDs** are equivocally effective in iritis but may have a steroid-sparing effect. They may also be successful in treatment of CME. **Current agents** include flurbiprofen 0.03% (Ocufen), suprofen 1% (Profenal), diclofenac 0.1% (Voltaren), and ketorolac 0.5% (Acular), the last three drugs in dosages of three to four drops per day for CME (see Appendix A for U.S. Food and Drug Administration [FDA]-approved use).

D. **Immunosuppressive agents.** Immunosuppressive drugs usually should not be prescribed by an ophthalmologist alone, but in concert with an oncologist or hematologist who is familiar with them and confident in their management. In making a decision as to which patient should receive immunosuppressive therapy, the physician must remember that the use of these drugs for nonneoplastic and non-life-threatening illness is a great clinical responsibility. To date there appear to have been very few severe complications from the combined regimen of corticosteroids and immunosuppressive agents, probably because of the lower dosages used and the better general health of the ophthalmic patients receiving them. Patients should be fully informed as to potential risks and benefits. A signed consent form or chart note to that effect is advisable.

1. **Selection of patients** involves choosing those who:
   a. Have Wegener's granulomatosis, polyarteritis nodosa, or Behçet's disease (immunosuppressive agents are the drugs of first choice).
   b. Failed to respond to conventional corticosteroid therapy or have an unacceptable side effect from the drugs.
   c. Have progressive, usually bilateral vision-threatening disease.
   d. Have adequate follow-up.
   e. Are reliable about following instructions.
   f. Are willing to undergo therapy with full knowledge of the possible deleterious side effects.
   g. May potentially benefit from the use of the drugs.
   h. Have no unequivocal contraindication such as active TBC, toxoplasmosis, or other infectious process.

2. **Three classes of immunosuppressive agents** are used in ocular inflammatory disease: alkylating agents, antimetabolites, and antibiotics.
   a. **The alkylating agents cyclophosphamide and chlorambucil** work by suppression of lymphocyte T-cell (cell-mediated immunity) and, to a lesser extent, B-cell (antibodies) function.
      (1) **Clinical indications** are most commonly Behçet's disease, sympathetic ophthalmia, Wegener granulomatosis, rheumatoid arthritis, polyarteritis nodosa, relapsing polychondritis, severe systemic lupus erythematosus, bullous pemphigoid, and malignancy. These medications can induce long-term remission in some patients with severe uveitis.
      (2) **Cyclophosphamide dosage** in adult patients starts at 150 to 200 mg per day (1 mg/kg/day) taken on an empty stomach, in the morning and followed with hydration of 3 L of fluid daily. The aim of the therapy is to lower the lymphocyte count to 1.0×10^9 per L (normal 1.3 to 3.5×10^9 per L). The total white cell count should not fall below 3.5×10^9 per L. The white cell count and differential are obtained at baseline and then followed twice weekly for the first 2 to 3 weeks. Once stabilized, laboratory tests are performed q4 weeks.
      (3) **Chlorambucil dosage** is begun at 0.1 to 0.2 mg/kg/day (usual dose 2 mg per day) and increased every 3 to 4 days to total dosage of 10 to 12 mg per day if there is no idiosyncratic reaction. The white cell count and differential are followed as for cyclophosphamide.
      (4) **Adverse side effects** of alkylating agents are uncontrolled leukopenia, thrombocytopenia, anemia, opportunistic infections, gastrointestinal disturbances, alopecia, jaundice, pulmonary interstitial fibrosis, renal toxicity, sterility, and testicular atrophy. Hemorrhagic cystitis is an indication for discontinuing the medication. An increased incidence of myeloproliferative and lymphoproliferative malignancy in patients taking these drugs is debatable, especially at the lower doses used for the treatment of uveitis.
   b. **The antimetabolite azathioprine** interferes with purine metabolism and **methotrexate** interferes with folate action; both functions are essential to nucleic acid synthesis. **Mycophenolate mofetil** (Cellcept) is a new antimetabolite that inhibits the enzyme inosine monophosphate dehydrogenase in activated T and B cells and blocks their production of guanine and thereby their function.
      (1) **Clinical indications** are in therapy of rheumatoid arthritis, pemphigoid, and regional ileitis. Azathioprine has also been used successfully in some cases of sympathetic ophthalmia, VKH syndrome, pars-planitis, and Behçet's disease. Methotrexate has been

effective in certain recalcitrant cases of intermediate uveitis and sympathetic ophthalmia, but ineffective in Behçet's disease and iridocyclitis. Cellcept has been used in the management of solid organ transplantation, and has been found to be useful in the treatment of uveitis.

(2) **Azathioprine dosage** is taken at doses ranging from 1 to 2.5 mg/kg/day. The usual dose range is 100 mg per day, divided in two doses.

(3) **Adverse side effects of azathioprine** are uncontrolled leukopenia, thrombocytopenia, hyperuricemia, and gastrointestinal disturbances.

(4) **Methotrexate dosage** is variable due to high drug toxicity. Generally, the dose is 0.2 mg/kg p.o. or subcutaneous weekly with reevaluation in 2 weeks and then q 4–6 weeks if parameters are normal. Treatment is continued until a therapeutic response is noted and then maintained per hematologic and renal and hepatic monitoring q 4–6 weeks. Maximum dose is 15–25 mg/wk.

(5) **Adverse side effects of methotrexate** include leukopenia, thrombocytopenia, hepatic and renal toxicity, gastrointestinal disturbances, interstitial pneumonitis, CNS toxicity, and sterility.

(6) **Hematologic monitoring** for both antimetabolites is similar to that of cyclophosphamide (alkylating agents).

c. **The antibiotic cyclosporin A** probably interferes with T-cell lymphocyte activation and interleukin activity, and **dapsone** may work by lysosomal stabilization.

(1) **The clinical indications** for **cyclosporine** are Behçet's disease (for which corticosteroids are contraindicated by many investigators), birdshot chorioretinopathy, sarcoid, VKH, and sympathetic ophthalmia. Relative indications are all noninfectious cases of uveitis unresponsive to maximum tolerated steroid therapy, Eales's disease, retinal vasculitis (noninfectious), and serpiginous choroiditis. Anterior segment disease responsive to this drug includes pemphigoid, Mooren ulcer, and high-risk corneal transplant rejection.

(2) **Cyclosporin A dosage** is 2.5 to 5 mg/kg/day given orally in an olive oil–ethanol solution with milk or juice. Maximum dosage is 10 mg/kg/day.

(3) **Adverse side effects** of the given **cyclosporin A** dosage are systemic hypertension, partially reversible **renal toxicity,** opportunistic infection, gastrointestinal disturbances, breast tenderness, neurotoxicity, nausea, vomiting, hyperuricemia, and hepatotoxicity. Monthly and, if warranted, weekly blood tests should monitor these effects.

(4) **Dapsone** is discussed in Chapter 5, sec. **IV.M.**

d. **Combination steroid and cyclosporin A therapy.** These drugs augment each other such that addition of prednisone (10 to 20 mg per day or short-term 1 mg/kg/day) may allow a lowering of the cyclosporin A dosage (4 to 6 mg/kg/day) with no loss of therapeutic efficacy.

e. **Chlorambucil or cyclophosphamide–steroid management technique** involves initial treatment with prednisone, 1 mg/kg/day, along with the cytotoxic drug at an appropriate dose. This treatment continues about 1 month until the disease is suppressed, then steroids are tapered and stopped over 2 months. The cytotoxic drug dose is adjusted to keep the white blood cell count (WBC) at 3,000 to 4,000 per mL and continued for 1 year to induce remission before being stopped. Monitor the CBC and urinalysis (cyclophosphamide only) weekly until stable, then every 2 weeks (see specific cytotoxic drugs above).

E. **Photocoagulation** in toxoplasmic chorioretinitis has not been confirmed as valuable therapy either in the acute or atrophic stage. It is, however, the treatment of choice in ocular histoplasmosis in which a neovascular net has developed under the retina. Coagulation of the net usually leads to obliteration of capillaries and some recovery of vision (see Chapter 8, secs. **III.** and **XI.**)

F. **Monoclonal antibody** therapy has been used in the treatment of autoimmune disorders. This form of therapy targets specific receptors in cells of the immune system that are important in modulating immune responses. These include antibodies against TNF receptor, IL-2 receptor, adhesion molecules, and T-cell receptor. The use of these agents is still experimental in the treatment of uveitis, and should be performed by centers familiar with this form of treatment.

VII. Complications of uveitis

A. **Corneal band keratopathy** usually indicates that the individual has had chronic uveitis. The calcified opacity at the level of Bowman membrane and the palpebral fissure is separated from the limbus by a clear zone and has disk-shaped holes corresponding to nerve channels. This band may be *removed for visual or cosmetic reasons* by the use of chelating agents such as, 0.5 to 1.0% sodium ethylenediaminetetraacetic acid (EDTA). The corneal epithelium is gently removed with cocaine 4% on a sterile cotton-tipped applicator and mild scraping with the edge of a Bard-Parker blade if necessary. A Weck-cell sponge cut to the shape of the band is soaked in the chelating agent and applied over the area of the band for 5 to 10 minutes. It is then removed and the band wiped again with a sterile cotton-tipped applicator or blade. The Weck-cell may need to be reapplied to complete removal of the calcium. EDTA may also be dropped onto the cornea but will produce a significant chemical conjunctivitis postoperatively. Antibiotic ointment and a short-acting cycloplegic should be instilled and mild pressure patching or a therapeutic soft contact lens is applied for 24 to 48 hours postoperatively.

B. **Cataracts** (see Chapter 7, sec. **V.E,G.**)

C. **Macular surface wrinkling** is an increased shagreen or reflection and crinkled cellophane-like appearance that have given rise to the term *cellophane maculopathy*. Various types of cells growing on the internal limiting membrane may produce this wrinkling. No specific therapy is available, although retrobulbar depot steroids may retard progression of macular traction. Surgical peeling of membranes may be successful.

D. **Edema of the disk and macula** may be seen in the more severe posterior uveitides and panuveitides. Edema of the disk does not result in much visual impairment, but macular edema is a major cause of reduced vision. Whenever vision is reduced in uveitic patients, this entity should be suspected and is probably best established diagnostically (in decreasing order) by the photo-stress test, by fluorescein angiography, by slitlamp microscopy of the macula using a +78 D lens, and least well by direct ophthalmoscopy. Systemic and posterior periocular **steroid** therapy or, if necessary, **immunosuppressive** therapy may be of significant use in reversing or limiting macular damage in appropriately selected cases. **Antiprostaglandin drugs** such as p.o. naproxen 250 to 375 mg bid, or diflunisal 500 mg qd to bid, may be of use in limiting macular edema in certain cases and may be used with **greater safety** than steroids or immunosuppressives for prolonged therapy or after a course of steroid. **Topical indomethacin** (one tablet per 5 mL saline), **flurbiprofen** 0.03%, **diclofenac** 0.1%, or **suprofen** 1% qid are often useful. The **carbonic anhydrase inhibitor** acetazolamide 250 mg p.o. qd for several weeks may also be effective. Optic disk swelling could be an indicator of CNS involvement and an appropriate workup is necessary, especially if clinical symptoms are present.

E. **Corneal edema** is proportionate to the degree of damaged corneal endothelium and to the height of IOP. Topical steroids should be used q2 to 6h as needed to quiet inflammation in the vicinity of the endothelium, and measures should be taken to reduce IOP. Carbonic anhydrase inhibitors, with or without topical beta-blockers, are effective.

F. Secondary glaucoma
1. Etiology
   a. **Debris blockage** is probably the most common cause of secondary glaucoma. The uveal meshwork becomes blocked by inflammatory material. The IOP may not increase until the ciliary body is recovering function and secreting normal amounts of aqueous again.
   b. **Anterior synechiae** result from inflammatory adhesions between cornea and iris, usually due to nodules or infiltration of the trabeculum, thereby closing the angle.
   c. In **rubeosis iridis** a fibrovascular membrane in the angle contracts like a zipper, causing angle-closure glaucoma. Rubeosis signifies an ischemic retina and conveys a poor prognosis.
   d. **Corticosteroids** themselves frequently result in an increase in IOP and may aggravate primary glaucoma. If the patient is a steroid responder, and the pressure cannot be controlled below 25 mm Hg or there is progressive cupping or field loss despite acetazolamide or methazolamide pills and beta-blocker, the physician may reduce the level of steroid to increase the degree of uveitis and effect a lowered pressure. If the problem is posterior, e.g., toxoplasmic chorioretinitis, prednisone tablets rather than depot injections or corticosteroid drops should be used.
   e. **Iris bombé.** If the iris becomes bound to the lens all around the pupil, **iris bombé** may develop, preventing flow of aqueous in the ciliary body into the anterior chamber and trabecular area. If pressure becomes too high, yttrium, aluminum, garnet (YAG) or argon **laser iridotomy** can be used or, if these fail because of iris edema and inflammation, surgery to produce a peripheral iridectomy opening is necessary.
   f. **Sclerosis** of the trabecular meshwork may follow chronic uveitis.
   g. A **hyaline membrane** may form over the trabeculum, blocking outflow.
   h. **Swelling** of the trabeculum from inflammation (trabeculitis) may reduce its porosity.
2. Treatment contraindications
   a. **Miotics are avoided in secondary glaucoma due to uveitis** because they increase the discomfort from the sphincter pupillae and increase inflammation.
   b. **Laser trabeculoplasty is not useful** and not indicated in uveitis glaucoma (see Chapter 10).
G. Retinal detachment
may be exudative, as in VKH syndrome. Uveitis may also give rise to detachment by producing shrinkage in the vitreous, with resultant traction and tears in the retina. In patients without uveitis, such a tear in the retina often gives rise to anterior segment changes that simulate uveitis.
H. Hypotony
is caused by the cyclitic membrane of the ciliary body, which surrounds the ciliary processes and compromises their secretory function. This is commonly seen in patients with JRA and poorly controlled chronic uveitis.
VIII. Infectious uveitides
A. Viral infections
1. **Adenovirus** may produce subepithelial corneal infiltrates, and rarely a nongranulomatous iritis appears 7 to 10 days after the onset of infection. Iritis will improve spontaneously with time, although mild cycloplegia with tropicamide can be used. Prednisolone (Pred Forte) 1.0% bid may be advisable during the acute phases. For particularly severe disease, prednisolone 0.125%, bid or tid topically for 7 to 10 days, may make the patient more comfortable and resolve the intraocular inflammation more quickly. Corticosteroids may prolong the persistence of the corneal infiltrates, however (see Chapter 5, sec. **IV.G.**).
2. **HSV iridocyclitis and chorioretinitis.** Iridocyclitis is a nongranulomatous anterior uveitis that may occur with or without active herpetic

keratitis or evidence of facial blistering. Type I HSV is associated with ocular involvement, and it is transmitted by direct contact with infected secretions. Eighty percent of infected individuals are asymptomatic. With the AIDS epidemic and increasing numbers of iatrogenically immunosuppressed patients in the population (e.g., organ transplant recipients, blood dyscrasia patients), there is a rapidly increasing incidence of HSV **chorioretinitis**, previously a rare form of posterior inflammation. HSV is also one etiologic agent in **acute retinal necrosis (ARN)**.

a. **Clinically, iridocyclitis** presents as a red, photophobic, often painful eye with tearing, blurred vision, miosis, and not infrequently active herpetic keratitis and immune stromal or ulcerative infections. There are cells and flare in the aqueous, often KPs, posterior synechiae, secondary glaucoma, and occasionally hypopyon. The etiology is unclear but thought to be primarily an immune reaction to viral antigen, although live or intact virus has occasionally been isolated from these eyes. **Chorioretinitis** is a direct invasion of the retina by HSV with a secondary choroiditis and vitritis. Although rare in immunocompetent individuals, chorioretinitis is more likely to occur in immunosuppressed patients. There are large white retinal infiltrates, vascular sheathing, and hemorrhages. Healing leaves areas of scarred, atrophic retina.

b. **Diagnosis** is based on clinical evidence of herpetic disease such as keratitis, decreased corneal sensation, iris sectorial transillumination defects or skin lesions and, if possible, viral cultures or enzyme-linked immunosorbent assay (ELISA) testing of scrapings taken from active corneal or skin lesions (see Chapter 5). PCR assay of the aqueous is positive for viral DNA. Serology for HSV antibodies is useful only if taken 3 to 4 weeks apart and demonstrating a four-fold increase in titer. Therapy cannot be delayed for the results of such tests, however.

c. **Therapy of HSV iridocyclitis** is mydriasis only, e.g., homatropine bid for mild cell and flare. For more marked disease, the mydriatic–cycloplegic therapy is coupled with topical steroid drops using the lowest dosage necessary to control the inflammation and tapering slowly over several weeks to months, *reducing the steroid dosage by no more than 50% at any given time,* e.g., 1% prednisolone tid for 1 week, bid for 2 weeks, qd for 3 weeks, and then switching to 0.05% prednisolone qid and tapering even more slowly until minimal maintenance level is achieved or the drops may be stopped altogether. If the patient is taking the equivalent of 1% prednisolone qd or higher, it is advisable to add oral acyclovir (Zovirax) or famciclovir (see Appendix A) prophylaxis. Antibiotic ointment qd is also advisable. Systemic oral acyclovir 400 mg bid can also be used for prophylaxis. If there is cornea ulceration present at the time steroid therapy is to be started or if it develops during therapy, topical steroids should be reduced or stopped, specific treatment for the ulcer given (see Chapter 5, sec. **IV.D.**), and, if necessary, a short course of systemic steroids give, e.g., prednisone, 30 to 40 mg p.o. each morning for 10 days.

d. **Systemic acyclovir** trials of oral drug therapy of *active* **stromal keratitis** or **iritis** showed no significant effect, although prophylaxis of *recurrent* stromal disease was significantly effective.

e. **Therapy of HSV chorioretinitis** is not established, but current evidence indicates that the disease responds to acyclovir 200 mg p.o. five times daily for 10 days or, in immunocompromised patients, 5 to 10 mg per kg or 500 mg/m^2/day i.v. q8h for 5 to 7 days. Neither regimen is FDA approved for this use, but there is little else to be offered these patients except to reduce, where possible, factors contributing to the immunosuppression. **Acyclovir-resistant** HSV is treated with foscarnet 40 mg per kg i.v. q8h for 7 to 10 days.

3. **VZV** may also cause nongranulomatous **anterior uveitis, panuveitis, and chorioretinitis** and probably is the main cause of acute retinal necrosis **(ARN).**

   a. **Clinical findings and treatment** of zoster ophthalmicus are as described in Chapter 5, sec. **IV.E.**

   The uveitis is a vasculitis due to live virus invasion and may result in hypopyon, hyphema, posterior synechiae, glaucoma, iris sector atrophy, heterochromia iridis, chorioretinal exudates, vascular sheathing and hemorrhages, and serous retinal detachment. **ARN** is defined by definite clinical characteristics: focal, defined areas of retinal necrosis in the peripheral retina outside of the temporal vascular arcades, rapid circumferential progression (untreated), occlusive vasculopathy, marked vitritis, and iritis. Supportive but not required criteria are optic atrophy, scleritis, and pain. It is distinguished from **peripheral outer retinal necrosis syndrome (PORN)** seen only in AIDS patients and also largely caused by VZV, which has multifocal retinal opacification initially in the outer layers, little inflammation, rapid progression to confluent lesions (untreated), and total retinal necrosis.

   b. **Diagnosis** is based on clinical evidence or history of zoster ophthalmicus. The virus is fastidious in its tissue culture requirements (human cells), and serial serology takes too long to be of use in deciding therapy. It may confirm a clinical diagnosis, however. Because zoster is associated with deficiency in cell-mediated immunity, **AIDS** (HIV infection) must be considered an underlying risk factor in the absence of other reasons for immunosuppression such as malignancy or organ transplantation, especially in patients less than 45 years old.

   c. **Therapy of VZV acute anterior segment and facial inflammation** is **acyclovir** 800 mg p.o. five times daily for 7 days, preferably started within 72 hours of onset of rash. *New p.o. antivirals, famciclovir (Famvir) 500 mg p.o. tid for 7 days and valacyclovir (Valtrex) 1 g p.o. tid for 7 days, are given in lower doses, less frequently, and have greater effect on postherpetic neuralgia.* Their efficacy in VZV chorioretinitis is under study. They are as effective as acyclovir in acute disease with more convenient dosing. Mydriatic–cycloplegics such as 1% to 2% atropine or 2% to 5% homatropine qd to tid should be used until only 0 to 2 cells per 0.2-mm slitlamp beam are seen and only mild to no flare is present. Topical steroids may be instituted if the iridocyclitis persists despite acyclovir therapy. These are used as described under sec. **VI.A.,** above. Topical antivirals are not used except for persistent pseudodentritic keratitis. Vidarabine 3% ointment qid is most effective. Topical antibiotics such as erythromycin or bacitracin should be used if ulcerative keratitis is present. Therapy is controversial with regard to *systemic corticosteroids.* Except for 1 to 2 days of p.o. prednisone 40 to 60 mg for the immunocompetent patient with orbital apex syndrome (edematous pressure on nerves and vessels entering here), corticosteroids are no longer used. In general, mild or no pain requires no drug except a mydriatic–cycloplegic such as cyclopentolate or homatropine bid. Nonnarcotic or narcotic analgesics for neuralgia may be used. Frequent monitoring for dissemination of disease should be carried out.

   d. **Therapy of VZV chorioretinitis and ARN** is not established, but current data indicate that effective treatment is acyclovir 5 to 10 mg per kg or 500 mg per m^2 i.v. q8h for 5 to 7 days. Intravitreal injection of 10 to 40 μg per 0.1 mL coupled with vitrectomy and scleral buckle has been reported as successful therapy of acute retinal disease. None of this treatment is as yet FDA approved for these indications. Famciclovir or valacyclovir in the doses noted above may become the drugs of choice. *Acyclovir-resistant* VZV is treated with i.v. foscarnet or vidarabine, as is HSV. Retinal vasoocclusive disease is an important component of the disease that justifies the use of antiplatelet drugs, such as aspirin 300 mg per day.

4. **Cytomegalic inclusion disease (CID)** is a multisystemic viral infection caused by CMV. There are three means of acquiring infection: (a) transplacentally in utero, (b) during the birth process from an infected maternal cervix, and (c) at any time in life by oronasal droplet infection, sexual transmission, or transfusion of fresh blood or organ transplant that contains infected white cells. Congenital infection is found in 1% of all live births, but of these only 10% will manifest the disease early in life. Over a period of several years, up to 50% of all patients may manifest sensorineural hearing loss and mental retardation. More than 80% of the adult population older than 35 years test positive serologically for CMV.

   a. **Clinical findings.** In generalized **congenital** CMV infection, ocular involvement may range from mild, less retinal or choroidal blood vessels involved, to total bilateral retinal necrosis, in which few islands of retinal tissue remain intact. Involvement may be peripheral, central, or all-inclusive. There may be an overlying peripheral vitreous haze resembling peripheral uveitis. With resolution of these lesions, the underlying RPE is clumped and mottled. More commonly, the posterior pole is affected and the lesions seen may be identical to those found with congenital toxoplasmosis. The lesions may include necrotizing chorioretinitis, which may be located just in the macula and resolve to a hyperplastic pigmented macular scar, or multiple focal lesions resolving into many small, rounded, pigmented chorioretinal scars. Retinal involvement with CMV may occur without signs of generalized CID. **Differential diagnosis** includes congenital toxoplasmosis or nematode infection. In the **acquired adult infection,** the eye is not involved despite presence of virus elsewhere in the body. In **immunosuppressed** patients, however, the physician must suspect CMV with the finding of retinal lesions. Clinically, there may be retinal cotton-wool spots (infarcts), extensive retinal hemorrhage and necrosis associated with vitreous haze, and a major retinal vasculitis. Not infrequently, multiple small, yellowish-white granular lesions are scattered along the course of the retinal vessels or in the peripheral retina. CMV retinitis develops in more than one-third of **AIDS patients** and patients with absolute CD4$^+$ T-lymphocyte counts of less than 50 per mL, and frequently is the presenting illness as opportunistic infection.

   b. **Diagnosis** is made on clinical findings, throat and urine cultures, and leukocyte culture. Serum antibodies should be drawn at the time disease is suspected and 8 weeks later in an attempt to establish an increase in titer as well as to differentiate from toxoplasmosis.

   c. **Therapy** of CMV is only partially satisfactory in that drug must be maintained indefinitely or until the basic immunosuppression can be resolved, if possible. Therapeutic breakthroughs are not infrequent. Currently recommended, FDA-approved treatments for CMV retinitis are the antiviral antimetabolites: **valganciclovir (VGCV)** (Valcyte), which is a newly synthesized prodrug of **ganciclovir (GCV)** (Cytovene), **cidofovir** (Vistide), **foscarnet** (Foscavir), and the antisense nucleotide **fomivirsen** (Vitravene).

      (1) Oral **VGCV** is the newly synthesized prodrug of GCV. It is rapidly absorbed from the gut and hydrolyzed to GCV with very high bioavailability comparable to i.v. GCV. The common regimen is VGCV 900 mg p.o. bid for 3 weeks, then 900 mg p.o. qd maintenance. Therapeutic efficacy is similar to that of i.v. GCV 5 mg per kg qd, with similar tolerability. Side effects of both drugs include hematologic suppression, gastrointestinal disturbance, fever, headache, and peripheral neuropathy. Because of its efficacy and ease of administration, VGCV is often the drug of choice in CMV retinitis in HIV-positive patients (FDA approved). Studies

are underway for use in extraocular CMV infection in immunosuppressed patients.

(2) **GCV** is given initially as 2.5 mg per kg i.v. q8h for 10 days and then
changed to a maintenance dosage of 5 mg/kg/day i.v. for 5 days
weekly or **orally** as 500 mg p.o. six times per day or 1,000 mg
p.o. tid. Bioavailability of oral GCV is one-tenth that of p.o. VGCV.
Recurrent breakthrough CMV retinitis is treated by VGCV or the
initial GCV therapy again and maintenance therapy 7 days per
week. Hematologic (WBC) toxicity is monitored q2 to 4 weeks. **Intravitreal** GCV has been used successfully in a limited number of
patients intolerant of systemic GCV. Dosage is 400 μg per 0.1 mL
(or higher), which has been repeated up to 58 times over several
months in some patients, as drug titers fall below therapeutic levels (10 mg per L) over 48 hours. There is little discernible toxicity,
but the usual frequency of injection is 5 to 8 times over 2 to 3 weeks.
An FDA-approved **GCV intraocular device** releasing 1 μg per
hour for 8 months is highly effective in preventing local disease,
but survival time of patients not receiving i.v. GCV or foscarnet is
25% that of those who are systemically treated.

(3) **Cidofovir,** because of its high in vivo potency and excellent therapeutic index, is now used as a first-line drug against CMV retinitis
using either i.v. infusions (5 mg per kg once weekly) for 2 weeks
and then maintenance low dose (3 mg per kg) or high dose (5 mg
per kg weekly). Signs of nephrotoxicity should be monitored.

(4) **Foscarnet** induction is i.v. 60 mg per kg every 8 hours for 2 to
4 weeks until clinical response followed by either low maintenance
at 90 mg per kg q24h or high maintenance at 120 mg per kg q24h
indefinitely, depending on any drug-induced **renal** toxicity, with
reinduction doses used as needed for breakthrough retinitis. Because foscarnet does not share hematologic toxicity with anti-AIDS
drugs, it may be used concurrently with them, whereas GCV usually may not be used concomitantly for long. **Combination GCV–
foscarnet** therapy is useful in patients that are poorly responsive
to single-drug therapy and inhibits emergence of resistant virus.
Doses are not FDA approved. The drugs are physically incompat-
ible. Infusions should be sequential, not simultaneous.

(5) **Fomivirsen** is FDA approved for intravitreal injection for CMV
retinitis in HIV-positive patients. It is given as 0.33 mg every other
week for two doses, then maintenance of 0.33 mg every month.

5. **AIDS** is caused by HIV-1. The virus destroys the T-lymphocyte (and
probably other) immune cells, thus progressively and severely immuno-
compromising the patient and enhancing susceptibility to a plethora of
viral, fungal, and parasitic infections.

a. **Clinically** the ocular findings in AIDS and AIDS-related complex
include punctate or geographic ulcerative keratitis (which may mimic
herpesvirus), follicular conjunctivitis, Kaposi sarcoma, nongranulomatous iritis, secondary glaucoma, retinal cotton-wool spots (white,
fluffy nerve fiber layer microinfarctions), retinal vasculitis, intraretinal hemorrhages, microaneurysms, Roth spots, ischemic maculopathy,
retinal periphlebitis, and papilledema. The HIV appears able to produce all of these diseases itself through direct viral invasion and
through deposition of immune complexes that clog the vasculature.
The opportunistic infections that may be superimposed include HSV,
VZV, CMV, *Cryptococcus, Pneumocystis, Toxoplasma, Candida,* and
Mycobacterium (choroidal granulomas). Several of these may occur
simultaneously, e.g., HSV, CMV, and HIV chorioretinitis.

b. **Diagnosis** is made by serologic testing (ELISA and Western blot) for
HIV antibody, assessment of the ratio of T-helper to T-suppressor lymphocytes, and, if available, culture of virus from blood, tears, or other
body secretions.

    c. Therapy is palliative only, but more recently has been often highly successful using combinations of protease inhibitors and antimetabolites.

  6. EBV is a herpesvirus and the cause of infectious mononucleosis and probably Burkitt African lymphoma, nasopharyngeal carcinoma, and some chronic fatigue syndromes.

    a. Clinical findings in the eye include follicular conjunctivitis, epithelial punctate or microdendritic keratitis, immune anterior stromal pleomorphic *nummular or ring-shaped keratitis*, acute or chronic nongranulomatous iritis, panchorioretinitis, optic neuritis, papilledema, convergence insufficiency, and extraocular muscle palsy.

    b. Diagnosis is by heterophile or Monostat serology for EBV antibodies.

    c. Therapy is still not established. Response to oral antivirals is unproven.

  7. Embryopathic pigmentary retinopathy presents as a salt-and-pepper chorioretinitis as seen in patients with **congenital syphilis, congenital rubella, varicella, influenza,** and **radiation during the first trimester.** Rubella retinitis is present in 50% of infants with maternal rubella syndrome. Peppering is usually limited to the posterior pole but may involve any or all sectors. Retinal vessels are always normal, but the optic disk may be pale. Rubella chorioretinopathy does not interfere with visual function unless a neovascular net develops in the macula. Occasionally, it may simulate toxoplasmosis.

  8. Other viral infections that may produce nongranulomatous iridocyclitis or chorioretinitis that are generally self-limited and usually bilateral are inclusion conjunctivitis (iritis), infectious mononucleosis (iridocyclitis), influenza (iridocyclitis or neuroretinitis), lymphogranuloma venereum (no characteristic pattern), measles (chorioretinopathy), mumps (iridocyclitis and neuroretinitis), and ornithosis and psittacosis (chorioretinitis). **Subacute sclerosing panencephalitis** produces a chorioretinitis of low-grade inflammation characterized by ground-glass whitening of the retina with occasional cotton-wool spots (infarctions), disturbances of the underlying pigment epithelium, and opalescent swelling of the macula. There is no hemorrhage.

B. Bacterial infections

  1. Lyme disease, caused by the spirochete *Borrelia burgdorfi,* may cause iritis or panophthalmitis (see Chapter 5, sec. **IV.L.2.**).

  2. TBC uveitis is probably caused by immune reaction to or very rarely by direct ocular invasion by the bacterium *M. tuberculosis.* It should be suspected in any case of chronic iritis, especially in the older patient, AIDS patients, individuals from endemic areas or those at high risk of exposure, and in any granulomatous disease of the anterior or posterior segment that is not explained by some other agent. Associated lesions are phlyctenules, conjunctival nodules, scleritis, and optic neuritis.

    a. Clinical types. Iritis may appear in four forms: (a) acute nongranulomatous uveitis, intense but brief; (b) mild nonspecific uveitis with tendency to chronic recurrence; (c) smoldering low-grade granulomatous inflammation resulting in synechiae formation, cataracts, glaucoma, or phthisis bulbi; and (d) fulminating, granulomatous caseating tubercles. In miliary tuberculosis, choroidal tubercles appear as yellow-white nodules 1.6- to 1.2-disk diameter (dd) in size with blurred borders. They are similar to the disseminated lesions of histoplasmosis, but their occurrence with fever is of diagnostic importance. A retinal periphlebitis and subretinal neovascularization may be present. The **differential diagnosis** of choroidal lesions includes syphilis, coccidioidomycosis, sarcoidosis, and cryptococcosis. With specific therapy, the choroidal lesions quiet down and in many cases disappear completely.

    b. Diagnosis

      (1) Chest x-ray and ESR. Diagnosis is made in part by these tests and by **skin testing** using the purified protein derivative of tuberculin (PPD-I) (5TU) (tuberculin units). If the skin reaction to 5TU is completely negative, the 250TU (PPD-2) should be used. In extremely rare cases, the skin test may be negative and live bacilli may be present in the eye. Any reaction (even erythema only) suggests that the uveitis could be due to tuberculosis. If there is enough inflammation in the eye, one proceeds to the isoniazid (INH) therapeutic test. Underlying **AIDS** should be considered.

(2) **INH** may also be used as a *therapeutic test in suggesting the diagnosis* of TBC. One 300-mg tablet is given qd for 3 weeks, and the ophthalmologist observes the eye at weekly intervals to check for improvement. Other therapy is kept constant. After the diagnosis of TBC is strongly suspected, one of the other anti-TBC agents should be added to the regimen. Weaknesses in this mode of diagnosis are the natural waxing and waning of the disease, the concomitant use of steroids, which also cause improvement in most uveitis cases, and drug resistance.

c. **Therapy.** The principle of therapy followed is the concomitant use of two or more drugs to prevent the emergence of bacterial resistance to any of the drugs used, without a break of more than 1 or 2 weeks to protect against relapse, for at least 1 year to prevent relapse of active TBC. The primary drugs (isoniazid and rifampin) are the most effective and have the least toxicity. The tertiary drugs (e.g., ethambutol, streptomycin) are the least effective and the most toxic. Severe chorioretinitis is treated with systemic steroids combined with anti-TBC therapy.

(1) **INH** is given as one 300-mg tablet per day (5 mg per kg). Because children tolerate large doses, the dosage does not need to be reduced unless the child's weight is less than 27.3 kg (60 lb). Administering pyridoxine, 25 mg per day, may prevent peripheral neuritis. Intolerance to INH, resulting in hepatitis, increases with age and occurs often. The FDA has recommended monthly monitoring of patients for liver toxicity. INH should be discontinued at least temporarily in patients whose values exceed three times the upper limit of normal.

(2) **Rifampin.** After the presumptive diagnosis of tuberculosis uveitis has been made, rifampin is usually used as the second drug. The dosage is two 300-mg tablets (10 mg per kg) a day, 1 or 2 hours before or after a meal.

(3) **Ethambutol.** In patients with a danger of hepatitis, ethambutol may be a better choice than rifampin. It is given once a day with food, if desired, in a dosage of 15 mg per kg body weight. Patients with decreased renal function need the dosage reduced as determined by serum levels. Ethambutol may produce an optic neuritis. Each eye should be monitored separately.

(4) The increasing emergence of **INH-resistant strains** leads many experts to start with a four-drug combination INH, rifampin, **pyrazinamide** 1.5 to 2.5 g p.o. qd (15 to 30 mg per kg), and either ethambutol or streptomycin 15 mg per kg i.m. qd. If INH sensitivity is shown, the last two drugs are stopped, **pyrazinamide** is given for 2 months and the first two drugs are given for 6 to 12 months.

3. **Syphilitic uveitis and neurosyphilis** caused by the bacterial spirochete *Treponema pallidum* are becoming more common due to the AIDS epidemic. These conditions may be congenital and quiescent, active at birth or in the teenage years, or, most commonly, may be acquired in adult life.

a. **Clinical manifestations of congenital syphilis** include the salt-and-pepper appearance of the fundus on a yellowish-red background. This salt-and-peppering may be found just at the periphery and is invariably bilateral. It may involve the posterior pole or only isolated quadrants. Vision is usually unimpaired. This form of the disease is nonprogressive. Anterior segment manifestations include bilateral interstitial keratitis. Physical findings associated with congenital syphilis are saddle nose deformity, Hutchinson teeth, and sensory hearing loss.

(1) The **differential diagnosis of salt-and-pepper fundus** includes prenatal rubella or influenza, rubeola, variola, varicella, mumps, vaccination, poliomyelitis, HSV, panuveitis, Cockayne's disease, cystinosis, choroideremia in males, and Leber congenital tapetoretinal amaurosis.

(2) **Secondary retinal pigmentary degeneration** is manifested by narrowing and sclerosis of choroidal and retinal vessels. There is optic nerve atrophy characterized by a pale disk with sharp margins. Pigment configurations are round, star-shaped, or bone corpuscle formation. Many areas of chorioretinal atrophy differentiate it from retinitis pigmentosa. It is always bilateral and may be either in the posterior pole or in the peripheral retina. Vision may be affected.

b. **Secondary acquired syphilis** may be present as an **acute iritis** or diffuse **chorioretinitis.** Three types of secondary syphilitic iritis are iritis roseata (small nets of capillaries), iritis papulosa (highly vascular papules), and iritis nodosa (large, well-defined, yellowish-red nodules the size of a pinhead or larger). The chorioretinitis of acquired syphilis is bilateral 50% of the time and presents with intermittent photopsia, metamorphopsia, and occasional central scotoma. Fundus examinations reveal fine punctate haze in the vitreous and diffuse gray-yellow areas of exudation. These exudates and subsequent pigmentation accumulate along blood vessels and around the nerve head. The choroiditis is particularly noted in the midzone of the fundus and may have scattered superficial flame-shaped hemorrhages and generalized chorioretinal edema. The midfundal localization of the most intense disease results in a partial or complete ring scotoma.

c. **Tertiary syphilis.** A recent survey of patients diagnosed as having presumptive syphilitic uveitis revealed that two-thirds of these patients had negative VDRL tests, but positive FTA-ABS tests. This finding suggests the possibility that some of these patients may be in the tertiary stage. Although syphilis may mimic most types of uveitis, the most common forms seem to be a diffuse or a disseminated chorioretinitis. In **neuroretinitis** the nerve head and adjacent retina are swollen in late stages post therapy, appearing as arteriolar narrowing and sheathing with pigment migration and bone corpuscle formation.

d. **Diagnosis** is made by the FTA-ABS test (98% sensitive), which may detect syphilis earlier than the VDRL test and rules out almost all biologic false-positives as well as allowing diagnosis of late latent syphilis. The VDRL test becomes negative in two-thirds of cases of late syphilis and in treated syphilis, but the FTA-ABS test never becomes negative. Lumbar puncture for cerebrospinal fluid (CSF) serology and cytology should be performed in patients with signs of late-stage syphilis. HIV testing is frequently positive.

e. **Treatment.** No conclusive data are available regarding the best treatment for ocular syphilis. Some physicians have recommended probenecid, which raises the level of penicillin in the aqueous. Probenecid may be helpful not only by its effect on the kidney, leading to higher blood concentrations, but also by its effect on the ciliary body. Ocular cases should be treated as neurosyphilis. Penicillin G, 2 to 4 million units (mU) q4h i.v. for 10 days, then 2 to 4 mU i.m. benzathine penicillin G every week for 3 weeks should be given to patients with neuroretinitis but no CSF abnormalities. If the CSF is also positive, 12 to 24 mu of crystalline penicillin G i.v. should be given qd for 10 to 15 days along with the probenecid to increase blood and aqueous drug levels. Such doses will also produce treponemicidal levels in the CSF. Do follow up VDRLs (see Chapter 5, sec. **IV.L.1.** for other regimen).

C. **Parasitic infections.** The following parasitic diseases have been considered causes of intraocular inflammation: amebiasis, angiostrongyliasis, ascariasis, cestodiasis, filariasis, giardiasis, gnathostomiasis, ophthalmomyiasis, onchocericiasis, porocephaliasis, schistosomiasis, trematodiasis, trypanosomiasis, toxoplasmosis, and toxocariasis.

1. **Toxoplasmosis** is the most common proven cause of chorioretinitis in the world. It is almost always congenital, but may be acquired through inhalation of oocytes in cat waste or ingestion of contaminated undercooked lamb, pork, or rarely beef and unpasteurized cheeses. Systemic toxoplasmosis is a benign disease unless the patient is pregnant or immunosuppressed. If a pregnant female becomes infected with *Toxoplasma gondii*, there is a 40% chance that her infant will be affected. **All women should have a serologic test for toxoplasmosis before they are married or become pregnant.** If positive, these women can be assured that they are immune and not able to pass toxoplasmosis to any of their children. If negative, they will need to be cautious during pregnancy to avoid infection of the fetus. The probability of a mother having a child with toxoplasmosis is 1 in 10,000 in the United States.

   a. **Congenital systemic toxoplasmosis** may or may not be active at the time of birth. The symptoms and signs of congenital toxoplasmosis are convulsions, scattered intracranial calcification, and chorioretinitis. The latter is present in 80% of children with congenital toxoplasmosis and is bilateral in 85% of these, with a predilection for the macular area. In children who have been spared the CNS damage of toxoplasmosis, the retinitis may become apparent to an ophthalmologist either by an esotropia or exotropia from macular scarring or by reduced vision at the time of an initial school vision test.

   b. The **etiology** of the initial disease is the protozoan *T. gondii,* but reaction of disease may be due to a number of mechanisms, including local proliferation of free forms following rupture of a retinal cyst, delayed hypersensitivity specific for *Toxoplasma* cyst content, hypersensitivity to retinal proteins from tissue breakdown, recurrent parasitemia, and wandering cells that liberate *Toxoplasma* into ocular tissues, allowing invasion of susceptible cells. A change in immune status due to AIDS or immunosuppression should be considered in these patients. The vitritis is much more severe than that seen with CMV retinitis in these patients.

   c. **Clinically,** in both the **congenital ocular** form and the **acquired ocular disease,** there is an *acute focal chorioretinitis* having its active onset of recurrence between ages 11 and 40 years. Lesions may be single and variable in size and are usually posterior to the equator. There is exudation into the vitreous and flare and cells in the anterior chamber. The vitreous may detach from the retina, with hemispheric collections of cells looking like KPs deposited on the back of the vitreous body and dubbed **vitreous precipitates.** The active disease often occurs next to an old scar to produce the so-called **satellite lesion.** It is usually 1 dd in size, although it may vary from pinpoint to extremely large. Activity in the lesion persists for about 4 months. It is less frequent in African-Americans and most frequent in teenage girls. Papillitis and papilledema are not uncommon. A rare type of vitreous reaction with the development of "grapevines" in the vitreous covered with "wet snow" may be seen.

   d. The **differential diagnosis** of congenital toxoplasmosis includes macular coloboma, cytomegalic inclusion disease, herpes simplex chorioretinitis, neonatal hemolysis, torulosis, cerebral trauma, and foci of retinoblastoma. In adults, TBC, candidiasis, and histoplasmosis need to be considered as well.

   e. **Diagnosis** is based on the clinical picture plus fluorescein angiography and serologic tests. The indirect fluorescent antibody test and the ELISA test are now the two most commonly employed methods. A single positive test even on undiluted serum is considered diagnostically supportive. The presence of IgM antibody titers indicates a recent infection. The chances of this test being positive in the population at large are roughly equal to a patient's age. A 50-year-old person has about a 50% chance of having a positive test; therefore, the test can be false positive, especially in older individuals. Serology is supportive but not definitive. Acquired toxoplasmosis is characterized by fever, myalgia, and lymphadenopathy. In such rare cases, an increasing antibody titer is seen.

   f. **Treatment** is a combination of systemic corticosteroids and at least one antitoxoplasmic agent (preferably two or three).

   (1) **Corticosteroid therapy is avoided without antitoxoplasmic prophylaxis.** It is indicated when severe vitritis is present or when the lesions are close to the optic nerve, next to a major retinal vessel, or in the macular area inside or straddling the temporal vascular arcades. The initiating dose is 50 to 150 mg p.o. every other breakfast and tapered over 3 to 6 weeks. If relapse occurs, dosage is increased just enough to handle the relapse and then tapered again.

   (2) **Antitoxoplasmic agents** include sulfadiazine, pyrimethamine, tetracycline, clindamycin, and atovaquone.

   (a) **Sulfadiazine and pyrimethamine** are the first drug treatments of choice. Sulfadiazine (triple sulfa) is given as two 500-mg tablets p.o. q6h for 4 to 6 weeks along with pyrimethamine. Pyrimethamine is used at levels of 100 mg p.o. bid the first day and 25 mg p.o. bid for 6 weeks or until activity subsides. Because pyrimethamine acts only on actively dividing *Toxoplasma,* only active cases are treated with this drug. To avoid toxic depression of the bone marrow, **folinic acid** (leucovorin, 3 mg) once or twice weekly counteracts development of thrombocytopenia without interfering with therapeutics. Leucovorin comes in an ampule that may be given by injection, but the patient may be taught to put it in any liquid except alcohol and take it orally. The patient should **not** take folic acid, which would counteract the effect of sulfadiazine or pyrimethamine. *In pregnancy, pyrimethamine should be avoided because of induced congenital malformation.*

   (b) **Clindamycin** 150 to 300 mg p.o. every 6 hours, combined with **sulfadiazine,** is a synergistic therapy of second choice. Patients should be warned that if they have four bowel movements a day more than normal they should stop taking clindamycin. In about 1% of patients, severe pseudomembranous colitis develops. The concomitant use of triple sulfa acts to prevent this colitis. If clostridial colitis develops, it is best treated with oral vancomycin.

   (c) **Tetracycline** is used with a loading dose of 1,000 mg, followed by 500 mg p.o. qid for 3 to 4 weeks. For bowel complications, Lactinex is helpful.

   (d) **Atovaquone (Mepron)** is an antiparasitic that inhibits mitochondrial activity in protozoa. It has been used in the treatment of *Pneumocystis* and toxoplasmosis infection in HIV patients, and it is believed to directly affect *Toxoplasma* cysts. It can be used as single therapy or as a substitute for the other agents if they are not tolerated. Atovaquone is taken orally at a dosage of 750 mg tid for 4 to 6 weeks.

   (e) **Platelet count** should be checked once weekly if pyrimethamine is used. If it decreases to below 100,000, pyrimethamine should be stopped but steroids not discontinued. Leucovorin 3 mg i.m. daily should be instituted until platelet count returns to normal.

(3) **Cryosurgery** and **photocoagulation** are reserved for patients with persistent recurrences. Activity of a lesion is manifested by its softness and elevation, and by the presence of cells in the vitreous over it, although the latter may persist in the vitreous for months. Their presence, therefore, is not an absolute guide.

(4) **Fluorescein angiography** is not of great help in following the progress of toxoplasmic chorioretinitis.

2. **Toxocariasis** is the most common parasitic disease in the United States. It is caused by the ascarid *Toxocara canis,* a frequent infestation of puppies. Although 14 types of ocular toxocariasis have been described, only posterior pole and peripheral granulomas in a quiet eye are common.

a. The **systemic disease** of visceral larvae migrans usually occurs before the age of 3 years; therefore, by the time the child sees the ophthalmologist, systemic manifestations are no longer present. Prophylaxis includes the avoidance of both dirt eating and the handling of cats and dogs. Puppies, especially, should be dewormed with piperazine.

b. **Differential diagnosis** includes *Toxoplasma* and retinoblastoma, which has been the most common erroneous diagnosis. No intraocular calcification has been observed, in contrast with retinoblastoma, which has an incidence of calcification of 75%. Other possible diagnoses are toxoplasmosis, primary hyperplastic vitreous, Coats's disease, sarcoid, and retrolental fibroplasia.

c. **Children with diffuse chronic endophthalmitis** are usually 2 to 9 years of age. They present with chronic unilateral uveitis with cloudy vitreous. There may be an exudative detachment, posterior synechiae, and cyclitic membrane.

d. **Posterior pole granulomas** are usually seen in children 6 to 14 years of age. The lesion is usually hemispheric, with a diameter roughly equal to or larger than the disk. It seems to be primarily retinal in location. Tension lines radiate out from the granuloma, and fibrous bands may extend into the vitreous and to the pars plana. These granulomas are usually solitary and unilateral. Those at the posterior pole usually lie at the macula or between the macula and the disk.

e. **Patients with peripheral granulomas** in a quiet eye range in age from approximately 6 to 40 years. These peripheral hemispheric masses are usually associated with dense connective tissue strands in the vitreous cavities that often connect to the disk. Bilateral cases are rare. Heterotopia of the macula may result from the tug of these peripheral masses. These patients need to be differentiated from those with retinopathy of prematurity, which occurs bilaterally.

f. **Diagnosis** is made on the basis of clinical findings, the ELISA blood test, vitreous and aqueous taps for eosinophils, ocular x-rays or B-scan for calcium, ESR, and CBC (eosinophilia are not seen with ocular disease).

g. **Treatment** of choice is periocular depot methylprednisolone (40 to 60 mg) in the area of greatest involvement. This may be repeated weekly or every other week until the process resolves itself. Short-term systemic prednisone may also be used in severe cases. Most inflammation does not start until the larva dies. Antihelminthic therapy is of equivocal use. If used, it should always be coupled with steroids. A common combination is thiabendazole 500 mg p.o. qid or 20 mg/kg/day in divided doses for 5 days, plus 40 mg of prednisone p.o. qd for 10 days, followed by taper as warranted by resolving intraocular inflammation. Cryocoagulation and photocoagulation also kill the larva effectively, but should not be used within the foveal area.

D. Fungal infections

1. **Histoplasmosis** in its ocular form is almost never associated with symptomatic pulmonary histoplasmosis or exposure to *Histoplasma* spores or bird droppings. More than 99% of histoplasmic infections are benign and asymptomatic, with about 2% of adults in the endemic Midwest having *"histo spots"* disseminated in the fundus. These spots begin to appear during late childhood and are important as a nidus for future maculopathy. The syndrome has been found occasionally to occur in Europe and in other areas where histoplasmosis is nonexistent; therefore, the best term is *"presumed ocular histoplasmosis syndrome"* (POHS). In endemic areas, at least 90% of the cases that are seen are probably the result of interaction between the eye's immune response and the exogenous organism, *Histoplasma capsulatum.*

   a. The **clinical findings** include disseminated **choroiditis** producing histo spots. These spots vary in number from 1 to 70, with a mean of eight per eye. They are more frequent in the left than in the right eye and are bilateral in two-thirds of patients. The majority is found behind the equator and spots are slightly irregular, round, deeply pigmented, 0.2 to 0.7 dd in size, and yellow in color. The *macular lesion* is typified in an active stage by a pigment ring and detachment of the overlying sensory retina. This serous and hemorrhagic maculopathy is the result of histo scars that are granulomas eating a hole in Bruch membrane, which then allows an ingrowth of capillaries. The maculopathy causes legal blindness in 60% of patients having ocular histoplasmosis syndrome. If blood and elevation of the sensory retina are present, the physician may assume the presence of a *neovascular net,* best demonstrated by fluorescein angiography. Changes around the nerve head are similar to histo scars in the periphery except that they may be confluent. Typically, there is a pigmented line next to the nerve, with a depigmented zone outside this line representing old choroiditis. The clinical course is one of exacerbation and recurrence of preexistent histo spots. If spots are present in the disk–macular area, the chances of a symptomatic attack are approximately 20% over the next 3 years. If none is present, the chances of a visually significant attack are reduced to 2%. Occasionally, however, fresh areas of choroiditis may appear; new lesions arise from the edge of old scars.

   b. **Differential diagnosis** is aided by the finding in histoplasmosis syndrome of a **clear vitreous,** which immediately differentiates it from most other types of uveitis. Other causes of granulomatous fundus lesions include TBC, coccidioidomycosis, cryptococcosis, and sarcoid. Fuchs spot of high myopia, the diskiform degeneration of old age, or maculopathy from angioid streaks may simulate the maculopathy. Hemorrhagic circumpapillary histoplasmosis is simulated by drusen of the optic disk with hemorrhage.

   c. **Diagnosis** is assisted but not confirmed by complement-fixation testing (negative in more than two-thirds of typical cases), calcification on chest x-ray (previous histoplasma pneumonitis), a positive histoplasmin skin test, and primarily the clinical findings described. Skin testing should not be done in patients with maculopathy, because the test may reactivate the ocular lesions. There is significant association between presence of maculopathy and positive HLA-B27 testing.

   d. **Treatment** is not conclusively established. Antifungals have no effect, and peripheral retinopathy is not treated.

      (1) **For acute maculopathy,** the patient should be started on 50 to 150 mg of **prednisone** every other breakfast with retrobulbar injection of long-acting steroid, e.g., 40 mg of depomethylprednisolone acetate about every 2 weeks for 1 to 2 doses. Tapering of steroids is done over several weeks proportionate to the improvement in maculopathy. Fluorescein angiography may assist

the physician with regard to decisions concerning tapering of medications and use of laser therapy.

(2) **Photocoagulation** with argon is used to coagulate capillaries and to eradicate the exudation from a neovascular net that produces a serous hemorrhagic detachment. The laser is the best therapy, but is indicated only if the neovascular net is still outside the fovea. The use of photodynamic therapy (PDT) in the treatment of subfoveal lesions is under investigation. Development of nets is not affected by use or nonuse of steroid therapy.

(3) **To decrease leakage into the macula,** aspirin, coughing, and other Valsalva maneuvers should be avoided. Because hemorrhages may appear in the fundus at high altitudes, it is not recommended that patients with an active maculopathy ascend unpressurized to heights above 800 feet. Riding on commercial air flights has not proved detrimental.

2. **Other fungal uveitides.** Although not as common as histoplasmosis, the other fungal infections reported to infect the eye are aspergillosis, blastomycosis, candidiasis, coccidioidomycosis, cryptococcosis, mucormycosis, nocardiosis, and sporotrichosis. Of these, only aspergillosis and candidiasis are common enough to warrant further discussion **(see endophthalmitis section,** sec. **XII.G.,** below).

IX. **Noninfectious/autoimmune uveitides**

A. **Anterior uveitides**

1. **Idiopathic anterior uveitis** is the most common form of anterior segment inflammation, with about 50% of patients having ocular findings only, about 30% iridocyclitis plus a positive HLA-B27 test, and the remainder having associated systemic disease such as Reiter syndrome, ankylosing spondylitis, inflammatory bowel disease, psoriasis, and JRA.

    a. **Clinical findings** may involve both eyes but usually only one eye at any given time. Findings include any or all of the following: pain, photophobia, diffuse redness with predominant circumlimbal flush, tearing, blurred vision, a nongranulomatous anterior chamber cell and flare reaction, and occasional aqueous fibrin, miosis, posterior synechiae, and secondary glaucoma.

    b. **Diagnostic tests** are usually not done for a single easily controlled attack unless there are systemic symptoms such as backache on a carefully taken review of systems (ROS). For a second recurrence or prolonged attack, repeat the ROS and obtain an ESR, CBC with differential, urinalysis, and FTA-ABS test. Expanded evaluation is done for three or more attacks, granulomatous uveitis, specific leads on the ROS, posterior disease, or retinal vasculitis (see Tables 9.2 and 9.3 and specific disease entities).

    c. **Therapy** is initial intensive topical steroids to control the attack, e.g., 1.0% prednisolone acetate q1 to 2 hrs in combination with cycloplegia such as homatropine one to three times per day for the first week. Once the inflammation is completely quiet, drops are tapered over several weeks. If **macular edema** develops, a short course of systemic steroid or periocular steroid injection may be needed. The addition of systemic oral NSAIDs can be considered for recalcitrant cases.

2. **Ankylosing spondylitis** is a chronic axial arthropathy with predominant involvement of the lower spine and sacroiliac joints. About 95% of patients with ankylosing spondylitis are HLA-B27 positive, and a 25% incidence of anterior uveitis is observed. Of these uveitis patients, 80% will have both eyes involved but usually at different times.

    a. **Clinical findings** in the ophthalmic examination are the same as in idiopathic anterior uveitis. Recurrences may occur monthly or less than annually. Systemic symptoms include intermittent buttock or lower back pain, sciatica, spinal stiffness and thoracic kyphosis. The onset is insidious. Unrecognized and untreated disease will progress to spinal fusion and complete disability.

  b. **Diagnostic tests** are listed in Table 9.3, the most important being lumbosacral spine x-rays for sacroiliitis and spinal fusion. The ESR is elevated and many patients are HLA-B27 positive. However, recurrent, bilateral-alternating, nongranulomatous, acute anterior uveitis in a young man with lower back pain, is suggestive of the diagnosis. Some have family histories of ankylosing spondylitis.

  c. **Therapy** is similar to that for idiopathic iridocyclitis with topical steroids used q1h initially to control the inflammation, followed with a slow tapered schedule once the inflammation is under complete control. NSAIDs, such as diflunisal 500 mg p.o. bid or naproxen 375 mg p.o. bid, will alleviate joint symptoms and can also help to maintain the ocular disease under control. The use of COX-2 inhibitors can also be used to treat both systemic and ocular manifestations. Consultation with a rheumatologist and physical therapist for the development of an appropriate stretching and exercise program should also be performed.

3. **Reiter syndrome** is rare in the United States, being seen most often in men and rarely in children. There is a nongonococcal triad of **arthritis, urethritis,** and **conjunctivitis.** It has been suggested that Reiter syndrome occurs in predisposed individuals, most being HLA-B27 positive, who have an unusual host response to an infection with certain organisms. Among the organisms suspected of having a possible etiologic role are *Chlamydia (Compylobacter), Ureaplasm, Yersinia,* and some *Salmonella* and *Shigella* sp. The post venereal form occurs exclusively in men, but a Gram-negative postdysenteric form has been observed in families.

  a. **Clinical findings** include the above triad plus a scaling skin eruption (keratoderma blennorrhagicum), balanitis, and aphthous stomatitis. Arthritis will develop in 95% of patients at some point and may involve joints of the hands, wrists, feet, knees, or sacroiliac area. Urethritis occurs in about 75% and conjunctivitis in 30% to 60% of patients. Acute, recurring nongranulomatous iridocyclitis occurs in up to 12% of patients, especially in HLA-B27-positive individuals. It may occur during or after the acute stage of the disease. A nebulous keratitis, multifocal punctate subepithelial, and anterior stromal infiltrative keratitis with or without pannus, pupillary synechiae, and CME may develop. Glaucoma or cataracts can be caused with the excessive use of topical steroids.

  b. **Diagnostic tests** of key importance are HLA-B27 and joint x-rays. Rheumatoid factor and autoantibody tests are usually negative (Table 9.3).

  c. **Therapy** of the ocular disease is topical, regional, or oral steroids as required. Oral NSAIDs can be used to treat systemic and ocular manifestations as well. In steroid-resistant patients, low-dose weekly immunosuppresion can be initiated in consultation with a rheumatologist. Systemic tetracycline 250 mg p.o. qid or doxycycline 100 mg p.o. bid for 3 weeks should be given if *Chlamydia* is suspected. The disease usually resolves completely between episodes.

4. **Inflammatory bowel disease (ulcerative colitis and Crohn's disease).** Ocular involvement in these gastrointestinal diseases occurs in less than 5% of patients. In both ulcerative colitis and Crohn's disease, HLA-B27 and ankylosing spondylitis seem to be associated. The iritis, colitis, and arthritis should be considered manifestations of the same immune process rather than as one resulting from the other. HLA-B27 individuals will exhibit the typical acute anterior uveitis, however, posterior segment involvement and retinal vasculitis can also occur. Other ophthalmic manifestations include episcleritis and scleritis. Topical corticosteroids are the **treatment** of choice for the iritis and appropriate systemic treatment of the intestinal disease.

5. **Psoriasis,** a skin disease caused by epidermal hyperproliferation, is strongly HLA-B27 gene-associated. An anterior uveitis similar to that

seen in other HLA-B27-positive idiopathic iridocyclitis patients may be seen in these patients with or without arthritis of the hands, feet, and sacroileum. The diagnosis of psoriatic uveitis is a clinical one, and may be made in that subset of patients capable of mounting multiple immune-mediated processes. **Treatment** is mydriasis, topical steroids, and oral NSAIDs as previously described for the other HLA-B27-associated diseases.

6. **Juvenile rheumatoid arthritis (JRA)** is broadly defined as arthritis of onset before the age of 16 years, which lasts for 6 months or more. It has a 20% incidence of anterior uveitis. There are three forms of JRA: (I) the acute toxic form *(Still's disease)* (10%), (II) the polyarticular form (40%), and (III) the pauciarticular form (50%). Patients at highest risk of ocular disease (14%) are young (4 years to teens) female JRA patients with fewer than four joints involved (pauciarticular), no wrist involvement, and positive ANA testing. Teenage males with pauciarticular disease and positive HLA-B27 testing form another high-risk group (75%) for developing ocular disease. Arthritis usually precedes ocular inflammation by several years, but occasionally the situation may be reversed.

   a. **Clinical findings** in the eye may be similar to those of idiopathic anterior uveitis (acute and symptomatic), especially in males. More dangerous is the insidious chronic smoldering iritis seen in more than 50% of the predominantly female HLA-B27-negative, ANA-positive group who develop iritis. This "silent" anterior uveitis is characterized by a white and quiet, initially asymptomatic eye with 1 to 2+ cells and flare. The ocular disease tends to progress despite therapy even after the joint disease has become quiescent as the patients mature. Long-term complications include band keratopathy, posterior synechiae, cataract, secondary glaucoma, hypotony, and occasionally vitritis and macular edema.

   b. **Diagnostic tests.** The joint distribution, elevated ESR, positive ANA on two substrates, primarily anterior nongranulomatous uveitis, and normal serum and urine calcium help to differentiate JRA from ocular **sarcoidosis** in children. Positive HLA-B27 and frequently negative rheumatoid factor also support a diagnosis of JRA anterior uveitis.

   c. **Therapy.** Mydriatic drops to prevent posterior synechia formation and topical steroids to eliminate ocular inflammation are the initial main treatment. Most of these patients will have permanent breakdown of the blood–ocular barrier, resulting in flare. Therefore, flare should not be used as an indicator of ocular inflammation and should not be used as a guide for treatment. Steroids should be used as little as possible because of drug cataractogenesis, but in some patients repeated periocular deposteroid injections may be needed to control chronic, active inflammation. Except in the most severe cases, long-term use of oral corticosteroids should be avoided. Children especially suffer adverse effects on growth and bone formation. Alternate-day therapy should be used if possible. Steroid-sparing systemic medications should be used to minimize the long-term use of steroids. This involves the use of NSAIDs initially and moving on to immunosuppressive therapy with low-dose methotrexate and possibly other agents for complete control of the inflammation. *A pediatrician or rheumatologist should comonitor any child taking periocular steroid injection, systemic steroid therapy for adverse drug effect. More importantly, immunosuppressive therapy needs to be prescribed by specially trained ophthalmologists or in collaboration with a rheumatologist* (see sec. **VI.D.**).

7. **Other anterior uveitides syndromes**

   a. **Fuchs heterochromic iridocyclitis** is found in about 2% to 5% of uveitis patients. The major complaint is blurred vision, which results from the development of a posterior subcapsular cataract or vitreous veils. Fuchs heterochromic uveitis is unilateral, painless, white, and quiet. The affected iris stroma looks less dense, and the pigment layer often has a moth-eaten appearance at the pupil margin. Unless the condition is bilateral, there is heterochromia, with a brown eye becoming less brown and a blue eye becoming a more saturated blue. Iris nodules are common and the anterior segment vasculature is abnormal, fragile, and can lead to easy bleeding. Posterior synechiae never develop. The KPs are most distinctive, being round or star-shaped and usually of medium size. Their most striking feature is that they are not confined to the lower part of the cornea but cover the entire back of the cornea. They do not conglomerate or become pigmented, and filaments are often seen between the precipitates. White dots are adherent to the framework of the vitreous. The cataract is the typical complicated posterior subcapsular type. The prognosis for cataract extraction is good, although there is an increased likelihood of progressive recalcitrant glaucoma. In the past, Fuchs iridocyclitis was considered a degenerative process, but it is now thought to be inflammatory because of the presence of plasma cells on histological sections. **Treatment** with short-term topical steroids is rarely used to reduce inflammation that results in the accumulation of dense KPs, which may affect vision and appears at the time of intraocular surgery. In general, the mild degree of inflammation in patients with Fuchs heterochromic uveitis can be left untreated and the use of topical steroids should be restrained in order to prevent undesirable side effects, such as glaucoma and cataract formation.

b. **Glaucomatocyclitic crisis (Posner-Schlossman syndrome)** is characterized by intermittent unilateral acute glaucoma with mild anterior uveitis. In some cases the result of HSV testing (positive aqueous viral DNA by PCR) can be positive. HLA-Bw54 is positive in 40% of patients. The crisis is unilateral, recurrent, and typified by a dilated pupil instead of the constricted pupil that is normally seen in iritis. The mild symptoms are those of blurred vision from corneal edema. Attacks last from a few hours to, rarely, more than 2 weeks. Although posterior synechiae do not form, small KPs usually appear with each attack, especially on the trabecular meshwork, and heterochromia may be present. Cells in the vitreous are usually not seen. **Treatment** consists of mild cycloplegia (homatropine 2% at bedtime), topical steroids, and systemic carbonic anhydrase inhibitors (ethoxyzolamide 50 mg p.o. tid or acetazolamide 250 mg p.o. tid to qid). The role of acyclovir p.o. is under study.

c. **Lens-induced uveitis** is an immune response to proteins of the crystalline lens exposed to the ocular environment after surgical or traumatic rupture of the lens capsule, or when a hypermature cataract is retained. Patients with lens-induced uveitis are healthy, and present with an acute, severe unilateral anterior uveitis, that can be nongranulomatous at the beginning, but becomes granulomatous during its chronic course. The **diagnosis** of unilateral granulomatous uveitis is made in a patient with a history of surgical or traumatic insult to the lens. Infectious endophthalmitis needs to be ruled out in most instances. Initially, **the treatment** of this condition consists of topical corticosteroids to control the inflammation, but the surgical removal of all lens material present is required as definite treatment. Vitrectomy techniques are used to achieve this goal and cataract surgery is performed in cases where a hypermature cataract is the source of the uveitis.

d. **Anticholinesterase agents** include glaucoma drops such as echothiophate iodide and eserine and may produce the rare complications of fibrinous iritis. The miotics, especially the stronger ones, appear to predispose to an increased postoperative iritis and should be discontinued several days before surgery. In addition, they should not ordinarily be used in the glaucoma found with uveitis, because they may aggravate the inflammation and lead to synechiae and a small pupil. Mydriatic cycloplegia with **cyclopentolate** may also aggravate iritis due to its neutrophil chemoattractant effect.

e. **Ischemic ocular syndrome.** Many patients with ischemic ocular syndrome are more than 55 years of age and have familial or medical histories of generalized vascular disease. They may have **fade-outs of vision** on arising or postprandially. Vision may be poor. The corneas may have mild edema and striate keratopathy. There is a moderate flare in the anterior chamber with some cells. The iris is usually abnormal, with matted stroma, and the pupil irregularly oval. The fundus may have dilated congested veins and mild retinal edema. The retinal artery frequently pulsates with the slightest pressure on the globe. Frequently, no carotid pulse is palpable. These eyes usually develop further iris atrophy and mature cataracts in 2 to 4 months. The clinician's efforts should be directed toward assessment of the **cardiovascular** system.

f. **Acute angle-closure glaucoma** is a cause of fibrinous iritis. The greater the fibrinous iritis, the greater the probability of adhesions. If medical treatment is effective, the IOP in the involved eye decreases below that of the uninvolved eye, perhaps because of a reduced capacity of the ciliary body to secrete aqueous. **Corticosteroid** drops are indicated for the fibrinous iritis (see Chapter 10, sec. **IX.**).

B. **Intermediate uveitis (pars-planitis, peripheral uveitis, chronic cyclitis)** is an inflammatory process of the peripheral retina and vitreous.

1. **Clinical findings.** This disease of children (ages 5 to 15 years) and young adults (ages 25 to 35 years) is typically bilateral and accounts for about 8% to 15% of all uveitis cases in office practice. *Multiple sclerosis* is strongly associated with intermediate uveitis. However, sarcoidosis, Fuchs heterochromic iridocyclitis, tuberculosis, syphilis, and Lyme disease should be considered in the differential diagnosis. Symptoms are blurred vision or floaters without pain or photophobia. Children may have some anterior chamber cells and flare and posterior synechiae, but such anterior inflammation is rare in adults. There may be peripheral corneal edema with KPs. The key findings are peripheral retinitis, perivasculitis, and vitritis, often with white snowbanking or snowballs, especially over the inferior peripheral retina. If there is snowbanking, areas of neovascular abnormality should be checked as potential sites of hemorrhage. Macular edema is frequently found (28%) and is the most important visual threat of this condition. There are five reported clinical courses:

   a. Benign smoldering and resolution with no loss of visual acuity.
   b. Inflammatory choroidal and serous retinal detachments.
   c. Vascularized high snowbanks and ultimately cyclitic membranes.
   d. Significant vascular obliteration with field loss and optic atrophy.
   e. Chronic smoldering inflammation with macular edema.

   Any of these groups may be seen in combination as well. Long-term visual disability develops in more than one-third of patients, and only 5% remit spontaneously.

2. **Diagnostic tests** are useful only in ruling out other causes of uveitis that may involve this area: sarcoidosis (chest x-ray, gallium scan, systemic symptoms, erythema nodosum, and elevated serum and urine calcium), toxocariasis (*Toxocara* serology), Lyme disease (Lyme serology), and idiopathic iridocyclitis (Table 9.3; see sec. **VIII.**). MRI and neurological consult are to rule out **multiple sclerosis.** There is no associated HLA phenotype. Fluorescein angiography will reveal periphlebitis, perifoveal capillary leak with CME, and optic disk staining.

3. **Therapy** may be deferred in a minority of patients who are asymptomatic with old pigmented cells and no evidence of active inflammation. *Active inflammation should be treated.* Oral NSAIDs can be used as first line of therapy in patients with mild inflammation. Significant vitritis and CME will require more aggressive therapy, beginning with periocular

steroid injections, using triamcinolone (40 mg periocular depot), if the patient is not a steroid responder. Improvement of the vitritis and CME occurs over a period of 4 to 6 weeks and the injections can be repeated every 2 to 6 months. If the injection is not tolerated, is ineffective, or the patient has bilateral macular edema, systemic corticosteroids are recommended. Oral prednisone 1 mg/kg/day (or equivalent steroid dose [Table 9.4]) is begun daily and tapered 5 to 10 mg per week until the minimum maintenance dose for control of the disease is achieved. Periods of exacerbation may require intermittent increase in dosing. A few patients will develop intractable inflammation or macular edema despite maximum tolerable steroid therapy. Other treatment options for these cases include pars plana cryopexy, therapeutic vitrectomy, and immunosuppression. Cryotherapy would be the next treatment, especially in patients with evidence of neovascularization of the pars plana. One or two rows of single-freeze cryotherapy spots are placed along the areas of snowbanking to eliminate the abnormal vascular permeability in the area. Patients that fail this treatment should then be treated with systemic immunosuppression, in combination with vitrectomy in severe cases. A stepladder approach should be used to decide the optimal medication that will achieve control of the intraocular inflammation.

C. **Autoimmune retinochoroiditis (multifocal or zonal)**
  1. **Acute posterior multifocal placoid pigment epitheliopathy (APMPPE).** Young healthy adults are affected and may have cerebral vasculitis, thyroiditis, erythema nodosum, enteritis, and positive HLA-B7. Eye findings are multiple, discrete, flat, grayish lesions scattered posteriorly; vitritis and occasional papillitis; retrobulbar neuritis; periphlebitis; iridocyclitis; and episcleritis. The picture on fluorescein angiography differs in the active and inactive stages. In the active stage there is blockage of dye by swollen opalescent plaques. In the inactive stage there is early transmission of background fluorescence through areas of depigmentation. Vision tends to fall to the region of 20/200 as a result of macular involvement. There is *often a dramatic return of vision* in the first 2 weeks. After 10 weeks the vision has usually improved about as much as it will. Examination of the posterior segment is significant for the presence of multiple "placoid" creamy-yellow lesions, with blurred edges and confluent. The etiology is unknown, but it may be related to an inflammatory obstruction of the feeding artery to a segment of the choriocapillaris. No **treatment** has been demonstrated to be of value.
  2. **Serpiginous or geographic peripapillary choroiditis** affects healthy young adults with no systemic findings except HLA-B7. It is usually unilateral but may be bilateral years later, with vitritis (30%), occasional focal phlebitis, contiguous APMPPE-like lesions, and is characterized by a cream-colored lesion moving in tongue-like spread from the disk area and lasting up to 18 months. If this tongue involves the macula, the vision is usually irreparably lost. The overlying retinal vessels are normal, and there may be a few cells in the vitreous. Intravenous fluorescein enters the extension very slowly. Once the fluorescein appears, it remains in a diffuse pattern for several hours. This entity is difficult to differentiate from a degenerative syndrome known as "areolar sclerosis" or choroidal vascular abiotrophy, which has a similar pathology. The use of aggressive immunosuppression (prednisone, azathioprine, and cyclosporin combination) have resulted in the remission of some cases, however, its role in definite cure is still under investigation. Successful treatment of subretinal neovascular membranes with laser photocoagulation is dependent on the location of the lesion.
  3. **Acute retinal pigment epitheliitis (Krill's disease)** is a minor macular disease of young adults characterized by an acute onset, with fairly rapid resolution in 6 to 12 weeks. A typical lesion is a deep, fine, dark gray, sometimes black spot that, in the acute stages and sometimes afterward, is surrounded by a pale yellow halo. These lesions usually appear in

clusters of two to four in the macula and may be unilateral or bilateral. There is no treatment.

4. **Multiple evanescent white dot syndrome** is of unknown etiology and occurs in healthy, young, usually female patients with prodromal viral symptoms in 30% and photopsia in 75%. Eye findings are enlarged blind spot, multiple grayish spots (1 to 3 dd) scattered in the peripapillary and peripheral macular area, orange foveal lesion, vitritis, and mild afferent pupillary defect. Fluorescein angiography shows an early circular pattern of hyperfluorescent dots that stain late along with the optic nerve. Dots resolve over days to weeks, but symptoms may persist for months with occasional recurrences. There is no treatment.

5. **Multifocal choroiditis and panuveitis syndrome** typically affects myopic women of any age, becoming bilateral in 82% of patients. Eye findings may include iritis, vitritis, and acute multifocal, discrete, yellowish lesions at the RPE–inner choroid in the macula or scattered. Late punched-out chorioretinal scars are left, simulating POHS (histoplasma), but ICG angiography may show multiple hypofluorescent lesions unlike POHS. Sarcoid, TBC, and syphilis must also be ruled out. Systemic steroids are useful for active macular lesions and in visual field and acuity loss. Photocoagulation may be needed for subretinal neovascularization.

6. **Birdshot retinochoroidopathy** is an uncommon uveitic syndrome most frequently found in white, middle-aged females. Eye findings are quiet anterior chamber, vitritis without snowbanking, multiple cream-colored circular or oval lesions deep to the retina, retinal vascular narrowing, optic atrophy, and macular edema. Diagnosis is assisted by fluorescein angiography, ERG, EOG, and positive HLA-A29. Therapy is initiated if vision starts to decrease and consists of systemic and periocular steroids (see sec. **VI.A.,** above). Treatment with cyclosporin A 2.5 to 5.0 mg/kg/day alone, or with azathioprine 1.5 to 2.0 mg/kg/day, is effective in controlling the disease.

7. **Sympathetic ophthalmia** is a bilateral granulomatous panuveitis that may develop about 4 to 12 weeks after either an injury or rarely intraocular surgery on one eye involving uveal tissue. It may occur as early as 5 days and as late as 66 years, but the majority commences between 1 and 12 months after injury. The etiology is unknown, but it is thought to be that injury to one eye results in programming of the body to produce ocular disease autoimmune in nature and predominantly a T-cell lymphocyte reaction in the injured and the sympathizing other eye. Antiretinal antibodies (photoreceptor and Müller cells) have been found in a few patients.

   a. **Clinically,** the external eyes are not inflamed, but both uveal tracts are massively thickened by granulomatous lymphocytic infiltration. Patients will complain of photophobia, decreased accommodation, and eye pain. The iris may be very edematous, and deep nodules and papillitis are common. Disseminated yellow-white spots may appear in the fundus **(Dalen-Fuchs nodules).** There may also be associated signs of vitiligo, poliosis, and alopecia, but these signs are less common than in the VKH syndrome. Sympathetic ophthalmia is extremely rare and may be similar to or associated with phakoantigenic (lens-induced) uveitis. Differentiation is important because removal of lens material will cure the phakoantigenic uveitis.

   b. **Diagnosis** is based on the history of injury or ocular surgery and the clinical findings. Fluorescein angiography, ERGs, and EOGs will indicate severity of disease and guide therapeutic response.

   c. **Treatment** of sympathetic ophthalmia involves cycloplegia, periocular injections daily to every 6 weeks depending on severity, and systemic medication of 100 to 200 mg of prednisone or equivalent every morning with breakfast for 7 to 10 days. Once disease is controlled, dosage may be reduced to a maintenance level (1.0 to 1.5 mg/kg/day) for at least 3 months, at which time success of the therapy should be reevaluated. If successful, therapy may be continued with 15 to 20 mg per day of prednisone. The immunosuppressive drugs—cyclosporin A, 6-mercaptopurine, methotrexate, azathioprine, or cyclophosphamide—have been used either when corticosteroids are not effective or when they are contraindicated (see sec. **VI.c.,** above). *Enucleation of the impaired eye should prevent sympathetic ophthalmia if done within 9 to 14 days after injury or surgery. After 14 days, enucleation should be performed if the eye has no potential for recovery, because this eye may aggravate the inflammation in the sympathizing eye.* If sympathetic ophthalmia develops, there is some evidence that the clinical course can be influenced if the inciting eye is enucleated within 2 weeks of disease onset. *This should not be performed if the inciting eye has useful vision or if the disease has been present for more than 2 weeks.*

8. **Vogt-Koyanagi-Harada (VKH) disease** is a bilateral granulomatous panuveitis, affecting individuals between the ages of 20 and 50 years. Clinically, these patients present with bilateral diffuse vitritis and choroiditis, beginning with bilateral visual failure, often accompanied by headache and nausea. In the fundus there are multiple foci of unevenly elevated cloudy patches that form circumscribed oval detachments within a few days. Gradual sinking of the fluid results in bilateral inferior serous retinal detachment that tends to reabsorb spontaneously with resultant reattachment of the retina. Retinal and optic nerve neovascularization and papillitis are not uncommon. Anteriorly, mutton fat KP cells and flare, perilimbal vitiligo, pupillary nodules, and anterior chamber shallowing are often noted. The disease is identical to sympathetic ophthalmia, with the exception of a history of penetrating injury. The associated signs of exudative retinal *detachment—poliosis* (whitening of the eyebrows), *vitiligo* (depigmentation of the skin), *alopecia* (focal baldness), and *hearing difficulties (meningismus)* plus typical findings on fluorescein angiography—are useful diagnostically. Cranial neuropathy is demonstrated by optic neuritis, tinnitus, hearing loss, nystagmus, ataxia, vertigo, and extraocular muscle palsy. Other ocular complications of VKH are secondary glaucoma from peripheral anterior synechiae formation, cataracta complicata, and phthisis bulbi from severe involvement of the ciliary body. VKH is most common in Japanese and Latin American patients, and the clinical course is variable from mild and self-limited to severe and progressing to blindness. Systemic complications may be fatal; hence it is essential to include an internist in the evaluation and management of VKH.

   a. **Differential diagnosis** is sympathetic ophthalmia and, in late cases, acute posterior multifocal placoid pigment epitheliopathy or sarcoid.

   b. **Diagnosis** is based primarily on clinical findings. HLA-MT3, HLA-Dr4, and HLA-Bw54 testing is positive in Japanese and HLA-DRw52 testing is positive in Native American patients. Abnormalities of the immune system such as high titers of antiretinal antibodies and high levels of circulating interferon gamma in the serum of patients have been described. However, these are not diagnostic of the VKH. Fluorescein angiography reveals characteristic multiple pinpoint leaks at the RPE level, disk staining, subretinal neovascularization, and, in some patients, arteriovenous anastomoses. ERGs and EOGs are abnormal.

   c. **Treatment** of VKH is difficult but rewarding if carried out assiduously. It includes prednisone 200 mg every morning with breakfast, plus periocular injections of soluble corticosteroid such as 4 mg of dexamethasone once or twice weekly during the acute phases. After 7 to 10 days, prednisone may be decreased to every other breakfast, and 2 weeks later to 100 mg p.o. every morning for 1 to 2 weeks, with continuing decrease in every other day corticosteroid over the ensuing weeks. Length of therapy varies with severity, with some patients receiving gradually tapering treatment for a year. The second line of therapy is an immunosuppressive agent: azathioprine, cyclophosphamide, or cyclosporin A. These have been successfully used as an alternative form of treatment and may be combined synergistically with systemic steroids, allowing lowering of the steroid dose. Laser therapy of neovascular nets is important adjunctive therapy.

9. **Sarcoidosis** is a multisystemic, granulomatous inflammatory condition (noncaseating granulomas) that can affect the eye. It accounts for about 2% of uveitis patients, and 25% to 50% of patients with sarcoidosis will develop ocular problems, usually uveitis. There is a concentration of sarcoidosis in Sweden and in the South Atlantic and Gulf regions of the United States. It is more common in black Americans than in black Africans, and 10 to 15 times as common in black Americans (usually females) as in white Americans. It has occurred concordantly in uniovular twins. It usually occurs in the middle years (age 20 to 50 years) and lasts about 2 years. The uveitis develops during the silent stage of systemic sarcoidosis in approximately 80% of patients.

   a. **Clinically,** sarcoidosis affects the upper and lower respiratory tracts, lymph nodes, skin, liver, spleen, and CNS. All the parts of the eye can be affected. Although sarcoidosis is typically assumed to be granulomatous in character, it presents equally often in a nongranulomatous form, so the iris may or may not have nodules similar to those seen in TBC uveitis. The following types of posterior involvement have been reported: a characteristic chorioretinitis, periphlebitis retinae (candle wax drippings), large chorioretinal granulomas, nonspecific chorioretinitis, optic nerve involvement, including atrophy, edema, and tumor, vitreous opacities, and preretinal infiltrates. The vitreous may have "snowball" opacities inferiorly. CNS manifestations occur in 10% to 15% of patients with systemic sarcoidosis, but this figure doubles when the fundus is involved.

   b. **Diagnosis** is aided by a chest x-ray and spiral CT scan of the chest, which are abnormal (hilar adenopathy) in approximately 80% of cases of ocular sarcoidosis. A gallium scan may show increased uptake in areas of inflammation in the parotid and lacrimal glands. Histologic proof is best obtained by biopsy of the conjunctiva, salivary or lacrimal gland, granulomas, skin lesions, or enlarged lymph nodes. Biopsy may be performed on the liver, gastrocnemius, or transbronchial. There is lack of a positive tuberculin reaction in approximately 50% of patients with sarcoidosis as well as a tendency toward hyporeaction on other skin tests (anergy). Other pertinent tests are serum and urine calcium, and angiotensin converting enzyme, all of which are elevated in active sarcoidosis. The serum albumin–globulin ratio, pulmonary function, and liver enzymes are also frequently abnormal. Children may have ocular and joint sarcoidosis but no lung involvement. Hand, knee, and foot films may be useful.

   c. **Patients diagnosed and treated early** have a favorable outcome and are left with little residual ocular disability. *Active sarcoid uveitis requires treatment.* Topical steroids are not always adequate, and periocular steroid injection of 20 to 40 mg of depomethylprednisolone may be needed to supplement drops for anterior nodular iritis and glaucoma. Systemic corticosteroids in high initial doses are often necessary as well, e.g., prednisone, 40 to 60 mg p.o. qd with taper over several weeks. Cycloplegics (atropine, homatropine) are continued throughout the steroid course. The use cyclosporin A and other immunosuppressive agents have been used successfully in recalcitrant cases, but no regimen has been established.

X. **Vasculitis** can be caused by systemic and intraocular inflammatory conditions. The differential diagnosis is extensive and a thorough history, review of systems and physical examination is essential in making a diagnosis. Retinal vasculitis can be characteristic of certain diseases such as Adamantiades-Behçet disease, but can also be part of other systemic conditions and infections (Table 9.5). The

TABLE 9.5. CAUSES OF VASCULITIS

Primary Systemic Vasculitis	Secondary Vasculitides
Small vessel vasculitis Henoch-Schönlein purpura Wegener granulomatosis Churg-Strauss syndrome Microscopic polyangiitis (microscopic polyarteritis) *Medium-seized vessel vasculitis* Polyarteritis nodosa (classic polyarteritis) Kawasaki disease *Large vessel vasculitis* Giant cell (temporal) arteritis Takayasu arteritis	*Infectious diseases* Viruses: human immunodeficiency virus, cytomegalovirus Bacteria: spirochaetales, mycobacteria, streptococci, whippeli Parasites: *Ascaris* Fungi: *Aspergillus* *Neoplasia* Non-Hodgkin lymphoma Myeloproliferative diseases Solid tumors Atrial myxomas *Drug induced* Opioids Antihypertensive (hydralazine) Antithyroid drugs (propylthiouracil, methimazole, carbamizole) Antibiotics (azithromycin, minocylcine) Atifibrotics (penicillamine) Leukotriene receptor antagonist (zafirlukast, montelukast, pranlukast) *Autoimmune diseases with secondary vasculitis* Rheumatoid vasculitis Adamantiades–Behçet's disease Behçet's disease Systemic lupus erythematosus Sjögren syndrome Ulcerative coliti Crohn disease Sarcoidosis Relapsing polychondritis Cogan syndrome

association of ocular inflammation and these systemic vasculitides can be the first manifestation of the disease and prompt diagnosis can be life saving.

A. **Behçet's (Adamantiades-Behçet) disease (recurrent uveitis of young adults)** is a multisystemic vasculitis typified by attacks of nongranulomatous usually posterior or panuveitis with hypopyon (66%), aphthous lesions in the mouth (100%), and genital ulceration (84%). It is especially common in the Far East and Mediterranean basin (8 cases per 1 million people). Loss of visual field occurs from widespread retinal vasculitis. Skin lesions include erythema nodosum, acne, cutaneous hypersensitivity, and thrombophlebitis. Other findings may include arthritis, gastrointestinal ulcers, aneurysms, and neuropsychiatric symptoms. The disease characteristically follows a chronic recurrent pattern of spontaneous remissions and exacerbations of 1 week to 3 years with intervals between attacks lengthening so that after 15 to 20 years there are no further attacks, but the average period from onset to blindness from retinal vasculitis is 3 years. In the United States, males and females are equally affected, but males are far more commonly affected in the Middle East and Japan. Both eyes almost always develop disease, sometimes simultaneously, sometimes separately. Age of onset is usually 17 to 37 years.

1. The **differential diagnosis** includes acute idiopathic anterior uveitis, but unlike Behçet's disease these uveitides are usually unilateral in any given attack and often HLA-B27 positive. Sarcoid may simulate the posterior uveitis but differs in that it is far more indolent than the explosive retinal vasculitis of Behçet's disease. The latter is, in fact, difficult to differentiate from the rapidly progressive viral vasculitic chorioretinitis infections. Other causes of **retinal vasculitis** include Eales's disease, birdshot retinopathy, lupus, multiple sclerosis, postvaccination, Wegener granulomatosis, Takayasu's and Buerger's diseases, polyarteritis nodosa, polymyositis, Whipple's disease, Crohn's disease, Sjögren A antigen, and numerous fungal, parasitic, viral, bacterial, and rickettsial diseases.

2. **Diagnosis** is based primarily on the clinical findings of uveitis and oral and genital ulcers with or without the other findings described. Japanese patients (not American born) are HLA-B51 positive nearly 60% of the time and Mediterranean patients are HLA-B5 positive more than 50% of the time. Skin hyperreactivity (pathergy) is common in these patient groups but not frequently in Americans. In contradistinction to the usual uveitis, cells in the anterior chamber are neutrophils. Fluorescein angiography will reveal the extent of retinal vascular occlusive disease and assist in monitoring therapeutic response.

3. **Therapy** is effective but not fully satisfactory. It is critical that these patients be treated in association with an internist familiar with the drugs and disease. Behçet's disease not only blinds but it may also be fatal. Currently, treatment in the United States is high-dose systemic steroids, e.g., prednisone 80 to 100 mg p.o. qd for several days until improved and then tapered to maintenance levels that control the disease, or until the diagnosis is made, at which point **immunosuppressives** are the drugs of choice if disease is posterior or there are systemic signs: cyclosporin A, cyclophosphamide, chlorambucil, or azathioprine. This is frequently coupled with colchicine therapy, 0.6 mg p.o. bid, between attacks or during attacks in 16-week courses. Colchicine inhibits the enhanced polymononuclear cell migration noted in Behçet's disease. It appears to be useful in preventing recurrent attacks among Japanese but is probably of marginal use in whites. Over the long run, *steroids* will reduce inflammation but *not prevent blindness or death.* For a moderate to severe first attack or for bilateral recurrent attack, the drug of first choice used by some centers is cyclosporin A in dosages discussed in sec. **VI.D.,** above, for at least 16 weeks and in many patients indefinitely at maintenance dosages. The Japanese almost never use steroids, because they feel it worsens the disease. In other clinical settings, the use immunosuppressive alkylating agents such as cyclophosphamide or chlorambucil are the drugs of first choice. For acute exacerbations on azathioprine, 1,000 mg i.v. of methylprednisolone every day for 3 days (or oral equivalent), may be added to the regimen and bring disease under control. Cytotoxic agents, particularly the alkylating agents cyclophosphamide or chlorambucil in dosages discussed in sec. **VI.D.,** above, may be tried and have been shown to be therapeutically effective in a number of patients. If disease is **unilateral** (rare), it is probably better just to observe or, if vision is being lost, to intervene only with colchicine and injected periocular steroids. Patients should be monitored closely for all the potential drug adverse side effects reviewed in sec. **VI.D.,** above.

B. **Systemic vasculitis and uveitis**

1. **Giant cell arteritis (GCA)** typically presents with acute posterior segment ischemia due to the occlusion of the central retinal artery or in the form of an ischemic optic neuropathy. Nevertheless, chronic ocular ischemia can mimic uveitis and cases of intraocular inflammation caused by GCA have also been reported. The diagnosis and treatment of GCA are discussed in Chapter 13.

2. **Polyarteritis nodosa (PAN)** is a vasculitis that affects medium-sized vessels, resulting in arterial occlusion and end-organ infarction. Men

between the ages of 40 to 60 years are affected more than women (2:1). Patients present with nonspecific symptoms such as fatigue, weight loss, myalgia, fever, and arthralgia. Organs that are commonly involved include the skin, heart, kidney, intestines, and CNS. The eye is involved in 10% to 20% of patients and the ocular manifestations include peripheral ulcerative keratitis, scleritis, and acute nongranulomatous iritis. Fundus examination reveals retinal vasculitis with intraretinal hemorrhages, retinal edema, and cotton wool spots. The **diagnosis** is confirmed with tissue biopsy from the skin, kidney, or ocular tissue showing evidence of vascular inflammation. Laboratory tests will reveal an elevated ESR, elevated immune complexes, and a positive p-ANCA in 14% to 16% of patients with uveitis without systemic symptoms. In 10% to 50% of patients hepatitis B surface antigen can be positive. **The outcome of PAN without treatment is fatal (5-year mortality rate in 80% to 90% of patients). The combination of systemic corticosteroids with cyclophosphamide is the treatment of choice for this condition.** The proper treatment of this condition will improve the 5-year mortality rate to 80%.

3. **Wegener's granulomatosis** is a systemic granulomatous necrotizing vasculitis of small vessels that predominantly involves the kidneys and respiratory tract circulation. Both sexes are equally affected and the disease can occur between the ages of 8 and 80 years. Similar to other vasculitides, patients with Wegener will present with nonspecific symptoms and cutaneous vasculitic lesions. Half of the patients with Wegener will have ocular manifestations, and these include pseudotumor, peripheral ulcerative keratopathies, scleritis retinal vasculitis, ischemic neuropathy, and uveitis. Uveitis is usually associated with scleritis, but can also occur primarily. A positive c-ANCA (PR3) serology is strongly indicative of Wegener. The treatment of choice is a combination of systemic corticosteroids with cyclophosphamide.

4. **Kawasaki's disease (mucocutaneous lymph node syndrome)** is a systemic vasculitis of children, two-thirds of which develop a nongranulomatous anterior uveitis in the first week. Systemic findings include fever, lymphadenopathy, erythematous skin rash, oral mucosal erythema, conjunctivitis, disk edema, vascular engorgement, and cardiac abnormalities. ANCA is often positive. Because the uveitis is self-limited, a short course of topical steroid and mydriatic or mydriatic alone usually suffices.

5. **Other vasculitides** that should be considered in the differential diagnosis of patients with systemic manifestations suggestive of vasculitis include Churg-Strauss, Henoch-Schönlein purpura, microscopic polyarteritis, and Takayasu's disease **(Table 9.5).** The presence of primary uveitis in these conditions is rare, however, many of them can present as a uveitis caused by chronic ocular ischemia from involvement of the ophthalmic and carotid circulation.

XI. **Masquerade syndromes** are systemic conditions that mimic uveitis and these include neoplasm. Intraocular lymphoma is a non-Hodgkin large cell lymphoma (NHL) that can arise primarily from the eye, the CNS, or both. Its potential for distance metastasis outside the eye and CNS is rare, however, it presents as a uveitis and can be fatal if the diagnosis is not made.

A. **Clinically,** patients with intraocular NHL are older with an average age of 64 years, and men are more commonly affected than women. The most common symptom described by patients with intraocular NHL is bilateral decreased vision associated with floaters. The anterior segment is quiet and evaluation of the posterior segment will reveal clumped vitreous cells. In advanced cases, multifocal, deep yellow solid subretinal infiltrates are seen. Optic nerve swelling, vasculitis, retinitis, and vitreous hemorrhage can also occur.

B. **Diagnosis** of intraocular NHL can be difficult and a high level of clinical suspicion must be maintained. Chronic uveitis that fails to respond to treatment, in an older patient with vitritis, should raise the diagnosis of intraocular NHL, especially if subretinal lesions are also present. *Fluorescein angiography* can be helpful in detecting early subretinal lesions, and a *brain MRI* may show CNS involvement. A *lumbar puncture* for histological analysis should be performed if there is radiological evidence or clinical signs suggestive of CNS diseases. A pars plana diagnostic vitrectomy can be extremely helpful to make the diagnosis and should be performed to confirm the diagnosis as a primary technique or in cases where other diagnostic modalities are unequivocal. Analysis of the vitreous biopsy should include cytology, flow cytometry, cytokine measurement, and PCR testing for Ig heavy-chain rearrangement (see sec. **V.G.3.**, below).

   C. **The differential diagnosis** of intraocular NHL lymphoma is infection (syphilis, tuberculosis, Lyme, or endogenous endophthalmitis), sarcoidosis, and birdshot retinochoroidopathy.

   D. **Treatment** should be coordinated by a hematologist–oncologist, who will first perform a systemic workup to determine extent of the disease. There is presently not a uniform consensus of the optimal treatment for this condition and treatment will vary among institutions. Treatment modalities include irradiation (ocular and/or brain, spinal cord if CNS is primarily involved), intrathecal or intraocular methotrexate, and systemic chemotherapy. Intraocular inflammation can be initially treated with corticosteroids, but eventually will resolve if the treatment of the lymphoma is effective.

XII. **Endophthalmitis** is a devastating clinical entity that may be most easily defined as purulent inflammation of the intraocular tissues in response to insult from infection (exogenous or endogenous), trauma, immune reaction, physical or chemical changes, vasculitis, or neoplasm.

   A. **Classification**

   1. The most common endophthalmitis is **acute postoperative endophthalmitis,** which may be **infectious** secondary to bacterial or fungal invasion. This condition is seen most commonly in debilitated patients such as diabetics, patients with immunosuppressive disease, or patients with alcoholism. Acute postoperative **sterile** endophthalmitis can be caused by chemical insult such as the use of irrigating agents, the retention of foreign bodies such as sponges or powder from gloves, or manipulation of the vitreous.

   2. **Long-term postoperative inflammation** is commonly associated with filtering blebs, either intentional or unintentional, that allow access to the external organisms directly into the eye through a very thin and tenuous conjunctival covering. The vitreous wick fistula, which is the result of externalization of the vitreous with no protective covering by conjunctiva, affords direct access to the inside of the eye for any external organisms as well. The fistulas seen with epithelial downgrowth are, of course, notoriously difficult to seal off. They also leave the eye open to direct invasion from the outside by whatever organism may be in the conjunctival cul-de-sac.

   3. **Trauma** to the eye, particularly lacerating injuries, is the least common cause of intraocular infection, possibly because intensive antibiotic therapy is started before infection is established.

   4. **Endogenous (metastatic) endophthalmitis** is from infectious loci elsewhere in the body, the most common causes being dermatitis, meningitis, otitis, urinary infection, septic arthritis, and following surgery, particularly of the abdomen, or associated with endocarditis or chronic obstructive pulmonary disease. Drug addicts who mainline heroin introduce into the vascular system fairly significant doses of both bacteria and fungi. Patients with **AIDS** or taking **immunosuppressive drugs** for lymphomatous disease, leukemia, or organ transplant are also susceptible to endogenous endophthalmitis, particularly that due to *Candida albicans.* CMV, herpes and zoster viruses, *Pneumocystis,* and numerous other opportunistic infections are also seen more commonly now and should be suspected in any immunosuppressed patient who has blurring of vision.

B. The **etiologic agents** involved in endophthalmitis in general order of frequency are as follows:
1. **Bacterial—postoperative**
   a. Acute
      (1) *Staphylococcus epidermidis.*
      (2) *Staphylococcus aureus.*
      (3) Gram-negative species:
         (a) *Pseudomonas.*
         (b) *Proteus.*
         (c) *Escherichia coli.*
         (d) Miscellaneous *(Serratia, Klebsiella, Bacillus).*
      (4) Streptococcal species.
   b. Chronic low grade
      (1) *Staphylococcus epidermidis.*
      (2) *Propionibacterium acnes.*
2. **Bacterial—endogenous**
   a. *Streptococcus* sp. *(pneumococcus, viridens).*
   b. *S. aureus.*
3. **Bacterial—posttraumatic:** *Bacillus cereus.*
4. **Bacterial—post filter bleb**
   a. *Haemophilus influenzae.*
   b. *Streptococcus* sp.
5. **Fungal—postoperative**
   a. *Volutella.*
   b. *Neurospora.*
   c. *Fusarium.*
   d. *Candida.*
6. **Fungal—endogenous:** *Candida*—yeast.
7. **Fungal—trauma:** *Fusarium and Aspergillus*
C. Clinically, the earliest sign is an unexpected change or exaggeration of the expected **postoperative inflammation.** Patients often, but not always, complain of pain. There is obvious increased hyperemia. Conjunctival chemosis may be considerable. Lid edema may be so severe as to shut the eye completely, and there may also be spasm. Decreasing vision is invariably part of the process, and corneal edema may be the very first objective sign of an intraocular process gone wrong. Ultimately and often early in the process, there will be considerable anterior chamber and vitreous reaction. *S. epidermidis* and *P. acnes* may, however, incite only a *low-grade inflammatory reaction lasting for weeks. P. acnes* is particularly *associated with intraocular lenses (IOLs)* and patients with rosacea–blepharitis. Endogenous endophthalmitis may be acute or slow in onset.

The *clinical manifestations* of endophthalmitis may sometimes be used to *differentiate* bacterial, fungal, and sterile etiologic agents. These manifestations are as follows:
1. **Bacterial**
   a. Sudden onset (1 to 7 days postoperatively), rapid progression.
   b. Pain, very red, chemosis.
   c. Lid edema and spasm.
   d. Rapid loss of vision and good light perception.
   e. Hypopyon and diffuse glaucoma.
2. **Fungal or low-grade bacterial**
   a. Delayed onset (8 to 14 days or more).
   b. Some pain and redness.
   c. Transient hypopyon.
   d. Localized anterior vitreous gray-white patch extending over face.
   e. Satellite lesions.
   f. Good light perception.
   g. Rare explosive exudation into anterior chamber.
3. **Sterile**
   a. May mimic bacterial or fungal infection.

  b. Undue surgical trauma.
  c. Incarceration of intraocular contents (lens, vitreous, iris) in wound.
  d. Foreign body (sponge, powder) retention.
      Vitrectomy.
D. The **differential diagnosis** of **sterile endophthalmitis** is late rupture of the anterior vitreous face. This rupture is frequently associated with nonexposed vitreous in the wound. It should be differentiated from vitreous wick syndrome, in which there is actual exposure to vitreous extraocularly. This late rupture is associated with the onset of redness and decreased vision, with anterior chamber and vitreous reaction several months postoperatively. Cystoid macular edema may present with decreased vision and increased vitreous inflammatory reaction. This syndrome can be differentiated from a true endophthalmitis by fluorescein angiography.
E. **Workup** for endophthalmitis includes **hospitalization** of the patient, a careful history regarding any predisposing events, and a clinical examination for some of the previously mentioned predisposing factors.
  1. **Cultures** obviously are of critical importance. Numerous studies have shown that conjunctival cultures are probably of very little use, because there seems to be little relationship between the flora growing outside the eye and that growing inside the eye in endophthalmitis.
  2. An **anterior chamber paracentesis** (0.2 mL) and a diagnostic and (in some cases) therapeutic core **vitrectomy** should be done. Approximately 30% of all anterior chamber paracenteses will be positive for organisms. Results of the paracentesis may be correlated fairly well with the prognosis; i.e., eyes with positive cultures have a poor prognosis, whereas those with negative cultures usually regain useful vision. In **vitrectomy,** approximately 40% to 50% of the cultures are positive. In aphakic eyes the vitreous may be taken through the limbal incision made for the aqueous sample and on through the pupil. In phakic eyes a pars plana incision should be made. A vitreous suction-cutting instrument should be used.
  3. The sample should be used for both **culture** and **smears** for staining.
      a. **Culture.** For **bacterial** culture, sheep blood agar plate, chocolate agar plate, beef heart infusion, and thioglycolate broth should be inoculated. These are stored at 37°C and will usually be positive within 12 hours. **Fungal** cultures should be placed on Sabouraud medium and blood agar plates, as well as beef heart infusion broth with gentamicin in it, to suppress bacterial growth. These are stored at 30°C or room temperature and will be positive in 36 to 72 hours as a rule.
      b. The **smears** should be Gram stained; any organisms that are found should be classified as positive, Gram-positive, or Gram-negative. The Giemsa stain smear, although it does not reveal whether the organism is Gram-positive or -negative, is superior for determining the actual morphology of any organism. Calcofluor white stain can be used to facilitate the detection of fungal filaments or hyphae in the sample.
F. **Therapy of bacterial endophthalmitis. After planting the culture, the physician should immediately start treatment** regardless of whether there have been any results on the smear. Broad-spectrum therapy should be maintained until definitive culture reports are obtained. The three main forms of therapy for endophthalmitis involve the use of antibiotics, mydriatic–cycloplegics (such as atropine), corticosteroids, and possibly *core vitrectomy.* Antibiotics are delivered by three to four routes: (a) intravitreal; (b) subtenon or subconjunctival injection; (c) systemic (i.v., i.m., or occasionally p.o.) and, if point of entry is anterior, trauma, wound leak or ulcer; and (d) topical (see **XII.F.1** below and Table 9.6 for intravitreal doses; Chapter 5, Table 5.7 for topical and subconjunctival doses, and Appendix B for systemic doses).
  1. **Therapy before culture data are known**
      a. **Immediately** following diagnosis of bacterial endophthalmitis and anterior chamber and vitreous aspiration for diagnostic purposes, commence **therapy** as follows in the **operating room.**

TABLE 9.6. INTRAVITREOUS ANTIBIOTIC AND STEROID PREPARATIONS

Drug	Initial Solution Mix		Final Solution Mix			Injected Dose (0.1 mL)
	Commercial Preparation (i.v.)	First Diluent Added to 1.0-mL Commercial Preparation[a]	Initial Solution (mL) Plus	Second Diluent[a] (mL)	Final Drug Concentration	
Amikacin	100 mg/2 mL	—	1.0	11.5	4 mg/mL	400 μgm
Carbenicillin	5 g/10 mL	1.0	1.0	9.0	25 mg/mL	2.5 mg
Cefamandole	1 g/5 mL	1.0	1.0	4.0	20 mg/mL	2.0 mg
Cefazolin	500 mg/mL	1.0	1.0	9.0	25 mg/mL	2.5 mg
Ceftazidime	1 g/mL	3.0–9.0	—	—	25 mg/mL	2.5 mg
Ceftriaxone	1 g/5 mL	1.0	1.0	4.0	20 mg/mL	2.0 mg
Clindamycin	150 mg/mL	2.0	1.0	9.0	5 mg/mL	0.5 mg
Gentamicin	80 mg/2 mL	3.0	1.0	9.0	1.0 mg/mL	0.1 mg
Tobramycin	80 mg/2 mL	3.0	1.0	9.0	1.0 mg/mL	0.1 mg
Vancomycin	500 mg/10 mL	—	1.0	4.0	10 mg/mL	1.0 mg
Vancomycin[b]	500 mg/10 mL	—	0.4	0.6	20 mg/mL	2.0 mg
Aqueous dexamethasone for steroid injection	24 mg/mL	1.0–5.0	—	—	4 mg/mL	400 μg

i.v., intravenous.

[a]With the exception of carbenicillin, vancomycin, and dexamethasone (sterile water for injection only), diluent may be sterile water or saline for injection (USP).

[b]If posterior lens capsule not intact.

(Adapted from Pavan-Langston D, Dunkel E. *Handbook of ocular drug therapy and ocular side effects of systemic drugs.* Boston: Little, Brown, 1991.)

(1) **Intravitreal** 400 μg amikacin or 2.25 mg ceftazidime plus 1.0 mg of vancomycin for postoperative endophthalmitis, 1.0 mg of vancomycin plus 0.5 mg of clindamycin or 400 μg amikacin for posttraumatic cases, and 1.0 mg of vancomycin plus 2.25 mg ceftazidime or 2.0 mg of ceftriaxone for postglaucoma filter bleb infections. Dexamethasone 400 μg is also usually given (see sec. **XII.F.3,** Table 9.6, and Appendix B for dosages, mixtures, and other drugs). Tobramycin or gentamicin 100 μg may replace amikacin or ceftazidime, but may be more retinotoxic. All are in 0.1 mL volumes and may be repeated in 24 to 48 hours if necessary. After aspiration of vitreous for diagnostic purposes, two tuberculin syringes, each containing antibiotic, are exchanged consecutively and the material slowly injected into midvitreous. The small volume of antibiotic delivered into the vitreous should not remain in the bore of the needle. In phakic eyes, both the diagnostic and therapeutic vitreal aspiration and injections are performed behind the lens through a tract made in the sclera 4.0 mm behind the corneal limbus.

(2) **Periocular injection** should be either subconjunctival (anterior subtenons) or retrobulbar (posterior subtenons).

(a) Gentamicin or tobramycin 40 mg (1 mL) treats most Gram-positive and Gram-negative organisms.

(b) Cefazolin 100 mg (1.0 mL) or vancomycin 50 mg per mL treats pneumococcus and streptococci not covered by the aminoglycosides.

b. **Systemic.** In the operating room or once the patient is back in the **hospital room,** if **topical** antibiotics are to be used, start fortified tobramycin or gentamicin 14 mg per mL, and cefazolin 133 mg per mL, two drops q1h around the clock. **Systemic** amikacin 15 mg per kg i.v. or i.m. q8h, coupled with cefazolin 1 g i.v. q6h for 2 to 5 days, or ceftriaxone for penicillinase or beta-lactamase producers, is broad initial therapy until organisms are known or if they are never identified (see Appendix B for dose and alternative drugs). Before the systemic treatment is started, a blood urea nitrogen and creatinine levels should be drawn. These should be monitored every 3 days because of the **_nephrotoxicity_** of these drugs. If the smears show Gram-positive organisms, bacitracin drops at a level of 10,000 units per mL (two drops q2h) should be added. If the smear shows Gram-negative organisms, carbenicillin 4 to 6 g p.o. or ticarcillin 200 to 300 mg per kg i.v. q6h should be added for extra protection against _Pseudomonas_ and _Proteus._ **Probenecid** 0.5 g p.o. qid is given to enhance cefazolin, carbenicillin, or other penicillin or cephalosporin levels.

c. **Quinolones** are ineffective as single agents.

2. **Once the cultures have returned,** the physician adjusts the topical regimen according to the organism found (see Appendix B for specific therapy).

a. **If the organism is a Gram-positive coccus,** the systemic therapy may be adjusted in that direction by vancomycin i.v. or cephalexin i.m. or i.v. qd for 7 to 10 days and subconjunctivally qd for two injections.

b. **If a gram-negative rod** is found on the culture, the physician should continue to administer either ceftazidime and tobramycin (synergistic), ticarcillin i.m. or i.v., or carbenicillin i.v. qid for 7 to 10 days and subconjunctivally qd for one to two injections.

c. **_Propionibacterium acnes_** is treated by a two-compartment approach: 1 mg vancomycin intravitreally and 0.5 mg intracamerally. Semisynthetic penicillins or cephalosporins may also be used. Surgical removal of an IOL and capsule may be needed.

3. Steroids

a. **Twenty-four hours after the antibiotic therapy** mentioned in **sec. XII.F.3.** is started, steroids may be initiated if intravitreal therapy was not given.

  (1) Dexamethasone phosphate 4 to 12 mg (1 mL), or prednisolone succinate, 25 mg (1 mL) subconjunctivally every other day, one to two times.

  2 Prednisone 40 mg p.o. qd for 10 days.

b. **The role of corticosteroids** in endophthalmitis is aimed at limiting inflammatory damage to the intraocular structures and improving visual outcome. If **fungus is not suspected,** the physician may safely and justifiably start these drugs. If a sterile endophthalmitis is suspected, the physician should continue the steroids at higher levels for a longer period of time.

4. **Vitrectomy** (plus all of the aforementioned therapy) is used in patients with moderately advanced or advanced disease. For patients with milder disease, intravitreal, periocular injected, systemic, and topical antibiotics are preferred after vitreous biopsy. If there is no improvement in 36 to 48 hours or if a virulent organism such as *Pseudomonas* or fungus is isolated, total vitrectomy is recommended along with more intravitreal antibiotic or antifungal agents and appropriate systemic drug adjustment.

G. Fungal uveitis and endophthalmitis

1. **Aspergillosis.** Most of the recognized aspergillosis infections have occurred in patients who showed no evidence of fungal infection elsewhere. This uveitis should be suspected in drug addicts who infect themselves with contaminated needles or in immunosuppressed patients.

  a. **Clinically,** there are vitritis with fluff balls and yellow-white fundus lesions similar to *Candida* chorioretinitis, intraretinal hemorrhages, and occasional hypopyon.

2. **Candidiasis** is the most common of the other fungal infections. It occurs in immunosuppressed and in hospitalized patients who receive systemic antibiotics, especially patients with indwelling i.v. catheters. A blood culture is valuable in establishing the diagnosis. The chorioretinitis may begin either in the choroid or in the retina. In mild cases it appears to remain localized in the choroid.

  a. The **clinical picture** simulates that seen in toxoplasmosis. Lesions are usually fluffy, yellow-white elevations, varying in size from those simulating cotton-wool spots to those measuring several dd in breadth. Unlike those seen in toxoplasmosis, these lesions are often multiple and unassociated with previous scars. They often have an overlying vitreous haze, as do the lesions of toxoplasmosis, but unlike toxoplasmosis the process may actually grow into the vitreous.

H. Therapy of fungal uveitis and endophthalmitis.

The general evaluation procedures followed are similar to those described in secs. **V.A.–F.,** above. The drug of first choice for fungal *endophthalmitis* is still amphotericin B given systemically and intravitreally (Table 9.7). **Synergistic** efficacy is obtained by adding oral flucytosine to systemic and intravitreal amphotericin B and continuing maintenance doses of both for 2 to 4 weeks before tapering. It should also be noted that ketoconazole is **antagonistic** to amphotericin B and should not be used with it. Topical natamycin q1h or amphotericin B q1 to 2h should be given in addition to systemic and intravitreal drug if the point of entry is anterior and accessible to topical therapy (see Chapter 5, sec. **IV.N.**). The role of subconjunctival drug is not well established but may be useful in poorly cooperative patients for pulsing high doses. Toxic sloughing may occur, however. Vitrectomy is discussed in sec. **XII.F.1,4.** and is generally the rule for fungal endophthalmitis.

I. Prophylaxis

1. **Preoperative antibiotics** are useful in decreasing the incidence of postoperative endophthalmitis from 0.71% to 3.05%, to 0.05% to 0.11%. In addition, the physician should not perform elective surgery if either the

TABLE 9.7. ANTIFUNGAL SYSTEMIC AND INTRAVITREAL THERAPEUTIC REGIMEN

Drug*	Intravitreal	Systemic	Effective in
Amphoteracin B (Fungizone)	5–10 μg	1 mg in 500 ml 5% D/W IV over 2–4 hr test dose. Work up by 5–10 mg total dose/d to maintenance of 0.5–1.2 mg/kg/d in 4–6 h infusions. Synergistic with flucytosine PO. See Table 5.8.	*Candida, Aspergillus, Cryptococcus, Coccidioides, Sporothrix, Paracoccidioides, Mucor*
Fluconazole (Diflucan)		400–800 mg PO or IV once daily.	*Candida, Cryptococcus, Cocciodioides*
Flucytosine (5 FC, Ancobon)		100–150 mg/day PO in 4 divided doses (q 6 h). Synergistic with fluconazole.	*Candida, Aspergillus, Cryptococcus, Cladosporium*
Ketoconazole (Nizoral)		200–400 mg PO qd–bid.	*Candida, Fusarium, Penicillium, Aspergillus, Alternaria, Rhodoturula, Histoplasma, Cladosporium, Coccidioides, Mucor, Paracoccidioides, Phialophora, Actinomyces*
Itraconazole (Sporanox)		200 mg PO qd or bid.	*Aspergillus, Cryptococcus, Histoplasma, Candida, Blastomyces, Paracoccidiomycosis, Sporotrichosis*

*Duration of treatment determined by organism and severity (weeks to months).

    lids or lacrimal sac appear inflamed or infected. Culture should be taken and these areas appropriately treated before any surgery is undertaken. The physician should also take great caution and use plentiful preoperative antibiotics in any patients who have keratoconjunctivitis sicca, acne rosacea, or atopic dermatitis, because all of these patients are more prone than normal to carrying highly infectious organisms in the external ocular tissues.

2. If the physician observes inadvertent **filtering blebs postoperatively,** an attempt should be made to seal these either with cryotherapy or, if necessary, with a secondary surgical procedure. If it is not possible to seal the bleb or in those patients who have intentional filtering blebs for glaucoma, it is advisable to use some form of chronic antibiotic therapy such as sulfacetamide drops or erythromycin ointment daily to protect patients from building up high levels of Gram-positive organisms in the conjunctival cul-de-sac.

XIII. Uveal trauma. Injury to the uvea may be either direct or countercoup. Direct contusion of the cornea can produce a rather marked posterior displacement, first of the cornea and then of the iris–lens diaphragm. This displacement places great stress on the area of the iris root and the zonules. In addition, the sclera expands in circumference in the area of the ciliary body. The ciliary body follows suit, but with some lag, resulting in possible separation within the uveal tissues or between the uveal tract and the sclera. After trauma, the endothelium of the cornea may show a fine dusting of pigment, especially near the trabecular meshwork, on the lens capsule, on the iris surface, and occasionally in the vitreous. A **Vossius pigment ring** on the anterior surface of the lens gives evidence of previous ocular trauma. This ring is located at the site of pupillary margin at the time of injury. The following entities seen after uveal trauma are discussed in Chapter 2 (see secs. **VIII.** and **IX.**): traumatic iritis, sphincter alterations (miosis and mydriasis), iridodialysis, angle recession, traumatic hyphema, choroidal trauma, traumatic choroiditis, and uveal effusion (ciliochoroidal). **Uveal effusion syndrome** may also occur under several other conditions (see Chapter 2, sec. **IX.C.5.**).

XIV. **Iris atrophy and degeneration.** There is a generalized thinning of the iris stroma with a flattening of the architecture and disappearance of crypts, especially in the pupillary zone. The brown sphincter muscle becomes visible, and the entire pigment epithelial layer is easily seen. The pupillary ruff often develops a moth-eaten appearance; granules of pigment may seem to be scattered over the anterior iris surface and the anterior lens capsule, as well as the back of the cornea and the trabecular meshwork.

  A. **Senile changes**
    1. So-called **senile miosis** is probably related to sclerosis and hyalinization of the vessels as well as of stroma, although preferential atrophy of the dilator muscle may play a role. Atrophy of both stroma and pigment epithelium occur as part of aging. The iris may become more blue or gray.
    2. **Iridoschisis** is a bilateral atrophy affecting mostly patients more than 65 years of age. The cleft forms between anterior and posterior stroma. Stromal fibers and blood vessels remain attached to a portion of the iris, with their loose ends floating freely in the anterior chamber. The avascular necrosis that may occur in angle-closure glaucoma predisposes to iridoschisis.
  B. **Essential iris atrophy.** Multiple vascular occlusions may be responsible for essential iris atrophy, which is characterized by unilateral progressive atrophy of the iris. It is five times more common in women, commencing in the third decade and almost always complicated by glaucoma. The patient complains of a displaced pupil. The pupil is displaced away from the atrophic zone. This atrophy progresses over a period of 1 to 3 years. With dissolution of additional areas, a pseudopolycoria develops. Peripheral anterior synechiae develop on both sides of the holes, and the IOP starts to increase.
  C. **Postinflammatory.** Although iritis can give rise to atrophy, it is seldom seen except in entities such as herpes zoster ophthalmicus.
  D. **Glaucomatous.** Slight dilation and irregularity of the pupil as well as a more segmental atrophy may follow an acute angle-closure glaucoma, due to necrosis of the sphincter muscle.
  E. **Neurogenic.** Depigmentation or focal hyperpigmentation may develop with an irregular pupil. This is seen in conditions such as neurosyphilis or lesions of the ciliary ganglion.

XV. **Choroidal atrophies and degenerations.** Atrophy is a loss of tissue mass. Degeneration may be slight and possibly even reversible. The affected tissue may be viable, but the metabolism is disturbed and the end process is the death of the cells.

  A. **Senile changes.** The most important senile changes occurring in the choroid, as in other parts of the uvea, occur in the blood vessels. These changes are especially evident at the posterior pole and about the optic disk. Associated hyperplasia and degeneration of the pigment epithelium may lead to an increase in deposition of hyaline material on Bruch membrane. This deposition may result in small focal thickenings in the cuticular portion. These drusen or translucent colloid bodies are homogeneous, dome-shaped, and sometimes calcified excrescences covered by damaged RPE. There is a diffuse thickening and basophilic staining of Bruch membrane. Cracks of Bruch membrane may develop.

B. Choroidal sclerosis. The clinical appearance of sclerosis of the larger choroidal vessels is mostly due to their prominence and easy visibility, with atrophy of the choriocapillaris and surrounding tissues. This process occurs in three regions: the extreme periphery of the fundus, the peripapillary zone, and the posterior polar region.

1. The **diffuse type of sclerosis** is rare. It usually commences in the fourth decade with an edematous appearance of the fundus, pigmentary migration, and small yellow or cream-colored spots. It slowly advances until the sixth decade, when the fundus develops a brownish tigroid appearance that is associated with extensive destruction of the RPE. The larger choroidal vessels are exposed and stand out as a prominent whitish network. The result is an exposure of the sclera, with complete atrophy. Transmission is usually autosomal dominant. Visual fields are contracted, but the visual acuity does not fail until the macula is involved. **Night blindness** is an early sign, and the ERG is subnormal. In the early stages, the differential diagnosis is difficult, and in later stages it simulates choroideremia.

2. **Peripapillary choroidal sclerosis** begins around the optic disk and is similar to the senile peripapillary halo. In the early stages differential diagnosis includes senile peripapillary halo, central areolar sclerosis, senile macular degeneration, and posterior polar inflammation.

3. Central choroidal sclerosis begins in the macula and remains stationary or spreads. It may be seen as early as age 15 years and may resemble uveitis because of the appearance of edema and exudation.

C. Gyrate atrophy of the choroid is characterized by a progressive atrophy of the choroid and retina, including the pigment epithelium. It usually begins in the third decade. Irregular atrophic areas develop, over which the retinal vessels appear normal, near the periphery. The atrophic areas enlarge, coalesce, and spread centrally. The macula is frequently preserved until late. **Night blindness** is a constant feature. The visual fields are usually concentrically contracted. Most of the hereditary patterns are recessive. Patients have an increased plasma, CSF, and aqueous humor ornithine concentration from 10 to 20 times higher than normal. These findings suggest an inborn error of amino acid metabolism, possibly a defective activity in the enzyme ornithine ketoacid aminotransferase.

D. Choroideremia is a bilateral, hereditary choroidal degeneration characterized by **night blindness** from childhood. The typical and fully developed form with a progressive course toward blindness occurs in males, whereas females have a mild and nonprogressive course. It is transmitted in a recessive sex-linked manner. The earliest change is often seen in late childhood. In males, this change consists of degeneration of the peripheral RPE, giving a salt-and-pepper appearance. This is followed by progressive atrophy with exposure of the choroidal vessels, until the sclera is bared. The process continues both peripherally and centrally, leaving a small patch of retina and choroid in the macula. The retinal vessels and optic disk retain their normal appearance until late.

In female carriers the appearance resembles that seen in very young males, with a combination of pigmentation and depigmentation or salt-and-pepper atrophy most marked in the midperiphery. In females the condition is benign and does not progress. Night blindness begins in early youth in males and progresses to total night blindness after a period of about 10 years. The ERG shows an absence of rod (non-color vision) scotopic activity and a progressive loss of photopic (color vision) activity.

E. Angioid streaks are reddish to dark-brown streaks of irregular contour, usually somewhat wider than retinal blood vessels. They extend outward from the disk toward the equator in a more or less circular pattern, and they lie underneath the retinal vessels. Later, a gray-white border representing proliferated fibrous tissue may bind them. Angioid streaks are almost always bilateral and are usually seen in middle-aged persons, more commonly in males. A stippled appearance of the fundus, resembling the cutaneous changes in pseudoxanthoma elasticum, has been called "peau d'orange." Several small, round, yellowish-white spots called "salmon spots" may also be seen in association with angioid streaks. Although the angioid streaks are asymptomatic, these breaks in Bruch membrane allow the ingrowth of capillaries from the choroid that leak and produce a diskiform degeneration similar to that seen in senile patients. Angioid streaks signify the frequent association of widespread degenerative changes of a similar nature involving elastic tissue elsewhere, in **systemic conditions** such as pseudoxanthoma elasticum (Gröenblad-Strandberg syndrome), osteitis deformans, Paget's disease, senile elastosis of the skin, sickle cell anemia, some hypertensive cardiovascular disorders, lead poisoning, thrombocytopenic purpura, and familial hyperphosphatemia. By far the most common association is that of pseudoxanthoma elasticum. Occasionally, photocoagulation of the neovascular net may be of value.

F. **Myopic choroidal atrophy.** In pathologic progressive myopia, a primary choroidal atrophy develops in which the sclera is thin and the choroid becomes atrophic. This degenerative myopia is usually associated with axial lengthening of the globe in the anteroposterior axis. The degree of myopia is usually genetically determined. It is more common in women and in some groups, such as Chinese, Japanese, Arabs, and Jews.

  Myopic degeneration often starts with the appearance of a temporal crescent at the optic disk that may spread to become a circumpapillary zone of atrophy. As the posterior eye enlarges, the sclera becomes thin and ectatic. The sclera may be exposed because the choroid does not reach the disk. Nasally, the choroid, Bruch membrane, and RPE may overlap the optic nerve head. Clefts resembling lacquer cracks may develop in Bruch membrane. These clefts are branching, irregular, yellow-white lines that take a horizontal course. Melanocytes disappear in the choroid, and there may be a widespread loss of the choriocapillaris. Breaks in Bruch membrane may give rise to a Fuchs spot at the macula that is similar to the maculopathy seen in angioid streaks and senile macular degeneration. The length of the eyeball should be determined with A-scan ultrasonography. If lengthening is documented, support for the stretching sclera can be gained by *surgical insertion of autographs* of fascia lata or homographs of sclera. This reinforcement surgery should be completed before severe degenerative changes take place.

G. **Pseudoinflammatory macular dystrophy of Sorsby** is a rare disease. To make the diagnosis, the physician should demonstrate dominant inheritance and lack of any signs of the presumed ocular histoplasmosis syndrome, angioid streaks, and high myopia. The onset is between the third and fifth decade.

H. **Secondary atrophy and dystrophy**
  1. **Ischemic.** Atrophy of choroidal tissues occurs when the blood supply to a given area is cut off or significantly diminished. Wedge-shaped areas of depigmentation are seen with their apices pointing toward the disk.
  2. **Glaucomatous.** In chronic glaucoma, atrophy of the uveal tract may result. Atrophy may be so extensive that only a thin line of flattened pigmented tissue may be seen histologically.

XVI. **Uveal tumors**
  A. **Epithelial hyperplasia of the pigmented iris epithelium** is common in response to long-standing inflammation, degeneration, or glaucoma, and consists of pigmented cells extending through the pupil over the anterior surface of the iris.
  B. **Embryonal medulloepitheliomas (dictyomas)** arise from the nonpigmented epithelium of the ciliary body. Although distant metastasis has not been recorded, they are locally invasive. They occur in young children and appear as a grayish-white mass in the ciliary body, eventually presenting in the pupil. **Enucleation** is advised.

C. **Medulloepithelioma** in an adult form usually arises from the pigmented epithelium of the ciliary body, but may also originate from the iris pigment epithelium. It occurs in previously traumatized or inflamed eyes, grows slowly, and appears as a dark mass. It is locally invasive and **enucleation** is suggested. *A- and B-scan ultrasonography and phosphorus-32 studies should be done before any surgical solution.*

D. **Nevi (freckles)** are a cluster of normal uveal melanocytes. A nevus is a highly cellular mass composed of "nevus cells" that are plump and that have few cytoplasmic processes. These cells are arranged in a nest-like manner. Although congenital, a nevus may not become recognizable until puberty, when it acquires pigment. It may be associated with ectropion uvea. Nevi may occasionally undergo malignant change. In the choroid they are bluish gray and flat with blurred margins, usually near the courses of the long posterior ciliary nerves. They are not usually associated with visual field defects.

E. **Malignant melanomas** are the most frequently occurring intraocular tumors in adults. The incidence in all eye patients is 0.4%. They are infrequent in African-Americans, occur usually after the fifth decade, and are rarely bilateral. The seriousness of the prognosis is directly related to tumor size and cell type. Spindle A cells are long cells with long, slender nuclei in which nuclear chromatin is arranged in a linear fashion along the long axis of the nucleus. There is some question as to whether these cells are malignant. Spindle B cells are oblong in shape; their nuclei are larger and plumper and have prominent nucleoli. Epithelioid cells are large and irregular in shape, and their nuclei are dense with prominent nucleoli. Usually there is a combination of cell types. Pigmentation can vary greatly from amelanotic to heavily pigmented lesions. The epithelioid cell type, pigmentation, and larger size suggest greater malignancy. Malignant melanomas spread by direct extension, local metastasis, or generalized metastasis.

1. **Differential diagnosis** includes hemorrhagic detachment of the pigment epithelium or retina (or both), choroidal detachment (serous), ciliary body or retinal inflammatory disease (or both), pigment epithelial proliferation, hemangioma, and metastatic lesions.

2. **Clinical diagnosis** is based on several features. A small-pigmented tumor **without retinal detachment** is most likely benign but should be photographed and reobserved for changes indicating growth in 3 months, and every 6 months after that if no growth is detected. Localized **retinal detachment** in the macula causing loss of central vision may be caused by either benign or malignant melanotic tumor. Photopsia is a warning, however, that there may be acute retinal damage resulting from rapid tumor expansion. Visual field testing cannot differentiate between visual loss due to a chronic nongrowing tumor and acute damage from a rapidly growing tumor. **Tumor elevation** of 2 mm or more is indicative of an actively growing tumor. **Drusen** over the tumor surface are indicative of a minimally to totally inactive lesion. Scattered plaques and orange pigment **without drusen** suggest active growth. Serous **retinal detachment,** clear or cloudy, indicates toxic changes due to nutritional deficiency but not necessarily growth. Choroidal neovascularization, in the form of fine fan-shaped flat tufts over the tumor surface, suggests long-standing chronicity and lack of growth, whereas large-caliber vessels are seen in active tumors.

3. **Diagnostic tests.** If a lesion is classified as a dormant small melanoma (<3 mm thick), baseline fundus photos, fluorescein angiography, and A- and B-scan ultrasonography should be done and repeated in 3 to 4 months. If there is no change, clinical observation and fundus photos should be repeated every 6 months and therapy started if changes appear. Medium-size (<10 mm thick), dormant-appearing melanomas have the same baseline examination, but because of a greater tendency for growth, photos and ultrasound should be repeated every 3 to 6 months and evaluated.

   Fluorescein angiography is useful in differentiating acute from chronic inactive lesions. Chronic signs are drusen, cystic retinal degeneration, and flat, fine neovascularization. More acute changes indicating growth are multiple pinpoint areas of dye leakage, widespread destruction of pigment epithelium, and an irregular pattern of moderate size vessels.

4. **Therapy** may be by laser photocoagulation for small melanomas not on the ciliary body and more than 2 mm from the macula or disk. More widely employed therapy currently for active tumors less than 10 mm in elevation is the use of surgically placed, low-energy, episcleral radioactive plaques. Isotopes used are cobalt-60, iridium-192, iodine-125, and ruthenium-106, depending on the size and virulence of the tumor. The plaques are left in place until 8,000 to 10,000 cGy is delivered to the tumor apex and are then removed. Special plaques are used for peripapillary or subfoveal melanomas. Alternative radiotherapy is use of heavy ion bombardment using proton beam or helium ions. Tantalum clips are required on the sclera for accurate localization. Treatment of choice is yet to be determined.

Local resection may be used in some cases of ciliary body or small to medium ciliary-choroidal melanomas and, of course, iris melanomas. Plaques may also be used, however, for the ciliary body tumors. Enucleation is generally reserved for eyes with tumors too large to manage with radiotherapy in a patient with another seeing eye, eyes with hopeless visual loss (e.g., total retinal detachment), or eyes with invasion of the optic disk. If there is only one eye or the patient is old or already showing evidence of metastatic disease, surgery may be deferred in favor of radiotherapy, which may be palliative rather than curative. Exenteration is indicated only for extensive extraocular involvement, but no evidence of metastases at the time of initial evaluation, or if there is orbital recurrence after enucleation.

F. **Neurilemoma** is a rare benign lesion that cannot be differentiated clinically from malignant melanoma but is extremely slow growing and, therefore, may be followed periodically for evidence of the notable growth indicative of melanoma.

G. **Neurofibroma** may appear only in the eye or may be a part of von Recklinghausen's disease. It is frequently associated with glaucoma, possibly because of chamber angle anomalies. It clinically resembles malignant melanoma and may be clinically confused with it.

H. **Leiomyoma** is a rare neoplasm and is difficult to differentiate from nevi and malignant melanoma of the iris. It appears as a grayish-white vascularized nodule, most frequently located in the inferior iris near the pupillary border. It is slow growing, and treatment is local excision.

I. **Hemangiomas** should be considered hamartomas and not true neoplasms. They can occur anywhere in the uvea, most frequently in the choroid. They may be associated with other angiomas and be a part of the **Sturge-Weber syndrome.** The choroidal lesions are usually in the posterior pole. The overlying retina shows microcystic changes. The lesions are not pigmented and are slow growing. They are usually associated with arcuate field defects. The tumors are endothelial-lined spaces engorged with blood and, because they lack a capsule, blend into the surrounding choroid. They are relatively flat and have a yellowish color. The diagnosis is improved with the use of fluorescein angiography, thermography, and ultrasonography. Photocoagulation can be used **therapeutically.**

J. **Secondary tumors.** Although any portion of the uveal tract can be the site of metastasis, the posterior choroid is the site of predilection because of its rich blood supply in the short posterior ciliary arteries. The breast is the most frequent primary site, with the lung second. The lesions clinically appear flat, diffuse, with an overlying shallow retinal detachment. The rapidity of growth is greater than that of malignant melanomas. **Radiation** may be used.

10. GLAUCOMA

Deborah Pavan-Langston and Cynthia L. Grosskreutz

I. **Definition, incidence, and risk factors.** *Glaucoma* is a condition in which the pressure inside the eye is sufficiently elevated to result ultimately in optic nerve damage and potential visual field loss via capillary microinfarction causing optic nerve ischemia. This combines with mechanical damage to the nerve by slippage of the lamina cribrosa. Glaucoma is the third leading cause of blindness worldwide behind cataract and trachoma, and in the United States, it is the third leading cause of blindness behind cataract and macular degeneration. Approximately 1.25 million Americans have the diagnosed condition, but another 1 million Americans have glaucoma and are unaware of it. Nearly 120,000 are bilaterally blind, and 1.6 million have visual field defects. It is the single most frequent irreversible cause of blindness among African-Americans and it affects more than 2% of all whites. Detection of glaucoma patients is, therefore, an important public health problem. There are more than 40 different types of glaucoma. Glaucoma can also affect younger people, and measurement of eye pressure is an important part of a routine eye examination. **Risk factors** for glaucoma include high intraocular pressure (IOP), old age, African-American race, family history of glaucoma, myopia, diabetes, and high blood pressure. The disease in primary form is hereditary by a yet-undefined polygenic mechanism.

II. **Physiologic mechanisms of various glaucomas.** Aqueous humor is produced by the ciliary body and flows into the posterior chamber, then between the posterior iris surface and lens, around the pupil edge, into the anterior chamber. It exits from the anterior chamber via *trabecular* and *nontrabecular* routes. The trabecular route is at the angle of the anterior chamber, formed by the iris base and peripheral cornea, flowing through the **trabecular meshwork (TM)** of the sclera, into Schlemm's canal (Fig. 10.1F). Via the collector channels in the sclera, the aqueous is carried to the episcleral vessels, where aqueous mixes with blood. On slitlamp examination, clear limbal aqueous veins can often be observed carrying aqueous into blood-filled episcleral veins. The latter can be identified by a laminated appearance of the blood–aqueous mixture. The level of IOP at any time represents a balance between the rate of formation of aqueous humor and the amount of resistance to its flow out of the anterior chamber. In almost every case of glaucoma, increased IOP is due to an abnormality in outflow from the anterior chamber, rather than to above-normal rates of aqueous humor formation. The nontrabecular aqueous route occurs through *uveoscleral outflow* via the supraciliary and suprachoroidal spaces and out along nerves and vessels coursing through the sclera. This route may be as important as the TM exit.

A. **In open-angle glaucoma,** the aqueous humor has unimpeded access to the TM in the angle of the anterior chamber, but there is abnormally high resistance to the fluid flow through the TM (uveal, corneoscleral, and juxtacanalicular—the last being the site of primary outflow resistance), into Schlemm's canal, and then into the scleral venous plexus. The peripheral iris does not interfere with the access of aqueous humor to the draining angle structures.

1. **Primary open-angle glaucoma (POAG)** is the most common form of glaucoma. The underlying abnormality in the trabecular angle tissue causing abnormal resistance to fluid flow is not known. The disease is not secondary to another eye disease or condition. POAG is a silent, surreptitious process. Usually there are no symptoms. Gradual loss of peripheral vision occurs. Loss of central vision is usually the last to occur. Only actual measurement of the IOP and inspection of the

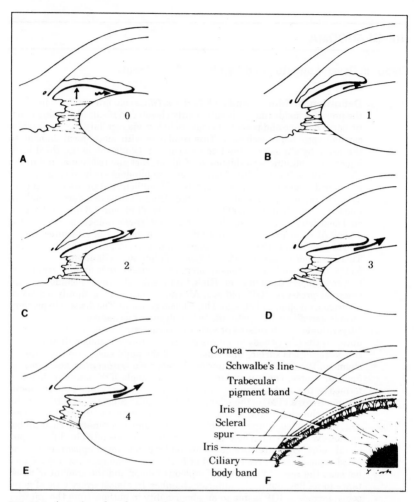

FIG. 10.1. Anterior chamber angle depth and anatomic structures of the angle. **A:** Grade O: Slit or closed angle. **B:** Grade 1: extremely narrow angle; closure probable. I-C (iris–corneal angle) = 10 degrees. **C:** Grade 2: moderately narrow angle; closure possible. I-C = 20 degrees. **D:** Grade 3: moderately open angle; no closure possible. I-C = 20 to 35 degrees. **E:** Angle wide open; no closure possible. I-C = 35 to 45 degrees. **F:** Anatomic landmarks of wide open angle as seen by gonioscopy. (Adapted from Anterior Chamber Angle Estimation Card, Allergan Pharmaceutical Co., Irvine, California.)

       optic nerve head with an ophthalmoscope can detect POAG in its early stages.

    2. **Secondary open-angle glaucoma** occurs as a result of or in association with another eye disease or condition such as uveitis or trauma, resulting in secondary blockage or damage to the canals and collector channels.

  B. **In angle-closure glaucoma,** the peripheral iris tissue covers the TM, preventing access of the aqueous humor to the TM. This type of glaucoma is often intermittent, with acute symptoms that are reversible when the peripheral iris is moved away from draining angle structures. In pure angle-closure glaucoma, the TM and Schlemm's canal angle tissue have inherently normal resistance to fluid flow. The IOP is elevated only when the peripheral iris covers the TM, preventing egress of the aqueous.

1. In **primary angle-closure glaucoma,** relative **pupillary block** is the mechanism of angle closure. This means that there is relative resistance to fluid flow of aqueous humor between the posterior iris surface and lens due to an abnormally close approximation at the pupil. This tends to occur in eyes with small anterior segments or short axial length. Relative pupillary block increases the pressure of aqueous in the posterior chamber, forcing the peripheral iris forward over the TM (Fig. 10.1). The state of relative pupillary block depends greatly on pupillary size and rigidity of the peripheral iris. For example, relative pupillary block may be increased and angle-closure glaucoma produced by putting a patient in a dark room or by using dilating medications that move the pupil into a middilated state. Drug-induced miosis may produce a very small pupil, blocking posterior chamber aqueous passage and thus pushing the iris forward to close the angle. Most eyes subject to possible angle-closure glaucoma can be recognized by the shallowness of their axial anterior chamber depth.

2. **Secondary angle-closure glaucoma** occurs as a result of or in association with another eye disease or condition, such as a swollen cataract or diabetic neovascularization pushing or pulling the iris over the TM.

III. **Methods of examination**

A. **Flashlight.** After examining pupillary light reactions, the physician should direct the flashlight to the temporal side of each eye, perpendicular to the corneal limbus, and note the shadow produced by the nasal peripheral iris against the cornea. In eyes with shallow anterior chambers that might be subject to angle-closure glaucoma, the relatively forward position of the iris will cause the nasal side to be in shadow. This flashlight examination should be performed in all patients before routine pupillary dilation. In eyes with shallow anterior chambers, the pupil should not be dilated until IOP is checked and gonioscopy is performed.

B. **Slitlamp examination**

1. The **axial and peripheral anterior chamber depth** may be measured and expressed in terms of corneal thickness. Direct a narrow slit beam onto the cornea at 60° just anterior to the limbus (Van Herick method). If the distance between the posterior corneal surface and the anterior iris surface is less than one-fourth the corneal thickness, the chamber is shallow. Anterior chamber depths less than three corneal thicknesses axially are also suspect and gonioscopy should be performed to assess angle narrowing.

2. **Other diagnostic signs** during slitlamp examination may be noted: for example, the presence of inflammatory cell deposits (keratic precipitates [KPs]) on the corneal epithelium, anterior chamber cells and flare, Krukenberg pigmented spindle on corneal endothelium, dandruff-like dusting on the lens capsule, iris heterochromia and transillumination (by placing the vertically narrowed beam coaxially in the pupil to create a red reflex back through the pupil), and abnormal iris vessels.

C. **Measurement of IOP** may be taken by Goldmann slitlamp or handheld applanation tonometry, other electronic or pneumotonometry, finger tension (estimate), Schiötz tonometry, applanation, or air-puff noncontact tonometry (see Chapter 1, sec. II.F.). Mean normal IOP is 16± mm Hg, although some eyes may sustain damage with IOP in the teens and other have none with IOP in the 30s. **An IOP greater than 22 mm Hg should be considered suspicious,** if not frankly abnormal, and the patient should be followed. Schiötz readings are falsely low in high myopes and in thyroidopathy due to low scleral rigidity. Considerable diurnal variation of IOP occurs normally (2 to 6 mm Hg), but IOP is greater in glaucoma patients (even down to normal levels); therefore, inspection of the optic disk and neural rim is just as important as the actual measurement of the IOP.

D. **Ophthalmoscopy of the optic nerve cup.** Atrophy of connective tissue associated with the hyaloid artery during embryogenesis results in a depression of the internal (vitreous) surface of the optic disk termed the *cup*.

1. **The normal physiologic disk cup** varies considerably. Large physiologic cups are usually round in shape, unlike the vertical elongation that occurs in glaucoma. The amount and the contour of disk tissue present in the rim of the optic disk between the end of the cup and the edge of the disk proper are important (Fig. 10.2). Not until the cup extends toward the edge of the disk does frank glaucomatous field loss occur. It is important to recognize that many glaucomatous and normal patients have a circular halo around the optic disk in which the retinal pigment epithelium and choroidal pigment is deficient, so that the physician is actually viewing the sclera underneath. The end of this peripapillary halo should not be misinterpreted as the edge of the disk in assessing the disk rim tissue. Statistically, *patients with large, round physiologic cups with a cup-to-disk ratio exceeding 0.6 are more at risk of developing glaucoma,* and they should be followed. Round cups with intact disk rim tissue, however, are not necessarily abnormal in the absence of other changes.

2. **The glaucomatous disk (nerve head)** may be recognized by certain changes in contour of the optic nerve cup. **Cupping** appears to be the result of faulty autoregulation of blood flow to the optic disk in the face of IOP. *Early signs of glaucomatous optic neuropathy include generalized or focal enlargement of the cup (vertical elongation or rim notching), asymmetry of cupping between the two eyes, superficial splinter hemorrhages, loss of nerve fiber layer (NFL), neuroretinal rim translucency, and nasalization of vessels.*

   a. **Parallax** should be used in monocular (direct ophthalmoscope) examination of the optic disk to assess the contour of the disk tissue. **Stereo viewing** through a dilated pupil with a fundus contact lens, a +78 or +90 diopter (D) handheld lens, or Hruby lens at the slit-lamp is critical. With glaucomatous damage to the nerve, actual loss of nerve tissue and its vascular and glial supporting tissue occurs. Such atrophy results in both contour (cupping) and color (pallor) changes in disk appearance. The **optic disk rim** is made up of ganglion cell nerve fibers and is best evaluated by viewing the fundus with a **green light (red-free)**. The **nerve fiber** bundles appear as radiating striations toward the disk and may be best documented with high-contrast black and white photos. Their loss may be diffuse or focal. Decreased visibility or white-out areas of the NFL at the rim and entering the retina are detectable in 90% of glaucomatous nerves before or during early visual field loss. In elderly people, however, nuclear sclerotic changes (early cataracts) often impart a rosy color to the disk and may be confusing. In primary optic atrophy, not due to glaucoma, change in pallor of the disk occurs with no change in contour.

   b. **In glaucoma, the cup usually enlarges vertically.** The increased cupping commonly progresses first toward the inferior pole of the disk and then enlarges superiorly, but there is considerable variation. Very rarely, the optic cup may extend straight temporally first rather than vertically. In such cases, **macular fibers may be affected early** in the course of the disease, with resulting *loss of*

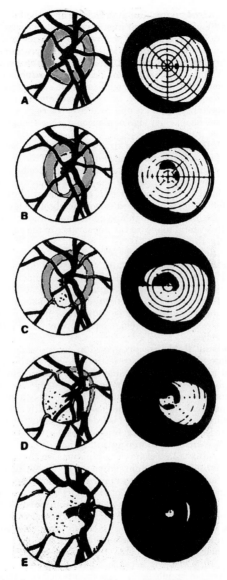

FIG. 10.2. Progressive glaucomatous atrophic cupping of the optic nerve head with commonly associated visual field defects. **A:** Early enlargement of physiologic cup. Field normal. **B:** Inferotemporal notching of the cup. Field shows enlarged blind spot and superonasal Bjerrum scotoma. **C:** Increased notching, thinning of rim of cup, and visible lamina cribrosa. Field shows constriction of superonasal field and advancing superior Bjerrum scotoma. **D:** Advanced generalized thinning of rim of cup with nasalization of vessels. Field shows further superior constriction and new inferior field defect resulting from damage to superior retinal nerve fibers. **E:** Total atrophy of the rim; pale, deep cup. Vessels disappear under rim. Field shows small central and temporal island of vision remaining. (Adapted from Paton D, Craig J. *Glaucomas: diagnosis and management.* Clinical Symposia. Summit, NJ: Ciba Pharmaceutical Co., 1976.)

central vision. Cupping close to or at the inferior pole of the disk will, of course, result in superior field loss; cupping close to the superior pole of the disk will result in inferior field loss. Occasionally, glaucomatous damage to the optic disk produces a shallower background bowing of disk tissue rather than excavation. The latter is called *saucerization. Temporal pallor* is rarely seen in glaucoma and, if noted, should raise the suspicion of an *intracranial compressive lesion, arteritic ischemia,* or old *trauma.*

  c. **Asymmetry** in the appearance of the right and left optic disk cups may be an early sign of glaucoma, even though each is within normal limits.

  d. **Enlargement** in the size of the cup occurs before visual field loss results. Inspection of the appearance of the optic disk cup is an important part of glaucoma screening procedures. During long-term follow-up, the size and shape of the cup are noted in addition to the IOP and visual field. If enlargement of the cup occurs during follow-up, then, regardless of the absolute level of IOP, that pressure level is too high and additional glaucoma therapy is initiated. It is useful to record the appearance of the cup size and shape on a diagram (Fig. 10.2).

E. **Visual fields**

  1. **Techniques** include confrontation (usually bedside examination) and various forms of automated static and kinetic perimetry (see Chapter 1, sec. **II.I.** and Chapter 13, secs. **I.A.–F.**). Glaucoma patients are followed with visual field examinations every 6–12 months as a routine; the latter time period is reasonable if the optic nerves are healthy, if no known field defect is present, and if the pressure is well controlled.

  2. If **visual field loss progression** occurs while the patient is being followed, then, regardless of the level of IOP, that pressure is too high and glaucoma therapy should be adjusted. Similar considerations apply to progression of optic disk cupping. Except in myopes or in glaucoma patients with episodes of extremely high pressure elevation, visual field changes should correspond with optic disk cupping. For example, superior field loss does not occur unless the disk shows increased cupping to the inferior pole.

  3. **Follow-up field examination** should be done with the pupil at the same size as in baseline examinations, so that a similar condition of retinal test object illumination exists for the follow-up fields added. Miotic glaucoma therapy may need to be reversed by dilation for field examinations with 2.5% phenylephrine or 1.0% tropicamide. Should the patient develop lens opacities, continued examination with the smaller test objects may produce artifactual field defects. The **size of the test object** should be graded to the visual acuity.

  4. **Glaucoma field defects** characteristically respect the horizontal meridian (unlike chiasmal lesions, which respect the vertical) (Fig 10.2). This is because glaucoma characteristically produces a nerve fiber bundle defect—an arcuate defect or Bjerrum scotoma, or a variant of these, such as a nasal step. The temporal nerve fibers in the retina sweep either superiorly or inferiorly around the macula and do not cross the horizontal raphe. Because it would be purely chance that exactly symmetric nerve fibers in the superior and inferior fields would be similarly affected, glaucoma defects characteristically show some discontinuity at the horizontal meridian, such as a nasal step. The papillomacular fibers are usually relatively resistant to chronic pressure effects until late in the disease, and visual acuity changes do not occur early. After central vision is lost from glaucoma, typically all that is left is a temporal island of vision. Automated perimetry or Goldmann fields may be the first to detect early defects. **Patterns of**

glaucomatous field loss include:

(a) **Paracentral scotoma**—an island of relative or absolute loss within 10° of fixation.

(b) **Arcuate scotoma**—arc-shaped loss 10 to 20° above or below fixation (nerve fiber bundle damage).

(c) **Nasal step**—relative depression of one horizontal hemifield compared to the other (damage to superior or inferior nerve fibers outside paracentral area).

(d) **Temporal wedge or step**—a wedge-shaped defect from blind spot toward the periphery (damage to nerve fibers serving retina above or below optic nerve head blind spot).

(e) **Loss of all but small central and temporal islands of vision.**

F. **Gonioscopy.** The angle is viewed by indirect slitlamp gonioscopy with a Goldmann two- to three-mirror lens using a viscous contact gel, or a Zeiss four-mirror lens with an Unger handle and no gel. Direct gonioscopy is done with the patient recumbent with use of a Koeppe-type dome lens and handheld microscope (see Chapter 1, sec. **II.Q.**). The angle is assessed for shallowness and possible susceptibility to angle-closure glaucoma, as well as for other abnormalities such as pigment, synechiae, exfoliation, new blood vessels, inflammatory deposits, and evidence of old injury such as angle recession. Generally, if the scleral spur can be seen through the entire circumference and the iris is not excessively convex, the eye is not likely to be susceptible to angle closure and the pupil can be safely dilated. One commonly used **angle rating system** adapted from *Schaeffer* is depicted in Fig. 10.1. The *Spaeth* system expands this to include description of the peripheral iris contour, insertion of the iris root, and the effects of indentation gonioscopy on the angle configuration. It should be noted that narrow-angle eyes can look distinctly different at different examinations, perhaps reflecting different rates of aqueous production and differing relative pupillary block. Repeat examination in such narrow-angle eyes is usually indicated. The Zeiss gonioscopic lens is useful for rapidly viewing the angle, although it readily causes indentation of the eye and artificial deepening of the anterior chamber. The latter is deliberately utilized to *differentiate appositional from synechial angle closure* in the Spaeth system.

G. **Optic nerve head and nerve fiber layer (NFL) imaging.** The most common method of imaging the optic nerve is by conventional photography. This is a useful means by which to document optic nerve head appearance and to perform longitudinal comparison to look for onset or progression of optic nerve cupping. Newer methods for imaging the nerve head and NFL include *optical coherence tomography (OCT, NFL), scanning laser polarimetry (NFL), and confocal laser scanning ophthalmoscopy* (three-dimensional imaging of optic nerve head and NFL using tomography) (see Chapter 1, secs. **II.I.** and **J.**). NFL imaging takes advantage of the fact that the loss of retinal ganglion cells, and hence their axons, will result in a thinning of the NFL in the peripapillary region. Because the density of nerve fibers is less in the peripapillary region than at the optic nerve head itself, NFL imaging is likely to pick up earlier changes in thickness. The Nerve Fiber Analyzer (I and II) and the Gdx (Laser Diagnostic Technologies) combine polarimetry with scanning laser ophthalmoscopy to quantitate the thickness of the NFL. It is hoped that the use and development of NFL imaging will allow earlier detection of damage and progression before functional changes have occurred. These methods should be considered as adjunctive to visual field testing, however, and will likely not replace the visual field as a method for evaluating and diagnosing glaucoma. In the end, the visual field is the only means by which the physician can truly determine what the patient sees.

IV. **Principles of therapy. In all cases of glaucoma it is essential to establish whether the glaucoma is open or closed angle.** This is accomplished by placing a gonioscopic contact lens on the eye and actually viewing the angle structures.

    A. In the therapy of **open-angle glaucoma** the physician usually first treats the condition medically to lower the IOP. This pressure may be lowered by increasing the facility of aqueous outflow from the anterior chamber through the angle tissues, or by decreasing the rate of aqueous humor formation by the ciliary body, or both. Laser trabeculoplasty (LTP) is usually used alone or in conjunction with medical therapy to control IOP, nerve cupping, or progressive visual loss. Studies have shown that LTP is effective as primary medical therapy or to minimize use of medical treatment. Surgery is used when all other methods have failed.

    B. **Angle-closure glaucoma** may initially be treated medically, but it is primarily a surgical (laser) disease, requiring peripheral iridotomy (placing a hole through the peripheral iris) to relieve pupillary block permanently. Posterior chamber aqueous pressure is thus relieved by aqueous flowing through this extra opening, and the peripheral iris falls away from the meshwork.

V. Medical treatments and side effects. Studies indicate that most ocular hypotensive drugs may achieve maximal effect with less frequent administration and lower concentrations if **nasolacrimal occlusion** is applied (finger pressure) for 3 minutes during and after drug instillation. This may also result in fewer side effects. (See Appendix A for listings of drugs, dosages, and commercial names.)

    A. Beta-adrenergic blockers (timolol, betaxolol, carteolol, levobunolol, metipranolol)

        1. Mechanism of action. Timolol, levobunolol, carteolol, and metipranolol are **nonselective** $beta_1$- (cardiac) and $beta_2$- (smooth muscle, pulmonary) receptor blocking agents. Betaxolol has 100 times more affinity for $beta_1$- than $beta_2$-receptors.

        2. Physiologic effects. The nonselective drugs decrease IOP by blockade of $beta_2$-receptors in the ciliary processes, resulting in decreased aqueous production. The mechanism for betaxolol is unknown because there are so few $beta_1$-receptors in the eye, but there may be "spill over" to bind $beta_2$-receptors as well. There is no effect on facility of outflow. The drug molecule timolol (and probably betaxolol and levobunolol) releases from the beta-receptor site as early as 3 hours after topical administration, yet clinical effect may last up to 2 weeks. This prolonged effect may result from rerelease of beta-blocker from depots in the iris pigment epithelial melanin. Carteolol, unlike the other beta-blockers, has intrinsic sympathomimetic activity, possibly resulting in fewer side effects. It also **lacks** timolol's tendency to **increase** serum **cholesterol** and **decrease high-density lipoproteins,** a factor to consider in cardiovascular patients.

        3. Indications are primary and secondary open-angle glaucomas including inflammatory glaucomas, acute and chronic primary and secondary angle-closure glaucomas, ocular hypertension, and childhood glaucomas.

        4. Precautions and contraindications include known drug allergy. These drugs should be used with caution or not at all, depending on severity of disease, in patients with asthma, emphysema, chronic obstructive pulmonary disease, bronchitis, heart block, congestive heart failure, cardiovascular disease, or cardiomyopathy. Although betaxolol is the blocker of choice in patients at risk for pulmonary reaction because of its greater $beta_1$ (cardiac) selectivity, the drug may induce bronchospasm in some patients.

        5. Available preparations. Timolol, 0.25% to 0.50%; betaxolol and levobunolol, 0.25%; metipranolol, 0.3%; carteolol, 1% eye drops. Timolol XE 0.25% or 0.50% gel qd is equivalent in effect to bid drops.

6. **Recommended dosage** is qd or q12h topically. All beta-blockers may be used with significant additive effect in **combination** with miotic agents, alpha$_2$-agonists, prostaglandin analogs, or carbonic anhydrase inhibitors (CAIs).
7. **Side effects**
   a. Bradycardia, cardiac arrest, acute asthma, and pulmonary edema have all been reported in susceptible individuals and result from systemic absorption of topical drug. **Lacrimal canalicular compression** should be practiced by patients at any risk, and the drug used with caution or not at all in those patients with moderate to severe cardiac or pulmonary disease.
   b. Full adult dosage should be **avoided** in **children** because **apnea** may result; 0.25% qd to bid with canalicular compression is the lower advisable dosage.
   c. **Nursing mothers** will excrete the drugs in breast milk; beta-blocker treatment of the mother should be considered carefully if she is breast-feeding.
   d. **Other side effects are lethargy, depression, impotence, hallucinations, and gastrointestinal symptoms.**
   e. **Ocular effects** include allergy, punctate keratitis, and diplopia. Corneal anesthesia may result from the membrane-stabilizing effects of timolol, but is less with the other beta-blockers.
B. **Alpha$_2$-adrenergic agonists** (apraclonidine and brimonidine).
   1. The **mechanism of action** and **physiologic effects** are unclear but appear to be alpha$_2$-receptor stimulation that results in decreased aqueous humor formation.
   2. **Indications** are to control increases in IOP after anterior segment laser surgery (U.S. Food and Drug Administration [FDA] approved), acute short-term pressure spikes, and in chronic primary or secondary glaucomas.
   3. **Contraindications** include known allergy to the drug and cardiac disease with untreated arteriovenous block or bradycardia.
   4. **Available preparations.** Apraclonidine is available as a 0.5% and 1% solution and brimonidine is available as a 0.2% solution.
   5. **Usual dosage.** One drop 1 hour before laser surgery and one drop immediately after the procedure or just one drop immediately post-laser appears equally effective and superior to any other glaucoma drug. This dose decreases the incidence of postlaser pressure spikes of 10 mm Hg or more to less than 2% and lasts 12 hours. **Chronic glaucoma treatment** is one drop of 0.5% apraclonidine or one drop of 0.2% brimonidine bid. There is a 30% allergic response to the 0.50% apraclonidine and approximately 10% to 15% allergy rate for brimonidine. A new preparation of brimonidine, utilizing a different preservative, promises to have a lower allergy rate. Beta-adrenergic blockers are the usual concomitant drugs, but prostaglandin analogs, miotics, epinephrine, and CAIs may be added as well for additive effect.
   6. **Side effects** include possible transient upper lid retraction, conjunctival blanching, mydriasis, burning or itching sensation, and subconjunctival hemorrhage. Systemically, there may be gastrointestinal reaction and cardiovascular effect such as bradycardia, vasovagal attack, palpitations, or orthostatic hypotension. Central nervous system disturbances include somnolence, insomnia, irritability, and decreased libido, all of which are transient.
C. **Prostaglandin analogs** (latanoprost, bimatoprost, travoprost, and unoprostone)
   1. **Mechanism of action.** Lowering of IOP by increasing uveoscleral outflow through a prostaglandin F_2 α-mediated mechanism.

2. **Indications.** Additive therapy for lowering of high IOP.
3. **Preparation and dosage.** Latanoprost (Xalatan) 0.005%, bimato-prost (Lumigan) 0.03%, and travoprost (Travatan) 0.004% are each given once daily, usually at bedtime. Unoprostone (Rescula) 0.15% is given twice daily. Latanoprost is temperature sensitive and needs to be refrigerated prior to and after opening.
4. **Side effects** include increased iris pigmentation, darkening of the eyelid skin, increased thickness and number of eyelashes, ocular irritation (redness, itching, etc.), uveitis, cystoid macular edema, and probable reactivation of *herpes simplex* virus.

D. **Carbonic anhydrase inhibitors (CAIs).** Acetazolamide, methazolamide and dichlorphenamide are oral agents. Acetazolamide is an intravenous (i.v.) agent as well, and dorzolamide and brinzolamide are topical agents.

1. **Mechanism of action.** CAIs inhibit the enzyme carbonic anhydrase.
2. **Physiologic effects.** The ciliary body enzyme, carbonic anhydrase, is related to the process of aqueous humor formation, most likely via active secretion of bicarbonate. CAIs decrease the rate of aqueous humor formation.
3. **Indications.** CAIs are additive therapy in the management of various acute glaucomas, but also in the chronic management of primary and secondary open-angle and angle-closure glaucomas not adequately controlled by topical medication.
4. **Contraindications.** Because of the metabolic and possible respiratory acidosis effects, patients with significant respiratory disease should be given oral CAIs cautiously and in lower dosages. Patients with a history of calcium phosphate kidney stone formation should be given the oral medication cautiously and only after consultation with their primary care provider. Known allergy is a contraindication. Patients with allergies to other sulfonamides should be given these agents with caution.
5. **Available preparations** include acetazolamide (Diamox, generic) 125 and 250 mg tablets, 500 mg capsules, 500 mg per 5 mL i.v.; methazolamide tablets (Neptazane, Glauctabs, MZM, generic) 25 mg and 50 mg tablets; dichlorphenamide (Daranide) 50 mg tablets bid to qid; dorzolamide (Trusopt) 2% drops; and brinzolamide (Azopt) 1% drops (see Appendix A).
6. **Recommended dosage.** Established dosages for near-maximum effect are acetazolamide tablets 250 mg q6h; methazolamide tablets 50 to 100 mg bid to tid; acetazolamide sustained-release capsules 500 mg q12h; and dichlorphenamide tablets 50 mg bid to qid. Because acetazolamide is excreted unchanged by the kidneys, patients with renal disease such as diabetic nephropathy should be started on lower than standard dosages. Methazolamide or dichlorphenamide may be used more safely in this situation. Dorzolamide 2% drops and brinzolamide 1% tid decrease IOP by $\approx$20%.
7. **Side effects.** Unfortunately, 40% to 50% of glaucoma patients are unable to tolerate systemic CAIs long term because of various disabling side effects. A symptom complex of **malaise, fatigue, depression, anorexia,** and **weight loss** is the most frequent side effect. **Loss of libido,** especially in young males, may also occur. These symptoms show some correlation with the degree of systemic metabolic acidosis on therapy. They may have a gradual, insidious onset over several months. Often neither the patient nor the physician relates these symptoms to the systemic CAI therapy. **Frequently, patients erroneously undergo extensive medical evaluations searching for occult malignancies.**
   a. **Simultaneous CAI and chlorothiazide** systemic hypertensive therapy may produce frank **hypokalemia,** and the patient

should have potassium supplementation. In the absence of this concomitant chlorothiazide therapy, changes in serum potassium tend to be small and there is no symptomatic benefit from potassium supplementation.

b. **Gastrointestinal** side effects occurring with oral CAI therapy tend to behave as local irritative phenomena, sometimes responding to administering the CAI with food, switching to a sustained-release preparation, or simultaneous mild alkali therapy.

c. **Malaise** symptoms occur in some patients. Decreasing the dosage will sometimes improve tolerance. In particular, using one 500-mg acetazolamide capsule a day (which has an effect for more than 18 hours) is very useful. In many of these patients this dosage will result in an undertreatment of their glaucoma, but in others, near-maximum effects will be maintained.

d. **Kidney stones** developing during oral CAI therapy are believed to be a result of calcium precipitation secondary to a decrease of citrate or magnesium excretion or both in the urine. The former is believed to be a direct consequence of the drugs making normally acid urine alkaline, which, with reduced citrate, induces calcium carbonate stone formation. There is a far *lower incidence of kidney stone formation with methazolamide* than with acetazolamide. Methazolamide has minimal action on citrate concentration or on the kidney. Management of kidney stone patients involves use of methazolamide in as low a dosage as the severity of the glaucoma permits, restriction of dietary calcium, and possibly concomitant use of chlorothiazide diuretics to alter the calcium–magnesium ratio in the urine. Electrolyte imbalance should be watched for in patients taking diuretics. Nephrologic consultation and measurement of urinary pH, calcium, and citrate should be obtained if stone formation is suspected.

e. **Blood dyscrasias** are rare. Thrombocytopenia, agranulocytosis, and aplastic anemia may occur as idiosyncratic reactions. Periodic blood tests would not be expected to anticipate these reactions and are not routinely performed. A history of a mouth or body sore that does not heal may be a clue to the occurrence of a blood dyscrasia.

f. **Myopia** occurs rarely as an idiosyncratic acute reversible phenomenon. It is believed to be due either to a change in hydration of the lens or shallow choroidal effusions, and it may be associated with a shallowing of the anterior chamber.

E. **Miotics**

1. **Pilocarpine**

   a. **Mechanism of action.** Pilocarpine is a direct-acting parasympathomimetic (muscarinic) **cholinergic** drug.

   b. **Physiologic effects.** The drug is used in chronic open-angle glaucoma to increase the facility of aqueous outflow. The mechanism of action is probably exclusively mechanical, via ciliary muscle contraction and pull on the scleral spur and TM. It is used in acute angle-closure glaucoma to move the iris away from the angle. Miosis is a side effect and is of no therapeutic benefit.

   c. **Indications** are chronic open-angle glaucoma, acute angle-closure glaucoma, chronic synechial angle-closure glaucoma (following peripheral iridectomy), and following cyclodialysis surgery.

   d. **Contraindications** are inflammatory glaucoma, malignant glaucoma, or known allergy.

   e. **Available preparations** are 0.25% to 10.0% eye drops, Ocusert P-20 diffusion membranes, and 4% gel (see Appendix A).

   f. **Recommended dosage**

      (1) **Eye drops.** Except in very darkly pigmented irides, maximum effect is probably obtained with a 4% solution. In milder

open-angle glaucoma, therapy is usually initiated with a 1% concentration. Duration of effect is 4 to 6 hours. It is usually prescribed for use every 6 hours.

(2) **Ocuserts** are changed once weekly. P-20s are generally used in patients controlled with 2% drops or less.

(3) **The gel** can be used alone at bedtime or as an adjunct to daytime medication.

g. **Combination.** Pilocarpine can be used in conjunction with other glaucoma medications and, in most instances, confers additional pressure-lowering effects.

h. **Side effects**

(1) **Ocular**

(a) **Contact allergy** is fairly rare.

(b) Contraction of the ciliary muscle results in accommodation and ensuing **fluctuating myopia.** In younger patients this is usually a disabling visual side effect that prevents use of pilocarpine. Continuous low-level, **constant-delivery ocular insert devices,** such as the Ocusert, are very effective in young patients with glaucoma who require pilocarpine therapy. These low levels of continuous delivery result in small amounts of myopia that tend to be steady and correctable, if necessary, with spectacles. Most patients above the age of 50 years do not develop such pilocarpine-induced myopia, presumably because of an inelasticity of their lens that is also responsible for their presbyopia.

(c) Pupillary **miosis** is a definite side effect of pilocarpine, which again exerts its antiglaucoma effect via ciliary muscle traction on the angle structures. This miosis results in **diminished night vision** and often some **contraction in peripheral visual field.** If the patient has early axial lens opacities, this miosis may result in **diminished visual acuity.** On the other hand, the miosis may result in a pinhole effect and an actual improvement in visual acuity.

(d) **Shallowing of the anterior chamber** may occur with higher doses of pilocarpine by forward movement of the lens–iris diaphragm subsequent to ciliary muscle contraction and relaxation of zonular tension. This shallowing may result in an increase in relative pupillary block, and it may convert an open-angle glaucoma with narrow angles into **partial angle-closure glaucoma.** This is true for all the standard miotic glaucoma therapies (carbachol, echothiophate iodide, demecarium bromide). In susceptible individuals, it seems to be dose related. There may be varying amounts of anterior chamber shallowing on miotic therapy. Similarly, in angle-closure glaucoma, lower concentrations of pilocarpine are used initially to minimize this axial shallowing and possible increase in relative pupillary block.

(2) **Systemic side effects.** Occasional patients are particularly sensitive and may develop sweating and gastrointestinal overactivity with usual dosages. **Sweating, salivation, nausea, tremor, headache, brow pain, bradycardia,** and **hypotension** have sometimes been observed as results of too vigorous treatment of angle-closure glaucoma with pilocarpine.

2. **Carbachol**

a. **Mechanism of action.** A **cholinergic** similar to pilocarpine.

b. **Physiologic effects.** Similar to pilocarpine.

c. **Indications.** Carbachol eye drops are longer acting that pilocarpine, thus having a greater stabilizing effect on diurnal pressure and myopia fluctuation. It may also be used in patients allergic to pilocarpine; otherwise, the indications are similar to pilocarpine. An intracameral preparation for intraoperative use induces miosis and inhibits postoperative pressure increase.

   d. Contraindications. Similar to pilocarpine.
   e. Available preparations are 0.75%, 1.5%, and 3.0% eye drops and 0.01% for intraocular use.
   f. Recommended dosage. Carbachol 3% is approximately equivalent to pilocarpine 4%, and 1.5% carbachol is roughly equivalent to 2% pilocarpine. The effect is reported to last up to 8 hours. Dosage tid (compared to qid with pilocarpine) may be a distinct advantage in certain patients.
   g. Side effects. Similar to pilocarpine.
3. **Anticholinesterase agents** (echothiophate iodide, demecarium bromide, physostigmine, isofluorphate 0.025%). Echothiophate is currently out of production but may become available again soon.
   a. Mechanism of action. Indirect-acting parasympathomimetic activity by virtue of binding to the enzyme, acetylcholinesterase, allows endogenous acetylcholine to accumulate.
   b. Physiologic effects. Ciliary muscle and iris sphincter muscle contraction occur similar to and possibly more marked than that occurring with other miotics, e.g., pilocarpine and carbachol. Miosis is a side effect of no therapeutic benefit.
   c. Indications are chronic open-angle glaucoma (especially with aphakia), chronic synechial angle-closure glaucoma (following peripheral iridectomy), and following cyclodialysis surgery. These agents are more potent than pilocarpine or carbachol and should be used only when pilocarpine 4% is no longer effective.
   d. Contraindications. Anticholinesterase agents should never be used in narrow-angle glaucoma without an iridototomy because of the extreme miosis they produce, as well as possible forward lens movement, which may actually increase pupillary block. Similarly, open-angle glaucoma with open but narrow angles may worsen because of partial-angle closure as a result of this therapy. Repeat gonioscopy on therapy is indicated. Other contraindications are inflammatory glaucoma or known allergy. These agents should be used cautiously in patients who are predisposed to **retinal detachment,** e.g., patients with lattice degeneration or family history of nontraumatic detachments.
   e. Preparations include echothiophate iodide 0.03% to 0.25%, demecarium bromide 0.25% and 0.50%, isofluorphate 0.025%, and physostigmine 0.25% to 0.5%. Physostigmine ointment 0.25% is available for bedtime use.
   f. Usual dosage. Anticholinesterase agents are administered twice a day. Because side effects are dose related, the lower concentration should be tried initially for pressure control.
   g. Side effects
      (1) Ocular
         (a) Possible side effects include **accommodative spasm** and **shallowing of the anterior chamber** as well as **diminished night vision** and **peripheral field,** similar to and possibly more marked than that occurring with other miotics, e.g., pilocarpine and carbachol. These **cataractous** changes are related to drug concentration, frequency of dosage, age of the patient, and patient susceptibility. These agents should be used only when pilocarpine 4% is no longer effective, and the lower concentrations should be tried initially for pressure control. The lens changes have been

classically described as mossy anterior subcapsular opacities, but posterior subcapsular opacities and progression of nuclear sclerosis have also been described.

   (b) Pupillary cysts may occur with anticholinesterase therapy and may lessen with concomitant daily phenylephrine 2.5% eye drop therapy. These agents may induce a breakdown of the blood–aqueous barrier and **increase anterior chamber flare.** They should not be used in the presence of active uveitis. There seems to be some small risk of **retinal detachment** with this therapy, possibly resulting from traction and forward movement of the ora serrata as a result of intense ciliary muscle contraction. If feasible, glaucoma patients should have dilated indirect ophthalmoscopy with scleral depression before initiation of strong miotic therapy. **Lacrimal punctal stenosis, conjunctival goblet cell,** and **tear abnormalities** have been reported.

   (2) Systemic

   (a) Anticholinesterase agents may cause **diarrhea, nausea,** and **abdominal cramps** if excessively absorbed. These toxic symptoms are cumulative and therefore appear only after many months of therapy. Patients should be instructed in lacrimal occlusion with digital pressure when taking drops to minimize systemic absorption and pharyngeal–alimentary passage of these agents. **Internists should be especially suspicious of gastrointestinal or systemic malaise complaints in glaucoma patients under chronic therapy with anticholinesterase or CAI agents (see sec. V.D.7, above). Because both of these agents frequently produce undesired systemic effects only after months of therapy, the correct diagnosis is too frequently missed.**

   (b) Serum pseudocholinesterase, which hydrolyzes succinylcholine and procaine, is often **decreased** in patients taking chronic topical anticholinesterase therapy, and therefore prolonged apnea may occur following use of succinylcholine in surgical procedures. It takes 4 to 6 weeks after cessation of topical anticholinesterase therapy for serum enzyme levels to return to normal, so **succinylcholine anesthesia should be avoided, if possible, in patients recently taking these agents.**

F. Epinephrine and dipivefrin hydrochloride (epinephrine [DPE]). **DPE** is an epinephrine prodrug in which the two pivalic acids are cleaved from an epinephrine molecule in the eye. It was synthesized for use on epinephrine-allergic as well as nonsensitized glaucoma patients.

   1. The **mechanism of action** is unclear, but appears to be a function of both alpha- and beta-receptor stimulation.

   2. **Physiologic effects.** Epinephrine both increases aqueous outflow (alpha- and beta-receptor stimulation) and decreases aqueous humor formation (alpha-receptor stimulation in the ciliary body). It is additive to the cholinergics, anticholinesterases, and CAIs in pressure-lowering effects.

   3. **Indications.** It is primarily used in open-angle glaucoma or in conjunction with miotics with mildly shallowed chambers. Certain patients show a greater pressure lowering following several weeks of epinephrine therapy than following a single, acute dosage.

   4. **Contraindications** include narrow-angle glaucoma or known allergy.

   5. **Available preparations.** Epinephrine is available in strengths 0.5% to 2.0% to treat open-angle glaucoma as a borate, bitartrate, or

hydrochloride eye drop. There is no significant difference in the clinical efficacy of the preparations. The bitartrate has only 50% drug available as free base, however. DPE is available as a 0.1% solution.

6. **Usual dosage** is epinephrine 1% bid to tid. There is some evidence that, at least in patients with dark irides, epinephrine 2% may be more potent than 1%. DPE 0.1% is used once every 12 to 24 hours and is roughly equivalent to the effect of 2% epinephrine. DPE should probably not be used with anticholinesterases such as echothiophate iodide because the latter may inhibit the esterases necessary for cleavage of the pivalic acid groups. DPE should probably not be used until at least 4 hours after instillation of beta-blockers, as noted under epinephrine.

7. **Side effects**
   a. Occasionally, paradoxic **pressure increase** may occur with epinephrine (with open angles); certain patients, for unknown reasons, have minimum pressure lowering on epinephrine therapy.
   b. Approximately 10% to 15% of patients are unable to tolerate long-term epinephrine therapy because of the development of **topical allergy.** Switching brands of epinephrine is rarely effective, and usually epinephrine must be discontinued.
   c. Epinephrine causes **cystoid macular edema (CME)** in 20% to 30% of aphakic patients after 1 week to months of therapy. This is almost always reversible on cessation of therapy.
   d. Oxidation products of epinephrine can result in **dark pigmented conjunctival deposits** as well as a **canalicular (tear duct) obstruction.**
   e. Occasional complaints of **palpitation, tachycardia, headache,** and **faintness** have been recorded in patients after topical usage. Although theoretically a concern (one drop of epinephrine 2% = 0.1 mg), epinephrine can almost always be given safely to patients with cardiovascular disease, especially if patients are taught how to **perform nasolacrimal compression** following topical administration to decrease systemic absorption by pressing over the medial lid area for 5 minutes.
   f. With DPE the incidence of adrenochrome deposits or CME, especially if the posterior capsule is intact, is unclear, but appears to be notably lower than that with epinephrine.

G. **Hyperosmotic agents** (mannitol, glycerin, isosorbide).
   1. **Mechanism of action.** Reduction of IOP by increasing plasma tonicity sufficiently to draw water out of the eye.
   2. **Indications.** Additive therapy for rapid reduction of high IOP. Onset of action is 30 minutes and lasts 4 to 6 hours.
   3. **Preparation and dosage**
      a. **Glycerin** (Osmoglyn) dosage is 1.0 to 1.5 g of glycerin per kg body weight given orally (p.o.). Osmoglyn is a 50%, lime-flavored solution with dosage 2 to 3 mL per kg (4 to 6 oz per patient). It is better tolerated served on cracked ice and may be given qd to tid. Topical glycerin (Ophthalgan) is a viscous solution used to clear corneal edema for a better view of the intraocular structures.
      b. **Isosorbide** is a 45%, mint-flavored solution with dosage of 1 to 2 g per kg (1.5 to 3.0 mL per lb body weight) given p.o. over ice qd to qid.
      c. **Mannitol** is a 5% to 20% hyperosmotic given warm (38 to 39°C to dissolve crystals) i.v., in dosage of 0.5 to 2 g per kg body weight. Most common is 25 to 50 mL of 25% solution given by slow i.v. push.
   4. **Side effects** may include severe systemic hypertension aggravation, nausea, vomiting, confusion, congestive heart failure, pulmonary edema, or diabetic hyperglycemia (mannitol). The drugs are contraindicated in oliguria or anuria.

H. Calcium channel blockers such as diltiazem, nifedipine, and vera-pamil inhibit calcium influx in vascular smooth muscle, decrease vascular tone, and increase blood flow. Studies have not proven that these oral drugs are effective in **low-tension glaucoma** by increasing optic nerve blood flow.

VI. **Argon and neodymium:yttrium, aluminum, and garnet (Nd:YAG) laser therapy** (see also Chapter 8, sec. XI.).

A. **General considerations.** The **argon laser** uses the heating, coagulative (less bleeding), and disrupting effect of the laser energy to create tissue burns or openings. The **Nd:YAG laser** produces a sudden focal expansion with tearing and disruption of tissue by delivering high-powered near-infrared irradiances in small, focused spots. In open-angle glaucomas, **argon laser trabeculoplasty (ALT)** application of nonpenetrating laser burns to the TM often results in improvement in the outflow of aqueous humor by an undetermined mechanism. Both mechanical and biologic effects have been postulated. In angle-closure glaucoma, the argon laser, YAG laser, or both have been used to create a small opening in the peripheral iris, thus alleviating pupillary block, which is the mechanism for angle-closure glaucoma.

B. **Argon laser trabeculoplasty (ALT)**

1. **Indications.** ALT should be attempted in almost all forms of open-angle glaucoma not adequately controlled with maximum tolerated medical therapy and prior to considering filtration surgery: phakic, aphakic, pseudophakic, pseudoexfoliative, pigmentary, and in noncompliant patients. Eyes with poor prognosis for beneficial laser effects (0% to 15% success) have steroid, neovascular, juvenile, or inflammatory glaucomas. In the chronic treatment of open-angle glaucoma, evaluating the benefit–risk ratio, ALT should probably be employed prior to the use of cholinesterase inhibitors or even p.o. CAIs because of their side effects. Because ALT seems to be more effective in phakic eyes, it should be performed prior to cataract surgery in patients with borderline control. **ALT as a primary procedure** is also a good approach. After 2 years, eyes treated with ALT first, and medications added later as needed, had lower mean IOPs and fewer medicines needed than medicine-only treated eyes. At 5 and 10 years post-ALT, 50% and 66% of the eyes, respectively, required further laser treatment or surgery for adequate control.

2. **Contraindications** to ALT are total angle closure and hazy media obscuring angle structures. Relative contraindications are: secondary open-angle glaucomas (such as inflammatory or neovascular) because there is negligible effect but risk of pressure spike, a serious complication, such as high-pressure spike after ALT in the first eye, uncooperative patients, and the need for urgent IOP control where filtration surgery would have a more rapid effect.

3. **Technique.** Continue all glaucoma drugs before ALT. Instill 1% apraclonidine or 0.2% brimonidine 1 hour before ALT and immediately postlaser. For narrowed angles, use 1% pilocarpine. If apraclonidine is contraindicated, CAIs and hyperosmotic agents are alternatives. Use topical 0.5% proparacaine anesthesia (retrobulbar block for nystagmus or poor cooperation). An antireflective Goldmann mirrored gonioscopic lens is applied with goniogel and using the 25× oculars on the slitlamp. The beam is focused on the **anterior** region of the TM to minimize post-ALT IOP increase and synechiae. The desired reaction of focal blanching on the TM is achieved with a 0.1-second duration, 50 μm spot size, and power between 700 and 1,200 mW. Bubble formation or pigment scatter means the power is too high. Forty to 50 burns over 180 degrees or 80 to 100 burns over 360 degrees are placed.

4. **Follow-up.** Acute pressure elevations (>10 mm Hg) occur in 10% to 15% of patients within 1 to 2 hours of ALT. IOP increase should be

prevented or lessened by a second 1% apraclonidine drop immediately post-ALT (see sec. **V.F.,** above) and CAIs. Current antiglaucomatous therapy is maintained and topical steroids tid to qid added and tapered over 1 to 2 weeks. The first post-ALT visit should be at 24 to 48 hours, 5 to 7 days after treatment, and at 4 to 6 weeks, at which time the IOP lowering effect is assessed. IOP and anterior segment inflammatory signs should be assessed. If inflamed, the patient should be examined with a gonioscope (for which the Zeiss lens is convenient) to look for inflammatory deposits in the angle or beginning peripheral anterior synechiae, and the steroid dosage thereby adjusted.

5. **Complications**
   a. **Peripheral anterior synechiae**
      (1) Usually low and not functional, but if "high" can cause worsening of glaucoma (convert open-angle to combined chronic angle-closure glaucoma).
      (2) If observed, decrease number and power of applications for any second treatment, and increase steroid dosage.
   b. **Corneal burns** (usually transient).
   c. **Hyphema**
      (1) Caused by blood in Schlemm's canal or wandering vessel (rule out undiagnosed neovascular glaucoma or increased episcleral venous pressure).
      (2) If encountered at time of ALT, increase pressure in eye by indenting with goniolens or decrease limbal compression in involved segment by tilting goniolens.
   d. **Iritis,** especially in patients under 40 years of age, should be treated with topical steroids.
   e. **Worsening of open-angle glaucoma,** about 3% incidence.
   f. **Closure of the peripheral iridotomy (PI)** is more frequent (up to 40%) with argon than Nd-YAG PI.
6. **Repeat ALT** is generally not effective for long-term IOP control, is more a temporizing measure for 1 to 2 years, and has the usual risks of ALT. Retreatment using 50 μm spot, 700 to 900 mW power, 0.1-second duration, 40 to 50 burns over 180 degrees or 80 to 100 burns over 360 degrees to the treated area has resulted in a second hypotensive response for at least a year in about 21% of patients.

C. **Selective laser trabeculoplasty (SLT)**
   1. **Indications.** SLT is a newly approved method of performing laser trabeculoplasty with a Q-switched, frequency-doubled Nd:YAG laser. Indications are similar to conventional ALT. It may be considered in patients who have a history of failed ALT, patients who have had their full complement of ALT, patients with poor compliance, and most types of open-angle glaucoma (POAG, pigmentary, pseudoexfoliation, juvenile, and angle recession). This technique specifically targets the pigmented TM cells in the absence of thermal or structural damage to nonpigmented TM cells and surrounding tissue.
   2. **Contraindications.** SLT is contraindicated in inflammatory glaucomas, congenital glaucoma, narrow-angle disease, or inability to adequately view the TM (corneal opacification, lack of cooperation).
   3. **Technique** is similar to ALT, with 180 degrees of the angle being treated at each session.
   4. **Complications.** IOP spikes and inflammation.
   5. **Repeat SLT.** Repeat treatment with SLT may be performed without increasing the failure rate of the surgery.
D. **Laser iridotomy (LI)**
   1. **Indications.** Argon, YAG LI, or both should always be attempted before considering surgical peripheral iridectomy. Except in chronic inflammation or rubeosis, in which a large surgical PI is less likely to close, indications for LI are a narrow "occludable" angle, postoperative

pupillary (iridovitreal) block, imperforate surgical iridectomy, malignant "ciliary" block glaucoma, nanophthalmos, and combined-mechanism (open and narrow) glaucoma.

2. **Technique of argon LI.** It is often helpful to treat the patient with pilocarpine 1% to 2% before LI to stretch and thin the iris and to maintain miosis. Instill topical anesthetic and 1% apraclonidine or 0.2% brimonidine 1 hour prelaser and immediately postlaser, to prevent a spike in pressure. A contact lens with a +66-D button such as the Abraham Wise lens dramatically improves the ease of the procedure. On the slitlamp, 25× ocular power should be used. Many methods involve pretreatment of the iris with **gonioplasty,** a peripheral arc of 100- to 300-mW, 0.2-second, 250-mm spots about 1.5 to 2.5 mm from the iris root deepen the chamber by stretching or thinning the iris. The LI is then done around 11 or 1 o'clock sites by the "chipping away technique," in which applications are superimposed with 50-mm, 0.2-second, 700- to 1500-mW settings for light irides and 0.02- to 0.05-second, 1,000- to 1,500-mW for dark irides until the iris is penetrated with 1 to 100 applications, more for darker eyes (a puff or pigment debris heralds this). The aiming beam must be crisply focused on the iris. If corneal endothelial clouding occurs, succeeding applications will have less effect, and laser applications must be immediately stopped in this area. When "pigment clouds" are dispersed into the anterior chamber, the treating surgeon should pause to allow their clearance before continuing with more laser applications. The lens capsule must be visualized to ensure that a full-thickness opening in the iris has been achieved. Transillumination can be misleading. In enlarging the opening, the circumference of the opening should be treated rather than strands bridging across the opening. Less laser energy will thus be absorbed by the crystalline lens. The procedure is performed ideally without causing any lens "whitening."

   If the cornea is hazy from elevated IOP, medical therapy should be used to decrease IOP and topical glycerin should be used to clear the cornea. With the "chipping away" method, one is usually able to penetrate the iris, although these "acute" LIs may close more commonly than those done in quiet eyes. If penetration of the iris is not achieved with attempted LI in an acute angle-closure eye, pupillary distortion induced by one or two 500 μm midiris laser spots often relieves pupillary block acutely with subsequent placement of the LI.

3. **Technique of YAG LI.** Premedication and lens use are the same as for argon LI. Power settings are 4 to 6 mJ and bursts of one to four pulses per shot should create the iridotomy. More pulses may increase the chances of lens damage. The beam is aimed on the iris in an area that will be covered by the upper lid and fired at a site about two-thirds of the distance between the pupil margin and the visible periphery. Blue irides perforate more readily than brown. Additional pulses should be delivered to the edge of the opening if enlargement is needed not directly over the lens capsule. Failure to penetrate the iris is usually the result of poor focus (e.g., corneal edema), iris edema, or use of insufficient laser energy. Another area may be tried. **Combined argon and Nd:YAG** is performed (argon 0.02 to 0.05 second, 1,000 mW, 50 μm, 5 to 25 applications followed by Nd:YAG 4 to 6 mJ and one burst of two to four pulses) or the procedure is terminated and retreatment is performed later after additional therapy, as indicated, has been given.

4. **Follow-up.** An acute increase in IOP within 1 to 2 hours of LI may occur and should be managed as discussed under ALT (see sec. **VI.B.,** above). LI can close anytime during a 6-week period (less often with YAG than argon). Therefore, it is best not to treat patients with

dilating drops at home, but rather to dilate the pupil in the physician's office at follow-up visits if necessary. Topical steroids should be used approximately tid to qid for 1 to 2 weeks and then tapered. At follow-up visits, the patency of the iridectomy should be documented by visualizing the lens capsule, and gonioscopy should be performed to document relief of pupillary block by observing deepening of the angle access. If the iridotomy closes, retreatment is necessary. At the 6-week office visit, the pupil should always be dilated to conclude that the iridectomy is patent and to rule out plateau iris.

    5. **Complications**

        a. **Lens injury.** No long-term adverse effect on the lens has been documented, even in eyes with areas of lens whitening post-LI.

        b. **Elevated IOP.** This elevation is usually controlled with mild antiglaucomatous therapy. Occasionally, IOP can be elevated to very high levels, sometimes shortly after the procedure. This should be monitored and appropriately treated. Often, increased steroid dosage is beneficial.

        c. **Iritis,** spontaneous angle closure from iridectomy closing, corneal burns (especially endothelial), and corectopia may occur and require therapy as indicated.

        d. **Bleeding** is more common with Nd:YAG than argon, because it is noncoagulative. Patients should not be taking anticoagulants, if possible, and iris vessels should be avoided at time of therapy.

VII. Surgical approaches. When medical or laser therapy fails, surgery is performed that results in a bypass of the conventional outflow pathways and allows drainage of aqueous humor from inside the eye. Antimetabolites are often used because they improve IOP lowering efficacy. These operations are called filtration procedures and are done before the other operations discussed below. Surgical outcomes vary by race, with African-Americans faring better with laser trabeculoplasty and whites doing better with trabeculectomy.

    A. **Filtering operations** were, in the past, full-thickness procedures (corneoscleral trephine, posterior lip, and thermal sclerectomies). Because of notably fewer complications (prolonged hypotony, flat anterior chamber, choroidal effusion), however, the development of guarded filtration has made **trabeculectomy** the most common of these procedures today, with full-thickness filtration used primarily in patients with advanced or low-tension glaucoma, requiring especially low IOP (6 to 10 mm). In trabeculectomy, a partial-thickness portion of the corneoscleral limbus is excised under a partial-thickness scleral flap. Five-year follow-up has shown a mean **IOP** of 15 mm Hg. Filtration surgery is generally associated with about 50% probability of preserving vision from progression to blindness. Those with poorest prognosis have more advanced field loss at the time of surgery.

        1. **Blebitis therapy.** Infection of a filtering bleb is an emergency. It is characterized by bleb purulence with or without anterior segment inflammation. If there is no clinical endophthalmitis, cultures are taken and topical ofloxacin or levofloxacin q1h round the clock is started. A systemic quinolone similar to the drops is therapeutically advisable. If there is vitritis or notable anterior chamber reaction, the approach should be the same as discussed in Chapter 9, VII, Endophthalmitis.

        Nonpenetrating filtration surgeries (**viscocanulostomy** and **deep sclerectomy** with collagen implant) have gained popularity over the past few years as alternatives to the trabeculectomy. In these procedures a partial thickness scleral flap is fashioned as in a trabeculectomy, and an additional scleral flap is dissected in the bed of the initial flap down to the level of Descemet's membrane and then excised. In viscocanulostomy, Schlemm's canal is entered and viscoelastic material is injected on both sides of the excised flap with the goal of clearing any resistance to outflow that exists in Schlemm canal. In deep sclerectomy with collagen implant, a collagen wick is placed in the bed of the scleral flap (with or without prior 5-fluorouracil [5-FU]) and dissolves over several months, leaving an area of filtration. Nonpenetrating filtration surgery has fewer immediate postoperative complications (hypotony, flat chamber, hyphema, or choroidal effusion), but the IOP control is not as good as with standard trabeculectomy. Up to one-third of the patients with nonpenetrating filtration surgery will require subsequent laser opening of Descemet's membrane for pressure control, converting the procedure to a conventional trabeculectomy.

B. Antimetabolites. Use of adjunctive mitomycin C or 5-FU (fluorouracil), both cidal to fibroblasts, usually yields IOPs lower than trabeculectomy alone and comparable to full-thickness procedures.

   1. **5-FU** is increasingly used as a single intraoperative application. A cellulose sponge soaked with 50 mg per mL 5-FU is held for up to 5 minutes in the bed and then rinsed off carefully before entering the eye. The drug may also be used at the first signs of filtering bleb failure or starting 1 day postoperatively with five 5-mg subconjunctival 5-FU injections administered 90 to 180 degrees away from the bleb over a 2-week period. It should **not** be given if a corneal graft was also done.

   2. **Mitomycin C** has replaced 5-FU as the antimetabolite used by a number of glaucoma surgeons, especially in darkly pigmented patients. It may be used when a corneal graft is also done, and is applied only once and at surgery. A cellulose sponge moistened with a 0.2 to 0.4 mg per mL (0.02% to 0.04%) mitomycin C is applied to the bed of the trabeculectomy flap for 1 to 5 minutes before the eye is opened, followed by profuse saline irrigation.

   3. **Adverse side effects** can occur with both drugs and are less at frequent at lower doses, e.g., leaks, epithelial defects, hypotony corneal haze, conjunctival congestion, and discomfort. A therapeutic soft contact lens will decrease 5-FU-induced discomfort, but the more serious side effects indicate treatment be stopped.

C. Procedures when standard filtration fails

   1. **Setons** include nonvalved devices such as the Baerveldt and Molteno, and valved devices such as Krupin and Ahmed implants. Each is a subconjunctival implant connected to a tube that enters the anterior chamber. Aqueous is shunted to the implant and diffuses away. These devices are used in refractory glaucoma or as a primary procedure in neovascular glaucoma with active iris neovascularization or keratoprosthesis, in which routine filtering surgery will likely fail.

   2. **Ciliodestructive procedures** to reduce aqueous production are often last-resort treatments for intractable glaucoma, including aphakic, pseudophakic, and neovascular disease and in patients unsuitable for standard filtration surgery (poor health, mental retardation, etc.).

      a. **Cyclocryothermy,** the transscleral freezing destruction of 180 degrees of ciliary body, has been used for decades with success, but can be associated with significant patient discomfort and ocular inflammation.

      b. **Transscleral** laser cyclophotocoagulation includes use of the solid-state ruby laser, and the Nd:YAG:glass laser for destruction of the ciliary body. Laser therapy is usually superior to cyclocryotherapy in visual and IOP outcome, postoperative pain, and need for retreatment. Complications are infrequent but include hypotony or phthisis. Retreatment is required in approximately half of the patients to control IOP.

D. Goniotomy in congenital glaucoma refers to an incision with a knife into the TM (see Chapter 11, sec. **XVII.**).

E. A surgical **peripheral iridectomy** is the removal of a peripheral portion of iris, alleviating pupillary block in angle-closure glaucoma by giving an extra opening for aqueous flow between chambers (see sec. **VI.D.,** above).

VIII. **Primary open angle glaucoma (POAG)**

A. **General considerations.** POAG is the most common form of glaucoma, affecting 1% to 2% of the world population; POAG is four to five times more common in African-Americans. In most cases, the disease develops in middle life or later and can be familial. The onset is usually gradual and asymptomatic, and tends to become progressively worse. The angle remains open at all times. Despite a normal appearance on gonioscopy, the TM outflow channels are functionally abnormal, and the facility of aqueous outflow from the anterior chamber is constantly subnormal in most cases (see sec. **II.A.,** above). The diurnal IOP may vary from normal to significantly elevated levels. This most likely represents variation in the rate of aqueous secretion, while the outflow facility remains subnormal. The facility of aqueous outflow usually becomes worse with time. Sometimes with age there is also a decline in the rate of aqueous production, and therefore this progressive impairment of outflow facility does not invariably result in further elevation of IOP. Nevertheless, in most cases, stronger medical therapy is required to control the IOP.

B. **Glaucoma detection**

1. A **spectrum** exists from normality to borderline abnormality to early glaucoma to frank glaucoma. The test of time is most useful in identifying patients with early glaucoma. Patients with an IOP of 22 mm Hg or greater, or those with optic disks with suspicious or asymmetric cupping regardless of the IOP (see sec. **XIV.,** below), should be followed as **glaucoma suspects** or **ocular hypertensives.** POAG differs from ocular hypertension in that the latter is a primary condition manifested by elevated IOP in the presence of open angles, but with no evidence of optic nerve damage or field loss. Approximately 2% of the population has ocular hypertension. About 5% of ocular hypertensives with IOP of 25 to 30 mm Hg will go on to develop nerve damage and field defects within 10 years. The diagnosis is then changed to POAG and appropriate therapy started. Therapy may also be started in the absence of damage if the IOP is sufficiently high, i.e., high 20s to low 30s, because it is likely that damage is inevitable should treatment be withheld.

2. **Glaucoma suspects** should be followed two to four times a year with IOP measurements and with careful inspection and drawing of the optic nerve cupping. Stereo disk photographs are useful. Visual fields should be performed once a year and optic nerve head and NFL analyses may also be performed on a periodic basis.

3. **Monocular glaucoma.** POAG always affects both eyes, although the disease may be more advanced in one eye. If glaucoma is truly monocular, other causes of secondary glaucoma must be investigated. Gonioscopy is often useful in diagnosis.

C. **Symptoms.** POAG is almost always a silent disease process with slowly progressive elevation of IOP. Occasionally, in younger patients, rapid increases in IOP may occur that result in corneal epithelial edema and symptoms of haloes, blurred vision, and pain, much as in pigmentary glaucoma (see sec. **XV.,** below).

D. **Indications for treatment**

1. **Early stage POAG.** The optic nerves of different patients differ in their susceptibility to the same level of IOP. For example, certain patients with NTG will show progression of disk cupping at ostensibly normal IOP (<22 mm Hg). It is generally believed that optic disks with thicker neuroretinal veins tolerate a given level of IOP better than those with thinner veins and glaucomatous damage. Patients off therapy generally require close follow-up. It is useful to check the IOP

at different times of day at different visits to detect significant diurnal peaks.

Often in early glaucoma, it is a borderline decision whether the patient should be treated. It is often useful to explain the situation and to let the patient have input into the decision. Often a trial of medical therapy to one eye is of value; if side effects occur, the patient may be followed off therapy a while longer. If therapy is efficacious and well tolerated, the patient often will prefer to have continued treatment, at least in one eye, often in both. In addition, by treating one eye initially, the efficacy of the therapy can be better evaluated.

2. **Change in disk cup appearance** indicates that medical therapy should be initiated. Different ophthalmologists have different cutoffs of IOP above which medical antiglaucoma therapy will be initiated regardless of disk appearance. With tensions chronically in the low 30s, glaucoma therapy should be routinely begun, provided there are not significant side effects. Certainly all patients with tensions in the upper 30s to 40s should be treated. Patients with wide cupping (even though it may be physiologic) with pressures in the upper 20s should also be treated. Patients with some glaucomatous damage to the nerve are treated to lower their IOP into the normal range (at least initially below 22 mm Hg).

3. **Progressive disk cupping or field changes in follow-up,** regardless of measured IOP, indicate that pressure is too high for the optic nerve and that further therapy should be added. Similarly, patients who present with extreme glaucomatous damage and IOP in the low 20s require vigorous therapy to achieve as low a pressure as possible (10 to 12 mm Hg). Even if the IOP is subnormal with medical and laser therapy, should future progression occur (as often may happen in patients with totally cupped disks and extensive field loss), then glaucoma filtering surgery is indicated to achieve as low an IOP as possible.

4. **Medical therapy** is usually begun with a beta-blocker, a topical CAI, an alpha-agonist, or a prostaglandin analog. *Miotics* are usually *avoided in younger patients* because of the accommodation and miosis. Allergies may occur with topical CAIs and alpha-agonists. Most but not all older patients tolerate pilocarpine well. With increased medical therapy, combinations of topical agents are often effective oral CAIs. Laser trabeculoplasty is usually reserved for patients not well controlled on maximum topical therapy, although it may reasonably be the initial treatment. It can be used at any point with medical treatment should IOP be inadequately controlled or if the patient cannot tolerate medical treatment.

5. **If maximum medical therapy** (i.e., that treatment the patient is able to tolerate locally and systemically) **fails** to control the IOP, glaucoma filtering surgery is indicated.

IX. **Primary acute angle-closure glaucoma**
  A. **Clinical findings**
    1. **Symptoms.** In acute angle-closure glaucoma, the relative pressure in the posterior chamber is increased as a result of pupillary block, and the peripheral iris is forced forward over the TM. The IOP increases rapidly because of the sudden blockage of aqueous outflow, resulting in the acute onset of severe pain, blurred vision, and perception of colored haloes about lights. The last two symptoms are from corneal epithelial edema that results from the rapidity of the IOP increase. The pain is usually quite severe. Often, it is not localized to the eye but involves the whole head and may be accompanied by nausea and vomiting. **The correct diagnosis may be missed by physicians who are not ophthalmologists, because they may misinterpret the headache and abdominal symptoms.**

2. **Signs.** Corneal epithelial edema can be detected on flashlight examination as a fine, rough haziness in the light reflex. The pupil is usually middilated (4 to 5 mm) and nonreactive to light, and the eye is red. Slitlamp examination reveals a shallowness of the axial and peripheral anterior chamber. There may be significant flare and a few cells as well in the anterior chamber. If the IOP has been elevated for a prolonged period during a previous attack, gray atrophy of the iris stroma and glaukomflecken (small white opacities in or under the anterior lens capsule) may be observed. Gonioscopy should be performed after clearing the corneal epithelial edema with topical glycerin (after a drop of topical anesthetic) and should confirm the angle closure (the peripheral iris covering over the TM).

B. Differential diagnosis

1. The physician should look carefully for the presence of new blood vessels or inflammatory cells on the iris and in the angle that would indicate a diagnosis of **neovascular or uveitis angle-closure glaucoma** rather than primary angle-closure glaucoma. The differential diagnosis also includes **acute open-angle glaucomas,** such as glaucomatocyclitis crisis or other uveitides, and pigmentary glaucoma. The physician should always examine the fellow eye with a gonioscope to confirm that it also is narrow and potentially closeable, with prominent iris convexity and the scleral spur not visible. If the fellow eye is not narrow, the physician should be careful that the correct diagnosis has in fact been made in the first eye and should then consider the differential diagnosis of true **monocular angle-closure glaucoma.** This includes acute central retinal vein occlusion, dislocated lens, phacomorphic glaucoma choroidal detachment or effusion, peripheral anterior synechiae secondary to uveitis, essential iris atrophy, and significant anisometropia (extreme difference in refractive error). In the emergency room, the diagnosis most commonly involves distinguishing primary angle-closure glaucoma from neovascular glaucoma.

2. **Inflamed red eyes** should always be suspicious for possible angle-closure glaucoma. In acute **conjunctivitis** there is usually a discharge with cells in the tear film, the cornea is clear, the vision is near normal, pupillary size and reaction are normal, and there is no true pain, unlike acute glaucoma. If the physician is suspicious of glaucoma in a red eye, it is important to measure the IOP. The Schiötz tonometer with a tonofilm cover is very valuable in these cases. In acute **anterior uveitis,** the pupil is usually small (unlike the middilation in acute glaucoma), the redness is more prominent in the area about the limbus, and the anterior chamber usually contains significantly more cells and flare than in acute angle-closure glaucoma. The cornea in uveitis is usually clear except for the presence of keratic precipitates. The vision is usually blurred and there may be considerable pain. All patients with uveitis should have their IOP measured, both to rule out angle-closure glaucoma and to detect the secondary open-angle glaucoma that may accompany uveitis, especially in the later stages.

C. Therapeutic implications of pupillary block. A coincidence of various physiologic and anatomic factors is responsible for an increase in pupillary block of posterior chamber aqueous flow to the anterior chamber, so that iris is pushed forward to cause angle closure. Pupillary size, rate of aqueous formation, rigidity of the iris, and axial position of the lens all influence the magnitude of pupillary block.

1. **Pupillary middilation** produces an increase in relative pupillary block. This middilated position may occur spontaneously because of illumination, e.g., an attack may occur when a patient visits a movie theater, or it may result from either topical or systemic administration of a pupillary dilating agent such as cyclopentolate, phenylephrine, or

atropine. Patients with narrow angles are asymptomatic before and after acute angle-closure attacks. The dilating agents must be used with care in patients found to have shallow anterior chambers on routine flashlight or slitlamp examination (see secs. **III.A. and B.,** above). The importance of assessing anterior chamber depth in ostensibly normal patients before use of these agents needs to be emphasized. In suspicious cases gonioscopy should be performed. Although topical agents are more frequently involved, cases of angle-closure glaucoma have been precipitated by **systemic** use of **atropine-like drugs** and inhalation of **bronchodilators.**

2. **Treatment of acute angle-closure glaucoma with miotics** moves the pupil from the middilated state to a smaller size, where there is less relative pupillary block. With excessive miosis, however, as may occur with use of **anticholinesterase agents,** an increase in relative pupillary block may actually occur, and thus these agents are **contraindicated in angle-closure glaucoma.** In addition, use of higher strengths of pilocarpine (4% to 6%) and other stronger miotics may move the lens forward because of zonular relaxation subsequent to ciliary muscle contraction, and this may actually increase relative pupillary block. For this reason, lower concentrations of pilocarpine (1% to 2%) are used initially to treat angle-closure glaucoma. Thus, in treatment of angle-closure glaucoma, ciliary muscle contraction may be an undesired side effect of pilocarpine therapy.

3. **Maximum pupillary dilation** pulls the iris sphincter away from the lens, and this relieves pupillary block. Attacks of angle closure may actually be broken by maximum pupillary dilation, although for surgical and laser considerations this is less desirable than miosis. After use of a topical mydriatic, the pupil may rapidly pass through the stage of middilation without angle closure, only to have a full-blown attack occur as the pupil returns from the widely dilated state toward a more normal size.

4. By **decreasing aqueous production, beta-blockers, alpha-agonists, and CAIs** may decrease the relative pressure force in the posterior chamber and lessen relative pupillary block. It is important to perform gonioscopy in the fellow eye before administration of CAIs or osmotic agents, which dehydrate the vitreous, because these agents may effect a temporary deepening of the anterior chamber.

5. **Small attacks of angle-closure glaucoma** may be spontaneously arrested by spontaneous movement of the pupil and by decrease in the rate of aqueous formation. The latter may occur temporarily as a result of the sudden elevation of IOP. Following an attack the eye may become hypotonous, and with the presence of some cells and flare, a mistaken diagnosis of uveitis may be made. Clues to the presence of previous attacks are areas of gray iris stromal atrophy, glaukomflecken, and shallow anterior chamber depth (also in the fellow eye). A history of episodes of colored haloes, pain, and blurred vision should be sought. Provocative tests, such as the dark room prone test, should be performed (see sec. **X.C.,** below).

D. **Treatment of acute angle-closure glaucoma**
   1. Topical aqueous suppressants, miotics, and CAIs (either orally or i.v.).
   2. **Systemic hyperosmotics** (glycerol or isosorbide p.o., or mannitol i.v. [see sec. **V.I.,** above, for dosage]) and i.v. acetazolamide (250 to 500 mg) should be given initially to lower the IOP below 50 to 60 mm Hg. Topical medications should be updated to lower the pressure further. At higher pressures the iris sphincter is ischemic and unresponsive to pilocarpine. Because miotics may allow forward lens movement by relaxation of zonular tension, a reduction in vitreous volume via the use of osmotics is probably useful in most cases. **Pilocarpine 1%** should be administered initially q15min. If the attack fails to respond to this

therapy, higher strengths of pilocarpine, up to 2% *(not higher, or pupillary block may increase),* may be substituted.

Once the IOP is lowered, it is important to examine the patient with a gonioscope to ensure the angle has opened. Use of osmotics, beta-blockers, and CAIs may result in a temporarily lowered IOP despite persistent angle closure.

3. **Once the attack is broken,** LI should be performed (see sec. **VI.C.,** above). If this procedure is delayed, the patient is usually maintained on pilocarpine 1% q4 to 6h until LI. The fellow asymptomatic eye may also be treated prophylactically. It is often useful to treat the patient with topical PF in addition to glaucoma medications for 1 to 2 hours before PI to allow the cornea to clear and to quiet the eye.

4. If medical therapy fails to break the attack, then LI should be performed as an emergency procedure. The use of osmotics almost always results in a temporarily sufficient IOP lowering and in less need for emergency surgery. The IOP, however, should not be allowed to remain above 60 mm Hg for more than a few hours, because permanent loss of vision from optic atrophy may result. If LI cannot be performed and if high pressure persists, surgical peripheral iridectomy should be performed.

5. **Prolonged attack** may result in permanent adhesions of the peripheral iris to the meshwork; i.e., **peripheral anterior synechiae** may form. In such cases, peripheral iridectomy will relieve pupillary block but will not restore normal IOP because of the residual chronic angle closure. LI with follow-up gonioscopy will help assess angle closure. If laser is unsuccessful, however, at the time of surgery a **chamber deepening technique** should be performed. The apparent angle closure viewed preoperatively may be due to a potentially reversible apposition of iris to TM or to true synechiae. In the chamber deepening technique, fluid is injected into the anterior chamber via a limbal paracentesis slit opening and gonioscopy performed to assess the extent of the peripheral anterior synechiae formation. If extensive peripheral anterior synechiae have formed (more than 90% of the angle), a filtering procedure rather than a peripheral iridectomy should be performed. (New techniques are being developed in which laser applications to the peripheral iris, termed *iridogonioplasty,* may break recently formed peripheral anterior synechiae with functional improvement in outflow) (see sec. **VI.C.2.,** above.)

6. **Prophylactic laser peripheral iridotomy** should be performed on the fellow asymptomatic eye within a few days after surgery on the first eye, unless there are circumstances of true monocular angle closure.

X. **Subacute and chronic primary angle-closure glaucoma**

A. **Subacute and chronic angle-closure glaucoma** result if the iris does not cover the TM in the full circumference of the angle. This may cause intermittent moderate elevation of IOP that is roughly proportional to the extent of closure. These subacute episodes may occur with mild symptoms of colored haloes, blurred vision, and red eye. A condition of continuous chronic partial-angle closure may occur and mimic open-angle glaucoma in its lack of symptoms and maintained elevation of IOP.

B. **Differentiation** of chronic angle-closure glaucoma from open-angle glaucoma with narrow but open angles in which full width of TM can be seen is important. In cases of suspected partial chronic angle-closure glaucoma, the relative effects of bright light, thymoxamine (alphablocker) drops, or weak (0.5% to 1.0%) pilocarpine on gonioscopic angle appearance and IOP may establish the correct diagnosis. **Thymoxamine** causes miosis but has no effect on facility of outflow.

C. **The dark room prone test** may be done on patients with suspiciously narrow angles who are not seen during an acute attack and who do not have glaukomflecken or gray iris stromal atrophy. This test may be utilized to identify dangerously narrow (but open at the time of examination) angles. In this test, IOP is measured and the patient is seated for 30 to 60 minutes in a darkened room with his or her head down on a cushioned table. The IOP is again measured in the darkened room. An increase of 6 to 8 mm Hg or greater or a significant asymmetric rise in pressure between the two eyes that is accompanied by gonioscopic confirmation of further angle closure is a positive test, and a prophylactic LI is indicated. It is important to perform all phases of this test in a darkened room. Miosis from external light or from the focal illuminator during gonioscopy may quickly reverse the angle closure. Placing the patient in a brightly lit room for 5 minutes after this test and observing a significant reduction of IOP will further confirm a positive test.

   D. A pharmacologic mydriatic test (2.5% phenylephrine) is sometimes used as a provocative test. Such a test is distinctly nonphysiologic and has significant false negatives. Most important, the angle may not close during the pupillary dilation, but rather may close many hours later as the pupil contracts. If such a test is performed, the patient should be kept under observation for several hours until the pupil returns to normal size.

XI. Plateau iris. Very rarely, a mechanism of primary angle closure may be the direct expansion of the peripheral iris against the TM as the peripheral iris thickens during pupillary dilation. This mechanism is independent of, but may coexist with, pupillary block and is called a *plateau iris*.

   A. Slitlamp examination reveals a discrepancy between the central anterior chamber which is deep and the peripheral anterior chamber which is narrow. On gonioscopy the iris plane is somewhat flat, and the peripheral iris is very close to the TM, with a characteristic small roll and trough just before the iris insertion on the ciliary body band.

   B. Therapy of patients with angle-closure glaucoma who have a plateau iris configuration includes an LI and, during convalescence, a provocative test with a weak mydriatic. A patient with true plateau iris will demonstrate a pressure elevation and gonioscopic angle closure. Such patients are managed successfully with long-term weak miotic therapy that prevents pupillary dilation and iris crowding of the angle. In those patients with a negative provocative test with pupillary dilation postiridectomy, it is believed that pupillary block was the mechanism of the preoperative angle closure despite the suspicious plateau configuration. The majority of plateau configuration patients fall into this latter category, which is why peripheral iridectomy should always be performed first in these patients.

XII. Differential diagnosis of pressure elevation following surgical peripheral iridectomy for angle closure

   A. Plateau iris. Treat with weak miotics.

   B. Imperforate peripheral iridectomy. Treat with a laser or repeat iridectomy.

   C. Malignant glaucoma is a condition in which there is maintained increase in total vitreous volume (or perhaps classically a pocket of aqueous trapped in or behind the vitreous) that results in flattening of the anterior chamber and closure of the angle. It occurs postoperatively after glaucoma or cataract surgery. Key to the diagnosis is a marked shallowing of the axial anterior chamber depth that results from the vitreous expansion. B-scan ultrasound will rule out choroidal detachment or suprachoroidal hemorrhage. A patent PI rules out pupillary block. **Treatment** consists of administration of daily 1% atropine drops used indefinitely, beta-blockers, CAIs, and short term systemic osmotics. If this is not successful, vitreous aspiration with puncture of the hyaloid is required. Aphakic eyes almost never respond to medical treatment.

   D. Topical cycloplegic and steroid postoperative medications may be responsible for elevated IOP through an ill-defined open-angle glaucoma mechanism. Such therapy may result in elevation of IOP in patients with POAG more characteristically. Axially, the anterior chamber is not flattened, and the glaucoma responds to cessation of the drops.

E. **Extensive peripheral anterior synechiae** may progress if iridotomy fails to break the attack because synechiae already exist. Filtering surgery should be performed following the chamber deepening procedure.

XIII. **Combined open-angle and angle-closure glaucoma**

A. **Angle-closure glaucoma** can occur occasionally in patients who have or subsequently develop **open-angle glaucoma.** Whether the latter is POAG or a result somehow of the episodes of high pressure elevation while the angle was closed is disputed. It has definitely been noted that some patients develop open-angle glaucoma several years after successfully treated angle-closure glaucoma.

B. **Gradual, progressive partial angle-closure glaucoma** may occur in some patients with well-documented, long-standing POAG. With aging, most individuals, both those with and without glaucoma, will show some tendency toward shallowing of the angle, most likely the result of an increase in size of the lens. The effect of miotic therapy on lens position may also be a factor. This partial angle closure will result in further chronic pressure elevation. Patients whose POAG worsens with therapy or age should always be **reexamined with a gonioscope** to rule out coexisting additive partial angle closure (or other unusual glaucoma, such as occult KPs in the meshwork). When 120 degrees or more of the angle is judged to be closed and the recent IOP course is consistent, LI is usually indicated.

C. **Subacute or chronic angle-closure glaucoma suspects** may, with the application of bright light, thymoxamine, or weak pilocarpine, have a dramatic lowering of IOP and total opening of the angle, although the IOP is still definitely above normal. Such patients should be suspected of having combined open-angle and angle-closure glaucoma and residual glaucoma after an LI.

XIV. **Normal-tension (low-tension) glaucoma (NTG).** The optic nerves of different patients have differing susceptibilities to similar levels of IOP. In the extreme, there are certain patients who demonstrate progressive disk cupping and field loss with normal or mildly elevated IOP. Such patients are generally referred to as having NTG and are usually elderly. About 10% to 50% of all POAGs fall into the low-tension glaucoma category. Factors predisposing to progressive nerve damage include preexisting wide physiologic cupping and factors affecting nerve perfusion such as faulty vascular autoregulation, arteriosclerotic vascular disease, systemic hypotension, carotid artery disease, arrhythmias, and diabetes mellitus. A cardinal sign of **optic nerve ischemia** is **flame-shaped hemorrhaging on the disk** in up to 40% of patients (rarer in POAG), making treatment all the more urgent. **Medical therapy** is aimed at rapidly reducing the IOP to the lowest level possible, not just at treating on the basis of current extent of cupping and field loss. A full medical evaluation should be carried out and systemic therapy, medical or surgical (e.g., carotid), to control problems relating to vascular perfusion initiated. Neuroimaging should be considered in patients with optic nerve pallor out of proportion to cupping or in patients with a significant color vision deficit. **Calcium channel blockers** are vasodilators and may have some favorable but unproven therapeutic effect on NTG (see sec. **V.J.,** above). **Laser trabeculoplasty** has only equivocal effects. Because of the low level of IOP that causes nerve damage, **filtration surgery** is frequently the only means of obtaining a low enough IOP.

XV. **Pigmentary dispersion syndrome and glaucoma** are the result of primary loss of pigment from the posterior surface (neuroepithelium) from the midperipheral iris. This pigment is disseminated intraocularly and deposited on various intraocular structures such as the corneal endothelium, where it may form a **Krukenberg spindle,** and in the TM, where it forms a dense continuous band of pigment throughout the circumference. The latter may occur with inconspicuous corneal endothelial pigmentation—a reason the condition may often be missed.

A. **Time of onset** is at a younger age than most other open-angle glaucomas; it appears in the 20- to 40-year-old group. The occurrence of this glaucoma in young myopic males is another good reason to perform routine applanation tonometry in all cooperative patients regardless of age.

B. **Wide fluctuations in IOP** may result in crises of high pressure elevation with corneal epithelial edema. Gonioscopy always shows the angle to be open and to contain the characteristic pigment band. Liberation of large amounts of circulating pigment into the anterior chamber is sometimes associated with these pressure elevations, and may be misinterpreted as cells of uveitis. In a few patients, exercise may induce such anterior chamber pigment liberation. During routine visits small numbers of circulating pigment particles can occasionally be seen in the anterior chamber in pigmentary dispersion syndrome patients. Because of the wide pressure fluctuations in this condition, a single normal IOP does not rule out the presence of pigmentary glaucoma. Approximately half of the patients with pigment dispersion syndrome will eventually develop glaucoma.

C. **Examination** by viewing the iris stroma directly will not reveal the loss of posterior iris pigment (although occasionally pigment can be deposited on the anterior iris surface). **Transillumination** using a fiberoptic light source applied to the lower lid or sclera, or pupillary transillumination on the slitlamp will demonstrate typical linear slit-like defects in the midperiphery of the iris, which is the key to the diagnosis. Gonioscopy often reveals significant backbowing of the peripheral iris, in addition to a dense pigment band covering the TM. In the presence of an elevated IOP, if sufficient backbowing of the iris is present, some authorities advocate laser iridotomy to relieve the "reverse" pupillary block that is postulated to exist in pigment dispersion.

D. **Treatment** is similar to that for POAG. Because of the patient's younger age and accommodation, however, there is poor tolerance to miotics, except perhaps the pilocarpine Ocusert.

XVI. **Pseudoexfoliation syndrome (PXF)**

A. **Clinical findings** in PXF include an amorphous gray **dandruff-like** material present on the pupillary border, anterior lens surface, posterior surface of the iris, zonules, and ciliary processes. This may represent basement membrane material from multiple ocular sites. The central area of the anterior lens capsule often has a dull, lusterless appearance through the undilated pupil; when the pupil is dilated the gray membrane is seen to end in the midperiphery in a scalloped border, often with curled edges. **Transillumination** of the iris frequently reveals loss of pigment from the posterior iris surface adjacent to the pupil, in contradistinction to pigmentary dispersion syndrome, in which defects occur in the midperiphery. This loss of pigment from the iris may result in an abnormal accumulation of pigment in the TM.

B. **Glaucoma may or may not occur in PXF.** Dandruff may be observed as an incidental finding during a routine examination in a patient with normal IOP. Such patients should be followed for possible future development of glaucoma, because exfoliation syndrome is often associated with a chronic open-angle glaucoma that may be initially monocular. Exfoliation glaucoma behaves similarly to and is **treated** like POAG. It may become more resistant to medical treatment with time than POAG, but fortunately is the type of glaucoma that usually responds best to laser trabeculoplasty.

XVII. **Glaucoma from contusion of the eye**

A. **Early onset**

1. **Acute glaucoma** may follow blunt trauma to the eye. This condition may be secondary to direct contusion injury to the trabecular angle

tissue, or it may be because of the deposition of inflammatory or blood elements from traumatic hyphema in the outflow pathways. The obstruction of aqueous outflow may be masked by coexisting hyposecretion of aqueous humor that may occur for a variable period following the injury.

2. **Treatment** of acute traumatic glaucoma consists of use of aqueous suppressants and oral CAIs. Topical **miotics** should be **avoided** because they possibly promote posterior synechiae and increase the inflammation in the eye. Should the IOP fail to be controlled with persistent pressures above the upper 40s, paracentesis and irrigation of the blood elements should be performed.

3. **Chronic erythroclastic (ghost cell) glaucoma** may be seen with prolonged hyphemas, but more commonly with vitreous hemorrhages in which the blood elements may remain in the vitreous for several days before passing into the anterior chamber. Red blood cells may degenerate into red cell ghosts with rigid cell membranes and **Heinz bodies** that are much more obstructive to aqueous outflow than the more pliable, fresh red cells, and a severe glaucoma may result. These red cell ghosts are khaki or off-white in color and must be distinguished from the white blood cells in inflammation. **Treatment** of chronic ghost cell glaucoma consists of use of topical aqueous suppressants and oral CAIs and, these failing, paracentesis and anterior chamber irrigation. If significant increased IOP persists, vitrectomy to remove hemorrhagic debris may be necessary.

4. **Uveitis** often accompanies the acute contusion injury and should be treated with topical cycloplegics and steroids. If there is a severe acute uveitis, the IOP is usually low due to hyposecretion. Occasionally, the glaucoma following within days of contusion injury may respond somewhat to topical steroids, and they should be attempted in this time period. In persistent glaucoma the physician should be careful to identify correctly the presence of ghost cell glaucoma, which does not respond to topical steroids.

B. **Late onset**

1. **Angle-recession glaucoma** may occur months to many years after blunt injury to the eye. It results from contusion to the trabecular angle tissue with associated tears in the uveal meshwork and ciliary muscle causing a more posterior, i.e., recessed, insertion of the iris onto the ciliary body band. This recession is not the cause of the glaucoma per se, but is associated with the glaucoma-producing trabecular injury. It is subtle, and **simultaneous gonioscopy in both eyes** is best to identify it correctly. Although acute tears may be observed in the TM, these heal with time. In chronic angle-recession glaucoma, the TM itself may not appear abnormal.

2. **Evaluation of patients with significant blunt trauma** to the eye that results in hyphema should include gonioscopy several weeks after the injury to identify possible angle recessions. Patients so identified, usually with greater than 180 degrees of recession, are at some risk of developing glaucoma in the future and should be so informed and followed. Fortunately, the majority of such patients will not develop glaucoma. Tonography may be of value in determining the frequency of follow-up.

3. **Differential diagnosis** of subtle angle recession must include other causes of true monocular glaucoma. Simultaneous gonioscopy must be performed to rule them out.

4. **Treatment** of angle-recession glaucoma is the same as that for POAG. It may become refractory in the later stages. It may also be associated with the histological development of a cuticular membrane in the angle.

XVIII. Glaucoma due to intraocular inflammation
  A. **Anterior uveitis**
    1. In **acute anterior uveitis** there is probably some obstruction to outflow that is masked at least initially by the more predominant hyposecretion of aqueous that results in hypotony. Later in the course, when with topical steroid treatment, aqueous production increases, this obstruction may become manifest with an elevation of IOP.
    2. **Steroid-induced open-angle glaucoma** may also be involved in certain patients. When faced with open-angle glaucoma in uveitis, it is usually unclear whether more or less topical steroid should be given. A trial of the former is usually useful to treat possible inflammation in the meshwork.
    3. **Angle-closure glaucoma** may also result from uveitis from posterior iris–lens synechiae formation causing **pupillary block with iris bombé.** Peripheral anterior synechiae may also form from primary inflammatory adhesions in the angle without pupillary block.
    4. **Treatment** consists of using topical aqueous suppressants and oral CAIs and increasing or decreasing the steroid dosage. Miotics are contraindicated. In treating inflammatory pupillary block, medications, usually intensive mydriatic–cycloplegic therapy, should be utilized to move the iris away from the lens into a dilated stage. If this fails, laser peripheral iridotomy will relieve the pupillary block.
  B. **Glaucomatocyclitic crisis (Posner-Schlossman syndrome)**
    1. **Crises of intermittent unilateral acute open-angle glaucoma** that are associated with very minimum but definite signs of anterior chamber inflammation characterize this disease of unknown etiology. Usually only a few cells and one or two areas of smudginess on the corneal endothelium are observed. Corneal epithelial edema may be present due to the sudden IOP increase. The eye is only mildly hyperemic and the patient has only slight discomfort. Repeated attacks may occur over the years and be benign. On the other hand, a patient may go on to develop chronic uveitis and open-angle glaucoma in later years. There is usually a great discrepancy between the acute glaucoma and the amount of anterior segment inflammation. Recent studies have shown **herpes simplex** antigen in the aqueous and therapeutic response to p.o. acyclovir.
    2. **Gonioscopy** always reveals the angle to be open, although occasionally KPs are seen. The disease must be distinguished by gonioscopy from acute angle-closure glaucoma.
    3. **Treatment** consists of beta-blockers, epinephrine, DPE, CAIs, or topical steroids, or any combination, and possibly a 10-day course of acyclovir. An attack may spontaneously abate without treatment within a few days to weeks.
  C. **Herpes simplex and zoster.** Open- or closed-angle glaucoma may occur in these diseases associated with uveitis. Either may have an early or late **trabeculitis** in a white and quiet eye, but with notable increase in IOP. Treatment is primarily high-dose topical steroids with taper and antiglaucoma drops as needed. If the pressure increase is not from trabeculitis but from steroids therapy, aqueous suppressants (not miotics) should be utilized to treat the IOP in addition to adjustments in steroid dosage discussed above (see sec. **XVIII.A.4.,** above; Chapter 5, secs. **IV.D. and E.;** and Chapter 9, secs. **VIII.A.2,3.**). Prostaglandin analogs should be used with care in patients with herpetic eye disease because they may cause uveitis. Patients with known ocular herpes simplex should be considered for prophylactic acyclovir 400 mg p.o. bid if taking prostaglandin analogs. Prostaglandin analogs should be used with some caution because they may exacerbate the underlying inflammation.
  D. **Fuchs heterochromic iridocyclitis** is characterized by chronic anterior uveitis in a white and quiet eye with no synechiae formation, but with

iris heterochromia (usually the lighter iris) and cataract formation. Filamentary precipitates on the corneal endothelium are also typical. This form of iridocyclitis is probably degenerative rather than inflammatory.

1. **Glaucoma** develops probably in a minority of such patients. It usually occurs late and develops gradually, although it often proves **refractory to topical medical therapy.** This may be due to a hyaline membrane histology.

2. **Treatment** is standard anti-open-angle glaucoma therapy and then LTP. If this fails, patients do well with filtration surgery. Cataract surgery is also uncomplicated, but does not influence the course of the glaucoma. Topical steroids do not influence the glaucoma.

E. **Keratic precipitate (KP) glaucoma** in the angle may occur occultly in a white and quiet eye with no apparent intraocular inflammation, but with elevated IOP that may mimic POAG. This condition is another reason to examine all glaucoma patients with a gonioscope. The precipitates may be very subtle and are best seen by retroillumination. With time they may organize and result in irregular peripheral anterior synechiae and an uneven insertion of the iris in the angle. This occult disease responds well to **topical steroid therapy,** but not to conventional topical antiglaucoma therapy, except perhaps timolol. Patients with presumed POAG who are placed on treatment and return with no apparent effect or even higher IOP should always be reexamined with a gonioscope to rule out this (and other) causes.

XIX. **Neovascular glaucoma**

A. **Clinical characteristics.** In certain patients with long-standing hypoxic retinopathy such as **diabetes, central retinal artery or vein occlusion, or carotid artery insufficiency,** a fibrovascular membrane will grow over the TM and ultimately result in total angle closure. Glaucoma may be present at a time when the membrane has not yet contracted and caused synechiae formation and the angle is still "open." Patients present with acute glaucoma that must be distinguished from primary angle-closure glaucoma by the presence of new blood vessels in the angle and almost always on the surface of the iris as well. Topical glycerin should be used to clear the corneal edema. A history of severe visual loss several months before the glaucoma may be helpful in identifying patients with central retinal vein occlusion. Other retinopathies and malignant melanoma may be associated with the development of neovascular glaucoma in rare cases.

B. **Treatment.** In eyes with total angle closure, treatment consists of use of aqueous suppressants and oral CAIs (methazolamide if renal function is impaired) to lower the IOP and topical steroids and cycloplegics for comfort. If the visual potential is good, filtration surgery or tube shunt placement often succeeds. Ciliodestructive procedures are now improved and often successful, although they are the last resort (see sec. **VII.C.3.,** above). In eyes with early neovascular glaucoma, panretinal photocoagulation will often lead to a regression or delay in the disease process.

XX. **Abnormal episcleral venous pressure**

A. **Intracranial vascular malformations,** such as those seen in patients with carotid–cavernous sinus fistulas and dural shunts in patients with Sturge-Weber disease, may produce an elevation of venous pressure that is transmitted back to the eye and results in a secondary open-angle glaucoma. This **elevated episcleral venous pressure** may also occur idiopathically in certain glaucoma patients. Usually a key to the diagnosis is the presence of prominent or abnormal episcleral vessels on slitlamp examination. These prominent episcleral vessels may be misinterpreted as indicating episcleritis or other inflammatory disease.

B. **Treatment** is standard open-angle glaucoma therapy, although the IOP cannot be lowered below true episcleral venous pressure, because the vessels constitute the draining bed for aqueous humor after it has passed through the angle tissue. Glaucoma filtering surgery may be successful, although these patients are at risk of developing **intraoperative choroidal effusions** due to the elevation of venous pressure. This should be anticipated and treated intraoperatively by a preliminary posterior sclerotomy.

XXI. **Corticosteroid glaucoma**

A. **Clinical characteristics.** Steroid glaucoma is anatomically indistinguishable from POAG: the pressure is elevated, angles are open and appear normal, outflow facility is decreased, and, with time, the nerves are progressively cupped and visual fields are compromised. Increased IOP may develop within 2 weeks of initiating steroid use or after many months or even years of use. The more potent agents such as dexamethasone and prednisolone are more likely to induce pressure increases sooner and higher than softer agents such as loteprednol, rimexolone, or fluorometholone. Patients who were formerly but no longer taking steroids and who had steroid glaucoma may be misdiagnosed as having low-tension glaucoma because of the presence of glaucomatous cupping, visual field defects, and normal pressures. Successfully controlled glaucoma patients may go out of control if steroid therapy is added to their drug regimen, and infants treated with steroid may develop a picture similar to that of primary congenital open-angle glaucoma. Close relatives of patients with POAG stand a significantly greater chance of developing steroid glaucoma (20%) than the rest of the population (4%). **The history of patient steroid drug therapy is essential to making the correct diagnosis.**

B. **Medical therapy** is first and foremost to stop or at least reduce the steroids or switch to loteprednol, rimexolone, or fluorometholone if possible. Reducing or discontinuing the drug will almost invariably result in spontaneous resolution of increased IOP within 2 to 6 weeks. If IOP does not return to normal but is reduced simply by discontinuing the steroid, it is likely that an underlying undiagnosed POAG was simply unmasked or aggravated by steroid usage. There is no definitive proof that these drugs cause permanent alterations in the ocular outflow channels. If steroids cannot be stopped or if the IOP is unacceptably high while waiting for spontaneous resolution, therapy as for POAG may be initiated to prevent progression of ocular damage. Alpha-agonists, CAIs, beta-blockers (except in asthmatics taking steroids), miotics (except in inflamed eyes), and sympathomimetics all may have a beneficial effect in this form of glaucoma.

C. **Surgical therapy** is rarely used for this condition and only in those cases where IOP does not return to acceptable levels despite stopping steroids and initiating antiglaucoma medical treatment. Subconjunctival depot injections may have to be resected, although they have usually washed out by 2 weeks. Laser trabeculoplasty is ineffective.

XXII. **Crystalline lens-induced glaucoma** (see also Chapter 7, sec. **V.H.3.**).

A. **Clinical characteristics.** An acute secondary open-angle glaucoma **(phacolytic glaucoma)** may result from a leaking hypermature or mature (rarely immature) cataract. There is usually rapid onset of ocular pain and redness with often very high pressures and corneal epithelial edema. Light projection may be faulty. Gonioscopy reveals the angle to be open, which distinguishes this disease from acute angle-closure glaucoma. Cellular reaction in the anterior chamber is usually minimal to moderate, although there is usually a heavy flare. Circulating white particles, which are larger than white cells and probably represent small portions of lens material, aggregated lens protein, or swollen macrophages can be seen frequently in the aqueous. The cataract often has patchy white deposits, which are probably macrophages, on the anterior lens capsule.

B. **Mechanism.** Phacolytic glaucoma is most likely the result of direct mechanical obstruction of the outflow pathways by the liberated lens proteins that leak from the cataract. Macrophages that act to clear lens material from the eye may also be involved in the obstruction to outflow. The **diagnosis** of phacolytic glaucoma is made by paracentesis and aspiration of aqueous humor, microscopic examination of which usually reveals the presence of engorged macrophages. Biochemical analysis for lens proteins may also be useful (see Chapter 1, sec. **III.L.**).

C. **Dislocated lenses.** In cases of cataractous lenses that are dislocated into the vitreous, the findings in phacolytic glaucoma may be quite subtle. The **differential diagnosis** includes angle-recession glaucoma, POAG, and an idiopathic type of chronic open-angle glaucoma apparently not related to lens reaction or obvious signs of angle recession.

D. **Retained lens cortex.** Glaucoma may result from the obstructive properties of liberated lens particles on the outflow pathways following extracapsular cataract surgery or lens injury. An inflammatory component may be additive.

E. **Differential diagnosis.** Phacolytic glaucoma must be distinguished from inflammatory glaucoma. Some KPs may be present on the cornea in phacolytic glaucoma. Consideration of the above factors will usually lead to the correct diagnosis but, especially in the rare cases of phacolytic glaucoma with immature cataracts, a trial of topical steroids may be useful. In phacolytic glaucoma, such steroid therapy will not result in a lasting improvement of IOP, and cataract surgery should then be contemplated. Again, diagnostic paracentesis will usually establish the correct diagnosis.

F. **Treatment** is cataract extraction. In general, the eyes show short-lived response to topical antiglaucoma or antiinflammatory therapy. There is usually significant reduction of IOP with use of a beta-blocker, alpha-agonists, CAIs, and osmotic agents, but the pressure frequently continues to increase again to high levels (40 to 80 mm Hg). All patients with presumed phacolytic glaucoma should have urgent cataract extraction, especially if the pressure continues to increase to these high levels. In the case of retained lens cortex, medical therapy with a beta-blocker, epinephrine, DPE, CAIs, cycloplegics, and possibly topical steroids should be tried, but if the glaucoma remains severe, the remaining lens material must be surgically removed.

XXIII. **Intraocular lens (IOL)-associated glaucoma** may stem from any of the previously mentioned causes such as exacerbation of preexistent POAG, pupillary block, malignant glaucoma following pupillary block, viscoelastic substance (see sec. **XXIV.**, below) or vitreous herniation into the anterior chamber blocking the TM, or chronic peripheral anterior synechiae. In addition, IOLs uniquely predispose to three other causes of glaucoma: smoldering chronic iridocyclitis, anterior chamber (and TM) mechanical distortion, and pseudophakic pigmentary dispersion. **Therapy** of all but the last three has already been discussed. For these three a decision must be made as to whether the IOL should be removed or medical therapy will suffice. IOL iritis is often associated with mechanical distortion of the anterior chamber due to improper lens sizing or placement. Steroid and, if needed, antiglaucoma therapy may control the process. If progressive adhesions or cystoid macular edema develop, however, the lens should probably be removed in the absence of other contraindications. In pigment dispersion (seen with iris plane and posterior chamber IOLs), the pupil and iris may be immobilized with longer-acting miotics to minimize mechanical rubbing against the lens. The IOL usually does not have to be removed.

XXIV. **Viscoelastic substance-induced glaucoma** is a secondary open-angle glaucoma seen postoperatively after use of these vitreous-stimulating materials. The newer such gels are much less prone to inducing IOP increase.

Clinical characteristics. Viscoelastic gels, although a great boon to anterior and posterior segment surgery, may have the undesirable side effect of transiently blocking the aqueous outflow system occasionally, with resulting severe increase in IOP.

Pressure increase may begin within an hour or two of closing the eye in the case of residual anterior chamber material, and at 72 hours in situations in which viscoelastic substance has been left in the posterior segment and has then moved forward. Symptoms may be absent or similar to acute IOP increase with ocular pain, steamy cornea, nausea, and vomiting. Posterior segment viscoelastic substance usually must be removed to control the glaucoma.

XXV. **Perforating injuries** may produce glaucoma as a result of peripheral anterior synechiae from the loss of the anterior chamber or may be the result of inflammation, lens material, or pupillary block. It is important to restore the anterior chamber in the treatment of such injuries.

XXVI. **Unusual secondary angle-closure glaucomas**

A. **Malignant glaucoma** (see sec. **XII.C.,** above)

B. **A dislocated lens** that is incarcerated in the pupil may cause angle-closure glaucoma by pupillary block. Treatment consists of laying the patient on his or her back, dilating the pupil, and attempting to force the lens back into the posterior chamber, following which the pupil is made miotic. If medical therapy fails, an LI (rather than lens extraction) should almost always be done. An exception would be a lens dislocated into the anterior chamber, close to or touching the cornea, that cannot be moved into the posterior chamber. Extraction of dislocated lenses is usually accompanied by vitreous loss and significant complications.

C. **Essential iris atrophy** is almost always a monocular condition of progressive iris atrophy with **distortion of the pupil** and **iris hole formation,** with glaucoma resulting from progressive peripheral anterior synechiae often extending anterior to Schwalbe's line. In **iridocorneal endothelial syndrome,** corneal endothelial dystrophy (beaten metal) and iris nodule formation may be observed. The disease may be due to progression and contraction of an endothelial cell membrane. In **Chandler syndrome,** corneal endothelial dystrophy is a predominant feature with corneal edema and haloes at mild elevations of IOP. Only mild iris atrophy without hole formation is characteristic of Chandler syndrome, although there is a disease spectrum. In addition to the iris and corneal changes, **diagnosis** is made on gonioscopy by the observation of peripheral anterior synechiae extending anterior to Schwalbe's line (unlike almost all other peripheral anterior synechiae). Differential diagnosis includes Axenfeld-Rieger syndrome and the corneal dystrophies. **Standard medical therapy** is employed, but this is a progressive disease and, especially in Chandler syndrome, in which a very low IOP is required, filtering surgery is frequently required.

D. **Multiple iris and ciliary body cysts** is a rare condition, though often familial, in which the cysts may directly push the iris over the TM and close the angle. They may be discovered after LI for angle closure. An uncommon bumpy contour of the peripheral iris on gonioscopy is characteristic. If accessible, the cysts may be ruptured by application of laser therapy through an iridectomy.

E. **Retinal detachment surgery.** Indentation of the eye by the buckle or suprachoroidal fluid or both may act as a force pushing the vitreous forward and increasing pupillary block. Rotation of ciliary processes forward against the iris with direct secondary angle closure may also be a factor. **Medical therapy** of cycloplegics to tighten the zonules and osmotics to dehydrate the vitreous may be tried, but most frequently **surgical therapy** of suprachoroidal fluid drainage and peripheral iridectomy are required.

F. Central retinal vein occlusion may rarely result in a reversible secondary angle-closure glaucoma, presumably the result of increased fluid volume in the vitreous or retina. The key to the diagnosis is the presence of true monocular angle closure and the severe impairment of vision from the vein occlusion. Because it is reversible after a few weeks, **standard medical therapy** for angle-closure glaucoma should be employed, except that maintained cycloplegics should be tried rather than miotics initially to tighten the zonules and reverse forward lens movement, as well as to dilate the pupil away from the lens.

XXVII. Glaucoma in children (see Chapter 11, sec. **XVII.**). Congenital glaucoma must be suspected in all babies with photophobia and excessive tearing. The cornea becomes hazy, and the eye often enlarges in size. In addition to this acute glaucoma, glaucoma in children may develop silently, as in adults. Whenever possible, measurement of IOP and inspection of the optic nerve head should be performed as a routine part of all ophthalmologic examinations.

XXVIII. Nonophthalmologic systemic medication in glaucoma patients. The physician must first differentiate between open-angle glaucoma and angle-closure glaucoma patients.

A. Angle-closure glaucoma. If a systemic medication causes the pupil to dilate, angle-closure glaucoma can be precipitated. Therefore, both systemic adrenergic and systemic anticholinergic medications can precipitate angle-closure glaucoma. Most patients who have diagnosed angle-closure glaucoma, however, will have been treated with a peripheral iridectomy in both eyes, and, therefore, the pupillary dilation that ensues from systemic medication will not cause the angle to close (unless the patient has the rare condition of plateau iris).

The **risk group** includes those patients with shallow anterior chambers and undiagnosed, asymptomatic, narrow, closeable angles. In these patients, pupillary dilation from systemic medication could cause the angle to close; therefore, the physician should routinely examine the depth of the anterior chamber in all patients with a flashlight projected tangential to the cornea. Cerebral vasodilators can be used with impunity in patients with narrow-angle glaucoma on the basis of all present data.

B. Open-angle glaucoma

1. **Systemic anticholinergics.** If a systemic medication paralyzes the ciliary muscle (cycloplegic effect), then, theoretically at least, this medication may worsen open-angle glaucoma because of the effect of ciliary muscle contraction on aqueous outflow. Those open-angle glaucoma patients who respond to topical anticholinergic drugs with a significant increase in IOP (highest risk group) demonstrate only a slight increase in IOP when given systemic anticholinergic drugs. This increase is easily controlled by standard glaucoma therapy. Therefore, if open-angle glaucoma patients need systemic anticholinergic therapy, it is possible for them to have it, provided there is ophthalmologic consultation so that the ophthalmologist can adjust the glaucoma therapy, if necessary.

2. **Systemic adrenergic drugs.** Administration of systemic dextroamphetamine sulfate (Dexedrine) to patients with open-angle glaucoma does not affect the IOP one way or the other. From this it can be assumed that systemic adrenergic agents are safe to give to open-angle glaucoma patients; vasodilator drugs are also safe. Systemic corticosteroids can increase IOP, and therefore ophthalmologic consultation should be requested. There is no absolute contraindication to their use in open-angle glaucoma patients, however, and most likely the effect of systemic corticosteroids on IOP can be managed by adjustment of the glaucoma therapy.

11. PEDIATRIC OPHTHALMOLOGY

Robert A. Petersen and William P. Boger III

Many of the methods of examination and ocular disorders relevant to adults also pertain to children. This chapter emphasizes the examinations, ocular disorders, and therapies that are especially relevant to pediatric patients. Strabismus is very prevalent in childhood, and the development of amblyopia is a problem up to age 9 or 10 years. (See Chapter 12 for many issues that often must be considered simultaneously in the care of pediatric patients.)

I. **Vision testing and clinical examination of the young patient**
   A. **Well-baby examinations.** Evaluation of visual function and the structural integrity of the ocular structures should be an integral portion of the pediatrician's routine examinations. The well-baby examination should include the following:
      1. **Newborn period**
         a. Pupillary responses to light.
         b. Size and clarity of cornea.
         c. Eye movements full in response to passive head turning.
         d. Red reflex with ophthalmoscope. (This maneuver screens for opacities in the media such as cataract as well as for gross fundus lesions.)
      2. **Infancy**
         a. Visual function (see sec. **I.B.,** below).
         b. Pupils round and reactive.
         c. Size and clarity of cornea.
         d. Eye movements full in following objects.
         e. When the child looks attentively at a flashlight, does the light reflex on the cornea fall in the middle of both corneas?
         f. Red reflex with ophthalmoscope.
      3. **Childhood**
         a. Formal visual acuity testing with verbal or matching responses from child after age 2 or 3 years.
         b. Glimpse of fundus details, especially the optic nerve, with direct ophthalmoscope.
         c. Remainder of examination as in sec. **I.E.,** below.
   B. **Evaluation of visual acuity.** The physician should concentrate on each eye separately when assessing visual acuity. A child may have a blinding disorder that needs attention or a life-threatening tumor in one eye and yet function normally with the other eye. Therefore, the examiner must **put an adhesive patch over one eye to ensure that the child is not peeking when assessing the visual acuity in the fellow eye.**
      1. **Newborn period.** Pupillary responses to light.
      2. **Infancy.** By 4 to 6 weeks of age, most infants will follow a light or large objects over a short range. By 3 months of age, they should fix on an object and follow it over a wide range and evidence social response to the examiner's or mother's face. If one eye is constantly deviated (inward with esotropia, outward with exotropia), the examiner must assume that its acuity is abnormal. A child with an eye deviation but with equal vision in the two eyes will alternately fixate with one eye and then the other. If available, preferential looking tests for infant vision such as the Teller acuity cards are quantitative and helpful.
      3. **Childhood.** At 2 or 3 years of age, most children are sufficiently verbal that a subjective visual acuity can be obtained using picture cards, such as Allen cards, or matching games, such as Lea symbols. **Each eye must be tested separately, and the child must not be able to peek.**

One or 2 years later, most children will be able to identify the letter E in various positions. After 1 or 2 more years, letters or numbers can be used. It is easiest to identify isolated figures, but by 5 or 6 years of age children should be able to read rows or clusters of letters. Visual acuity assessment should be checked annually.

C. **Indications for referral to an ophthalmologist**

1. **Newborn period.** Some referrals at this age are dictated by abnormalities noted by the pediatrician during the examination before discharge from the maternity unit. The panoramic view of the fundus provided by the indirect ophthalmoscope through the dilated pupil can provide important information not otherwise obtainable. Critically ill newborns who may have a congenital infection (see sec. **II.,** below), those with multiple congenital anomalies, and those suspected of having a chromosomal abnormality (see sec. **VI.,** below) should have indirect ophthalmoscopy. Very premature infants (see sec. **XII.** below) should have an ophthalmic examination before or shortly after discharge from the hospital, beginning at 30 to 32 weeks postconception and continuing until the retinal vessels are mature.

2. **Infancy.** During the first few months of life, many youngsters have brief periods when the eyes do not appear to be aligned. It is abnormal at any age, however, to have a constant ocular deviation. An infant with a constant ocular deviation should be promptly and thoroughly evaluated by an ophthalmologist. The referral should not be delayed in the hope that the deviation will improve spontaneously. Most constant deviations do not improve with time; more important, a constant deviation may be the first sign of a serious ocular disorder, such as a **retinoblastoma** (see sec. **XI.,** below).

   If an intermittent deviation of the eyes persists past 3 to 4 months, the child should be referred to an ophthalmologist for evaluation. Infants with physical abnormalities such as asymmetric or large corneas, cloudy corneas, or a dark fundus reflex with the ophthalmoscope should be promptly referred for evaluation. Delay in referring a youngster with a large cornea resulting from glaucoma (see sec. **XV.,** below) may contribute to irreparable loss of vision.

3. **Childhood**

   a. **Visual acuity** should be comparable in the two eyes and should be testable to at least 20/40 in both eyes by the age of 3 years. If the vision is less than 20/40 in either eye or if there is more than one line difference on the Snellen chart between the two eyes, the child should be evaluated by an ophthalmologist.

   b. **Identification of the cause of visual asymmetry** is important. Serious ocular disease may be the cause, or there may be a marked difference in the refraction of the two eyes. In the latter case, glasses (perhaps with patching) may fully correct the situation if instituted in the early years. Amblyopia from asymmetric refractive errors discovered several years later may be irreversible or much more difficult to treat (see Chapter 12, sec. **VI.D.**). **An adequate refraction cannot be done in infancy and early childhood without cycloplegic medication.**

   c. **Age at examination.** The question is often raised, "What is the best time to have my child's eyes checked?" If the child has an evident ocular abnormality, it should be evaluated by the ophthalmologist regardless of the age of the child. Although the child has no evident ocular problem and the pediatrician has found no abnormality on routine well-baby examination, some parents still request a routine eye examination. Three years of age is an ideal time for this kind of screening examination. At this age the child is old enough to give a subjective response to visual acuity testing and yet still young enough for effective amblyopia therapy if such an abnormality is discovered.

D. Medications in the young patient. Medications administered as eye drops may be absorbed through the mucous membranes in significant amounts and exert systemic effects. This fact is particularly important in infants and small children when multiple eye drops are administered. Adequate cycloplegia and mydriasis are usually achieved within 30 minutes after one drop of cyclopentolate 1% is instilled into each eye along with one additional drop 5 minutes later. If dilation is insufficient after 30 minutes, an additional waiting period is advisable. The use of additional cycloplegic drops runs the risk of toxic side effects with disorientation and ataxia. Alternatively, atropine 1% *ointment* can be used for 3 nights preceding the next office visit to obtain adequate mydriasis and cycloplegia.

Some ophthalmologists routinely use atropine and accordingly defer the fundus examination and refraction until the patient's second visit. The use of the shorter-acting cycloplegic–mydriatic agents such as cyclopentolate allows the examiner to rule out the presence of a serious ocular disorder such as retinoblastoma and makes possible a more thorough evaluation at the first visit. Cyclopentolate administered as described in the preceding paragraph provides satisfactory and reproducible cycloplegia for refraction. Appropriate glasses can therefore be prescribed for a refractive error or for strabismus therapy after the first visit.

E. Differential diagnosis of clinical presentations in childhood
  1. Cloudy cornea
   a. Unilateral
     (1) Infantile glaucoma.
     (2) Trauma with rupture of Descemet's membrane (forceps injury).
   b. Bilateral
     (1) Infantile glaucoma.
     (2) Corneal endothelial dystrophy.
     (3) Mucopolysaccharidose (Hurler, Scheie, Morquio, and Maroteaux-Lamy syndromes).
     (4) Mucolipidoses.
     (5) Interstitial keratitis (IK).
  2. Tearing
   a. Infantile glaucoma.
   b. Dacryostenosis.
  3. Large cornea
   a. Infantile glaucoma.
   b. Megalocornea (less likely).
  4. Photophobia
   a. Keratitis (herpes simplex).
   b. Infantile glaucoma.
   c. Uveitis.
   d. Achromatopsia.
  5. Red eye in newborn period (rule out trauma, uveitis, keratitis)
   a. Chemical conjunctivitis, formerly common with $AgNO_3$ prophylaxis (usually mild with onset 1 to 2 days after birth).
   b. Gonorrhea (purulent conjunctivitis, usual onset 1 to 3 days after birth).
   c. Chlamydial infection (usual onset 5 to 14 days after birth).
   d. Bacterial infection (staphylococcal or pneumococcal; usual onset 3 to 30 days after birth).
  6. Strabismus. All eye deviations should be assumed to be due to an organic lesion in the deviating eye (e.g., retinoblastoma) involving the macula until proved otherwise (see Chapter 12).
  7. Nystagmus
   a. Sensory nystagmus (associated with poor visual acuity):
     (1) Macular scars, e.g., toxoplasmosis.
     (2) Macular hypoplasia, e.g., albinism, aniridia.

        (3) Achromatopsia.

        (4) Retinal degeneration, e.g., Leber congenital amaurosis.

        (5) Optic nerve hypoplasia.

    b. Motor nystagmus (visual acuity is maximum in position of least nystagmus—the null point).

    c. Latent or occlusional nystagmus (nystagmus is induced or aggravated by covering one eye).

    d. Spasmus nutans (uniocular or markedly asymmetric nystagmus, often associated with head nodding, head cocking, and strabismus).

8. Unusual, gross, or chaotic eye movements

    a. Opsoclonus:

        (1) Neuroblastoma.

        (2) Encephalitis.

    b. Diencephalic ("happy waif") syndrome.

    c. Subacute necrotizing encephalomyelopathy (Leigh's disease).

9. Optic atrophy

    a. Associated with central nervous system (CNS) degenerative disorders, such as multiple sclerosis, adrenoleukodystrophy, metachromatic leukodystrophy, and subacute necrotizing encephalomyelopathy.

    b. Associated with CNS tumor, such as craniopharyngioma.

    c. Hereditary optic atrophies may be inherited in an X-linked fashion (Leber optic atrophy) or in a recessive fashion (Behr optic atrophy); dominantly inherited forms have also been reported.

    d. Secondary to retinal degeneration, as seen in Tay-Sachs disease, Niemann-Pick disease, G_{M1} gangliosidosis, mucopolysaccharidoses, retinitis pigmentosa, and allied disorders.

10. Cherry-red maculae

    a. Commotio retinae (following blunt trauma to the eye).

    b. Central retinal artery occlusion.

    c. Metabolic storage diseases

        (1) Tay-Sachs and Sandhoff's disease (G_{M2} gangliosidosis) (100% of individuals evidence this macular change).

        (2) Niemann-Pick disease (50% of affected individuals evidence this macular change).

        (3) G_{M1} gangliosidosis, infantile form.

        (4) Farber lipogranulomatosis (subtle grayness around fovea, difficult to distinguish from normal).

        (5) Metachromatic leukodystrophy (subtle grayness around fovea, difficult to distinguish from normal).

        (6) Sialidosis.

11. Subluxed or dislocated lenses

    a. Marfan syndrome.

    b. Homocystinuria.

    c. Weill-Marchesani syndrome (short stature, brachycephaly, stubby fingers and toes with joint stiffness, spherophakia, myopia).

    d. Sulfite oxidase deficiency.

    e. Traumatic.

    f. Familial idiopathic.

12. White pupil (leukocoria)

    a. Retinoblastoma.

    b. Cataract.

    c. Retinal detachment.

    d. Severe posterior uveitis from any cause.

    e. Severe cicatricial retinopathy of prematurity (ROP).

    f. Persistent hyperplastic primary vitreous.

    g. Retinal dysplasia (Norrie's disease).

    h. Coats's disease.

13. **Proptosis**
   a. Rhabdomyosarcoma.
   b. Orbital cellulitis.
   c. Inflammatory pseudotumor of the orbit.
   d. Optic nerve glioma.
   e. Retrobulbar hemorrhage.
   f. Thyroid ophthalmopathy.
   g. Chloroma (granulocytic leukemia).
   h. Neuroblastoma.
   i. Histiocytosis.
14. **Lid ecchymosis**
   a. Trauma.
   b. Neuroblastoma.
15. **Hyphema**
   a. Trauma.
   b. Juvenile xanthogranuloma.
   c. Tumor (retinoblastoma, rare presentation).
   d. Herpes simplex uveitis (uncommon presentation).
16. **Microphthalmos**
   a. Developmental anomaly.
   b. Persistent hyperplastic primary vitreous.
   c. Chromosomal anomaly.
   d. Congenital rubella syndrome.

II. **Congenital and neonatal infection** (**TORCH titers:** *t*oxoplasmosis, *o*ther [syphilis and others], *r*ubella, *c*ytomegalovirus, *h*erpes simplex)
   A. **Infections that are usually congenital**
      1. **Congenital toxoplasmosis.** Although ocular lesions may occasionally be acquired during a primary infection in adulthood, the vast majority of ocular toxoplasmosis lesions result from congenital infections. The characteristic lesion is a focal necrotizing retinitis. It may be solitary or in small clusters and is commonly in the posterior pole. Juxtapapillary lesions are not uncommon.
         a. **Physical findings. Classic findings of congenital toxoplasmosis are** focal necrotizing retinitis, intracranial calcification, and hepatosplenomegaly, but there is a wide spectrum of presentations. **Severely affected children** have massive inflammation of the retina, choroid, and vitreous; cataract; strabismus; microphthalmos; and petechial hemorrhages in the newborn period. **Mildly affected children** may be left with only small inconspicuous retinal scars and positive serologic titers.
         b. **Treatment** (see Chapter 9, sec. **VIII.B.**).
      2. **Congenital syphilis.** The introduction of penicillin dramatically reduced the incidence of syphilis in general, with a concomitant reduction in the incidence of congenital syphilis. In recent years, however, there has been a resurgence of syphilis in the population as a whole, and in 1988 crude rates of primary and secondary syphilis reached their highest levels in 40 years. Reported rates of congenital syphilis in 1988 were also the highest for the past several decades. In contrast to the stages of acquired syphilis, congenital syphilis has no primary stage.
         a. **Early congenital syphilis.** The sequelae of focal inflammation in the intrauterine and early formative years become apparent in bony and structural malformation. Manifestations of the first 2 years of life are as follows:
            (1) **Inflammatory manifestations**
               (a) Dermal eruption, vesicular or pustular.
               (b) Mucous membrane involvement:
                  (i) Purulent snuffles.
                  (ii) **Conjunctivitis** (treponemes can be isolated).
               (c) Periostitis ("pseudoparalysis" of limb).

  (d) Generalized lymphadenopathy.
  (e) A severely affected infant may have
    (i) Hepatosplenomegaly.
    (ii) Hyperbilirubinemia.
    (iii) Anemia.
  (f) **Chorioretinitis**
    (i) More common: widespread, small, focal yellowish-white exudates leading to "salt-and-pepper" fundus—tends to be bilateral, heals spontaneously, and is said not to recur.
    (ii) Less common: isolated peripheral circumscribed lesions.
  (g) Rhagades (cracks or fissures about the mouth or nose resulting from infantile syphilitic rhinitis).
  (2) **Sequelae of focal inflammation**
    (a) Bone deformities:
      (i) Frontal bossing of skull.
      (ii) Saber shins.
      (iii) Scaphoid scapulas.
      (iv) Saddle nose.
      (v) Scoliosis.
      (vi) Perforation of hard palate.
      (vii) Clutton joints (painless hydroarthrosis, usually of the knees).
    (b) Teeth deformities:
      (i) Hutchinson teeth (notched and barrel-shaped central incisors).
      (ii) Mulberry or Moon molars (maldeveloped cusps of first molars).
    (c) Psychomotor retardation.
  b. **Late congenital syphilis** is more analogous to latent forms of acquired syphilis. Manifestations include:
    (1) **Neurosyphilis**
      (a) Optic atrophy.
      (b) Pupillary abnormalities.
      (c) Eighth nerve deafness.
    (2) **IK.** This condition usually results from congenital syphilis but may occur after acquired syphilis. With the former, the onset is usually between 5 and 20 years, although it has been observed at birth. Although IK often appears in later life, treponemes have been isolated from clear corneas in newborns. The pathogenesis of IK may be immunologic. IK has occasionally been reported after adequate treatments with penicillin in early years of life.
3. **Congenital rubella syndrome (CRS).** Formerly common, CRS has become rare in the United States since rubella vaccination was introduced in the late 1960s. CRS is now mostly seen in immigrants from nonimmunized populations. Approximately 50% of mothers with clinical evidence of rubella infection during the first month of gestation will bear offspring with malformations at birth. Slightly lower rates of malformation follow rubella infections during the second and third months of gestation. The **classic physical findings** are as follows:
a. **Ocular findings**
  (1) Nuclear cataract in newborn period with surrounding zone of clear cortex; gradual progression so lens becomes pearly white.
  (2) Microphthalmos closely associated with presence of cataract.
  (3) Congenital or infantile glaucoma. The infant may or may not have cataract as well; the cataracts and the infantile glaucoma are independent variables.
  (4) Corneas transiently hazy without increased intraocular pressure (IOP), possibly due to a keratitis or to an endothelial dysfunction, and may lead to permanent scarring.

        (5) Speckled retinitis of posterior pole "like a piece of coarse Scotch tweed over which pepper has been strewn," but not usually causing vision loss.

   b. Nonocular findings

        (1) Congenital heart disease.

        (2) Neurosensory deafness, may be acquired in early childhood and is not necessarily congenital, but may be an isolated abnormality from infection in the second trimester.

   c. Current knowledge about CRS was greatly increased by intensive study of the United States epidemic in 1964 and 1965. It is now clear that affected youngsters actively shed virus up until 2 years of age. Virus has been recovered from lens material as late as 3 years of age. It is still unclear how long virus persists within the congenitally infected individual. The persistence of virus in these individuals is not a matter of immunologic tolerance, because the rubella child's serologic and cell-mediated responses have been appropriate. During the 1960s, a multisystem disease, the **expanded rubella syndrome,** was identified during the first months of life. Signs of this expanded rubella syndrome include:

        (1) Thrombocytopenia and consequent purpura (blueberry muffin baby).

        (2) Bone lesions.

        (3) Hepatitis.

        (4) Hemolytic anemia.

        (5) CNS involvement.

   d. Late-onset disease. From 3 months of age until the end of the first year, several other clinical problems may arise. These problems include a generalized rash with seborrheic features, an interstitial pneumonitis that is responsive to corticosteroids, and lymphocytic infiltration of the pancreas. These manifestations of late-onset disease have been difficult to explain, and the question of an immunologic mechanism stimulated by the rubella virus has been raised.

   e. Intrauterine infection with rubella does not act simply as a teratogenic agent. It clearly stimulates an ongoing process that has neonatal features but may also cause continuing disease. Some youngsters with the congenital rubella syndrome have measurable hearing in early childhood, but when they are tested 2 years later they have become entirely deaf. The mechanism of this progressive loss is uncertain. A handful of youngsters born with maternal rubella syndrome have developed a panencephalitis at 10 or 12 years of age, with rubella virus recoverable from the brain at that time.

   f. Ophthalmologic care of these children starts with attention to cataracts and glaucoma in infancy. The glaucoma is treated as described under infantile glaucoma (see sec. **XVII.A.,** below). When cataracts are bilateral, they should be aspirated in the first few months of life. As much lens material as possible should be removed during the operation.

      Infants with congenital rubella syndrome who have had surgery for glaucoma or cataract *must* be followed regularly throughout life. The onset of intraocular inflammation or glaucoma (or both) has occurred even 10 or 15 years after initial successful and uneventful surgery. Late retinal detachment is also a complication of cataract surgery.

   g. Cytomegalovirus (CMV) belongs to the herpes group and is a common virus. Many women have complement-fixation titers to CMV by their childbearing years. Approximately 4% to 5% of pregnant women actively excrete CMV in their urine. Postnatal infections are also possible, because 25% of women with positive antibody of CMV have the virus in breast milk. Most neonates with congenital CMV are asymptomatic. Now that these youngsters can be identified serologically and followed longitudinally, it appears that there is an increased incidence of psychomotor retardation and microcephaly. A small subgroup of neonates with congenital CMV are very sick with hepatosplenomegaly, hyperbilirubinemia, thrombocytopenia, and petechiae. Intrauterine growth retardation and microcephaly may be evident at birth, and there may be encephalitis with or without hydrocephalus. Chorioretinitis similar to that seen with congenital toxoplasmosis has been reported. Intracranial calcification, hydrocephalus, hepatosplenomegaly, and focal chorioretinitis resulting from CMV may mimic congenital toxoplasmosis. The chorioretinitis reported in **congenital** CMV has been focal, in contrast to the widespread retinal necrosis and "smeary" hemorrhage described in adults in the context of an **acquired** CMV infection in an immunologically compromised host, e.g., following renal transplant or in human immunodeficiency virus-positive patients. Ganciclovir and foscarnet are U.S. Food and Drug Administration approved for use in progressive CMV retinitis in immunocompromised patients (see Chapter 9, sec. **VIII.A.**).

B. **Ophthalmia neonatorum.** These hyperacute infections are generally acquired after rupture of the membranes during the time the child is in contact with the mother's cervix and vaginal tract. They may occur anytime in the first month of life and be considered neonatal. Potential **etiologic agents** include chemical conjunctivitis from 1% silver nitrate antimicrobial instilled prophylactically at birth, *Chlamydia trachomatis* (inclusion blennorrhea), *Staphylococcus aureus, Streptococcus pneumoniae, Haemophilus* sp, *Pseudomonas* sp, *Neisseria gonorrhoeae,* and herpes simplex virus (HSV) (see Chapter 5, secs. **III.B.** and **IV.C,D.**; Table 5.2; and Chapter 9, sec. **X.B.** for additional discussion).

1. **Herpes simplex.** Rarely, a youngster may be born with evidence of infection acquired during pregnancy. Such evidence includes microcephaly, cerebral calcification, chorioretinitis, and mental retardation. The more usual form is acquired at the time of birth.

   a. **Neonatal herpes simplex**
      (1) **Cutaneous** manifestations may be present without systemic involvement. Cutaneous vesicles may be present with or without **conjunctivitis,** and with or without **keratitis.** The keratitis may present as a **classic dendrite.**
      (2) **The disseminated form** has an average onset of 1 week of age. The neonate may be severely ill with jaundice, fever, hepatosplenomegaly, encephalitis, and disseminated intravascular coagulopathy. There may be few or no skin lesions to help with the diagnosis.
      (3) The more localized form of **CNS involvement** without systemic visceral involvement has an average onset of 11 days. It is more likely to have herpetic skin vesicles. Apparently the virus is rarely isolated from the CNS in this form.

   b. Neonatal systemic infection with HSV is almost invariably symptomatic and often lethal; only rare cases of inapparent infection have been documented despite large-scale attempts to identify these patients. The role of brain biopsy for early diagnosis is controversial. The availability of antiviral agents such as vidarabine and acyclovir has provided new possibilities for systemic therapy. The risk of transmission to offspring when maternal genital lesions are present at birth has been estimated at 40%. Transmission to the offspring is common when delivery follows rupture of the membranes by more than 6 hours, whereas abdominal delivery within 4 hours of membrane breaking appears to reduce the risk of intrauterine spread.

2. **Gonorrhea.** It is wise to consider **all purulent conjunctivitis in the first few days of life as gonococcal until proved otherwise.** The

rapidity with which gonococcus can penetrate the cornea has been well documented, and gonococcal conjunctivitis presents a true ophthalmic emergency.

a. Once the diagnosis is made by Gram stain of conjunctival scraping, the child should be hospitalized and **treated** with high-dose parenteral and topical antibiotics. Confirmatory cultures should be planted on Thayer-Martin medium. Although prophylaxis with silver nitrate drops or antibiotic ointment is helpful against the organism, the current epidemic of gonococcal disease makes it prudent to maintain a high suspicion for gonococcal conjunctivitis not only in the newborn period but at all ages. The parents should be treated as well as the neonate.

b. Treatment guidelines for gonococcal disease are also described in Chapter 5, sec. **III.D.**

   (1) Infants born to mothers with untreated gonococcal infections are at high risk of infection (e.g., ophthalmia and disseminated gonococcal infection) and should be treated with a single injection of **ceftriaxone** (50 mg per kg intravenous [i.v.] or intramuscular [i.m.], not to exceed 125 mg). Ceftriaxone should be given cautiously to hyperbilirubinemic infants, especially premature infants. Topical prophylaxis for neonatal ophthalmia is not adequate treatment for documented infections of the eye or other sites.

   (2) Neonates with clinical gonococcal ophthalmia should be evaluated by a careful physical examination, especially of the joints, blood, and cerebrospinal fluid (CSF) cultures. Infants with gonococcal ophthalmia should be treated for 7 days (10 to 14 days if meningitis is present) with one of the following regimens:

   (a) Ceftriaxone 25 to 50 mg/kg/day i.v. or i.m. qd **or**

   (b) Cefotaxime 25 mg per kg i.v. or i.m. q12h. Children older than 8 years of age should also be given **doxycycline** 100 mg bid for 7 days. All patients should be evaluated for coinfection with syphilis and *C. trachomatis.* Follow-up cultures are necessary to ensure that treatment has been effective.

   (3) Alternative regimens

   (a) Limited data suggest that uncomplicated (no corneal involvement) gonococcal ophthalmia among infants may be cured with a single injection of **ceftriaxone** (50 up to 100 mg per kg). A few experts use this regimen for children who have no clinical or laboratory evidence of disseminated disease.

   (b) The quinolones, **ciprofloxacin** and **norfloxacin,** are highly active against gonococcus and may be given p.o. *with caution* to children, including the penicillin-allergic child, under the guidance of a pediatrician or infectious disease specialist. Adult dosage is 1.0 g p.o. q12h for ciprofloxacin, or 1.2 g p.o. for norfloxacin once if no corneal involvement or q12h for 7 to 14 days with corneal involvement. Pediatric dosage is per the guidance of the specialist.

   (c) If the gonococcal isolate is proved to be susceptible to penicillin, **crystalline penicillin G** may be given. The dosage is 100,000 units/kg/day given in two equal doses (four equal doses per day for infants more than 1 week old). The dosage should be increased to 150,000 units/kg/day for meningitis.

   (d) Infants with gonococcal ophthalmia should receive **eye irrigations** with buffered saline solutions until discharge has cleared. Topical antibiotic therapy alone is inadequate.

   (e) Simultaneous infection with *C. trachomatis* and syphilis has been reported and should be considered for patients who do not respond satisfactorily. Therefore, the mother and infant should be tested for chlamydial and syphilitic infection.

3. **Inclusion conjunctivitis (blennorrhea, chlamydial infection)** is caused by *Chlamydia trachomatis*. Credé 1% silver nitrate prophylaxis is not effective against inclusion blennorrhea. The conjunctivitis usually commences 5 to 12 days after birth.

   a. The **diagnosis** is made by observation of cytoplasmic inclusions on a Giemsa stain of conjunctival scrapings. There is a mixed cellular response in these scrapings, with both mononuclear cells and polymorphonuclear cells present. Culture and nonculture methods for diagnosis of *C. trachomatis* (Microtrak) are also now available. Results of chlamydial tests should be interpreted with care. The sensitivity of all currently available laboratory tests for *C. trachomatis* tests is substantially less than 100%; thus, false-negative and false-positive tests are possible.

   b. **Therapy.** Because the presence of chlamydial agents in the conjunctiva implies colonization of the upper respiratory tract as well, systemic erythromycin (125 mg p.o. qid for 3 weeks) should be given. Sulfisoxazole is the alternative drug (see Appendix B). The infant should also receive topical sulfonamide, erythromycin, or tetracycline qid for 3 weeks. Both parents should be treated (see Chapter 5, sec. **IV.C.**).

   c. **Long-term follow-up** has indicated that poorly treated individuals may develop a trachoma-like corneal pannus or vascularization. Appropriate **topical** antibiotic therapy appears to prevent this. Some children born to mothers with chlamydial infections do not have conjunctivitis but still develop antibodies to the organism, and the agent of inclusion blennorrhea has recently been implicated as the cause of a severe pneumonitis in infancy.

4. **Prevention of ophthalmia neonatorum.** Instillation of a prophylactic agent into the eyes of all newborn infants is recommended to prevent gonococcal ophthalmia neonatorum, and is required by law in most states. Although all regimens listed below effectively prevent gonococcal eye disease, their efficacy in preventing chlamydial eye disease is not clear. Furthermore, they do not eliminate nasopharyngeal colonization with *C. trachomatis*. Prophylaxis of gonococcal and chlamydial disease is

   a. **Erythromycin** (0.5%) ophthalmic ointment, once, **or**

   b. **Tetracycline** (1%) ophthalmic ointment once.

   c. **Silver nitrate** (1%) aqueous solution, is **not** effective against *Chlamydia* and causes unacceptable chemical conjunctivitis; antibiotics are the treatment of choice.

III. **Infections of childhood**

   A. **Orbital cellulitis versus preseptal (periorbital) cellulitis**

   1. **Preseptal cellulitis.** Facial cellulitis that happens to involve the lids may produce alarming swelling and closure of the lids. The eye itself, however, retains full range of movement, is not proptotic, and has good visual acuity and normal pupillary reactions. Like cellulitis elsewhere, staphylococcal or streptococcal etiology is most likely, and parenteral antibiotics are indicated.

   H. influenzae must also be considered, especially in young children.

   2. **Orbital cellulitis** denotes the infection of tissues behind the orbital septum, involving orbital structures, to produce proptosis, chemosis, limitation of eye movement, and possible loss of vision. The orbit is usually infected from a contiguous structure; often sinusitis is the cause, and in a young child *Haemophilus* infection must be considered. Blood cultures and consultation with an otolaryngologist are indicated. This is a life-threatening condition and requires emergency treatment.

Exploration of the orbit itself is not usually indicated immediately, but may be necessary later if an abscess forms. In addition to parenteral antibiotics, surgical drainage of the contiguous abscess or sinus infection by an otolaryngologist may be indicated.

B. *Toxocara canis* is a nematode infestation that may present as a large vitreoretinal mass. Pica has been implicated in the etiology, particularly when dirt has been contaminated by animal feces. Covers for sandboxes are highly recommended as a prophylactic measure. The diagnosis is difficult to establish conclusively on clinical grounds. Eosinophilia of the peripheral blood may be helpful. A serologic test, enzyme-linked immunosorbent assay, is available at the Centers for Disease Control (CDC) in Atlanta, Georgia, and in many state laboratories. Active systemic infestation with *T. canis* is almost never present when ocular involvement is noted. Presumably, the ocular lesion is a late sequela of systemic infestation (see Chapter 9, sec. **VIII.C.**).

C. **Subacute sclerosing panencephalitis (SSPE)** presents as an intellectual and behavioral deterioration in school-age children. There may be rhythmic myoclonic jerking. A focal chorioretinitis may be present. The chorioretinitis frequently, but not always, affects the macular region. Because SSPE is a panencephalitis, cortical blindness, optic atrophy, nystagmus on a neurologic basis, and papilledema may occur. SSPE is a slow virus disease that occurs after naturally acquired measles infection in 5 to 10 cases per million. It may more rarely follow live measles vaccination (0.5 to 1.1 cases per million). No specific therapy for the chorioretinal lesions is available.

IV. **Inflammations of childhood**

A. **Juvenile rheumatoid arthritis (JRA)**

1. The basic **ocular** lesion is iridocyclitis. In contrast to most other forms of iridocyclitis, ocular inflammation associated with JRA is chronic and insidious, with minimum or no injection or symptoms until complications have already set in. Cataract, glaucoma, band keratopathy, and synechiae are all consequences of the basic inflammation.

2. **Nonocular** aspects of JRA can be subdivided into (a) systemic disease with arthritic disease and (b) two forms of joint disease with less prominent systemic manifestations: polyarticular arthritis and pauciarticular arthritis. Ocular disease is extremely rare in systemic disease with arthritic disease. It is uncommon in the polyarticular variety and is most often seen in youngsters, especially girls, with only a few joints involved. It is associated with antinuclear antibody positivity and histocompatibility leukocyte antigen (HLA) class II antigens, e.g., HLA-DR5. The ocular inflammation may come long after the arthritis has completely resolved or may precede the onset of arthritis. Because the early stages of ocular inflammation are asymptomatic in JRA, it seems wisest to examine these youngsters routinely every 4 to 6 months. Therapy of the iritis involves the use of topical steroids and topical mydriatics (see Chapter 9, sec. **VIII.A.6.**).

B. **Ankylosing spondylitis**

1. **Iridocyclitis** of ankylosing spondylitis is usually highly symptomatic. When the inflammation begins, the patient has photophobia and discomfort in the eye, and the eye has a ciliary flush or perilimbal injection. The iridocyclitis is acute and remits with topical steroids and mydriatic–cycloplegics, but it may be recurrent (see Chapter 9, sec. **VIII.A.2.**).

2. **The tissue-type antigen HLA-B27** is relatively uncommon in the normal population (6%) but is very prevalent in the population with ankylosing spondylitis (90%). Fifty percent of all patients with acute anterior uveitis, regardless of cause, have positive HLA-B27. Patients with JRA do not differ significantly from the population with anterior uveitis in general, 42% of them being HLA-B27 positive.

C. **Peripheral uveitis–intermediate uveitis** (pars planitis, peripheral retinal vasculitis) is a chronic inflammation that may present as iridocyclitis. The diagnosis does not become apparent until a careful examination of the peripheral retina is performed and until cellular debris is found in "snowbanks" along the vitreous base. The etiology is not clear. Systemic corticosteroids or periocular steroid injections can reduce the inflammation, but in view of the chronic nature of the disorder, these therapies are usually reserved for microcystic edema of the macula or intense vitreous involvement that reduces vision (see Chapter 9, sec. **VIII.B.**).

D. **Erythema multiforme.** The conjunctiva along with other mucous membranes may become inflamed in severe erythema multiforme. Cleansing of the lids and lubrication with bland antibiotic ointments are recommended. Topical steroids and sweeping of the fornices have been advocated as therapies and have some theoretic justification, but conclusive evidence for their efficacy has not been presented. **Herpes simplex** must be thoroughly excluded in the differential diagnosis before topical steroid administration is considered.

E. **Inflammatory pseudotumor of the orbit** is a poorly understood cause of recurrent orbital inflammation and proptosis. The diagnosis is generally made only by exclusion of other causes. Regression of the orbital mass after systemic corticosteroids has been helpful diagnostically and therapeutically.

V. **Principles of genetics and genetic counseling**

A. **Basic genetic principles.** Hereditary characteristics are carried on loci on the chromosomes called *genes*. The normal number of human chromosomes is 46, one-half being inherited from the father and one-half from the mother. There are 22 pairs of autosomes plus, in the female, two X chromosomes and, in the male, an X and a Y chromosome. Deviations from the normal number of chromosomes, either extra chromosomal material or deficient chromosomal material, cause severe abnormalities.

1. **Alleles.** The alternative forms that genes in a particular locus on a chromosome may take are called *alleles*. An individual who inherits the same gene from both parents is called *homozygous*. If the two allelic genes are different, the individual is said to be *heterozygous*. The sex chromosomes are paired in the female (two X chromosomes), and the male has an X and a Y chromosome.

The X chromosome contains much more genetic material than the Y. In the male, the genetic material on his single X chromosome is not paired. The male is said to be *hemizygous* for the characteristics represented by the genes on his single X chromosome.

2. **Inheritance and expression of genetic traits.** The individual's genetic makeup as inherited from his or her parents is known as the *genotype*. These inherited characteristics may or may not be expressed in a way that affects the individual's appearance or functioning. The outward expression of the genotype is called the *phenotype*. The phenotype depends on the mode of inheritance of various characteristics. It may also be affected by the environment.

3. **Modes of inheritance.** The three modes of inheritance are dominant, recessive, and X-linked.

a. In **dominant inheritance,** the expression of a specific trait is determined by only one of the pair of genes and is not affected by its allele. Therefore, an individual with a dominantly inherited disease will be affected when one of the allelic genes is abnormal even if the other one is normal. Examples of dominantly inherited disorders are Marfan syndrome and neurofibromatosis. Both alleles may be expressed simultaneously, in which case they are called *codominant.* An example would be in the hemoglobinopathies, in which both members of the pair of genes will be expressed phenotypically. Thus, an individual may be AA (normal), SA (sickle trait), SS (sickle cell disease), or

SC (sickle-C disease). Dominantly inherited diseases are not expressed in all individuals who carry the gene, but may still be passed on to the offspring of unaffected carriers.

b. In **recessive inheritance,** the expression of the trait determined by a recessive gene is masked by the presence of its allele. An innocuous example would be a gene for blue eyes being masked by the gene for brown eyes, so that an individual who is heterozygous for eye color would have brown eyes. Many metabolic disorders are inherited recessively (see sec. **VII.,** below). Individuals who are heterozygous for recessively inherited disorders (carriers) generally have a normal phenotype but may be identifiable biochemically. For example, individuals heterozygous for Tay-Sachs disease may be identified because they have less than the normal concentration of the enzyme hexosaminidase-A, but this partial deficiency is not enough to cause abnormal function. The homozygote is severely and fatally affected by an almost total absence of the enzyme.

Patients who are homozygous for a recessively inherited disease may be protected by their environment from phenotypic expression of the disorder. This protection may, in fact, form the basis for treatment. Patients with galactosemia (deficiency of the enzyme galactose-1-phosphate uridyl transferase) who are not exposed to galactose in the diet will remain normal.

c. In **X-linked inheritance,** affected males manifest traits carried on the X chromosome, i.e., they are hemizygous. Carrier females have the normal allele on one of the paired X chromosomes. A classic example of X-linked inheritance is red-green **color blindness.** Carrier females, with only one abnormal gene for color blindness and a normal allele on the other X chromosome, have normal color vision. Affected males, having only the gene for protanopia (red blindness) or deuteranopia (green blindness), are "color blind" for certain colors but not all colors; they are really color anomalous rather than color blind. Heterozygote female carriers of X-linked disorders may sometimes be phenotypically identified or may express the disease in milder form than their hemizygous sons. An explanation of this phenomenon is the **Lyon hypothesis.** Each cell of a female acts as if one or the other of her X chromosomes is inactivated, so that only one of each of the allelic genes on the chromosomes can be expressed. This would make each female a mosaic in which about one-half of the cells have one X chromosome active and the other one-half have the other X chromosome active. Heterozygous females with Fabry's disease exhibit the ocular findings, but not such severe and ultimately fatal systemic manifestations as their hemizygous male relatives suffer (see sec. **VII.B.7.,** below).

B. **Genetic counseling.** The psychosocial aspects of genetic counseling are important. When an abnormal child is born to a set of parents, there is psychic trauma, including feelings of guilt, which may be aggravated if the disorder is inherited. If the parents want more children, they will need to be advised about the chances of producing another affected offspring. The physician's role is to advise the parents about the chances of having further affected offspring and to explain ways of preventing the birth of an unwanted affected offspring, if the parents so desire. The physician must refrain from advising the parents whether or not to have more children. The parents should make the decision, based on the best information the physician can give. In some straightforward cases, the ophthalmologist can provide the genetic counseling; in more complicated situations, the parents should be referred to a clinical geneticist.

1. **Autosomal-recessive disorders.** If a child has a disorder recognized to be recessively inherited, each of the parents must be phenotypically unaffected carriers of the abnormal recessive gene; i.e., each parent

must be heterozygous for the abnormality. Chances of future offspring being affected can be calculated by recognizing that one-half of the mother's eggs and one-half of the father's sperm will contain the normal gene and the other one-half the abnormal allele. There is a 25% chance that both normal genes will be present in the offspring, a 25% chance that both abnormal genes will be present in the offspring, producing an individual homozygous for the disease, and a 50% chance that the offspring will be heterozygous for the abnormal gene (25% of the offspring will get a normal gene from the father and an abnormal gene from the mother, and 25% will get an abnormal gene from the father and a normal gene from the mother). These heterozygotes will be phenotypically normal; therefore, it can be predicted that **each** future offspring will have a 25% chance of being abnormal and a 75% chance of being normal. It will depend on the family situation and the nature of the disorder whether the parents will find these odds acceptable or unacceptable for having further children.

Fortunately, in a few instances of recessively inherited diseases, diagnosis of the disease can be made antenatally in the fetus through **amniocentesis.** The classic example is **Tay-Sachs disease.** Genetic counseling may begin even before marriage. This gangliosidosis has a much higher incidence in individuals with Ashkenazic Jewish ancestry (4% are carriers) than in the general population. The deficiency of hexosaminidase-A can be identified in the heterozygous carriers, so Ashkenazic Jewish populations can be screened and individuals advised of their genotype for this illness. Heterozygous individuals may decide not to marry each other or to refrain from having children. In families where such premarital screening has not occurred, with the birth of a child affected with Tay-Sachs disease, **amniocentesis** can provide a way of avoiding the birth of future affected offspring. If further children are desired, cells from the fetus can be obtained by amniocentesis and grown in tissue culture so the level of hexosaminidase-A can be measured. If the fetus is identified as lacking the enzyme, the parents may elect therapeutic abortion. If the fetus is a heterozygote, or homozygous normal, the pregnancy can be carried to term. Unfortunately, biochemical assays that may be performed after amniocentesis are currently limited to only a few inherited diseases.

2. **Dominantly inherited disorders.** An individual who is affected with a dominantly inherited disorder is known to be carrying an abnormal gene that is presumably paired with a normal allele. Fifty percent of the gametes, i.e., eggs or sperm, of the affected individual will have the abnormal gene and 50% will be normal. Because all gametes from the other parent will presumably be normal, each offspring has a 50% chance of being born with the dominantly inherited gene. Because of partial penetrance of most dominant genes, somewhat less than 50% of the offspring will be phenotypically affected.

3. **X-linked recessive disorders.** Female carriers of X-linked recessively inherited disorders can often be identified because they have some phenotypic characteristic. They may also be identified by tracing the family tree. The daughter of a man affected with an X-linked recessive characteristic must be a carrier, because one of her X chromosomes to make her a female must have come from her father. Because a male must get his single X chromosome from his mother, he cannot inherit an X-linked recessive characteristic from his father. An affected maternal uncle or grandfather may help to identify a mother as a carrier. Each of a female carrier's sons will have a 50% chance of inheriting the X-linked recessive characteristic. When a woman is known to be a carrier of a severe X-linked recessive disorder, amniocentesis and therapeutic abortion may be used to prevent the birth of male offspring, each of which has a 50% chance of being affected. Chromosomal

analysis can be performed on the fetal cells to determine the sex of the fetus.

If the parents are opposed to the therapeutic abortion on religious grounds, amniocentesis should not be offered because the information gained would be of no therapeutic significance. Because the procedure carries a small risk to the mother and to the possibly normal fetus, it should be performed only if the information gathered will be used.

VI. **Chromosomal abnormalities**

A. **Basic principles.** Chromosomes are classified according to their microscopic morphology into eight groups, A through G, and numbered from 1 through 22, plus the X and Y chromosomes. Different chromosomes and different regions of each chromosome may be distinguished by staining techniques called *banding.* The centromere of each chromosome divides it into long and short arms. The short arm is represented by "p" and the long arm by "q." Chromosomes are prepared for analysis by culturing tissues (most commonly skin fibroblasts or leukocytes), arresting the cell division in metaphase by use of colchicine, and staining the chromosomes appropriately for microscopic examination.

Two kinds of abnormal occurrences during meiosis (cell division leading to gamete formation) may lead to chromosomal abnormalities: **nondysjunction** and **translocation.** In normal meiosis, each pair of chromosomes contributes one chromosome to each daughter cell so that each egg or sperm has 23 single chromosomes (the haploid number).

1. In **nondysjunction,** the two chromosomes of a specific pair remain together; as a result, one of the daughter cells gets both chromosomes and the other gets neither. If the gamete (daughter cell) receiving both chromosomes of a pair combines with a normal gamete during fertilization, the resulting zygotes will contain an extra chromosome. This is called **trisomy.** If the gamete that is missing the chromosome in question entirely combines with a normal gamete during fertilization, the resulting zygote will have only a single chromosome of the pair in question. This deletion produces **monosomy.**

2. **Translocation** can produce partial trisomies or deletions. During formation of the gamete, chromosomal breakage may occur and genetic material may be exchanged between chromosomes. If this exchange is uneven, part of the original chromosome will be duplicated in one of the new chromosomes, and part will be missing in the other. This leads to a **partial trisomy** or partial deletion. Trisomy 13 and trisomy 21 usually result from nondysjunction but sometimes translocation. Except for Turner syndrome, which is caused by deletion of an entire X chromosome, the major chromosomal deletion syndromes are due to partial deletion secondary to translocation. Balanced translocation results in a phenotypically normal individual. However, because the gametes of that individual have loss or duplication of genetic material, the offspring will suffer from partial deletion or partial trisomy.

3. **Chromosomal mosaicism** is the condition in which some of an individual's cells contain the trisomy or the deletion and others contain the normal number of chromosomes. These individuals may be less severely affected phenotypically.

B. The most common **trisomies that produce ocular abnormalities** are trisomy 21 (G trisomy or Down syndrome), trisomy 13 (D trisomy or Patau syndrome), and trisomy 18 (E trisomy or Edwards syndrome).

1. **Trisomy 21 (Down syndrome).** Patients with trisomy 21 have nearly normal life spans, and the ophthalmologist will be called on to follow the patients and to intervene when necessary. Correction of high refractive errors, treatment of blepharitis and amblyopia associated with esotropia, and surgical treatment of cataracts may all be necessary to help these patients function optimally.

a. The major **ocular findings** are
  (1) Upward slanting palpebral fissures.
  (2) Almond-shaped palpebral fissures.
  (3) Epicanthus.
  (4) Telecanthus.
  (5) Narrowed interpupillary distance.
  (6) Esotropia (35%).
  (7) Blepharitis.
  (8) High refractive errors.
  (9) Cataracts.
  (10) Brushfield spots.
  (11) Iris hypoplasia.
  (12) Keratoconus.
b. The major **systemic findings** are
  (1) Mental deficiency.
  (2) Small stature.
  (3) Defective, awkward gait.
  (4) Congenital heart disease.
  (5) Dry, rough skin.
  (6) Brachycephaly.
  (7) Small nose.
  (8) Small, round external ears.
  (9) Thick, protruding tongue.
  (10) Dental hypoplasia.
  (11) Short, thick neck.
  (12) Hypotonia.
  (13) Small, broad, stubby hands, and incurved little finger.
  (14) Transverse palmar crease.
  (15) Short, broad feet with gap between first and second toes.
  (16) Renal hemangiomas.
  (17) Infertility.
  (18) Undescended testes.
  (19) Duodenal atresia.
  (20) Cleft lip and palate.
2. **Trisomy 13 (D trisomy, Patau syndrome).** The life expectancy is only a few months, so even though the eyes are severely affected, the ophthalmologist's role is limited mainly to help in diagnosis.
  a. The **ocular findings** of trisomy 13 are
    (1) Microphthalmos.
    (2) Colobomas (almost 100%).
    (3) Communication of extraocular connective tissue with intraocular hyaloid system via scleral coloboma.
    (4) Intraocular cartilage.
    (5) Retinal dysplasia.
    (6) Cataracts.
    (7) Corneal opacities.
    (8) Optic nerve hypoplasia.
    (9) Cyclopia.
  b. The **systemic findings** are
    (1) Failure to thrive, death within first few months of life.
    (2) Congenital heart disease.
    (3) Hernias.
    (4) Cryptorchidism in males.
    (5) Bicornuate uterus in females.
    (6) Scalp defect.
    (7) Arrhinencephaly.
    (8) Mental retardation.
    (9) Wide fontanelles.

(10) Apneic spells.
(11) Seizures.
(12) Deafness.
(13) Microcephaly.
(14) Cleft lip and palate.
(15) Polydactyly.
(16) Transverse palmar crease.
(17) Hyperconvex, narrow fingernails.
(18) Posterior prominence of heel.

3. **Trisomy 18 (E trisomy, Edwards syndrome).** These patients survive less than 1 year, so the ophthalmologist's role is limited mainly to help in diagnosis.
   a. The major **ocular findings** are
      (1) Epicanthal folds.
      (2) Blepharophimosis.
      (3) Ptosis.
      (4) Hypertelorism.
      (5) Corneal opacities.
      (6) Microphthalmos.
      (7) Congenital glaucoma.
      (8) Uveal colobomas.
   b. The major **systemic findings** are
      (1) Death within first year.
      (2) Mental deficiency.
      (3) Decreased growth.
      (4) Congenital heart disease.
      (5) Cryptorchidism.
      (6) Hernias.
      (7) Hypoplasia of muscle and subcutaneous fat.
      (8) Prominent occiput, narrow bifrontal diameter.
      (9) Low-set, malformed ears.
      (10) Micrognathia.
      (11) Microstomia, narrow palatal arch.
      (12) Hypertonicity.
      (13) Camptodactyly.
      (14) Overlapping of index finger over third, and fifth finger over fourth.
      (15) Rocker-bottom feet, prominent heels.
      (16) Hypoplasia of nails.

C. The major **chromosomal deletions** that have been associated with ocular abnormalities include 5p syndrome (**cri du chat** syndrome), in which part of the short arm of the 5 chromosome is missing; 11p, in which part of the short arm of the 11 chromosome is missing; 13q, in which part of the long arm of the 13 chromosome is deleted; 18q (**DeGrouchy** syndrome), in which the long arm of the 18 chromosome is deleted; and XO syndrome (**Turner** syndrome), in which an entire X chromosome is missing. Ocular and systemic abnormalities of these syndromes are listed in Table 11.1.

Patients with 5p, 13q, and 18q are almost always severely retarded and require institutionalization. The ophthalmologist may help in the identification and diagnosis of these patients. (Rarely, patients with 13q have **retinoblastoma** as the only finding and are of normal intelligence.) Patients with Turner syndrome, however, are generally of normal intelligence and will benefit from treatment of their ophthalmologic defects.

D. **Genetic counseling in chromosomal anomalies.** Most trisomies are sporadic in their occurrence, although the chance of a future sibling of a child with Down syndrome being affected is slightly increased. The chance of giving birth to a child with Down syndrome increases with maternal age, approaching 1% by age 40. In translocation Down syndrome, chromosomal

TABLE 11.1. CHROMOSOMAL DELETION SYNDROMES

Syndrome	Chromosome	Ocular Signs	Systemic Signs
Cri du chat	Arm 5p-	Hypertelorism, epicanthus, antimongoloid slant, strabismus	Retardation, mewing cry, microcephaly, hypotonia, failure to thrive, low ears, round face, micrognathia, high palate, simian crease
	Arm 11p-	Aniridia, glaucoma, foveal hypoplasia nystagmus, ptosis	Wilms tumor, genitourinary anomalies, retardation, prominent bridge of nose
	Arm 13q-	Retinoblastoma, hypertelorism, microophthalmos, epicanthus, ptosis, coloboma, cataract	Retardation, microcephaly, trigonocephaly, low-set malformed ears, micrognathia, congenital heart disease, hypoplastic, low-set or absent thumb, foot anomalies
DeGrouchy	Arm 18q-	Hypertelorism, epicanthus, ptosis, strabismus, myopia, glaucoma, microphthalmos (with or without cyst), coloboma, optic atrophy, corneal opacity	Retardation, microcephaly, low birth weight, midface hypoplasia, prominent forehead and jaw, fish mouth
Turner	XO	Downslanting palpebral fissures, epicanthus, ptosis, strabismus, blue sclera, eccentric pupils, cataract, male incidence of red-green color defects, coloboma, retinitis pigmentosa-like fundus	Short, webbed neck, low posterior hairline, broad chest, widely spaced nipples, nevi, congenital heart disease, genitourinary anomalies

analysis on the parents may identify one of them as having a balanced translocation, with material missing from a 21 chromosome and attached to another chromosome. This greatly increases the chances of an offspring being affected. Similarly, parents of patients with partial deletions may be identified as having balanced translocations, increasing the risk for their future offspring. Parents with such translocations may decide to have no more children. Alternatively, parents may elect **amniocentesis** with chromosomal analysis on fetal cells to identify an affected fetus.

VII. **Inherited metabolic disorders**

A. **The mucopolysaccharidoses (MPS)** are caused by deficiencies of enzymes responsible for the turnover of mucopolysaccharides. These enzymopathies cause abnormal tissue accumulation and urinary excretion of certain mucopolysaccharides and a variety of systemic and ocular abnormalities. The MPS are classified by number and eponym. All but one are inherited as autosomal recessive disorders.

1. **MPS IH (Hurler syndrome)** is an autosomal recessively inherited disorder with skeletal and facial dysmorphism, mental retardation, and corneal clouding. Retinal pigmentary degeneration and optic atrophy have been reported. Activity of the enzyme alpha-L-iduronidase is deficient, and the patients excrete increased amounts of heparan sulfate and dermatan sulfate in the urine.

2. **MPS IS (Scheie syndrome,** formerly MPS V) is inherited as an autosomal recessive with the gene at the same locus as the gene for Hurler syndrome. The major difficulty in these patients is corneal clouding, which is accompanied by very mild facial and skeletal dysmorphism and usually normal intelligence. Retinal pigmentary degeneration and optic atrophy have been reported. Deficiency of alpha-L-iduronidase (the same enzyme as in Hurler syndrome) is less severe, and the same mucopolysaccharides are excreted in the urine. MPS IH/S is a genetic compound of MPS IH and MPS IS genes. The phenotype is intermediate.

3. **MPS II (Hunter syndrome)** is an X-linked recessive disorder that occurs in two phenotypes: A and B. In severely affected boys (MPS IIA), the skeletal and facial dysmorphism is milder but reminiscent of that in Hurler syndrome, but there is no corneal clouding. Mental retardation is present. In the milder phenotype (MPS IIB), there is less severe dysmorphism, and the intelligence is less handicapped. These patients have rarely been reported to develop mild corneal clouding later in life. Retinal pigmentary degeneration and optic atrophy have been reported in both phenotypes. The enzyme iduronate sulfatase is deficient, and heparan sulfate and dermatan sulfate are excreted in excessive amounts in the urine in both types.

4. **MPS III (Sanfilippo syndrome)** occurs in four forms: A, in which heparan N-sulfatase is the deficient enzyme; B, in which alpha-N-acetylglucosaminidase is the deficient enzyme; C, in which acetyl coenzyme A-alpha-glucosaminide-N-acetyltransferase is deficient; and D, in which N-acetylalpha-D-glucosaminide-6-sulfatase is deficient. They are all recessively inherited, but they are not allelic and are classified together only because of their phenotypic similarity. These children have a normal appearance with mild dysmorphism, but they are severely retarded and may have seizures. Corneal clouding has not been described, but retinal pigmentary degeneration and optic atrophy have been reported. There is excessive excretion of heparan sulfate in the urine in all four types.

5. **MPS IV (Morquio syndrome)** occurs in two autosomal recessively inherited forms, A and B. Skeletal dysplasia is a major feature in type A. Facial dysmorphism is unusual, and the patients are generally of normal intelligence. These children have corneal clouding that is generally less severe than that in the MPS I disorder. Retinal pigmentary degeneration has not been reported, but optic atrophy has been seen rarely. The deficient enzyme in type A is galactosamine-6-sulfate sulfatase. Patients with MPS IVB are deficient in the enzyme beta-galactosidase. They have mild skeletal dysplasia and corneal clouding. Patients of both types excrete an excessive amount of keratan sulfate.

6. **MPS V** classification is vacant now that Scheie syndrome has been reclassified (see sec. **VII.A.2.,** above).

7. **MPS VI (Maroteaux-Lamy syndrome)** occurs in three allelic phenotypes: severe, intermediate, and mild. All are inherited as autosomal-recessive characteristics. Facial and skeletal dysmorphism is prominent in the first two types and mild in the last. Patients with all types are generally of normal intelligence, and corneal clouding is a prominent feature. Optic atrophy is rare in the severe phenotype and has not been reported in the others, and retinal degeneration has not been reported. There is a deficiency of arylsulfatase B activity, and an excessive amount of dermatan sulfate is excreted in the urine.

8. **MPS VII (Sly syndrome)** is a rare autosomal recessively inherited disorder with facial and skeletal dysmorphism, mental retardation, and corneal clouding. The enzyme beta-glucuronidase is deficient, and dermatan sulfate, heparan sulfate, and chondroitin sulfate are excreted in the urine.

9. In summary, **corneal clouding** is a prominent feature of MPS IH and IS, and is less severe in MPS IV, VI, and VII. (It may occur to a mild degree in older individuals with MPS IIB.) Keratoplasty has been performed successfully in patients with Scheie syndrome. Pigmentary degeneration of the retina occurs in MPS IH, IS, II, and III, but not in IV or VI. Optic atrophy occurs in all types except VIB. Facial dysmorphism is prominent in MPS IH, II, VI, and VII; skeletal dysplasia is present in all of these as well as in MPS IV. Patients with MPS IH, IIA, III, and VII are severely mentally retarded, whereas patients with MPS IS, IIB, IV, and VI are generally of normal or near-normal intelligence.

B. **The sphingolipidoses** are characterized by enzyme deficiencies that interfere with the normal hydrolysis of certain sphingolipids. Because of this lack of ability to metabolize the lipid, it accumulates in abnormal amounts in the CNS, the viscera, or both. Metachromatic leukodystrophy, often considered with the sphingolipidoses, and G_{M1} gangliosidosis are discussed under the mucolipidoses (see sec. **VII.C.,** below).

1. **G_{M2} gangliosidosis type I (Tay-Sachs disease)** is the best known of the sphingolipidoses. Approximately 65% of the patients are of Ashkenazic Jewish ancestry. With the exception of unusual sensitivity to sound, infants with Tay-Sachs disease develop normally until the age of 6 or 7 months. A **cherry-red spot** in the macula can be seen as early as 2 months of age. It is caused by a deficiency of hexosaminidase A, which leads to accumulation of G_{M2} ganglioside in the ganglion cells of the retina. These cells occur in greater numbers around the macula. Severe CNS manifestations, including dementia, spasticity, blindness, and deafness, are caused by similar accumulation in the large neurons of the gray matter. As the ganglion cells die from the effects of excessive lipid accumulation, the cherry-red spot gradually fades and the optic disk develops atrophy. The patients are generally blind by 18 months of age and die by age 3 years.

2. A similar clinical course may be expected in **G_{M2} gangliosidosis type II (Sandhoff's disease).** In this disorder both globoside and G_{M2} ganglioside accumulate as a result of a lack of both hexosaminidase A and B enzymes. There is no specific ethnic predisposition in Sandhoff's disease.

3. In **G_{M2} gangliosidosis type III** there is no cherry-red spot in the macula, but there may be pigmentary retinopathy, and optic atrophy is usually present. These children become blind later in the course of the disease than in Tay-Sachs disease and Sandhoff's disease.

4. **Type A (infantile) Niemann-Pick disease.** This recessively inherited disease is characterized by accumulation of sphingomyelin and cholesterol in the viscera, causing hepatosplenomegaly, and in the brain, causing severely retarded psychomotor development. The enzyme sphingomyelinase is deficient. The cornea is slightly cloudy and there is a brown discoloration of the anterior lens capsule as well as a macular cherry-red spot in most cases. Patients with this infantile form of Niemann-Pick disease have a life span about the same as Tay-Sachs, i.e., 2 to 3 years. The other three or more phenotypes of Niemann-Pick disease are either much less common or do not become manifest in childhood.

5. **Globoid cell leukodystrophy (Krabbe's disease)** is a recessively inherited deficiency of beta-galactosidase that causes accumulation of galactocerebroside. It produces an early and rapidly progressive CNS degeneration and optic atrophy with blindness. A cherry-red spot is not a feature of Krabbe's disease. The life span is about 2 years.

6. **Gaucher's disease,** also recessively inherited, occurs in at least three types. A defect in beta-glucosidase causes accumulation of glucocerebroside in the viscera and probably the nervous system. The infantile variety usually leads to death within 1 or 2 years of age. The eyes are normal in the infantile type and in the extremely rare juvenile type.

7. **Angiokeratoma corporis diffusum universale (Fabry's disease)** is distinguished from the other sphingolipidoses by being inherited as an X-linked recessive, by having normal intelligence without the severe CNS effects of other sphingolipid accumulations, and by having systemic manifestations. Characteristic skin lesions (angiokeratomas) are present on the trunk, and hemizygous males are subject to recurrent fevers and episodes of severe abdominal and limb pain. The lipid accumulation in blood vessels causes severe renal disease and may cause cerebrovascular disease.

   The most characteristic eye manifestation, seen best with the slit-lamp, is a striking whorl-like corneal epithelial opacity radiating out in curved lines from a spot just inferior to the center of the cornea. Characteristic star-shaped radiating lines of opacity are found in the posterior lens as well as strikingly kinky conjunctival and retinal blood vessels. Heterozygous female carriers usually manifest these ocular findings. They may also suffer from the systemic manifestations, though much less severely than the hemizygous males.

C. **The mucolipidoses** present some phenotypic and chemical features that overlap the MPS on one hand and the sphingolipidoses on the other. The various disorders in this group may have the facial and skeletal dysmorphism of the MPS and accumulate mucopolysaccharides in the viscera, as well as exhibiting corneal clouding in some of the disorders. With the exception of juvenile sulfatidosis and G_{M1} gangliosidosis, however, these patients do not excrete excessive amounts of mucopolysaccharide in the urine. Features overlapping with the sphingolipidoses include early progressive neurologic deterioration and, in some of the disorders, a cherry-red spot in the macula. The mucolipidoses are all recessively inherited.

1. **G_{M1} gangliosidosis,** infantile form, is somewhat reminiscent of Hurler syndrome, with corneal clouding, facial and skeletal dysmorphism, but also usually a cherry-red spot and optic atrophy. Both keratan sulfate and G_{M1} ganglioside accumulate in the tissues because of a deficiency of lysosomal beta-galactosidase.

2. **Metachromatic leukodystrophy** may rarely have corneal clouding but commonly has a pigmentary change in the macula and optic atrophy. Because of the lack of the arylsulfatase enzymes, both sulfated acid mucopolysaccharides and sphingolipid sulfatide accumulate.

3. **Sialidosis** (formerly mucolipidosis I) exhibits a deficiency in alpha-neuraminidase.

   a. **Type I.** The patients have a cherry-red spot and myoclonus, but somatically appear normal.

   b. **Type II.** There are coarse features, cherry-red spot, myoclonus, and ataxia.

4. Two disorders of lysosomal synthesis have failure of acid hydrolase incorporation into lysosomes. **I-cell disease** exhibits Hurler-like features and mild corneal clouding, and **pseudo-Hurler polydystrophy** has stiff joints and mild peripheral corneal clouding later. These disorders were formerly classified as mucolipidosis II and III.

5. **Farber lipogranulomatosis** may produce ocular inflammation as well as macular pigmentary change. It is characterized most dramatically by arthropathy and subcutaneous swellings caused by formation of histocytic granulomas. An intracellular accumulation of a ceramide occurs in and around joints, viscera, retinal ganglion cells, and brain caused by a deficiency of acid ceramidase.

D. Neuronal ceroid lipofuscinosis (Batten-Mayou disease) is characterized by mental deterioration and by a pigmentary retinopathy involving most severely the macula, with loss of central vision. Optic atrophy also occurs.

Cherry-red spots are not seen. The onset is usually in the first decade, less commonly in the second decade. The peripheral leukocytes in both affected homozygous patients and unaffected heterozygotes may have characteristic abundant azurophilic granules. The pathologic changes include loss of the outer segments and pigment epithelium of the retina and accumulation of ceroidlipofuscin in various tissues (histologic examination of ganglion cells on rectal biopsy may help make the diagnosis), including the retinal pigment epithelium (RPE) and CNS. No specific enzyme defect has been identified, but there are lysosomal inclusions on electron microscopy. This disease occurs in four types:

1. **Infantile,** with blindness by age 2 and death by age 5 years.
2. **Late infantile.**
3. **Juvenile,** with optic atrophy and macular degeneration by age 4 to 8 years and death in adolescence.
4. **Adult,** with severe CNS deterioration, often with blindness, without clinical ocular signs.

E. Aminoacidurias. Most aminoacidurias are recessively inherited.

1. **Homocystinuria** is inherited as an autosomal recessive and is the result of absence of the enzyme cystathionine synthetase. Some affected individuals are helped by **pyridoxine therapy.** Subluxed lenses (ectopia lentis) are characteristic. Patients may also have myopia, retinal detachment, glaucoma, and optic atrophy. Patients are frequently hypopigmented and are usually mentally retarded or have a peculiar affect. They may suffer from osteoporosis. Special care must be taken if a patient requires ocular surgery with general anesthesia because of the tendency to arterial and venous thromboses.

2. **Cystinosis** is inherited as an autosomal recessive disorder. A lysosomal transport defect causes intracellular accumulation of cystine. The deposition of cystine crystals in the cornea causes photophobia. Such crystals are also deposited in the conjunctiva and choroid. They may be readily seen on slitlamp examination. Pigmentary and degenerative changes may occur in the retinal periphery. The disease has severe systemic manifestations of renal tubular acidosis, with renal rickets and eventual renal failure leading to death. Benign cystinosis is an unrelated adult disorder.

3. **Oculocerebrorenal syndrome (Lowe syndrome)** is an X-linked recessive characteristic with an unknown enzyme defect. It may result from deficient amino acid transport. The eye involvement is very severe and includes cataract, microphakia, and severe congenital glaucoma. The glaucoma results from malformation of the filtration angle or from subluxed lenses. The systemic abnormalities include metabolic acidosis (which makes anesthesia more difficult, complicating surgery of the cataracts and glaucoma), rickets, mental and growth retardation with hypotonia, and, usually, early death.

4. **Cerebrohepatorenal syndrome (Zellweger syndrome)** is autosomal recessively inherited. The specific enzyme defect is unknown, but aminoaciduria is a prominent feature. The eye involvement includes a characteristic hypoplasia of the superior orbital margins, with resultant flat brow and prominent eyes. The patient may also have a characteristic "leopard spot" peripheral retinal pigmentation, as well as cataracts, congenital glaucoma, and optic nerve hypoplasia. Patients are severely retarded secondary to cerebral dysgenesis, and they have microcystic kidneys and hepatic dysgenesis. Life expectancy is less than 1 year; therefore, ophthalmologic treatment is moot.

5. **Galactosemia** is an autosomal-recessive deficiency of galactose-1-phosphate uridyltransferase. It is included here because aminoaciduria is a prominent part of the picture. Accumulation of galactose causes sugar cataracts in infancy that, in their early stages, can be reversed by a galactose-free diet. The severe systemic manifestations include failure to thrive, vomiting, hepatomegaly, jaundice, and aminoaciduria, all of which can also be reversed by a galactose-free diet.

6. **Galactokinase deficiency** is an autosomal recessively inherited deficiency of the enzyme galactokinase. There are no systemic manifestations or aminoaciduria; the cataracts that form when the child is exposed to galactose are the presenting finding. If the problem is recognized early enough, the **cataracts are reversible** by a galactose-free diet.

F. **Miscellaneous disorders of connective tissue**

1. **Arachnodactyly (Marfan syndrome)** is inherited as an autosomal dominant. Patients exhibit skeletal abnormalities including arachnodactyly, laxity of the joints, tall stature, scoliosis, and sternal deformities. They may suffer from dissecting aneurysms of the thoracic aorta and aortic and mitral valvular disease. They are of normal intelligence. No chemical abnormality has been identified; therefore, no confirmatory laboratory tests are available. The most important ocular manifestation is ectopia lentis, which occurs in about 80% of the patients. The usual direction of dislocation is upward, but the lens may be dislocated in any direction. In contrast, dislocation of the lens in homocystinuria is usually downward. Other ocular abnormalities include strabismus, myopia (sometimes with retinal changes), glaucoma, filtration angle anomalies, retinal detachment, and blue sclerae. The subluxation of the lens may cause high degrees of astigmatism, and patients require frequent refractions. There is some **risk of dilating the pupils,** especially chronically, because of the danger of dislocation of the lens into the anterior chamber. Generally, the lens should not be extracted unless it becomes cataractous or unless it is dislocated into the anterior chamber and cannot be made to return posteriorly by dilating the pupil and positioning the patient supinely.

2. **Osteogenesis imperfecta** may be inherited as either an autosomal-dominant or autosomal-recessive disorder. Recessive inheritance generally is associated with more severe skeletal anomalies. The bones are fragile and fracture easily, sometimes spontaneously, causing deformities, especially of the long bones. Blue sclerae are characteristic because of the thinness of the sclerae. The corneas are also thin and vulnerable to laceration and rupture from relatively minor trauma. Keratoconus, megalocornea, embryotoxon, and glaucoma may occur. Protective spectacles with safety glass and sturdy frames should be prescribed for patients who are not bedridden.

3. **Disorders associated with angioid streaks of the retina. Angioid streaks** are cracks in Bruch membrane of the RPE. They may interfere with visual acuity if they involve the macular area. Generally, **no treatment** is indicated, but **photocoagulation** has been advocated for neovascularization in an angioid streak not yet involving the macula. The most common disorders associated with angioid streaks appear in the following list:

a. **Pseudoxanthoma elasticum** is a recessively inherited disorder. Affected areas of the skin have small yellow papules and plaques. Eventually, affected skin may hang in loose folds. The most commonly affected skin is the axillae, the antecubital and popliteal fossae, and the sides of the neck. Similar papules and plaques in the stomach may cause gastrointestinal bleeding.

b. **Ehlers-Danlos syndrome** is an autosomal-dominant condition with hyperelasticity of the skin, hyperextensibility of the joints, and fragility of the tissue, sometimes resulting in bleeding. Keratoconus, microcornea, blue sclera retinal hemorrhages, angioid streaks, and retinal detachments may occur.

   c. Paget's disease of the bone is dominantly inherited. Its major manifestation is thickening of the bones, most prominently of the skull. Angioid streaks usually occur relatively late in adult life.

   d. Sickle cell anemia is a codominantly inherited disease that causes severe anemia and multiple thromboembolic crises. Other eye manifestations are more prominent than the angioid streaks (see sec. **XIX.E.,** below).

G. Hepatolenticular degeneration (Wilson's disease) is inherited as an autosomal recessive. In children it usually presents as hepatic disease. In older adolescents and young adults, a more common presentation is progressive neurologic disease and ataxia from deposition of copper in the CNS, especially in the basal ganglia. Its major manifestation in the eye is the Kayser-Fleischer ring in the cornea. This is a brownish or golden deposition of copper in the peripheral portion of Descemet's membrane. In early cases it may be visible only on slitlamp examination. A brownish discoloration of the anterior lens capsule in a petal-like distribution (the sunflower cataract) may also be seen. Copper is deposited in many other tissues as well. Liver biopsies from affected homozygous individuals have 20 to 30 times the normal concentration of copper. Usually the level of ceruloplasmin, which binds copper in the serum, and the level of copper in serum are low. **Treatment** is necessary to avoid irreversible liver damage and basal ganglion damage. It consists of a low-copper diet and treatment with a chelating agent, penicillamine. As treatment progresses, the Kayser-Fleischer rings may diminish.

H. Albinism. The three most common and important types of albinism from an ophthalmologist's point of view are (a) tyrosinase-negative oculocutaneous albinism; (b) tyrosinase-positive oculocutaneous albinism, both of which are inherited as autosomal recessives; and (c) X-linked ocular albinism. Other, much rarer forms of albinism may be associated with a variety of other anomalies. All types are associated with abnormal crossing of nerve fibers in the chiasm.

   1. Tyrosinase-negative oculocutaneous albinism. These patients are generally almost completely devoid of pigment. They have pink skin and white hair, including the eyelashes and eyelids. Irides are light blue and transilluminate markedly. Transillumination is best accomplished by making the room completely dark and placing the tip of a shielded transilluminator against the lower eyelid with the patient's eye open. In normal individuals the light will come through the pupil only, but in albinos a red reflex will be seen through the iris as well. Patients with oculocutaneous albinism have macular hypoplasia or aplasia and generally have very poor vision and sensory nystagmus. They also have a tendency toward high refractive errors, especially myopia. They require correction of their refractive errors and help with low-vision aids. Their lack of pigmentation makes them sensitive to bright light, and they may require sunglasses for comfort. The skin is also sensitive to sun damage. Parents of affected children should be warned to avoid exposure of their children to sunlight.

   2. Tyrosinase-positive oculocutaneous albinism is nonallelic with the tyrosinase-negative variety. A mating between these two types of albinos would produce a normally pigmented child, because the child would be heterozygous for each form of albinism. The two forms can be distinguished by a simple test in which hairs epilated from the scalp are incubated in tyrosine. Tyrosinase-negative albinos will show no darkening of the hair bulb. In contrast, the hair bulbs of tyrosinase-positive albinos will become much darker when incubated in tyrosine. Patients with tyrosinase-positive oculocutaneous albinism tend to show some increasing pigmentation as they grow older, and there may be some improvement in visual acuity with time. There is no good evidence, however, that the decreased pigmentation per se is directly related to the decreased visual acuity. Rather, the poor vision and nystagmus seem to be associated with macular hypoplasia.

3. **Ocular albinism** is inherited as an X-linked recessive. The affected males have normal skin and hair pigmentation, but deficient pigmentation in the eyes and macular hypoplasia with poor visual acuity and sensory nystagmus. The carrier females are not entirely unaffected; they have abnormal iris transillumination and a blotchy pigmentary abnormality in the peripheral retina. They have normal visual acuity, however.

I. **Miscellaneous disorders**

1. **Achromatopsia** is a group of autosomal recessive disorders. Patients have absent or markedly abnormal cone function with poor visual acuity, sensory nystagmus, and virtually complete color blindness. These patients characteristically avoid bright lights. This is not true photophobia, but an attempt to keep their rods dark-adapted so they can see. The appearance of the fundus is normal. Achromatopsia can be diagnosed by the clinical picture and electroretinogram (ERG). **Treatment** consists of (a) correcting any refractive error, (b) fitting the patient with extra-dark sunglasses with side shields, and (c) the use of low-vision aids as required.

2. **Protan and deutan color blindness.** These two forms of color blindness are both X-linked recessive. The loci for the two forms are closely linked on the X chromosome but are not allelic. Approximately 8% to 10% of the male population is hemizygous for one of these two forms of color blindness. Homozygous females are rare. Each form of color blindness can exist in a relatively mild deficiency in red sensitivity (protanomaly) or green sensitivity (deuteranomaly) or in a more complete lack of sensitivity to red (protanopia) or green (deuteranopia). The eyes of these individuals are otherwise normal, with normal visual acuity. They should be counseled to avoid occupations that require good color vision, but otherwise they will suffer no disability.

3. **Norrie's disease** is inherited as an X-linked recessive. Boys with this disorder are usually born with bilateral complete detachments of severely dysplastic or undifferentiated retinas. Occasionally, the retinal detachment may occur in early infancy rather than being congenital. The affected males are normal mentally at birth, but about 25% of them become demented or psychotic sometime during life. **Amniocentesis** and therapeutic abortion of male fetuses may be offered to carrier females.

4. **Incontinentia pigmenti** as an X-linked trait that is lethal in affected male fetuses, resulting in spontaneous abortion; consequently, the disease is seen only in females. Its name comes from the whorls of pigmented lines in the skin of the trunk and limbs. Patients may also have skeletal, dental, cardiac, and CNS anomalies. About 25% of affected individuals have eye problems, including cataracts, strabismus, optic atrophy, intraocular inflammation, microphthalmos, and retinal detachment in infancy.

5. **Aicardi syndrome** is another disorder that is found only in females and is probably lethal in males. Its mode of inheritance is uncertain, because no familial cases have been described in the 120 cases so far reported. The fundus picture is quite striking, with lacunae of depigmented and pigmented areas of varying sizes in the fundus, mostly in the posterior pole. These lacunae may be confused with chorioretinal scars of toxoplasmosis, which they somewhat resemble, or with colobomas in atypical locations. The optic disk often exhibits a dark gray discoloration. These patients have infantile spasms with hypsarrhythmic electroencephalogram and are severely mentally retarded. The corpus collosum

is absent, and there are ectopic projections of abnormal brain tissue into the ventricles.

   6. **Familial dysautonomia (Riley-Day syndrome),** an autosomal recessive, is almost exclusively seen in individuals of Ashkenazic Jewish ancestry. A deficiency in the enzyme dopamine-beta-hydroxylase interferes with the synthesis of norepinephrine and epinephrine from dopamine. Affected individuals have marked vasomotor instability with paroxysmal hypertension, abnormal sweating, relative lack of sensation, and absent fungiform papillae on the tongue. Intradermal histamine injection produces less than the normal pain and erythema. Patients suffer also from recurrent fevers and have an increased susceptibility to infection. The eyes are involved with decreased tear production and corneal hypesthesia, which may lead to drying, exposure, and corneal scarring. Because of this susceptibility to exposure keratopathy, care must be taken to protect the corneas during the periodic crises of these patients. The pupil exhibits denervation **supersensitivity to parasympathomimetic drugs.** Methacholine 2.5% or pilocarpine 0.25% will cause pupillary constriction in a Riley-Day patient but not in the normal patient. The ophthalmologist can help in the **diagnosis** of Riley-Day syndrome with this pharmacologic test.

VIII. **Phacomatoses.** The term *phacomatosis* was introduced by van der Hoeve and colleagues in 1917 and 1923 to unify the diverse manifestations of tuberous sclerosis and neurofibromatosis. Both of these familial disorders involved tumors arising in multiple organs. The tumors could be present in the newborn child or might arise later in life. Because of the "in-born" nature of the tumors they were called phacomata from the Greek *phakos,* meaning mother spot. Inherent in the original concept was the recognition that some growths might become malignant, and van der Hoeve emphasized the inborn predisposition for individuals of these families to develop malignancy. Van der Hoeve subsequently included von Hippel-Lindau angiomatosis as a phacomatosis and with these three classical phacomatoses he had the powerful insight that the predisposition for cancers can be inherited, thus anticipating by many decades some of the recent genetic advances that provide more basic explanations for van der Hoeve clinical observations.

The usefulness of the term phacomatosis unfortunately was greatly diluted when van der Hoeve himself made the mistake of generalizing from a single rare case of Sturge-Weber syndrome in which a retinoblastoma developed. The Sturge-Weber syndrome is not as clearly hereditary as the three classical phacomatoses, the vascular tumors in Sturge-Weber are generally present at birth, rather than arising de novo in later life, and malignant transformation is rare. Hogan and Zimmerman and many subsequent ocular pathologists ignored the original emphasis on familial malignancy and emphasized disorders in which the basic lesions are hamartomas, that is, they are tumors consisting of those tissue components that are normally found at the involved site. This is in contrast with choristomas, which are tumors, such as dermoids, composed of elements not normally found at the involved site. It is in this context that ataxia–telangiectasia and the Wyburn-Mason syndrome are sometimes included in current discussions of the phacomatoses. The original concept has been so altered that occasionally additional neurocutaneous syndromes are also referred to as phacomatoses.

A. **Tuberous sclerosis (Bourneville's disease)**
   1. **Ocular lesions.** Retinal lesions may be either large with white concretions within their substance ("mulberry" lesions) or flat and gelatinous in appearance. Pathologically, they are astrocytic hamartomas of the nerve fiber layer. They may enlarge over the years.
   2. **Cutaneous manifestations** include:
       a. "Adenoma sebaceum," usually developing between 2 and 5 years of age; this is actually a misnomer because the lesion does not involve the sebaceous glands and is an angiofibroma.

      b. Ash-leaf spots of depigmentation, particularly evident under ultraviolet illumination, which may be present at birth.

      c. Periungual and subungual fibromas, often appearing after puberty.

    3. Systemic manifestations include:

      a. CNS involvement with variable mental deficiency, seizures, and intracranial calcifications.

      b. Hamartomatous lesions of heart and kidney.

 B. Neurofibromatosis (von Recklinghausen's disease, NF1) is one of the more common human autosomal-dominant disorders with an estimated prevalence of 1 in 3,000. Approximately 50% of cases are thought to be new mutations. NF1 is contrasted to the much less common (1 in 50,000) "central variant" **NF2** characterized by acoustic neuromas, and a relative lack of cutaneous findings. The gene for NF1 has been localized to chromosome 17, whereas the gene of NF2 is on 22. Both are thought to be tumor suppressor genes. The NF1 gene is very large and its large size is postulated to be responsible for the high mutation rate, thus inactivating the gene.

    1. Ocular lesions of NF1 include:

      a. Plexiform neuromas of the eyelids that may produce a characteristic S-shaped configuration of the lid margin.

      b. Optic nerve gliomas of optic nerve and chiasm.

      c. Nevoid hamartomas of the iris (Lisch nodules).

      d. Glaucoma (in some cases abnormal tissue in the filtration angle is the cause).

      e. Deficiency in sphenoid development, leading to pulsating exophthalmos.

      f. Retinal lesions (rarely).

    2. Cutaneous manifestations of NF1 include:

      a. Café au lait patches.

      b. Pedunculated skin lesions (fibrous molloscum).

      c. Plexiform neuromas.

    3. Systemic manifestations of NF1 include:

      a. CNS neurofibromas, gliomas, meningiomas, and ependymomas.

      b. Neurofibromas of the viscera.

      c. Skeletal deformities.

      d. Pheochromocytomas.

 C. Angiomatosis retinae (ocular lesion described by **von Hippel,** systemic aspects of the disease described by **Lindau**).

    1. Ocular manifestation is retinal hemangioma.

    2. Systemic manifestations include:

      a. Cystic cerebellar hemangiomas.

      b. A wide variety of visceral manifestations, such as renal cysts, association with renal cell carcinomas, tumors and cysts of the epididymis, pancreatic cysts, and pheochromocytomas.

IX. Multisystem vascular hamartomas causing local morbidity without malignancy (no definite hereditary influence)

 A. Encephalotrigeminal angiomatosis (Sturge-Weber syndrome). Although port-wine stains may occur anywhere on the body, Sturge observed that patients with unilateral **facial** port-wine stains (nevus flammeus) regularly had seizures and hemiparesis of the contralateral side, and speculated correctly that this was the result of an intracranial hemangioma. Weber described the characteristic linear calcifications seen on skull x-rays.

    1. Ocular manifestations include:

      a. Lid nevus flammeus.

      b. Conjunctival and episcleral vascular lesions.

      c. Glaucoma (both abnormal angle structures and increased episcleral venous pressure are possible etiologies).

    d. Choroidal hemangiomas, which give the fundus a "tomato-ketchup" appearance (suprachoroidal serous detachments may develop in these eyes during the hypotony of intraocular surgery).

    e. Heterochromia iridis.

    f. Megalocornea in the absence of glaucoma.

  2. Cutaneous manifestation is nevus flammeus or the port-wine stain.

  3. Systemic manifestations include jacksonian seizures, hemiparesis, hemianopia, and, at times, mental deficiency.

X. Recessively inherited multisystem disease with special mechanisms of malignancy

  A. Ataxia–telangiectasia (Louis-Barr syndrome)

    1. Ocular lesions. Bulbar conjunctival telangiectasis is an essential component of the disorder. It is not present at birth, but is usually noted between 4 and 7 years of age. Abnormalities of eye movements are consequent to the CNS abnormalities.

    2. Cutaneous manifestations have been reported but are not pathognomonic of the disorder.

    3. Systemic manifestations

      a. CNS. Progressive ataxia in childhood was the striking feature initially reported in 1941. At autopsy, degeneration of the cerebellar Purkinje cells is a prominent finding.

      b. Immune deficiency. Thymic hypoplasia is associated with a profound defect in cell-mediated immunity (T cells) and a selective humoral deficiency of immunoglobulin G21 (IgG21), IgG4, IgA, and IgE. This immune deficiency appears to be the reason for frequent pulmonary infections.

      c. More random chromosomal rearrangements and the inability to repair radiation-induced damage to DNA. Chromosomal breaks occur at sites responsible for the assembly of genes required for the synthesis of antibodies and T-cell antigen receptors, sites at which "cutting and splicing" of DNA naturally occur.

      d. Chromosome localization of the genes. The gene responsible for ataxia–telangiectasia has been localized to 11q22 to 23.

  B. Wyburn-Mason syndrome

    1. Ocular lesions. Racemose hemangioma of the retina is present on the ipsilateral side of midbrain involvement with racemose hemangioma.

    2. Cutaneous lesions. On occasion, these may be pulsatile vascular nevi in the distribution of the trigeminal nerve.

    3. Systemic manifestations. The racemose hemangioma of the midbrain is congenital and nonprogressive. Neurologic consequences develop as a result of direct-compression hemorrhage and infarction.

XI. Developmental disorders by anatomic region

  A. Abnormalities of the lacrimal drainage apparatus: lacrimal duct obstruction, dacryocystitis, congenital dacryocele

    1. Background. The watery component of tears is produced largely by the lacrimal glands in the conjunctival fornices. Tears are distributed across the cornea by the lids during blinking and then pass through the lacrimal drainage apparatus. Tears enter the puncta of the upper and lower lids, pass through the canaliculi, through the common canaliculus, and into the lacrimal sac. The lacrimal sac drains through the nasolacrimal duct into the nose. Lacrimal duct obstruction usually occurs at the lower end of this nasolacrimal duct where it enters the nasal cavity. In the presence of lacrimal duct obstruction, tears and mucus pool in the lacrimal sac above the obstruction. The mucoid material may reflux through the puncta when pressure is placed over the nasolacrimal sac. The stagnation of tears in this situation leads to chronic discharge on the eyelashes, and **dacryocystitis** (infection of the lacrimal sac itself) may occur.

In rare instances, the obstruction at the lower end of the nasolacrimal duct is associated with distention of the nasolacrimal sac (congenital dacryocele). The infant is born with a distended nasolacrimal sac full of a mucoid material but does not have an active infection in the lacrimal sac, at first.

2. **Physical findings**

   a. **Congenital lacrimal duct obstruction** will cause tearing and discharge. Characteristically, there will be some mucous discharge on the lashes, but the conjunctiva will be white and uninflamed. Injection of the conjunctiva indicates a concurrent conjunctivitis. Digital pressure over the nasolacrimal sac often produces a reflux of mucoid material.

   b. **Tearing without discharge** on the lashes or reflux from the nasolacrimal sac should make the clinician suspicious that **congenital glaucoma** rather than lacrimal duct obstruction may be causing the tearing.

   c. **Dacryocystitis** will produce redness, tenderness, and swelling medial to the inner canthus. It may be present at birth but characteristically develops after a period of stagnation and obstructed tear flow.

   d. A **congenital dacryocele** will produce swelling and bluish or purplish discoloration of the soft tissues medial to the inner canthus but is not inflamed. It is usually present at birth and occasionally may wax and wane in size if untreated.

3. **Treatment**

   a. **Congenital lacrimal duct obstructions.** Eighty percent of congenital lacrimal duct obstructions will remit during the first 6 to 9 months of life. The likelihood of spontaneous clearing over the next 2 to 3 months decreases as the infant gets older.

      (1) **Digital compression of the nasolacrimal sac** can minimize accumulation of mucoid material in the sac. The effort is made to minimize stagnation and to avoid infection. If infection occurs, **antibiotic ointment** (e.g., erythromycin or tobramycin) qid initially and then as frequently as necessary to control purulent discharge should be prescribed.

      (2) If tearing and discharge persist, **probing of the nasolacrimal sac** may be indicated. Although probing can sometimes be done in the office, a brief general anesthesia gives the surgeon better control and is preferable. Endotracheal intubation is not required, so the procedure can be done under mask insufflation anesthesia in an ambulatory surgery unit. Although there is no controversy with regard to the efficacy of probing, there is some variation in the recommended timing of the probing. Some ophthalmologists if presented with a family unhappy with a child's purulent, recurrently infected eye, probe at presentation regardless of age. An advantage of probing early is that youngsters are smaller and therefore weaker and require less restraint for probings done in the office. Most ophthalmologists who do office probings will tend to probe children early (e.g., at time of presentation), whereas most ophthalmologists who wait 9 to 12 months or longer to see if the child's problems will remit spontaneously will tend to use brief general anesthetics on an outpatient basis for the probing of the older child. If tearing persists or occurs after probing, another probing is indicated. If several probings have failed, the physician is dealing with an unusual situation, and intubation with Silastic tubing or a dacryocystorhinostomy may be indicated.

   b. **Dacryocystitis** should be treated with systemic antibiotics. The systemic antibiotic choice keeps changing and for these small infants needs to be calculated on a per weight basis (see Appendix B). Once the infection has cleared, the obstruction and cause of the problem can be relieved by probing the nasolacrimal duct.

   c. **Congenital dacryocele** should be relieved by probing promptly in the newborn period. At this age probing can be done without general anesthesia.

B. Ptosis may be present as an isolated anomaly, but there may be associated abnormalities. As soon as the diagnosis of ptosis is made, a complete ophthalmologic examination is indicated, even though surgical intervention to lift the lid may not be undertaken for several years.

   1. **Isolated congenital ptosis.** Even if it is severe, congenital ptosis rarely threatens visual development by covering the pupil. Children usually hold their heads back and peer out below the ptotic lid. Visual development may be threatened, however, by the astigmatism that may be present in the eye with a ptotic lid. These children are at risk for anisometropic **amblyopia** (see Chapter 12, sec. **VI.D.**). They should be seen early and given glasses and patching as indicated.

   Generally, it is best to wait for ptosis surgery until the child is at least 3 or 4 years old and until reliable measurements of levator function are obtainable. The choice of surgical procedure depends on the degree of levator function. Levator resection is indicated when reasonable levator function is present. Frontalis sling using fascia lata, preferably autogenous, is necessary in the absence of levator action.

   2. **Differential diagnosis.** In the evaluation of ptosis, special attention should be paid to pupillary size. A small pupil associated with ptosis may indicate **Horner syndrome.** A larger pupil associated with ptosis and appropriate extraocular muscle weakness would indicate a **third nerve palsy.** Occasionally, the amount of ptosis may be influenced by chewing through a synkinesis known as the **Marcus-Gunn "jaw-winking"** syndrome, in which the levator palpebrae is innervated by a branch of the motor division of cranial nerve V. As the patient chews or moves the jaw from side to side, the ptotic eyelid elevates, sometimes to a level higher than the normal position.

C. Colobomas along the optic fissure. A number of congenital anomalies appear to derive from localized failure of the optic fissure to close during intrauterine development. These anomalies may be of no visual consequence, as is the case with isolated inferior iris colobomas or small choroidal defects seen inferior to the disk. Although iris colobomas per se are of no visual consequence, they may be associated with more extensive colobomas in the back of the eye that are visually significant, or they may be associated with other systemic anomalies.

   Large chorioretinal colobomas may cause profound visual dysfunction if they involve the macula or the optic nerve. One of the more extreme examples of failure in fissure closure is microphthalmos with cyst. In this condition substantial portions of intraocular tissue are found in a colobomatous cyst, and useful vision is not possible.

D. Optic nerve anomalies (see Chapter 13, sec. **II.**). All visual information generated by the retina must pass through the optic nerve, so anomalies of the optic nerve may have profound effects on visual function. **Severe colobomas** and anomalous configurations such as **"morning glory" anomaly** and **profound hypoplasia** of the optic nerve may cause profound and irreparable defects in visual function and in pupillary reactions. Regional defects in the optic nerve such as **segmental optic nerve hypoplasia** or **optic nerve drusen** may give rise to visual field defects but leave good central vision and good visual acuity. **Optic nerve pits** are congenital defects that may be associated later in life with serous detachments of the macula and an acquired diminution of vision. One of the most common anomalies of the optic nerve is the presence of **medullated nerve fibers** in the nerve fiber layer of the retina. These feather-like white patches do not interfere with visual function except for localized visual field scotomas that correspond to their location. (The medullated nerve fibers are opaque and prevent light from stimulating the outer segments behind them.)

E. **Macular hypoplasia.** The embryologic defect that gives rise to macular hypoplasia is not known. In some cases it is inherited in association with albinism or aniridia. Macular hypoplasia may, however, also occur in isolation without other ocular or systemic findings. The diagnosis is made on the basis of clinical examination in the context of poor vision. No foveal reflex is seen, and blood vessels may course through the normally avascular macular region.

F. **Hyaloid system.** During embryologic life the hyaloid vasculature extends from the optic nerve through the vitreous and nourishes the developing lens. It normally regresses completely in later development, but in some individuals remnants remain at the surface of the optic disk as **Bergmeister papilla.** More rarely, a loop of vascular tissue extends some distance into the vitreous from the optic disk. Sometimes the hyaloid vascular system regresses completely at the optic disk, but a small opacity at the posterior surface of the lens (a Mittendorf dot) reminds one of its anterior location. These anomalies do not interfere with function and require no therapy.

If the hyaloid system does not regress at all and if tissue **(persistent hyperplastic primary vitreous [PHPV])** persists between the optic nerve and the posterior surface of the lens, the eye does not develop normally. These eyes are small, and the tissue behind the lens gives the eye a white pupil. Vision is poor because of occlusion by the opaque tissue and anomalous development. Surgery is indicated to prevent angle-closure glaucoma caused by progressive shallowing of the anterior chamber and to avoid recurrent vitreous hemorrhages. Some patients have achieved useful vision after clearing of the visual axis followed by aggressive amblyopia therapy. The term *posterior PHPV* has been used for a glial contracture of the retina **(falciform fold)** without a retrolental mass. These eyes also have evidence of anomalous development and are microphthalmic.

G. **Anterior chamber dysgenesis.** A spectrum of congenital malformations involve the iris, the iridocorneal or filtration angle, and the cornea. The etiology of these disorders is unclear. The most peripheral edge of Descemet's membrane of the cornea terminates at the upper edge of the trabecular meshwork (TM). This most peripheral edge is called Schwalbe's line. If Schwalbe's line is unusually thickened or prominent, it is called **posterior embryotoxon** (on the posterior surface of the cornea, it is a curved line; from the Greek word *toxon,* meaning *bow*). The term *Axenfeld anomaly* has been given to a prominent Schwalbe's line when it is associated with large peripheral anterior synechiae from the iris. **Axenfeld syndrome** includes glaucoma. **Rieger syndrome** includes the prominent Schwalbe's line, peripheral iris anomalies, iris atrophy, glaucoma, as well as nonocular skeletal and structural abnormalities. Although **Peters anomaly** is sometimes classified with these chamber angle anomalies, the characteristic features include (a) a central corneal opacity (leukoma), apparently the result of locally absent corneal endothelium; and (b) iridocorneal adhesions at the edge of the central leukoma. Glaucoma is frequently associated with these anomalies. **Therapeutic** efforts involve treatment of glaucoma when present and penetrating keratoplasty when Peter anomaly is bilateral (see Chapter 5, Fig. 5.2).

H. **Dermoids.** A rubbery, firm, subcutaneous mass along the orbital rim present since birth is most likely a dermoid tumor. Although dermoids are most common along the superotemporal orbital rim, they occur not infrequently in other quadrants. They may enlarge slowly. A dermoid is a choristoma and is composed of tissues not normally present in that region of the body. Dermoids can be removed satisfactorily by local dissection. In children this is best done with endotracheal intubation and general anesthesia. On occasion, a dermoid that appears to be localized to the orbital rim may have a significant posterior extension into the orbit or may extensively involve the bone of the orbital rim. It may be advisable to consider radiologic studies of the involved area before surgery if the extent of the mass cannot be determined with certainty by palpation alone.

I. **Hemangiomas** involving the eyelids pose special problems. Infants with such hemangiomas should be followed by an ophthalmologist from the earliest possible age. The mass of the hemangioma may cause total occlusion of the eye and produce irreparable **deprivation amblyopia.** Like hemangiomas elsewhere on the body, those that involve the lids have a tendency to grow during the first year of life and then tend to regress spontaneously. In terms of minimizing scarring and side effects of **therapy,** the physician should delay intervention as long as possible, but if the eye is completely occluded by a hemangioma, the physician must intervene, however young the infant. Injecting triamcinolone directly into the tumor may hasten regression, but has been associated with ocular complications including blindness, as well as cushingoid systemic effects because the dose is quite large and all is absorbed. Intralesional injection, therefore, has little advantage over oral administration of steroids. In addition to occlusion amblyopia, these eyes are at risk for anisometropic amblyopia, because the mass effect of the hemangioma produces an astigmatism in the involved eye. The involved eye may also develop high myopia. Whether or not the eye is completely occluded, it is essential that the child be refracted at an early age and appropriate attention be given to glasses and patching.

XII. **Developmental disorders by syndromes**

A. **Branchial arch syndromes versus Tessier clefting classification.** Specific ocular anomalies are regular features of certain syndromes with facial anomalies. Overlapping classification schemes have been proposed for these disorders, but knowledge of underlying mechanisms is still lacking. Tessier comprehensive classification of facial clefting syndromes based on morphology can be used for the **Treacher Collins syndrome and Goldenhar syndrome,** but the cause of the clefts is unknown. Another classification is based on the embryologic origin of many of the affected tissues (the branchial arch syndromes). Heredity plays a strong role in many families with Treacher Collins deformity, but appears to play less of a role in Goldenhar syndrome.

1. **Mandibulofacial dysostosis: Treacher Collins (Franceschetti-Klein) syndrome.** Maxillary hypoplasia and downward displacement of the lateral canthi give these individuals a highly characteristic appearance. Prominent ocular findings include notching of the inferior lids, deficient lashes on the lids medial to the notching, and astigmatism that seems to correlate with the clefting axis. Corneal irritation may result from misdirected lashes caused by lid notching. Deafness and ear anomalies often accompany the ocular and facial deformities.

2. **Oculoauriculovertebral dysplasia: Goldenhar syndrome.** Usually the ocular features (limbal corneal dermoids, orbital lipodermoids, and notching of the superior lid) and preauricular skin tags are the prominent features in childhood. The most frequent vertebral anomalies include fused cervical vertebrae, hemivertebrae, spina bifida, and occipitalization of the atlas. Occasionally, however, the associated systemic abnormalities (cardiovascular, renal, genitourinary, and gastrointestinal defects) may be so severe that they dominate the clinical picture. The limbal dermoid is amenable to local excision with a partial keratectomy, but the orbital lipodermoid should not be treated surgically. The orbital lipodermoid is much less disfiguring, and attempted excision may lead to scarring involving the extraocular muscles with restricted motility.

3. **Hallermann-Streiff-François syndrome.** Mandibular hypoplasia and feeding problems are prominent in the neonatal period. The characteristic ocular lesions are cataracts that mature rapidly in infancy,

becoming liquid, and may absorb spontaneously if left untreated. In general, however, it is advisable to proceed with cataract aspiration as soon as the child can tolerate general anesthesia, because the rate and completeness of spontaneous absorption cannot be predicted so that deprivation amblyopia may supervene, and the process of spontaneous absorption may be a causative factor in the late development of secondary glaucoma.

4. **Pierre Robin anomaly.** Mandibular hypoplasia with upper airway obstruction and feeding problems may be prominent in the neonatal period. Some also have Stickler syndrome (see sec. **XIX.C.4.,** below) and may have high myopia, glaucoma, and retinal detachment, so a complete ophthalmic examination at an early age and follow-up are advisable.

B. **Craniofacial dysostosis.** The most commonly seen disorders of this type are **Crouzon** syndrome and **Apert** syndrome. The syndactyly of Apert syndrome is the most clear-cut distinction between these two disorders, both of which have craniofacial deformities due to craniosynostosis. Both disorders have markedly shallow orbits with prominent globes, and the globes may prolapse in front of the lids spontaneously or with minimal trauma. This prolapse usually appears to do no harm to the globes, and the eyeball can be gently repositioned with the lids held open. Youngsters with both Apert and Crouzon syndromes have highly characteristic eye movements. They regularly have V patterns with eyes most divergent in upgaze, closer together in gaze straight ahead, and closest together in downgaze. They regularly have markedly underactive superior rectus muscles. They may also have underactive superior oblique muscles and overactive inferior oblique muscles. These individuals may have a V pattern **esotropia,** a V pattern **exotropia,** or mixed strabismus with a V pattern (exotropia in up gaze, esotropia in down gaze). Some individuals with Apert syndrome also have irides that transilluminate. Alignment may be changed by craniofacial surgery, so in general, strabismus surgery should be postponed until craniofacial surgery is completed.

Although children with craniostenosis were thought in the past to develop optic atrophy from bone encroachment on the optic nerve, this mechanism must be exceedingly rare. When these children with craniostenosis do have optic atrophy, it generally appears to be secondary to their hydrocephalus. In contrast, optic atrophy from abnormal bony overgrowth is a prominent feature of the rare disorder **craniometaphyseal dysplasia.** This dominantly inherited disorder appears to be the result of a deficiency in bone resorption and causes gradual narrowing of all cranial foramens. There is a characteristic facial disfigurement.

C. **Hypertelorism.** The term *hypertelorism* has somewhat different meanings, depending on whether the clinician is considering **ocular hypertelorism** or **orbital hypertelorism;** for this latter determination, craniofacial surgeons refer to the distance between the medial walls of the orbits as determined by orbital x-rays or computed tomography scan. The distance between the lateral orbital walls (outer orbital distance) is a traditional ophthalmic measurement. Interpupillary distance gives a clinical measure of **ocular hypertelorism.** The distance between medial canthi, if it is excessive, gives a measure of **telecanthus.**

Orbital hypertelorism may be part of a large number of craniofacial syndromes, but it also occurs in an isolated form. There is a high association of exotropia with isolated orbital hypertelorism. After craniofacial surgery, the degree of exotropia is often markedly reduced, and the patient may even be esotropic. If a patient with orbital hypertelorism were a candidate for craniofacial surgery, it would be prudent to postpone strabismus surgery until after the craniofacial surgery.

XIII. **Tumors of childhood**

A. **Retinoblastoma** is the most frequent ocular tumor of childhood. The incidence is about 1 in every 20,000 live births. It has one of the highest cure rates of any malignant tumor. Untreated, it is almost invariably fatal.

1. **Heredity.** Retinoblastoma acts like an autosomal dominant trait with greater than 90% penetrance. In fact, it is really recessively inherited because both retinoblastoma genes at the 13q14 locus must be abnormal before the cell becomes malignant. Individuals with the hereditary form have one abnormal gene in all of their cells. A mutation in the other gene allows expression of the tumor. In the nonhereditary form, both mutations occur only in the retinal cell that has become malignant. Of all cases of retinoblastoma, 60% are nonhereditary and 40% are hereditary. Because there is a high spontaneous mutation rate in retinoblastoma, even most of the hereditary, bilateral cases will have no previous family history of the tumor. Such sporadic, bilaterally affected individuals will nevertheless still have a 50% chance of passing the disease on to each offspring. All bilateral cases and about 10% to 20% of unilateral cases of retinoblastoma are hereditary. Again, because of the high spontaneous mutation rate, 94% of all cases of retinoblastoma are sporadic, i.e., there is no **previous** family history of the tumor.

   The risk estimates are important for **genetic counseling.** If one parent is affected with familial retinoblastoma or bilateral sporadic retinoblastoma, each of the offspring will have a 50% chance of inheriting the tumor. The risk of the offspring of healthy siblings or healthy children of a patient with familial retinoblastoma is 1 in 15. Once an affected child is born to such an individual, the chance becomes one in two because she or he is then known to be an unaffected carrier. Because unilateral sporadic cases of retinoblastoma are usually not hereditary, the risk to the offspring of such individuals is much less, variously estimated between 1% and 8%. The risk to siblings of sporadic cases of being affected has been revised downward over the years from 15% to 1%. That there is any risk at all stems from the fact that the first mutation may have occurred in one of the parents without being expressed, rather than in the affected child. Fortunately, risk estimation and genetic counseling have become much more accurate in most families through the use of DNA sequence analysis and polymorphisms.

2. **Presentation.** In families known to harbor retinoblastoma, the diagnosis should be made within a few days of birth by routine examination. In sporadic cases, those who are bilaterally affected usually present by the age of 15 months and those who have unilateral retinoblastoma by 20 to 30 months of age. The most common presenting sign is a **white reflex** in the pupil, detected by the parents or the pediatrician. **Strabismus** is the second most common mode of presentation. Apparent intraocular inflammation and glaucoma secondary either to the tumor pushing the lens iris diaphragm forward or to tumor cells clogging the TM are also seen. Much less common modes of presentation include proptosis (secondary to retrobulbar extraocular extension), the appearance of a pseudohypopyon of tumor cells in the anterior chamber, and evidence of distant metastases. These all indicate a poor prognosis for life.

3. **Appearance.** The tumor may be a single or multifocal, smooth, pinkish, rounded mass in the retina. It may grow in, on top of (endophytic), or under (exophytic) the retina. The tumor may seed into the vitreous and grow back into the optic nerve. As mentioned, it may extend to the anterior segment.

4. **Mode of spread.** The tumor most commonly metastasizes to the bone marrow or extends back through the optic nerve into the subarachnoid space and spreads, via the CSF, throughout the CNS. Less commonly, distant metastases may occur in bone, and direct extension through the sclera into the orbit may occur.

5. **Pineal malignancies,** histologically similar to the ocular tumors ("trilateral retinoblastoma"), have been uniformly fatal.

6. **Survivors** of a familial retinoblastoma are very prone to develop other malignancies, most notably osteosarcoma.

7. **Treatment**

a. For 60 years in eyes that could be saved with useful vision, **radiation therapy** was the treatment of choice. With external beam irradiation using supervoltage *x-ray,* the local control rate is about 95%. With this sharp-edged beam, the entire retina can be treated without irradiating the lens. Contraindications to the use of radiation therapy as a primary mode of treatment include invasion of the optic nerve, invasion of the anterior segment of the eye, extensive vitreous seeding, and irreversible loss of vision in the eye. The total tumor dose is about 4,000 to 5,000 cGy. All bilateral tumors that are favorable to radiation therapy should be subjected to this mode of treatment. Because of the risks of radiation therapy, including a 4% incidence of malignant tumors in the field of radiation, the use of radiation for unilateral retinoblastoma, even in favorable cases, is somewhat controversial. The traditional treatment is enucleation of the unilaterally affected eye. With small, solitary tumors, except those near the fovea or optic disk, photocoagulation or cryotherapy may be justified (see sec. **XIII.A.7.d.,** below). *Proton beam* therapy may have advantages over x-ray or chemoreduction.

b. If the tumor is unfavorable for radiation therapy, then **enucleation** is the treatment of choice. Especially if the optic nerve is involved ophthalmoscopically, a long piece of optic nerve should be included with the enucleation of the globe. The prognosis is poor when the tumor has extended beyond the lamina cribrosa, and even poorer if it extends to the cut end of the optic nerve, on histologic examination. Local orbital spread and the detection of tumor at the end of the optic nerve in an enucleated specimen are indications for radiation therapy to the orbit and remaining optic nerve back to the chiasm. Evisceration is probably not of value.

c. Recently, **multiagent chemotherapy** to reduce the size of the tumors **(chemoreduction)** followed by local treatment with laser photocoagulation, cryotherapy, or radioactive plaques of individual tumors which have not completely regressed has superseded x-ray therapy. Thermoreduction has the advantage of not causing the facial deformities or increasing the risk of other malignancies associated with external beam radiation therapy.

d. **If individual tumors recur** or if new tumors appear in an eye after radiation therapy, they may often be successfully treated with **cryotherapy** by repeated freeze and thaw cycles, or by **photocoagulation.** Because retinoblastoma is usually multicentric, cryotherapy and photocoagulation should not be depended on as the primary mode of therapy, except in the case of small, solitary, extrafoveal tumors.

e. Scleral plaques containing radioisotopes (e.g., iodine-131) may be used to deliver high doses of radiation locally to individual tumors not treatable by other techniques, resulting in salvaging of eyes and vision that otherwise would be lost.

B. **Rhabdomyosarcoma** is a rare tumor, but it is the most common primary orbital tumor in childhood. It usually presents with rapidly progressive proptosis and displacement of the globe either upward or downward depending on the location of the tumor. It may mimic inflammation because of its rapid course and attendant signs of inflammation. The **diagnosis** is made by biopsy. In the past, **therapy** involved radical evisceration, sometimes with removal of bones around the orbit, with a 35% to 40% long-term survival. Combined chemotherapy, with the addition of radiation therapy if necessary, offers an 85% long-term survival with more than

90% local tumor control, and the treatment is much less disfiguring. To completely treat the tumor, no attempt is made to shield the lens or cornea from the effects of radiation therapy if needed; 5,000 to 6,000 cGy are given to the orbit with supervoltage x-ray through an anterior port. With this dose of radiation, a cataract always develops, and radiation retinitis is frequently seen. Radiation keratitis is often a problem, and dry eye syndrome from loss of lacrimal glands usually occurs. Before radiation therapy, the child, if old enough to understand, and the parents should be informed of the inevitable loss of vision.

C. **Neuroblastoma** is a common childhood tumor, usually originating in the paraspinal sympathetic chain or in the adrenal glands. It often metastasizes to the orbit, frequently first presenting as proptosis of the globe or ecchymosis of the eyelids or both. These presentations must be distinguished from trauma. The **treatment** consists of local radiation therapy and systemic chemotherapy, both of which are primarily of palliative value, though some young infants survive.

D. **Optic glioma** is thought by some to be a relatively stable hamartoma of the optic nerve. It may occur anywhere along the length of the nerve, including the optic chiasm. Optic glioma is commonly associated with neurofibromatosis (see sec. **VIII.B.,** above). If it is in the intraorbital portion of the nerve, it may produce loss of vision and unilateral optic disk swelling. In the optic chiasm it may produce visual field defects (which may remain stable over long periods of time) and optic atrophy. Some tumors in this area behave aggressively, invading the third ventricle, causing hydrocephalus, or they may involve the hypothalamus. It is unclear in some of these instances whether the tumor originates in the optic chiasm or in the hypothalamus itself. Because of the benign course of many of these tumors, some clinicians have advocated simple observation. If an intraorbital optic glioma is causing marked proptosis and is endangering the cornea, the optic nerve containing the tumor can be excised either from an orbital or intracranial approach. Chiasmal gliomas generally do not respond well to surgical treatment and may be subjected to radiation therapy. There are conflicting opinions about the effectiveness of this mode of treatment of optic glioma.

E. **Leukemia.** The most common form of leukemia in childhood is acute lymphoblastic leukemia that, with modern techniques of chemotherapy, has a greater than 90% 5-year survival and apparent cure rate. Acute myelogenous and monocytic leukemias are less common and have a worse prognosis, with survival of about 50%. The ocular manifestations are similar. The most common manifestation in the eye is retinal hemorrhage, which generally occurs when the patient is quite anemic and thrombocytopenic. These hemorrhages often have white centers (**Roth spots).** The central white area is not evidence that the retina is involved with leukemic cells. The retina can be massively infiltrated with leukemic cells, but this is rare and usually occurs in a patient who has a relapse of leukemia. Leukemic infiltration of the optic nerve is an emergency situation, because vision may be lost within a period of a few hours. The optic nerve is swollen and infiltrated with leukemic cells and may resemble papillitis. Radiation therapy to the posterior globes and orbit on an emergency basis is indicated to preserve vision. Leukemic cells may infiltrate the iris and circulate in the anterior chamber, resembling iritis. Secondary glaucoma may ensue. Sometimes the anterior segment involvement will respond to topical steroid treatment, but usually a small dose of radiation therapy to the anterior segment is required. In acute myelogenous leukemia, local large infiltrates of leukemic cells may rarely occur in the orbit, causing proptosis. This uncommon manifestation has been called **chloroma.** It responds dramatically to radiation therapy.

F. **Craniopharyngioma** is a tumor arising from the anterior pituitary in children.

Posterior pituitary tumors occur only rarely in children. A craniopharyngioma frequently presents with visual field loss or loss of vision in one eye secondary to pressure on the optic chiasm or an optic nerve or tract. It may also involve the third ventricle, causing increased intracranial pressure or hydrocephalus. Calcification in the suprasellar region is seen on x-ray. Sometimes the tumor can be completely excised surgically. More commonly, the cysts that form in the tumor are decompressed neurosurgically and then the tumor is treated with radiation therapy. Patients who have rapidly evolving visual field loss sometimes have complete restoration of visual function if treatment is undertaken quickly. Another complication of craniopharyngioma is hypopituitarism from damage to the posterior pituitary by tumor, surgery, or radiation therapy.

G. **Medulloepithelioma (diktyoma)** is a rare embryonic epithelial tumor usually involving the ciliary body and sometimes the optic nerve. It may be benign or malignant and may contain heterotopic mesodermal elements (teratoma). The presentation in the ciliary body may grow into the pupillary area, becoming visible to the parents or interfering with the child's vision. Sometimes it presents as cysts in the pupil. Those in the optic nerve may cause proptosis. **Treatment** is enucleation.

H. **Juvenile xanthogranuloma** is a benign dermatologic disorder in which yellowish skin lesions ranging in size from a few millimeters to several centimeters in diameter appear in the first few months of life, increase in size gradually, and then gradually fade spontaneously by age 5 years. The iris may be involved with xanthomas, which may cause spontaneous hyphema. Generally, the blood absorbs without causing permanent damage, although secondary glaucoma and other complications of hyphema may occur. Sometimes the hyphemas are recurrent. The iris xanthomas usually resolve spontaneously as the child grows older, and the problem resolves. On rare occasions topical steroids or a small dose of radiation therapy to the iris may be required.

XIV. **Retinopathy of prematurity (ROP) (formerly retrolental fibroplasia)**

A. **Background.** ROP was the leading cause of blindness in children in the 1940s and 1950s. After oxygen was identified as an etiologic factor, ROP became relatively rare. The severe oxygen restriction that prevailed from the mid-1950s to the mid-1960s, however, resulted in a striking increase in neonatal death and brain damage in premature infants. Therefore, the use of oxygen was liberalized in the late 1960s. Very small premature infants, who previously had died, now survive in large numbers. These tiny infants are at great risk, and ROP has become more common again.

B. **Etiology.** Excessive oxygen in the newborn period in premature infants was certainly the important factor in ROP in the 1940s and 1950s. The occurrence of ROP correlates with the length of time in an increased oxygen environment and with higher oxygen saturation as measured by continuous transcutaneous monitoring. The danger of ROP increases with short gestational age and low birth weight. ROP has been reported rarely, however, in full-term infants and in premature infants who never received added oxygen. The possible explanation for the latter is the sudden increase in Po_2 from 40 mm Hg in utero to 100 mm Hg after birth in room air.

C. **Pathophysiology.** Normal retina is gradually vascularized from the optic disk to the periphery during the final half of gestation, the temporal periphery finally becoming vascularized shortly after term. The earlier in the gestational period an infant is born, the less the vessels have grown out. The developing vessels may be arrested in their growth by excessive oxygen in the developing peripheral retina, which obliterates the newly forming vessels. When normal blood vessel growth is interrupted in this way, the vanguard of mesenchymal tissue builds up and forms a ridge that may be interrupted or continuous. The capillaries posterior to this ridge are obliterated, and the ridge forms an arteriovenous (AV) shunt. Microaneurysms may form posterior to the ridge. The peripheral avascular retina becomes hypoxic and releases humoral agents, including vascular endothelial cell growth factor, which stimulate blood vessel growth. In more severe cases, extraretinal neovascular proliferation on the surface of the retina and in the vitreous may occur.

In milder cases, intraretinal capillaries may bud from the anterior edge of the ridge, resuming the normal vascularization of the retina with complete regression of the ROP. In more severe cases, scarring takes place, which may produce traction on the retina. This scarring may be localized to the previous area of the ridge or may produce distortion of the posterior retina, including the macula, with fixed folds, and, in the most severe cases, may produce total retinal detachment. Even in cases where the posterior retina is relatively intact, there may be persistent AV shunts and avascular peripheral retina. Up to the point at which scarring occurs, it is possible for acute, active ROP to regress, leaving no abnormalities or only minimum peripheral changes and normal function.

D. **Stages of ROP.** A generally accepted international classification of ROP has been developed to standardize communication and criteria for evaluating treatment.

1. **Stage 1** is the appearance of a distinct demarcation line separating the peripheral avascular retina from vascularized posterior retina.

2. **Stage 2** involves the formation of a ridge that is elevated and has width.

3. **Stage 3** includes extraretinal fibrovascular proliferative tissue growing off the posterior edge of the ridge into the vitreous or onto the surface of the retina.

4. **Stage 4** exhibits a subtotal retinal detachment without involving the fovea (4A) and a retinal attachment involving the fovea (4B).

5. **Stage 5** is a total retinal detachment.

6. Any of the stages of ROP may exhibit **dilation** and **tortuosity** of the posterior retinal blood vessels, in which case a "+" is added to the number of the stage.

E. **The location and extent of ROP** are described by dividing each retina into three zones with the disk, where the retinal blood vessels begin, at the center of concentric circles.

1. **Zone 1** has a radius that extends from the disk about twice as far as from the disk to the macula.

2. **Zone 2** extends all the way to the ora serrata on the nasal side and a little bit anterior to the equator on the temporal side.

3. **Zone 3** is a crescent that involves the remaining superior, inferior, and temporal retina. The retina is divided also into clock hours.

F. **Examination and treatment.** Premature infants who are born with a birth weight of less than 1,250 to 1,500 g or a gestational age less than 32 weeks should be examined beginning around 4 weeks of age and every 2 to 3 weeks thereafter until the vessels have reached the ora serrata. If ROP is discovered, the patient should be followed more closely, depending on the activity and severity of the abnormalities. If stage 3+ ROP is reached, involving 5 hours or more of the circumference of the retina continuously or 8 hours intermittently, one should consider treating with confluent cryotherapy or indirect diode laser therapy to the entire avascular retina. When ROP has reached this stage, about 50% will still regress spontaneously without loss of central vision, but with cryotherapy about 75% will regress. If the severe ROP occurs in zone 1 or posterior zone 2, the prognosis is much poorer with or without treatment. In stage 4A and 4B ROP, scleral buckling with drainage of subretinal fluid may be indicated, and with stage 5 ROP, vitrectomy with lensectomy and peeling of preretinal membranes will be necessary in an attempt to reattach the retina. The retina can be reattached in 50% to 60% of eyes that have reached stage 5 ROP, but useful vision may be obtained in only a small number of eyes. A collaborative study to determine potential benefits of treating at an earlier stage (ET [early treatment]-ROP study) in certain infants at higher risk of progression is underway.

G. **Late complications of cicatricial ROP** include angle-closure glaucoma from anterior displacement of the lens iris diaphragm and late rhegmatogenous retinal detachments from traction by the peripheral scarring, causing retinal holes. Patients with cicatricial ROP also have an increased incidence of high myopia, and those with visual disabilities may require low-vision aids and referral to special education programs for the visually handicapped.

XV. **Toxicity of systemic medications to ocular structures**

A. **Chloramphenicol** may cause **optic neuritis** as well as **peripheral neuritis** after chronic use. The toxic effect of the drug acts like retrobulbar neuritis, with loss of visual acuity of varying severity and development of a **central scotoma.** In the vast majority of patients, the visual acuity returns to normal when the chloramphenicol treatment is discontinued. If treatment is resumed to control infection, many patients will not suffer a recurrent attack of toxic optic neuritis. Papillitis with swelling of the optic nerve has not been noted in chloramphenicol toxicity.

B. **Systemic steroids**

1. **Cataracts.** Prolonged treatment with high-dose systemic steroids will eventually lead to posterior subcapsular cataract. The opacity may progress to involve the rest of the lens if the dose cannot be decreased. Steroid cataract may regress if the patient can be kept on a very low dose of systemic steroids or if the steroids can be stopped entirely. Cataracts will develop in most patients after the equivalent of 15 to 20 mg of prednisone a day for a period of 2 years. In children, two diseases that commonly require systemic steroids for periods long enough to produce cataracts are asthma and systemic lupus erythematosus. Other entities in which the use of long-term steroid therapy has caused cataracts include Crohn's disease, nephrotic syndrome, renal transplantation, scleroderma, and leukemia.

2. **Glaucoma** can be caused by long-term systemic corticosteroid therapy as well as by topical steroids in susceptible individuals (see Chapter 10, sec. **XXI.**).

XVI. **The management of cataract in infancy and childhood.** The etiology of cataract and associations with other disorders and syndromes are discussed in preceding sections of this chapter. The development of amblyopia when the vision is blurred or completely obscured by a cataract in infancy or childhood introduces additional factors into the management of these youngsters.

Even when it is opaque with cataract, the crystalline lens in infancy and childhood is soft compared with an adult lens. The lens in childhood can be readily broken up and aspirated through a needle. A variety of cutting–aspiration techniques are available (see Chapter 7, sec. **VII.D.**). The posterior capsule must be removed and a shallow anterior vitrectomy performed, because the infantile posterior capsule always opacifies. **Phacoemulsification** and other techniques that have been introduced to break up the hard nucleus of the adult lens are not necessary and are **contraindicated** for the removal of childhood cataracts (see Chapter 7, sec. **VII.D.**).

A. **Dense bilateral cataracts in infancy.** Dense cataracts early in life obscure vision and produce sensory nystagmus. Review of systems and systemic pediatric examinations may reveal additional abnormalities. These cataracts should be removed as early in infancy as possible, preferably within the first few weeks of life, the second eye being done within days after the first. If the 3-mm central axis is opaque, amblyopia will occur without surgical correction.

B. **Dense unilateral cataracts.** Marked asymmetry in the visual input to the CNS from the two eyes will lead to a dense amblyopia in the more handicapped eye. Unilateral cataracts may also be associated with other ocular abnormalities. The therapy of a unilateral cataract includes prolonged and vigorous amblyopia therapy after the surgical removal of the cataract within the first few weeks of life.

C. **Traumatic cataracts.** A cataract after trauma in early childhood may produce dense amblyopia. Deprivation of vision in this way may lead to loss of steady fixation in only a few months. Once the cataract is removed, continued attention is required to provide appropriate optical correction and vigorous amblyopia therapy with patching of the better eye. With an injury in early childhood, management of the amblyopia requires very close supervision at least until age 10 or 12 years. Late complications from severe trauma and cataract surgery, such as glaucoma or retinal detachment, may not manifest themselves until adult life, so the patient needs to be followed indefinitely.

D. **Zonular (or lamellar) developmental cataracts.** Developmental cataracts are present at birth and have a highly characteristic appearance (see Chapter 7, sec. **V.B.**). Usually they are present in both eyes and remain unchanged year to year. If they are quite symmetric in the two eyes and if the child's visual development seems to be satisfactory, it is often possible to delay surgery indefinitely or until the child has difficulty with schoolwork or some other specific visual task. Marked asymmetry in the opacities in the two eyes, however, may create amblyopia in the eye with the denser cataract, and might require intervention at an earlier age.

E. **Visual rehabilitation** after cataract surgery is achieved by fitting the infant or child with **contact lenses.** In the unusual case of contact lens intolerance, aphakic spectacles are a perfectly acceptable alternative when both eyes are aphakeic. There is **no indication** for **intraocular lenses** (IOLs) in congenital cataracts. An IOL may be justified in an older child with acquired cataract(s) or whose congenital cataract(s) becomes visually significant later in childhood. If sufficient support is present, a secondary IOL implant may be considered later in childhood.

F. **Amblyopia** is treated or prevented by patching the unaffected eye for 80% of the waking hours in an infant or for 4 to 5 hours daily up to full time in an older child. Once strong fixation is achieved with the contact lens-bearing aphakic eye, occlusion of the normal eye should be continued in young children, varying the length of time as necessary until vision can be measured (age 3 to 4 years) and occlusion times adjusted appropriately. Although not entirely comparable to Snellen (recognition) acuity, grating acuity tests, e.g., Teller acuity cards, are helpful in following the treatment of amblyopia in preverbal and preliterate infants.

XVII. **Glaucomas of infancy and childhood.** Public awareness of glaucoma has increased to the point that most people know that it affects a significant proportion of the adult population over 40 years of age (variably estimated as between 2% and 5%). Regrettably, there is not the same awareness that glaucoma exists in childhood. It is crucial to make this diagnosis early in life before vision has already been irreparably damaged or lost. To make the diagnosis, it is important to maintain a high index of suspicion and to consider it routinely in the differential diagnosis of ocular problems of childhood.

A. **Infantile glaucoma**

1. **Signs. Tearing, photophobia, cloudy cornea, and corneal enlargement** in one or both eyes are the classic signs of infantile glaucoma. The signs may be present at birth (truly congenital), they may develop early in the newborn period, or they may develop in the first few years of life. Only one sign may be present initially, and it is important not to wait for the full constellation before making a complete evaluation for glaucoma. It is worthy of note that after 2 years of age the corneas generally do **not** enlarge even if the IOP is elevated.

2. **Differential diagnosis of cloudy cornea**

a. **Congenital glaucoma.** Cloudy corneas from **congenital glaucoma** may be diffusely hazy with epithelial edema or may have more intense opacification of the cornea over breaks in the corneal endothelium (Haab striae). Characteristically, this break resulting from increased IOP and stretching will be circumferential or sometimes horizontal.

   b. **Forceps injury.** In contrast to Haab striae, an endothelial break due to **forceps injury** will usually be vertical in its orientation, there may be other signs of facial injury in the newborn period, and IOP will not be elevated.

   c. **Corneal endothelial dystrophy.** Infants with **corneal endothelial dystrophy** also have diffusely hazy corneas with epithelial edema. The endothelial surface of the cornea may have marked irregularities to help localize the difficulty at this level, but these changes are not always present. The IOP and the optic nerves are normal in corneal endothelial dystrophy.

   d. **MPS (Hurler, Scheie, Morquio, and Maroteaux-Lamy syndromes) and mucolipidoses.** The corneas are hazy, but there is no epithelial edema. The IOP is normal, and the optic nerves do not have glaucomatous cupping.

   e. **IK.** Although it has been reported at birth, IK rarely presents at such an early age.

   f. **Congenital rubella syndrome.** The corneas may be transiently or permanently hazy with normal IOP, or a true infantile glaucoma may be present.

3. **Examination.** Complete ophthalmologic examination includes assessment of IOP, inspection of the optic nerves, gonioscopic examination of the filtration angle, and examination of the cornea under magnification. In many infants, all of these examinations can be done in the office. Although some information may have to be obtained during anesthesia, especially in older children, the physician can usually narrow the differential diagnosis substantially at the time of the initial thorough examination in the office.

   a. **Assessment of IOP.** Measurement of IOP in the office is greatly facilitated if the infant is hungry at the time of examination and is given a bottle.

   After the infant is involved in feeding, a combination topical anesthetic and fluorescein (Fluress) can be applied and IOP measured. A handheld applanation device (e.g., Perkin tonometer) is very helpful in this situation. Several readings are taken, and it is the lowest consistent unsedated IOP that is usually the most relevant. Struggling or lid squeezing will tend to erroneously elevate the IOP.

   IOP measurements in the office are much more satisfactory than those under general anesthesia. *General anesthetics all decrease the IOP*, so that measurements in the operating room are helpful in diagnosis only if they are elevated.

   b. **Inspection of the optic nerves.** Optic disk cupping in childhood is a very sensitive indicator of IOP, especially in the stages before permanent visual field loss. Asymmetry in optic nerve cupping may be helpful in making the initial diagnosis, and evaluation of cupping may also be helpful in the postoperative management and long-term follow-up of the glaucoma patient. The optic cup may become smaller within hours of successful goniotomy or trabeculotomy.

   c. **Gonioscopic examination of the angle.** Koeppe lens examination may be possible in the unsedated infant without discomfort or struggling. In an older child this may have to await general anesthesia. Gonioscopy is an important initial step in making the differentiation between infantile glaucoma and other forms of angle anomalies such as Rieger syndrome. In follow-up, gonioscopy is helpful in understanding the success or failure of previous trabecular operations.

   d. **Examination of the cornea under magnification.** In cases of corneal cloudiness, close inspection is essential for proper diagnosis.

With the Koeppe lens in place, close inspection of the cornea may be done with the Barkan light and handheld microscope. Even small children can be held up to the slitlamp if sufficient personnel are mobilized. Standard slitlamp examination in the operating room with the anesthetized child lying on his or her side can be helpful. A handheld, portable slitlamp may also be useful.

4. **Special studies.** If the office ophthalmologic examination indicates infantile glaucoma, a prenatal and birth history, review of systems, and careful pediatric evaluation are worthwhile. It may be very helpful to identify a syndrome such as congenital rubella syndrome that up to age 2 years requires isolation during hospitalization. A systemic metabolic disorder such as Lowe syndrome will require considerable medical attention in addition to the ophthalmologic evaluation. Special studies are selected on the basis of the history and systemic examination.

5. **Treatment.** Once the diagnosis of infantile glaucoma has been made by office examination, acetazolamide, 15 mg/kg/day in three or four divided doses, is started. A cloudy cornea may clear significantly after a few days of acetazolamide therapy. Examination under anesthesia completes the diagnostic procedures. Surgery is directed to the trabecular tissues in the form of either goniotomy or trabeculotomy, both of which result in an incision into the TM. Goniotomy (or internal trabeculotomy) was the first major advance in therapy of this condition and remains a straightforward, low-risk procedure. Trabeculotomy (or external goniotomy) has advantages when the cornea is hazy, and apparently also develops filtration in some patients. Trabeculotomy scars the conjunctiva, making future filtration surgery in that area more difficult. Barkan observations regarding the effectiveness of trabecular surgery remain the major clues to the etiology of infantile glaucoma.

Goniotomies and trabeculotomies are not always successful, even when repeated several times. Long-term management of youngsters in whom surgery has not been successful is difficult and involves the use of chronic medications (see Chapter 10, sec. V.). Although miotics do not appear to be very effective in untreated infantile glaucoma, a youngster who has had a partially effective goniotomy or trabeculotomy procedure may subsequently be benefited by miotic agents. Filtration surgery can be tried, but it is more difficult to maintain filtration in children than in adults. Cyclocryotherapy may also be effective, but if undertaken it is essential to leave several hours of the circumference unfrozen to avoid hypotony. Transscleral diode laser cycloablation may also control elevated IOP.

6. **Follow-up.** Even if initial trabecular surgery appears to be effective, these youngsters must be followed indefinitely (several times a year initially and then at least annually for their lifetimes) because the elevated pressure may return even years after successful surgery. If the glaucoma recurs, another goniotomy or trabeculotomy may be effective.

B. **Aniridia**

1. **Physical findings.** The term *aniridia* is used for a multifaceted ocular disorder that involves much more than the underdevelopment of the iris. Despite the term, the iris is not totally absent, a small stump being visible 360 degrees by gonioscopy and sometimes by slitlamp. Also present at birth is the macular aplasia that correlates with the markedly diminished vision and sensory nystagmus. Congenital lens opacities are frequent. During the first and second decades these patients often develop a characteristic peripheral corneal pannus, readily seen at slitlamp examinations. Indirect ophthalmoscopy of the far peripheral retina may reveal small yellow dots circumferentially.

These children may or may not develop glaucoma. Because glaucoma does develop in a significant number of aniridia patients, close examination from infancy onward is warranted. The occurrence of glaucoma correlates with adhesion of the peripheral iris to the TM. The mechanism of this adhesion is not well understood. Once the peripheral iris covers the outflow channels and glaucoma is present, the condition is difficult to treat. Walton has advocated the use of prophylactic goniotomy when the peripheral iris starts to cover the TM and before the IOP is elevated.

2. **Heredity.** Aniridia may be inherited in a dominant fashion, or it may appear as the result of a spontaneous mutation. The eponym **Miller syndrome** has been given to the close association of sporadic aniridia and **Wilms tumor.** Accordingly, thorough evaluation of the abdomen should be done when the diagnosis of aniridia is first made in a child without family history of the condition. Studies of the abdomen should probably be repeated once or twice a year during the first few years of life. Some patients with aniridia and Wilms tumor apparently have a deletion of the short arm of the eleventh chromosome, 11p. It appears that a more extensive deletion involving the aniridia locus gives rise to the association of aniridia and Wilms tumor with mental retardation, hypogonadism, and other urogenital anomalies.

C. **Juvenile open-angle glaucoma.** On occasion, open-angle glaucoma may have its onset in the first decades of life. The diagnosis may be overlooked because the disorder is asymptomatic until irreversible visual damage has occurred. Certainly a family history of glaucoma, particularly early-onset glaucoma, is a strong indication to take routine IOP measurements in childhood. The only way to make this diagnosis in the very early stages is to check IOP routinely even in children. **Large cups** or **asymmetric cupping in childhood** is as valuable an early sign of glaucoma as it is in adults. Juvenile open-angle glaucoma is treated with the same medications and the same principles as adult open-angle glaucoma (see Chapter 10, sec **V.**).

D. **Childhood glaucomas secondary to inflammation.** Untreated ocular inflammation (uveitis) may cause glaucoma by producing an adhesion between the iris and the anterior surface of the lens (seclusion of the pupil). When the aqueous is no longer able to pass through the pupil into the anterior chamber, iris bombé and glaucoma result. Mydriatic therapy during episodes of uveitis is designed to avoid this.

Chronic iritis such as that associated with pauciarticular JRA or sympathetic ophthalmia, or following extracapsular cataract extraction on occasion can produce a secondary open-angle glaucoma with markedly diminished outflow facility. A delayed glaucoma several years following congenital cataract extraction in the absence of apparent inflammation is not unusual. The exact nature of the damage to the TM is not known. **Open-angle glaucoma secondary to inflammation is difficult to treat.** Miotic agents are often contraindicated because of the ongoing inflammation (see Chapter 10, sec. **XVIII.**). If medications cannot control the IOP, filtering surgery must be considered, but both the young age of the patient and the presence of active inflammation are adverse factors for achieving effective filtration. Trabecular surgery by goniotomy or a modified goniotomy "trabeculodialysis or trabeculotomy" has helped some individuals over short periods, but long-term successes from these procedures have not been reported.

The influence of steroid therapy on the IOP has to be evaluated in each patient. Steroids employed in the management of the uveitis may cause glaucoma in some individuals (steroid-induced glaucoma). In contrast, steroid therapy decreases the IOP in the condition of keratic precipitates in the angle (see Chapter 10, sec. **XXI.**). Iridocyclitis usually causes a reduction in aqueous production by the ciliary body, and, therefore, in some critical situations the decision may be made to reduce the steroid therapy and allow the inflammation to worsen. If it has been decided to do filtration surgery, however, it is important to suppress inflammation with steroids as much as possible in the pre- and postoperative periods.

   E. **Glaucoma following trauma.** Glaucoma following ocular trauma in childhood may occur promptly or years later by the same mechanisms as in the adult (see Chapter 10, sec. **XVII.**). In childhood it is important to include assessment of IOP in the initial and follow-up examinations of the traumatized eye because of the possibility of permanent trabecular damage following blunt trauma or hyphema.

XVIII. Special issues concerning trauma in childhood

   A. **History taking** from traumatized children is notoriously unreliable. Not infrequently, the child feels guilty about the circumstances of the injury and gives an inaccurate or incomplete account of the accident. The physician must not be misled by an innocuous sounding history, but should be guided by the **physical findings** and entertain a high degree of suspicion that the injury involves more than the presenting signs. For example, lid laceration must be assumed to involve an intraocular injury until specifically proved otherwise.

   B. **Penetrating ocular trauma.** A full-thickness lid laceration should be fully evaluated and repaired by an ophthalmologist. The likelihood of an accompanying penetrating injury to the globe is great; if any doubt remains after examination in the emergency room, it is best to treat the eye as if it were penetrated and resolve the issue in the operating room (see Chapter 2, sec. **VI.**). Although several routines for inducing sedation in the emergency room are available (pedimixes for i.m. injection or "soothing syrups" for drinking), the child is usually not sufficiently sedated for repair in this sensitive area. Heavy sedation runs the risk of serious respiratory depression, so it is generally safest and best to make the repair in the operating room with the aid of general anesthesia.

     If careful examination establishes that injury causing a lid laceration has not caused a penetration of the globe, it may still have involved sufficient force to cause intraocular damage.

   C. **Blunt ocular trauma.** Despite the slight, even jocular, attention often given to a "shiner," a black eye may be the prominent initial feature of serious ocular injury. Blowout fracture of the orbital floor, retinal detachment, hyphema, dislocated lens, traumatic iritis, and other ocular injuries may be overlooked because the lids are so swollen that insufficient attention is paid to the globe itself. All black eyes should be evaluated by an ophthalmologist. If there is any other sign of ocular abnormality such as conjunctival injection or diminished visual acuity, ophthalmic examination with dilated fundus examination is definitely indicated (see Chapter 2, sec. **VIII.**).

   D. **Patching in young children.** Young children often need an eye patch applied for a day or two after **treatment** of an ocular condition such as corneal abrasion, removal of a corneal foreign body, or an ultraviolet sunlamp burn. A pressure patch of this sort is sometimes prescribed for several days consecutively. In a very young child (especially in the first year or two), this may be a significant period of visual deprivation. In some cases, a patch has induced **strabismus** or **amblyopia.** Therefore, indications should be carefully weighed against risk when patching of very young children for more than a few days is being considered.

XIX. Retinal diseases in children

   A. **Retinal degenerations. Retinitis pigmentosa** and its allied disorders constitute a diffuse group of disorders in which the mechanism of retinal degeneration is not known although the loci of the defective genes have been identified in several families. Early loss of night vision, followed by loss of peripheral vision and eventual difficulty with central vision are characteristic. In classic retinitis pigmentosa, family history is prominent; the pattern of inheritance may be recessive, dominant, or X-linked. Some allied disorders, such as **albipunctate dystrophy,** have a distinctive fundus appearance; others, such as choroideremia, have characteristic fundus features and characteristic hereditary patterns (X-linked in the case of choroideremia). **Leber congenital amaurosis,** recessively inherited, may have little morphologic abnormality of the retina on fundus examination, but presents with severe visual loss in the newborn period or early childhood. Confirmation of this diagnosis is provided by a markedly abnormal ERG.

Although it is not currently possible to treat most retinal degenerations, it is nevertheless important that efforts be directed toward identifying affected individuals early in their diseases. One should rule out potentially correctable disorders as well as give genetic counseling. Therapeutic interventions cannot hope to recover vision from the damaged retinas of adults already blind from the disorders. **Therapy** should be directed toward individuals who are still functioning, in the hope of avoiding further retinal degeneration. Systemic biochemical abnormalities have recently been identified with **gyrate atrophy,** and treatment with vitamin B6 seems to have been beneficial in some patients. Previously, systemic biochemical abnormalities had been identified only in multisystem disorders that happened also to include retinal degeneration, e.g., **abetalipoproteinemia (Bassen-Kornzweig syndrome),** neuronal ceroid **lipofuscinosis (Batten-Mayou disease)** (see sec. **VII.D.,** above), and **Refsum's disease.** The findings of a specific biochemical disorder in an isolated retinal degeneration such as gyrate atrophy is particularly encouraging and gives hope of similar discoveries with regard to retinitis pigmentosa and its allied disorders.

B. **Childhood macular degenerations.** A number of dominantly inherited macular degenerations, such as **Best vitelliform dystrophy** and **butterfly dystrophy,** present in childhood. Family history is helpful in identifying these conditions.

   Stargardt macular degeneration (fundus flavimaculatus) may cause considerable reduction in central visual acuity with minimum funduscopic changes. These youngsters have on occasion been erroneously considered to be malingering, and only years later when the process had reached an advanced stage was it properly recognized. There is **no** specific **therapy** for these disorders, but funduscopic, psychophysic, and electrophysiologic testing should at least help characterize the disorder and improve early **diagnosis.**

C. **Vitreoretinal degenerations**

   1. **Juvenile retinoschisis.** Strabismus, poor visual acuity, nystagmus, or a "cart wheel" (spoke-like) macular region may be the presenting features of juvenile retinoschisis. Although the macular areas resemble microcystic edema on ophthalmoscopy, there is no leakage on fluorescein angiography. Schisis in the peripheral retina and X-linked heredity complete the clinical picture. Careful documentation of the fundus findings may be helpful because some of these youngsters subsequently lose vision acutely because of hemorrhaging from a retinal vessel or a retinal detachment. The family may benefit from genetic counseling.

   2. **The Goldmann-Favre syndrome** is a rare disorder that might be considered if peripheral retinoschisis were seen in a young girl or in a boy in whom autosomal-recessive inheritance seemed more likely than X-linked inheritance. There are preretinal membranes and a retinitis pigmentosa fundus picture.

   3. **Wagner vitreoretinal degeneration** has a dominant inheritance. Cataracts occur at an early age, and the vitreous contains dense membranes. Characteristic retinal pigmentation parallels the retinal vessels. Retinal detachments are frequent so periodic indirect ophthalmoscopic examinations to identify retinal breaks or early detachment are recommended.

4. **Stickler syndrome,** dominantly inherited, has high myopia, liquefied vitreous, retinal pigmentary changes, and retinal detachment, which may be very difficult to treat. Systemic manifestations include skeletal dysplasia, cleft palate, and characteristically flattened facies.

D. **Coats's disease (Leber miliary aneurysms).** The basic anomaly appears to be a congenital malformation of the retinal blood vessels leading to aneurysmal dilations that look like "light bulbs" in the peripheral retina on indirect ophthalmoscopy. The aneurysmal dilations are "leaky," so exudate accumulates in the subretinal space. This exudate tends to accumulate initially in the macular area, so a peripheral lesion should be considered when unexplained macular exudate, including a macular star figure, is seen. Obliteration of the peripheral vascular anomalies by **cryotherapy** or **photocoagulation** may be beneficial at this stage. With more exudation the retina may be completely detached. Total retinal detachment with fat and cholesterol in the subretinal fluid may create a white pupil (leukokoria). By that point vision is irretrievable, but it is very important to differentiate Coats's disease from retinoblastoma as the cause of the white pupil.

E. **Sickle cell anemia.** Although sickle cell SS disease is the more severe systemic disorder, sickle C and sickle thalassemia disease are the more frequent causes of retinal neovascularization. Perhaps the anemia of sickle cell disease partially protects the flow through the small vessels of the retina. Retinal detachment may follow neovascularization; patients with sickle cell, sickle C, and S thalassemia disease as a group do poorly with retinal detachment surgery. Prophylactic treatment of retinal breaks seems particularly prudent in these patients. Because retinal changes can be seen even in the first decade, it is advisable to begin periodic ocular examinations when the diagnosis of SC or S thalassemia is made.

12. EXTRAOCULAR MUSCLES, STRABISMUS, AND NYSTAGMUS

Deborah Pavan-Langston and Nathalie Azar

I. **Normal anatomy and physiology of the extraocular muscles**
   A. **Innervation and action.** All four recti muscles and the **superior oblique (SO) muscle** originate at the orbital apex (Fig. 12.1). The four recti muscles arise from the annulus of Zinn. The inferior oblique originates at the medial aspect of the interior orbital rim.
   1. The **medial rectus (MR)** muscle courses anteriorly along the medial aspect of the globe to insert 5.5 mm posterior to the limbus. Innervation is by the third cranial nerve. Contraction of the muscle causes the eye to **turn inward (adduct)** toward the nose.
   2. The **lateral rectus (LR)** muscle courses anteriorly along the temporal aspect of the globe to insert 7 mm posterior to the limbus. Innervation to this muscle is by the sixth cranial nerve. Contraction causes the eye to **turn outward (abduct)** horizontally.
   3. The **superior rectus (SR)** muscle runs over the dorsal aspect of the eye to insert 7.5 mm posterior to the limbus. Innervation is via the third cranial nerve. Contraction produces various combinations of **vertical, horizontal,** and **rotary** movement, depending on the angle of gaze of the eye. As the muscle runs forward at an angle of 23 degrees to the medial wall of the orbit and inserts anterior to the center of rotation of the eye, the movement produced by contraction of the muscle would be pure elevation if the eye were at a horizontal starting position of 23 degrees abduction. If the eye were adducted inward to a position of 67 degrees, the only movement on contraction of the SR would be intorsion of the globe. With the eye in the primary position of straight-ahead gaze, contraction of the muscle produces combined elevation and intorsion with slight adduction.
   4. The **inferior rectus (IR)** muscle courses along the ventral aspect of the globe to insert 6.5 mm posterior to the limbus. Innervation to this muscle is also via the third cranial nerve. Contraction produces various combinations of **vertical, horizontal,** and **rotary** movement, depending on the horizontal position of the eye. With the eye at a position of 23 degrees abduction, the only movement is depression. If the eye is adducted inward to a position of 67 degrees, the only movement is extorsion as the muscle inserts anterior to the center of rotation of the globe. When the eye is in the primary position, contraction of the IR produces depression and extorsion with minimum adduction.
   5. The **SO** muscle runs forward along the superomedial wall of the orbit to pass through the trochlea, where it turns backward temporally, traveling at an angle of 51 degrees from the medial wall of the orbit over the dorsal aspect of the globe but ventral to the SR muscle. It inserts on the posterotemporal surface. Innervation to this muscle is by the fourth cranial nerve. Contraction results in various combinations of **vertical, horizontal,** and **rotary** movements, depending on the location of the eye horizontally. With a starting position of 39 degrees of abduction, the only movement is intorsion. With a starting position of 51 degrees of adduction, the only movement is depression. If the eye is in the primary position of straight-ahead gaze, the motion is combined intorsion and depression with minimum abduction. Abduction is secondary to the muscle insertion, being posterior to the ocular rotation center when the eye is in the primary position.
   6. The **inferior oblique (IO)** muscle originates at the anterior nasal orbital floor and runs backward and temporally at an angle of 51 degrees

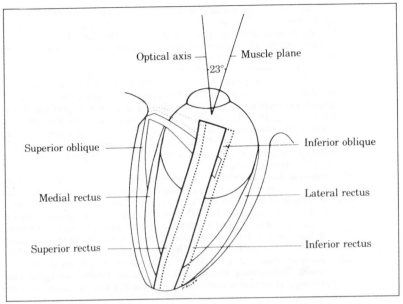

FIG. 12.1. Dorsal view of extraocular muscle attachments to the eye. Dotted lines are muscles inferior to the globe. (Adapted from von Noorden G, Manumenee AE. *Atlas of strabismus.* St. Louis: Mosby, 1967.)

from the nasal orbital wall to insert under the LR muscle in the macular area. Innervation to this muscle is by the third cranial nerve. Contraction produces various combinations of **vertical, rotary,** and **horizontal** movements. Starting from a 39-degree position of abduction, the only movement is extorsion. If the starting position is 51 degrees of adduction, the only movement is elevation. Contraction of the muscle with the eye in the primary position produces a combined extorsion and elevation with minimum abduction secondary to the insertion being posterior to the center of rotation.

    7. The **spiral of Tillaux** is a theoretic line connecting the insertions of the four rectus tendons. The medial rectus is closest to the limbus (5.5 mm posterior to it). The IR insertion is at 6.5 mm, the LR is at 6.9 mm, and the SR is at 7.7 mm.

B. Hering's law of equal innervation states that equal and simultaneous innervation is given to synergistic muscles or muscle groups concerned with a desired direction of gaze. The law is applicable to voluntary and some involuntary muscle movement.

    1. In **practical application,** during left gaze the right MR and left LR muscles receive equal innervation. If the head is tilted to the right, the muscle groups concerned with cycloduction (intorsion) of the right eye and excycloduction (extorsion) of the left eye will receive equal and simultaneous innervation.

    2. **Diagnosis of paralytic strabismus** is aided by knowledge of Herring law in determining **primary and secondary deviation.** Because the amount of innervation to both eyes is determined by the fixating eye, the angle of deviation will vary depending on the eye used for fixation. Primary deviation occurs when the nonaffected eye is fixing; secondary deviation occurs if fixation is with the paretic eye. The examiner may detect a paretic muscle or muscle group in **noncomitant strabismus**

(measured deviation unequal in different directions of gaze) by measuring the deviation of the eyes in diagnostic positions of gaze with each eye fixating in turn. For example, in paralysis of the right LR, normal innervation moves the normal left eye in adduction during right gaze. The paretic right eye does not follow outward beyond the midline, however, because the normal amount of innervation required by the paretic eye is not sufficient to overcome the paresis of the right LR. The resulting horizontal deviation is primary. When the paretic eye fixates, however, and an excessive amount of innervation is released in attempt to perform abduction on right gaze, by Herring law, the same increased level of innervation will be transmitted to the normal MR of the contralateral eye, resulting in an excessive adduction of that eye. This is secondary deviation and is greater in magnitude than the primary deviation. It points to the right LR as the paretic muscle.

C. **Sherrington law of reciprocal innervation** states that increased contraction of an extraocular muscle is associated normally by diminished contractile activity of its antagonist muscle. Therefore, on right gaze there is increased contraction of the left MR and the right LR, accompanied by decreased tone of the antagonistic left LR and right MR. During convergence, there is increased activity of both MR muscles with associated decreased activity of both LR muscles. When the head is tilted to the right shoulder there is contraction and relaxation of antagonistic muscle groups on levocycloversion. **Retractory nystagmus** and **Duane retraction syndrome** are pathologic examples of cocontraction of medial and lateral recti in the same eye.

D. **Ductions** refer to the movement of just one eye. **Abduction** is the horizontal movement away from the midline vertical axis and is a function of LR contraction and MR relaxation. **Adduction** is the horizontal movement toward the midline vertical axis and is accomplished by the contraction of the MR muscle and relaxation of the lateral muscle. **Infraduction** is a vertical movement or depression inferior to the horizontal axis of the eye and results from combined contraction of the IR and SO muscles. **Supraduction** is a vertical movement or elevation superior to the horizontal axis of the eye, and results from the combined contraction of the SO and IO muscles and the combined relaxation of the IR and SO muscles. **Incycloduction** or **intorsion** is a rotary movement of the eye about the anteroposterior (AP) axis such that the superior pole of the cornea is displaced medially and results from combined contraction of the SO and SR muscles with relaxation of the IO and IR muscles. **Excycloduction** or **extorsion** is a rotary movement of the eye around the AP axis displacing the superior pole of the cornea laterally and results from the combined contraction of the IO and IR muscles with concomitant relaxation of the SO and SR muscles.

E. **Binocular movements** are divided into two categories: **versions** and **vergences.**

1. A **version** refers to the simultaneous movement of both eyes in the same direction. Versions, like ductions, normally adhere to Herring and Sherrington laws, and include right and left lateral horizontal and vertical gaze.

   a. **Dextroversion** and **levoversion.** Dextroversion is the result of contraction of the right LR and left MR muscles. Levoversion is accomplished by contraction of the left LR and right MR with simultaneous relaxation of the left MR and the right LR.

   b. **Vertical versions** are supraversion or infraversion. **Supraversion** or **upgaze** is the result of bilateral contraction of the SR and IO muscles with simultaneous relaxation of the inferior recti and SO muscles in the primary position. **Infraversion** or **downgaze** in the primary position is the result of increased innervation to the IR and SO.

   c. **Cycloversion** is the simultaneous and equal tilt of the superior corneal poles to the right or left. **Dextrocycloversion** is the result of contraction of the extorters of the right eye (IR and IO) and the intortors of the left eye (SR and SO) with concomitant relaxation of their antagonist muscles. **Levocycloversion** is the mirror image of this action, with increased innervation to the extorters of the left eye and the intortors of the right eye and decreased innervation to their antagonistic muscle groups.

   2. A **vergence** is the equal simultaneous movement of the eyes in opposite directions. **Convergence** is inward movement; **divergence** is a simultaneous outward movement. Convergence is the result of contraction of both medial recti and relaxation of the lateral recti; divergence results from contraction of the lateral recti with concomitant relaxation of the medial recti. **Vertical vergences** result in contraction of the elevators of one eye and the depressors of the contralateral eye with subsequent opposing vertical movements. **Cyclovergence** is simultaneous equal tilting of the corneal superior poles inward or outward.

F. The **primary position of gaze** is the position assumed by the eyes when fixating a far distant object directly ahead. This position may be maintained with the head erect or with it tilted to either side. **Secondary positions** are any eye positions other than primary and include near-fixation, the cardinal positions, and midline vertical positions.

   1. The **near-fixation position** is usually taken at 0.33 m from the eyes. This reflex involves convergence and accommodative action.

   2. The **cardinal positions** are six positions of gaze that compare the horizontal and vertical eye alignment resulting from action by the six extraocular muscles (Fig. 12.2).

   3. The **midline positions** are vertical positions up and down from the primary positions.

II. **Single binocular vision** is a conditioned reflex, the prerequisites for which are straight eyes starting in the neonatal period and similar images presented

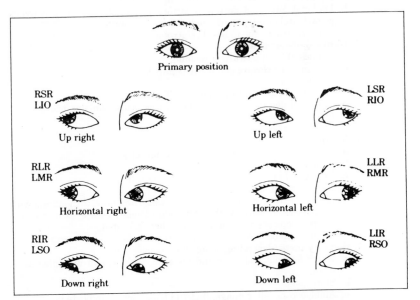

FIG. 12.2. Normal cardinal positions of gaze and extraocular muscles involved as primary movers in a given field of gaze. *R,* right; *L,* left; *SR,* superior rectus; *IO,* inferior oblique; *LR,* lateral rectus; *MR,* medial rectus; *IR,* inferior rectus; *SO,* superior oblique.

to each retina. Patients with congenital strabismus lack single binocular central vision, but early elimination of the strabismus may result in peripheral single binocular vision. The age at which congenitally strabismic patients may develop single binocular vision after surgical straightening is unknown, but the current maximum estimate is 2 years. **Simultaneous perception, fusion, and stereopsis** are three different perceptual phenomena comprising single binocular vision. They may function simultaneously or in decreasing degrees, with stereopsis being the most highly developed and simultaneous perception the least developed in normal eyes. *For each retinal point in one eye there is a corresponding area in the opposite eye, within which the same image must project if the two are to be fused into a single image.* The further this retinal point is from the fovea, the larger the corresponding area in the opposing eye. If the retinal sites are anatomically identical, **normal retinal correspondence (NRC)** is present (see sec. **VI.C.,** below).

A. In **simultaneous perception** all objects projecting their images outside of corresponding retinal areas are not fused, but they may be perceived simultaneously. This may result in double vision or diplopia unless the patient is inattentive to these images.

B. **Fusion** is the result of all objects projected onto corresponding retinal points, with their two images fused at the level of the central nervous system (CNS) into one perception.

C. **Stereopsis** is the perception of the third dimension, i.e., the relative nearness and distance of object points as obtained from fused but slightly disparate retinal images. The **Titmus test** for stereopsis is described under tests for retinal correspondence (see sec. **VI.C.3.a.,** below).

III. **Strabismus classification**
  A. **The general order of examination** for strabismus is as follows:
    1. **History**
      a. Deviation: age of onset, description of deviation, frequency and duration, symptoms, and previous treatment. A review of unposed photographs of the patient at various ages is useful.
      b. Personal: pre- and postnatal factors, course of pregnancy, delivery, growth and development, medications, and surgery.
      c. Family: strabismus in blood relatives.
    2. **General observation**
      a. Abnormal head posture or nodding.
      b. Spontaneous closure of one eye (squint).
    3. **Visual acuity**
      a. Without glasses and with glasses, if worn.
      b. Near and distance vision (oculus dexter, oculus sinister, oculus uterque).
      c. Amblyopia testing.
    4. **Motor**
      a. Ductions and versions of extraocular muscles.
      b. Near point of convergence.
      c. Near point of accommodation, where indicated.
      d. Measurement of deviation
        (1) Cover tests (phoria or tropia) distance and near, without and with glasses, if worn; with +3.00 add at near; with eyes in all nine positions of gaze and head tilt when indicated.
        (2) Accommodative convergence–accommodation (AC/A) ratio.
    5. **Sensory tests** (depending on age and cooperation)
      a. Worth four-dot test near and distance, without and with glasses, if worn.
      b. Stereopsis.
      c. Amblyoscope: after image, Bagolini lenses where indicated.
      d. Fusional vergence reserves.
      e. Double Maddox rods where indicated.

6. **Fixation**
   a. Monocular, alternating, binocular.
   b. Nystagmus type.
   c. Visuscope: foveal, or eccentric fixation.
7. **External examination.**
8. **Anterior segment examination.**
9. **Fundus examination**
   a. Assess fundus torsion.
10. **Cycloplegic refraction.**

B. **Pseudostrabismus**
   1. **Pseudoesotropia** or apparent **turning in** of the eyes may result from a prominent **epicanthal** skin fold that obscures part of the normally visible nasal aspects of the globe, thereby giving a false impression that esotropia is present. As the infantile flat nasal bridge develops, this excessive epicanthal skin is raised and the condition self-corrects.
   2. **Pseudoexotropia** is seen in hypertelorism, in which there is an abnormally wide separation of the eyes as a result of disproportionate growth of the facial bones, or as a primary deformity. Despite the physical appearance, the eyes are aligned normally.
   3. **Pseudohypertropia** may result from orbital or palpebral asymmetry simulating a vertical ocular deviation.
   4. **Angle kappa** is the angle between the line of sight that connects the point of fixation with the nodal points at the fovea and the pupillary axis with the line through the center of the pupil perpendicular to the cornea. The angle is **positive** when the corneal light reflex is displaced nasally and **negative** when it is displaced temporally. A positive angle kappa up to 5 degrees is considered physiologic in emmetropic eyes. The angle kappa is **measured on a perimeter** with the patient fixating on the central mark. A light is moved along the perimeter until its reflex is centered on the cornea. The difference in the position of the light and the center mark is indicated in degrees of arc on the perimeter and constitutes the angle kappa, which can also be measured with an amblyoscope using a special slide. This angle is significant in that a positive angle kappa may **simulate an exodeviation.** This is particularly common in retinopathy of prematurity where the macula is dragged temporally. A negative angle kappa may **simulate esodeviation** unless the cover test is performed. Ocular misalignment may be missed in an apparently normally alignment if a positive angle kappa is associated with a small angle esotropia or a negative angle kappa with a small exotropia.

C. **Orthophoria** indicates that the eyes are perfectly aligned with no latent deviation even when fusion is artificially disrupted by the examiner.
D. **Heterophoria** is a misalignment in which fusion keeps the deviation latent. It may be detected by the tests described in sec. **IV.,** below.
E. **Heterotropia** is the manifest misalignment of the eyes. The cover–uncover test is used to document the presence of a tropia (Fig. 12.3).
   1. **Horizontal deviations** include **esophoria** and **esotropia,** which are convergent (inward) deviations of the eyes, while **exophoria** and **exotropia** are divergent (outward) deviations of the eyes.
   2. **Vertical deviations** include hyperphorias or hypertropias, in which the fellow eye is higher than the fixing eye, and hypophoria or hypotropia, in which the fellow eye is lower than the fixing eye.
   3. **Torsional deviations** include incyclophoria or incyclotropia, in which the superior poles of the corneas are tilted medially, and excyclophoria or excyclotropia, in which the superior poles of the corneas are tilted temporally.

IV. **Diagnostic tests** in strabismus are many. The most commonly used tests fall into four basic categories: (a) the cover tests, which depend on the fixation reflex; (b) the corneal reflex tests, which are based on the ability of the corneal surface

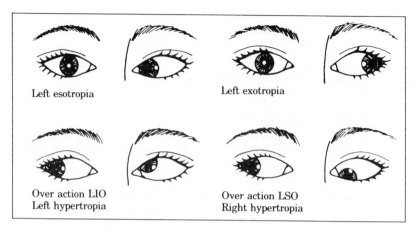

FIG. 12.3. Common heterotropic muscle imbalances. *LIO,* left inferior oblique; *LSO,* left superior oblique.

to reflect the examining light; (c) the dissimilar image tests, which are based on patient response to double vision produced by converting an isolated object of regard into separate images on each retina; and (d) the dissimilar target tests, which are based on patient response to dissimilar images when different targets are presented to each eye. Many of these tests involve eliciting **diplopia (double vision)** as a means of evaluation.

A. **Cover tests.** The cover test and cover–uncover test are qualitative tests used to determine whether a heterophoria or heterotropia is present. These tests are performed using fixation targets at both distance and near.

1. **Cover tests for detection of heterotropias.** If heterotropia is present, tests for fusion are negative because one eye is not aligned with the fixation target. Covering the fixating eye will require the deviated eye to move to take up fixation, and this movement in the **uncovered eye** is looked for by the observer. If the nonfixating deviated eye is covered, however, there will be no movement of the fixating eye. Consequently, each eye must be covered in turn and the fellow eye watched for a fixation shift to determine whether tropia is present or not. If the eye moves outward to fixate, esotropia is present; if the eye moves inward to fixate, exotropia is present. If the uncovered eye moves downward, a hypertropia exists. If the uncovered eye moves upward, a hypotropia exists. **Phorias** of any type may be **quantitated** by Maddox rod testing or by placing **prisms** of increasing strength before the deviating eye until no fixation movement occurs on uncover: **base-out for esodeviation, base-down for hyperdeviation, base-up for hypodeviation, and base-in for exodeviation** (Fig. 12.4).

2. **Cover–uncover tests for heterophoria detection.** Phoria deviations are kept latent by fusion mechanisms as long as both eyes are in simultaneous use. When fusion is disrupted by occluding one eye, the latent deviation will become evident. Each eye is covered separately in turn for 2 to 3 seconds and the occluder then quickly removed. The examiner must note whether or not the eye **under cover** makes a movement inward or outward to pick up fixation again. If there is no movement of either eye when it is covered and then uncovered, there is either no latent phoria present or a microtropia syndrome is present and must be tested for (see sec. **X.A.,** below). If, when uncovered, an eye moves outward to fixate, esophoria is present. If the eye moves inward to fixate, exophoria is present. A movement down to fixation reveals hyperphoria, and a

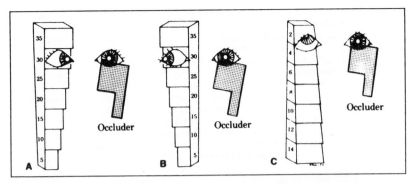

FIG. 12.4. Use of prism bar. **A:** Horizontal prism bar run base-out to measure esodeviations. **B:** Horizontal prism bar run base-in to measure exodeviations. **C:** Vertical prism bar base-down over hypertropic right eye (or base-up over hypotropic left eye alternative).

movement upward to fixate reveals hypophoria. A disadvantage of this test is that small-angle phorias may be missed, but these may be picked up later with the Maddox or base-out prism tests (see secs. **III.B.** and **C.,** below).

3. **The simultaneous prism–cover test** measures the manifest deviation and is most useful in patients with small-angle heterotropia. The examiner covers the fixating eye and simultaneously slips a prism of known power and appropriate base direction in front of the uncovered eye. This may need to be repeated until the prism power selected equals the heterotropic angle and no movement occurs as the eye behind the prism takes up fixation.

4. The prism alternate cover test quantifies the total deviation made up of the manifest and latent deviation together. The prism is placed over one eye and the cover is alternately placed in front of each eye. The uncovered eye is observed for movement and the prism power is increased until the eye movement is neutralized. The power of the neutralized prism corresponds to the amount of deviation present.

B. **Quantitative measurement of strabismic deviation by corneal reflex tests**

1. **Hirschberg test.** A fixation light is held 33 cm from the patient, and the deviation of the corneal light reflex from the center of the pupil in the nonfixating (turned) eye is estimated. **Each millimeter of decentration corresponds to 7 degrees of ocular deviation.** Therefore, a 3-mm **inward** deviation of the light reflex corresponds roughly to a 21-degree **exotropia,** whereas a 4-mm **outward** deviation of the light reflex corresponds roughly to 28 degrees of **esotropia. One degree equals two prism diopters (pds) of deviation.**

2. **Krimsky test.** Dissimilar positions of the corneal reflex in the pupils of each eye are indicative of strabismus, which may be measured by placing successively increasing prism power before the fixating eye until the reflection is similarly positioned in both eyes. Base-out prism is used for esotropia and base-in prism is used for exotropia (Fig. 12.4). This is a direct reading of the estimated squint angle.

3. **Perimeter method** requires that the patient steadily fixate the 0 mark on the perimeter with the preferred eye as the examiner moves a light along the back side of the perimeter arc until the corneal reflex of the light appears located in the pupillary center of the deviated eye. The angle of deviation may be read in degrees from the perimeter arc at the point at which

the flashlight is stopped. **One degree equals approximately 2 pds of deviation.**

4. **The major amblyoscope** is a haploscopic device that consists of a medial septum between the two eyes with angled mirrors that reflect separate targets for each eye. These targets are set at the focal distance of the lenses in the eyepiece; thus, viewing the targets simulates optical infinity or distance fixation. The addition of -3.00 spheres into the eyepiece stimulates accommodation and near convergence, so that a reading of the deviation at near can be made. Adjusting the tubes so that the corneal reflexes of illumination are centered in each pupil gives the examiner an approximation of the angle of deviation. By occluding the light sources alternately and having the patient fixate on the lighted target, the alternate cover test can be performed and the angle of deviation can be read directly.

C. **Dissimilar image tests**

1. **Maddox rod testing for heterophoria or tropia** is diplopia testing with dissimilar images of the same object. The Maddox rod is a red- or white-ribbed lens. A point source of light shined through this lens is seen as a red or white streak 90 degrees away from the axis of the multiple cylinders of the rod. Horizontal alignment may be checked by orienting the rod so that the streak is vertical, and vertical alignment checked by orienting the rod so that the streak is horizontal. The patient views the fixing light with both eyes open. If the streak appears to run through the center of the light both vertically and horizontally as the lens is turned, orthophoria is present in both directions. If the streak is displaced away from the light, misalignment is present. **A phoria cannot be distinguished from a tropia by this test.**

   a. **Horizontal deviations.** If the patient sees the vertical rod streak on the same side of the light as the eye that has the rod in front of it, **uncrossed** images are present and are indicative of esodeviation. If the patient sees the streak on the other side of the fixation light from the eye behind the Maddox rod, **crossed** images are present and are indicative of exophoria or exotropia. The degree of phoria or tropia may be **measured** directly by increasing the amount of prism power presented before one eye with **base-out for esodeviation** and **base-in for exodeviation** until the streak is aligned in the center of the light. The measurement may then be read directly from the prism power producing this effect. Maddox rod measurements are valid only with NRC.

   b. **Vertical deviation** may be measured by presenting **base-down prism to a hypertropic** eye or **base-up prism to a hypotropic** eye until the horizontal streak is aligned with the fixation light.

   c. **Cyclodeviations** may be checked by placing Maddox rods, one red and the other white, before each eye at the same axis setting for each eye. The axis settings of the rods are then adjusted until they appear parallel to the patient. The difference in degrees in cyclodeviation may then be measured directly from the trial frame in which the rods are set. Cyclodeviations may also be measured with an amblyoscope.

2. **The red glass test** is straightforward diplopia testing utilizing the image seen by the fovea of the fixating eye and the extrafoveal image of the deviated eye. It is performed by placing a plain red lens in front of one eye. This test is similar to the Maddox rod tests in horizontal and vertical deviations but is of no value in cyclodeviation measurement. Prisms with bases oriented toward the appropriate direction for the types of deviation (see sec. **III.C.1.**, above) are used to eliminate the horizontal or vertical diplopia of white light and red light when the patient is viewing the fixation bulb, thereby yielding a direct measure of the deviation in the presence of NRC. The Maddox rod and red glass tests can be used to measure deviations in the diagnostic positions of gaze.

D. Separate image tests. In the presence of NRC, the point at which two separate images, one presented to each eye, appear superimposed provides a direct reading of the patient's alignment.

   1. Lancaster red-green projection. The patient wears glasses with a red filter before one eye and a green filter before the other and views a white screen marked with a grid calibrated in squares of 7 degrees (14 pds) from a distance of 1 m. A linear red light and a linear green light are shined on the screen simultaneously, one light held by the patient and the other by the examiner (light held by the examiner determines the fixating eye), and adjusted until they are seen as superimposed by the patient. Any actual disparity between the location and angle of the red and green lights gives the examiner a direct reading in centimeters of any deviation—horizontal, vertical, and torsional.

   2. The **major amblyoscope** is used to show the patient dissimilar objects that are simultaneously seen, one with each eye. The patient is asked to adjust the angle of the tubes so that one image is superimposed on the other. In the presence of NRC, horizontal, vertical, and torsional deviations may be read directly from the scales on the instrument, which indicate the deflection of the tubes away from 0 in these three planes.

V. Measurement of fusional reserves (vergences). Patients with heterophoria and microtropia may be asymptomatic by virtue of their relative fusional reserves. These reserves may be measured using accommodative targets at near and distance on a major amblyoscope. To **measure divergence reserves,** the examiner increases base-in prism over one eye until the patient reports blurring or diplopia of the target. To **measure convergence reserves,** base-out prism is increased to a similar end point. Vertical fusional reserves, positive, are determined by placing prism base-down before the right eye and, negative, by placing prism base-down before the left eye. **Normal divergence reserves** are in the range of 6 D with rapid recovery at distance, 10 to 14 D at near. **Normal convergence reserves** are 20 to 30 D at distance with rapid recovery and slightly more at near. Vertical reserves average 2 to 4 D at near or distance.

VI. Sensory evaluation

   A. Visual acuity. Early determination of visual acuity is critical in evaluation of any patient with strabismus. An estimation of visual acuity may be obtained in infants by observing behavior as each eye is alternately covered. If vision is equal or nearly equal in either eye, an infant or very young child will not object to having either eye covered. If visual acuity is reduced in one eye, however, the child will cry or push the occluder away when the normal eye is covered. If this occurs, ocular disease, **amblyopia** (nonorganic visual loss), or high refractive error should be suspected.

   1. The preferential looking technique permits reliable measurements of visual acuity to be made in infants from birth to age 1 year. At present this technique, as well as **evoked potential estimates of acuity,** is still available at specialized university medical centers. Before assuming that amblyopia is present (see sec. **VI.D.,** below), it is essential that the examiner establish that visual loss is not the result of organic disease. This is done by taking a **past medical history** on the child, including any circumstances during or after pregnancy that may have contributed to ophthalmic disease in the child. An examination of the **ocular anterior segments under magnification** is essential. A dilated **fundus examination,** preferably with the indirect ophthalmoscope, to rule out retinal pathology is an essential part of every examination.

   2. Visual acuity may be determined in the **illiterate and in preschool children** (age 36 to 60 months) using the E game. The parent instructs the child at home to indicate with the hand, or with a test letter that he or she holds, the direction in which the three bars of a test letter E held by the examiner are pointing. The illiterate Es can also be projected. An alternate means is the use of Allen preschool vision test on cards or projected Allen figures, which are small animals and common images that the child age 18 to 36 months is asked to identify. Once the child understands the test, vision may be determined by finding the smallest letter E or Allen figure read with each eye at 20 feet or, alternately, if vision is very poor, designating the optotype read at a distance closer than 20 feet.

B. **Suppression testing.** Suppression **scotomas (areas of decreased retinal sensitivity)** are present both in eso- and exotropic patients. The esotropic patient has an area of suppressed vision extending nasally to the hemiretinal line, whereas the exotropic patient has an area of suppressed vision extending over a large area temporal to the hemiretinal line. These scotomas protect the patient from double vision (diplopia) when both eyes are open.

1. **The Worth four-dot test** will detect fusion, suppression, and anomalous retinal correspondence (see sec. **VI.C.,** below). The patient wears a red filter before one eye and a green filter before the other, mounted in the glasses frame, and views four lights at near and distance—two green, one red, and one white. Normally the white light is seen through both filters, the green lights are seen through only the green filter, and the red light through only the red filter. A patient who is fusing reports four lights, with the white light usually seen as a mixture of red and green. A patient suppressing the eye with the red filter will see only green, and the patient suppressing an eye with the green filter will see only red. The examiner may test the **macular area** by using very small Worth dots held at 0.33 m from the patient. This projects only a 6-degree angle, and the macular area is approximately 3 degrees. Fusion at this distance reveals normal bimacular or central fusion. Extramacular fusion (peripheral fusion) is detected by projecting larger Worth lights at a distance 6 m from the patient. Patients with an esotropia of 10 D or greater will not fuse the distant Worth four dots. **NRC** will be identified in strabismic patients if they report that they see five lights (two red and three green), if the position of the lights corresponds to the angle of deviation. The dots seen by the fixating eye will be clear, whereas those seen by the deviating eye will be blurred. **Anomalous retinal correspondence** is present if the patients report that they see four dots while displaying a manifested deviation or if they have a microstrabismus (see sec. **VI.C.,** below).

2. **The red glass test for suppression and detection of retinal correspondence.** A heterotropic patient with normal vision in each eye but no diplopia (double vision) may be suppressing or ignoring the image received by the retina of the turned eye. With the patient fixating on a bright white light, a red glass placed before the deviated eye will make the second image visible to the patient if it has been ignored. If there is deep suppression present, only the white light will be seen despite the presence of the red lens over the deviated eye. Some examiners prefer holding the red glass over the fixating eye to make the patient aware of diplopia more easily, thereby evaluating the depth of suppression. If NRC is present, the patient sees the red light on the same side as the eye behind the red glass; **uncrossed diplopia** is present, indicating esodeviation. In **crossed diplopia** the red image is seen on the opposite side of the eye behind the red glass and indicates an exodeviation. If the red image falls on a suppression scotoma in the deviating eye of an exotropic patient, it is not seen. If the red filter is then placed before the fixating eye, diplopia may be elicited despite the presence of deep suppression. **Suppression may be differentiated from anomalous retinal correspondence** by holding a prism base-down before the red glass, thereby displacing the retinal image upward and beyond the suppression scotoma. With NRC, the image will appear superiorly and to the right or left of the light. If anomalous retinal correspondence is present, the image will appear horizontally aligned but separated vertically from the fixation light.

3. **The 4-D base-out test** is used to determine whether central fusion (bifixation) or absence of central fusion (monofixation) is present in a patient whose **eyes appear straight.** With the patient reading letters on the distance vision chart, a 4-D base-out prism is slipped alternately before one eye and then the other. The prism-covered eye is watched for movement. If the prism is placed before the fixating eye and both eyes move toward the apex of the prism and **stay moved,** a microtropia is present. If the prism is placed before the nonfixating eye, **neither** eye will move. The absence of movement by one eye is proof of a relative macular scotoma on that side. Bifixation may be recognized by each eye moving inward to refixate in response to displacement of the image produced by the prism. Occasionally, a bifixating patient will not make the necessary convergence movement to pick up the moved image, thereby making the test variable in its accuracy.

4. **Blind spot syndrome** may be found in patients with an esotropia persistently between 25 and 35 D at near and distance fixations. These patients are utilizing the blind spot of the deviated eye as a mechanism of avoiding diplopia in binocular vision. The image of the deviated eye falls on the optic nerve head scotoma. This phenomenon may be detected by placing a **base-out prism** before the deviating eye, thereby moving the visual image to an area between the optic disk and the fovea. The patient will suddenly experience uncrossed diplopia.

C. **Retinal correspondence**

1. **Normal retinal correspondence (NRC)** is the occipital cortical integration of similar images projected onto anatomically corresponding areas of each retina into a single perception, producing normal single binocular vision. Once binocular vision of this nature is established, it will be retained as long as there is functional vision in both eyes.

2. **Abnormal retinal correspondence (ARC).** If there is a disruption of the alignment of the eye, normal binocular vision may produce an annoying diplopia or **visual confusion.** Very young children are able to adapt to this disturbed state of alignment by compensatory CNS occipital cortex adjustment such as suppression, or by development of anomalous retinal correspondence. ARC is the occipital cortical adjustment in the directional values that permits fusion of similar objects projected onto noncorresponding retinal areas. It may develop whether the strabismus is vertical or horizontal. ARC may be present whether there is foveal fixation in both eyes or eccentric fixation present in one eye. It is **manifest only during binocular viewing.** There is no abnormality in the directional values of the retina in either eye during monocular viewing. A patient who has developed ARC may be made aware of diplopia or may experience visual confusion again after surgical correction of strabismus. A new angle of ARC may be developed to rid the patient of these annoying symptoms.

3. **Tests for retinal correspondence.** All tests commonly used for retinal correspondence involve some degree of alteration in the normal conditions of seeing. With the exception of the Bagolini lenses, the eyes are dissociated in the tests, thereby creating an apparatus-induced situation that will influence the result.

   a. **The Titmus stereotest** for three-dimensional vision and retinal correspondence allows the examiner to quantitate a patient's ability to fuse similar images projected onto slightly noncorresponding retinal areas. The patient wears polarized glasses and view pictures of a large fly, three lines of animals, and nine four-circle sets, all with increasing refinement of projection on the noncorresponding retinal areas. Patients with NRC, good vision, and fusion will appreciate all nine sets of circles for three dimensions; patients with ARC may appreciate the three-dimensional aspect only of the large fly using their peripheral fusion mechanisms or up to six circles with microtropia.

b. The Bagolini striated lenses are optically plano lenses with barely perceptible striations that do not blur the view but do produce a luminous streak when the wearer looks at a point source of light. These lenses are mounted in a spectacle or trial frame with the patient's visual corrective lenses in place behind. The Bagolini lenses should be placed so that the axis variation is oriented at 45 degrees in the right eye and 135 degrees in the left eye. The test is carried out at 33 cm and at 6 m (20 ft) from the eye. If patients see only one line running downhill from left to right, they are suppressing their left eye. If they see an X and the cover test reveals no shift, fixation is central and NRC is present. If the cover test reveals a shift and they see an X, ARC is present.

c. The Hering-Bielschowsky afterimage test. With the fellow eye occluded, the better eye views a horizontal glowing linear filament for 20 seconds or an electronic flash in a darkened room. The better eye is then occluded and the contralateral eye views a vertically oriented glowing filament or an electronic flash for 20 seconds. Patients will continue to see these **afterimages** for some time after they have been turned off. They are asked to indicate the relative position of the two gaps in the center of each afterimage. These gaps correspond to the visual direction of each fovea in the presence of central fixation. The interpretation of the test, however, is dependent on the result of previously determined fixation behavior. If central fixation is present by visuscope examination, the patient may have NRC and will see a perfect cross with the two gaps superimposed. In the presence of ARC, the vertical line will be displaced nasally in an esotropic patient and temporally to the horizontal in an exotropic patient.

D. Amblyopia is impaired foveal vision in the absence of organic disease and is most likely the result of lack of continuous use of one or both foveas for visual fixation. It is basically a deprivation phenomenon caused by nonuse of fixation reflex. **The fixation must be developed early in life and used until a child is approximately 7 years old, or amblyopia may develop.**

1. Types of amblyopia

a. Strabismic amblyopia is most frequently encountered in the esotropic patient, but also may occur less frequently in exotropia. As a compensation to avoid diplopia, the patient will inhibit the foveal region of the deviating eye, which in turn will result in strabismic amblyopia of disuse.

b. Anisometropic (refractive) amblyopia is the result of a marked disparity in the refractive error. Small differences are tolerated, but a difference in refraction greater than 2.5 D between the eyes may disturb binocular function and cause a patient to develop either alternating vision, using the near-sighted eye for near vision and the contralateral eye for distance vision, or to suppress the blurred image of one eye, thereby causing amblyopia in that eye.

c. Isoametropic amblyopia. High refractive error in both eyes may cause bilateral amblyopia due to a bilateral blurred image. Refractive error of greater than +5.00 D or −10.00 D need to be corrected early in order to avoid amblyopia.

d. Deprivation amblyopia. Media opacities, congenital or acquired, will degrade the formed image and lead to amblyopia. This type of amblyopia is more severe in unilateral cases as compared to bilateral amblyopia from identical opacities.

2. Diagnostic tests in amblyopia

a. The visual acuity of the amblyopic eye is greater for isolated letters than for whole lines of letters. The acuity drops according to the degree that the letters are crowded together and is called the **crowding phenomenon.** As amblyopia responds to therapy, this phenomenon will be reduced or disappear altogether. Because the visual acuity obtained on the reading of entire lines of letters is a more sensitive indicator of the depth of amblyopia than the acuity obtained with isolated letters, linear Snellen or crowding should be used to follow the amblyopic patient's response to testing.

b. The **neutral density (ND) filter test** is used to differentiate between functional and organic amblyopia. Combined neutral density filters, such as Kodak no. 96, ND 2.00 and 0.50, of sufficient density to reduce vision in a normal eye from 20/20 to 20/40 are slipped before the amblyopic eye. Vision will be decreased by one or two lines, be unaffected, or be slightly improved if the impairment is functional and, therefore, reversible. If organic amblyopia is present, the vision is often markedly reduced.

c. Fixation behavior should be determined in patients with amblyopia. Central viewing is foveal; in eccentric fixation, parafoveal retinal areas are used for viewing—this is more commonly seen with strabismic amblyopia than with anisometropic amblyopia. The presence of eccentric fixation implies a visual acuity of 20/200 or worse. The following tests can aid in the diagnosis of fixation behavior:

(1) Visuscope motor test. The visuscope is a modified ophthalmoscopic device that projects an asterisk onto the patient's retina. The untested eye is occluded and the patient is requested to look directly at the asterisk while the examiner observes the fundus. In central fixation, the asterisk will fall on the fovea. In **eccentric fixation,** the eye will shift so that the asterisk moves immediately to the extrafoveal area of retinal fixation.

(2) Alternate cover test for bilateral eccentric fixation reveals that either eye remains in its exotropic position when the contralateral eye is covered and makes no attempt to pick up what appears to be refixation of the image. The visuscope test will be that of eccentric fixation in both eyes.

(3) Hering-Bielschowsky afterimage test in eccentric viewing and fixation. In eccentric viewing, the foveas retain their common visual direction, and the afterimage result will be similar to that in a patient with ARC. In eccentric fixation, the fovea of the better eye has a common visual direction with a noncorresponding retinal area in the contralateral eye, so the patient will see a perfect cross, as if NRC were present. The visuscope must be relied on for diagnosis of eccentric fixation.

3. Antisuppression therapy should be carried out only in selected cases, by an orthoptist under the direction of an ophthalmologist, because elicited awareness of diplopia may be the one result, producing new annoying symptoms in patients unable to fuse.

a. Suppression may be treated by placing a red filter over one eye to produce dissimilarly colored objects when the patient fixates on white light. The patient is then asked to fixate either the red or the white image but at the same time to try to view the other image. The deviated eye is then rapidly covered and uncovered with an occluder, so that the previously suppressed image may be seen alternately with the first. If the patient is unable to achieve diplopia using this method, a 4-D prism may be placed base-down before the deviating eye to lift the image out of the scotoma. Diplopia will then be apparent. Once the patient learns to recognize the diplopia, he or she must concentrate on maintaining it. The red filter is removed and the patient will, with good fortune, continue to see two different white lights alternately flashing on and off. When the occluder cover-and-uncover motion is stopped, the patient should see two sustained white lights. If a vertical prism is used, it may be withdrawn either abruptly or gradually. Once the two lights are maintained without alternate cover, the patient is taught to transfer fixation of the light from eye to eye, maintaining double vision while either eye fixates. Once this is accomplished, the patient may practice on other objects, such as a ball or matchbox. Between practice sessions, occlusion on the nonsuppressed eye is continued to prevent renewal of the suppression habit. **Other techniques** involve the use of the major amblyoscope rather than fixation light, red filter, occluder, and vertical prism to perform antisuppression treatment.

  b. **After a patient has been taught to recognize diplopia** and ARC is present, attempts are made to restore NRC, either by correcting for the angle of deviation with prisms or by placing the amblyoscope tubes at the objective setting. The patient is asked to try to fuse the identical targets or to superimpose larger dissimilar targets. The patient may experience monocular diplopia or binocular triplopia, which represents a transient stage in passage from ARC to NRC as retinal areas view with one another to localize the image in the nonfixating eye. Once the patient has achieved fusion with NRC, occlusion of one eye is maintained to prevent recurrence of ARC between practice sessions. The eyes may then be aligned by surgical means or by use of prisms.

4. **Treatment of amblyopia** is based on forcing the patient to depend on the amblyopic eye for vision.

  a. **Occlusion therapy with patching** of the preferred eye has been the treatment of choice. Adhesive patches should be used to discourage removal by the patient and to prevent peeking. Elastoplast eye occluders and Opticlude orthoptic eye patches are most commonly used. **A general rule of thumb is 1 week of full-time patching for each year of age between acuity checks of both eyes. Full-time patching refers to patching all waking hours or all but 1 hour.** Very young children should be seen every few weeks and vision or at least preferred fixation tested in **both eyes** to ascertain that **occlusion amblyopia** is not developing under the patch and that progress is or is not being made visually in the amblyopic eye. Once good visual acuity or alternating fixation is achieved, the patching is tapered and eventually discontinued. After the cessation of patching, the patient should be followed because **amblyopia may recur.**

  b. **Lens occlusion** of the preferred eye by either taping the back of a spectacle correction or using a Bangerter patch to force use of the amblyopic eye through the other lens may be used in children who are reliable and will not pull the spectacles down to peek over the covered lens. In general, the acuity in the amblyopic eye must be better than 20/60 (6/18) for this form of therapy to be successfully used.

  c. **Occluder contact lenses** have been used more frequently in patients with aphakia or high **anisometropia.**

  d. **Atropinization** of the preferred eye is effective only when the visual acuity in the amblyopic eye is 20/100 (6/32) or better. Atropine 1% is instilled in the preferred eye either daily or on 3 to 4 consecutive days per week. Atropine in the sound eye will paralyze accommodations and force the patient to use the amblyopic eye for near viewing. If hyperopia is present and uncorrected in the sound eye, the effect of atropinization is potentiated. If vision in the amblyopic eye is worse than 20/100, the patient will prefer the blurred image in the atropinized eye and continue to use it in favor of the amblyopic eye.

VII. **Motor evaluation**

  A. **Comitant esodeviations** may be defined as those in which the convergent angle of the eyes remains unchanged in any given direction of gaze within 5 D, using fixed accommodation. These deviations may be caused by seemingly unrelated factors, such as the near convergence reflex, congenital overaction of the medial recti, acquired hypotony of the lateral recti, and monocular loss of useful vision in infancy or childhood. **Noncomitant deviations** (horizontal or vertical) are deviations that measure differently in the different fields of gaze and are usually seen in situations in which there is paresis or restriction of one or more muscles or in A-V deviation (see sec. **IX.**, below).

1. **Accommodative esodeviations** are associated with overaction of the convergence reflex in its association with near accommodation. If this deviation is within the fusional range, it is **accommodative esophoria;** if the esodeviation is beyond fusional possibility, it is **accommodative esotropia.**

   a. The **etiology** of accommodative esodeviation may be one of two unrelated causes that may occur together or alone. The first is seen in the **hypermetropic** or farsighted patient in whom the retinal image remains blurred unless the patient clears it by increased accommodative effort. This is associated with an increased convergence of the eyes in the accommodation convergence reflex. The second cause is an abnormally high **AC/A ratio.** This may occur even in patients with no refractive error and represents an abnormal relationship between accommodation and the accommodative–convergence reflex elicited with focus at the near point. The amount of convergence associated with each diopter of accommodation is excessive.

   b. The **average age of onset** of accommodative esotropia regardless of etiology is 2.5 years, but ranges between 6 months and 7 years. If a high AC/A ratio is associated with hypermetropia, a larger-angle esotropia will be present at near as compared to distance fixation. If the patient is emmetropic (no refractive error) with a high AC/A ratio, esotropia will be present only on near fixation.

   c. **Clinical evaluation**

      (1) A **cycloplegic refraction** is an integral part of the evaluation of any strabismic patient, but is of critical value in the patient with accommodative esodeviation. A patient may be prepared for cycloplegic refraction with one drop of 1% cyclopentolate q10min three times within an hour of retinoscopic examination. Cyclopentolate 0.5% is recommended for infants—cyclopentolate is usually combined with phenylephrine for enhanced dilation. Similarly, 1% atropine drops in each eye at bedtime for 3 days immediately before retinoscopic examination is sufficient and preferable in preschool children. By paralyzing accommodation, the examiner may usually detect nearly the full amount of hypermetropia, although subsequent cycloplegic refraction may disclose more hypermetropia than detected during the first refraction. It is not uncommon for patients with a normal AC/A ratio to have more hypermetropia than those with a high AC/A ratio. The greater the degree of hypermetropia, the greater the tendency to accommodate to clear vision and secondarily to overconverge to an esodeviation state.

      (2) **The AC/A ratio** may be determined with one of two methods: the gradient method and the heterophoria method. In the gradient method, the change in deviation to an accommodative target is divided by the change in lens power. For example, the deviation with full correction to an accommodative target is measured, e.g., as esotropia 10 D. A 1.00 sphere is then placed over both eyes to stimulate 1 D of accommodation and the deviation is remeasured. The esotropia may now be 16 D. The AC/A in this example is 6 D of accommodative convergence to 1 D of accommodation. The heterophoric method looks at the distance–near relationship. Deviations should measure similarly at distance and near. If there is greater esotropia measured of near, then there is a high AC/A ratio.

      (3) **Sensory complications** seen in accommodative esotropia are those mentioned earlier (see sec. **VI.**, above). A nonaccommodative esotropia may be superimposed on the accommodative component.

(4) Therapy of accommodative esotropia is by correcting the hyperopic refractive error. Miotics are no longer used as a model of treatment of accommodative esotropia.

    (a) Bifocals are the *treatment of choice* in the accommodative esotropic child with a high AC/A ratio causing esotropia at near despite a full correction for any existing hypermetropia at distance. A child given his or her full cycloplegic refraction should be examined at 3 to 4 monthly intervals to ascertain that the glasses control the accommodative esotropia. If the esotropia persists at near despite the eyes being straight at distance, an additional +3.00 D bifocal segment should be prescribed. This lower segment should be set higher for children than is routinely done for adults, because segments that are too low will be overviewed by the child, or the child will have to raise his or her chin significantly to depress the eyes to see through the additional plus lens at near in primary gaze. The ideal level for the top of the bifocal segment is at the point of bisection of the pupil.

    (b) Miotic therapy. Echothiophate (phospholine iodide) is *rarely if ever used* in the treatment of accommodative esotropia. Concentrations of 0.06% to 0.12% may be used with one drop in each eye each morning. The drug will cause pupillary miosis and may be associated with pupillary cysts. The miotic works by "tricking" the eye into thinking that it is maximally accommodated, thereby preventing the convergence reflex. Occasionally, children, particularly older children, may be controlled with miotic therapy every other day. Side effects of echothiophate such as cataracts are rarely seen in children. **If surgery is anticipated, echothiophate must be discontinued** 2 to 3 weeks before any general anesthesia to allow restoration of the normal plasma and erythrocyte cholinesterase levels, thereby avoiding the **risk of prolonged postoperative apnea.** Because this drug cannot be considered harmless because of its systemic and possible cataractogenic effect, dosage should be reduced as soon as the accommodative esotropia is brought under control. This should be a progressive decrease to every other day and possibly to two or three times weekly dosage, with the final levels being determined by the minimum dosage necessary to control the deviation and to allow fusion.

    (c) In children less than 4 years of age the full cycloplegic hyperopic correction is prescribed as glasses. If the child initially refuses to wear the glasses, the instillation of atropine 1% drops in each eye each morning (see sec. **VI.D.4.,** above) for 2 to 4 consecutive days may be useful in encouraging use of the glasses, but miotics should not be used as alternative permanent therapy in place of the glasses. With time, the hyperopic power is decreased as long as the alignment and fusion are maintained.

    (d) Children 4 to 8 years of age need to wear only that amount of plus lens power required to maintain fusion and provide maximum visual acuity rather than wearing the full cycloplegic refractive correction. **The examiner should be able to demonstrate some esophoria by alternate cover tests with glasses on.** This indicates a high degree of tone and that the fusional divergence is being maintained. If orthophoria is maintained for several years with glasses without any stress on the patient's fusional divergence, eventual withdrawal of the glasses will cause only symptoms of asthenopia or blurred vision.

(e) **Children older than 8 years of age** may begin to show signs of spontaneous improvement. The hypermetropia usually decreases and the severity of the AC/A ratio diminishes spontaneously well into the teens. The power of the plus lenses may be decreased, and if bifocals were used to correct a condition that was primarily the result of a high AC/A ratio rather than hypermetropia, these may be discontinued as well. The other factors of concern in total withdrawal of glasses, e.g., astigmatism and severity of hypermetropia, must be taken into account.

2. **Nonaccommodative esodeviations** are the varying convergent forms of strabismus not associated with accommodation. The **etiology** may be either neurogenic or anatomic. Patients may have **partially accommodative** and **partially nonaccommodative** deviations, and therapy (surgical and medical) should be adjusted accordingly. The nonaccommodative deviation is that amount that remains when full therapy of the accommodative component is in effect.

   a. **Infantile esotropia** (or **congenital esotropia**) is an esodeviation noted within the first 6 months of age. It is commonly seen shortly after birth but may not become clinically apparent for 2 to 4 months. The angle of deviation is usually greater than 30 D with little variation in measurement in the otherwise healthy child.

   (1) **Diagnosis** of infantile esotropia is assisted not only by the time of discovery but also by the finding of alternate fixation in the primary position and **crossed fixation** on lateral gaze, such that the patient uses the right eye to view objects in the left field and the left eye to view objects in the right field. Those few who do not alternate are amblyopic in the nonpreferred eye and if left untreated, may develop eccentric fixation. Nystagmus blockage syndrome is discussed in sec. **XIII.D.7.,** below.

   (2) The **differential diagnoses** of infantile esotropia are the abduction limitation syndromes and LR paralysis problems including Duane and Möbius syndromes (see sec. **X.,** below).

   (3) **Tests for abduction**

   (a) **Spinning.** If the child is held and spun around the examiner's head, the labyrinth stimulation will create a nystagmus causing abducting movements of the eye on the side opposite to the direction of head acceleration. In this manner, the examiner may determine if there is, in fact, abduction potential of each LR. **Doll eye** movement may serve a similar purpose.

   (b) **Occlusion.** An alternate method of inducing abduction in the cross-fixating eye of an infantile esotrope is occlusion of one eye for several hours. Abduction will appear in the contralateral eye if true crossed fixation is present.

   (c) **Forced ductions** are of use in determining whether or not an ocular deviation is secondary to mechanical obstruction. It is most commonly used in infantile esotropes with crossed fixation who cannot be made to abduct despite the foregoing tests. Under general anesthesia the conjunctiva and episclera are grasped with forceps near the muscle in question, and the globe is moved in the direction away from that muscle. If the eye moves freely away from the location of the muscle, no mechanical obstruction exists. If the eye is moved only with difficulty, it is likely that there is scarring or fibrosis of the muscle that is the source of the deviation. This test may also be performed with local anesthesia in adults, but voluntary eye movement may affect the results. It is used in children and adults in **differentiating such entities** as traumatic paralysis of the IR muscle from an orbital floor fracture with entrapment of the muscle, a tight LR muscle after excessive surgical resection, congenital fibrosis syndrome, and thyroid myopathy.

   (4) The **esotropic angle is measured** by techniques discussed earlier (see sec. **IV.,** above).

   (5) **Therapy of infantile esotropia** in the absence of amblyopia involves surgical straightening of the eyes. Botulinum injection of the medial recti, has been used with varied success. If amblyopia is present or suspected, occlusion therapy should be started **before any surgical correction.** In the nonamblyopic child, surgery is performed early in life in an attempt to achieve at least peripheral fusion. More commonly, surgery is performed on both medial recti under general anesthesia.

 b. **Esotropia secondary to monocular impaired vision.** Any anomaly either preventing development of normal sight or interfering with normal sight once developed may produce an esotropia, usually about 6 months after the anomaly appeared.

   (1) The **esotropic angle** is not usually as large as that encountered in infantile deviations, but fixation is irretrievable in the involved eye, thereby making measurements of the angle of deviation difficult using prism and alternate cover test. The Krimsky test or the Hirschberg light reflex test must be used for evaluation of the angle of deviation.

   (2) **Management** includes careful ophthalmoscopy to elicit the etiology of decreased vision; i.e., retinoblastoma or chorioretinitis can be ruled out if no disease is apparent in the anterior segment. If the etiology is not life threatening and the visual anomaly cannot be corrected, surgical correction of the esodeviation is indicated. The object of surgery is to correct the angle of deviation to approximately 8 pds of esotropia. When the eyes are aligned, the patient will gain an increased binocular peripheral field on the side of the previous deviated eye. Secondary exotropia can develop as the eyes tend to drift outward as a child matures, and the initial esotropic correction may have to be reversed in subsequent years.

 c. **Divergence insufficiency** is an acquired comitant esodeviation that is maximum at distance, decreases to orthophoria on near fixation at 1 m or less, and remains unchanged in angle of deviation on lateral gaze. **Onset** may be at any age, and the initial symptom is homonymous diplopia at distance. Abduction is normal in each eye. The **etiology** is often obscure but may be rarely associated with intracranial disease. This must be ruled out. **Treatment** of divergence insufficiency is supportive, with the object being only to relieve diplopia using prisms or occlusion therapy after neuroophthalmologic evaluation has been completed. If the condition persists for more than 6 months without change, surgical intervention may be justified. The prognosis is good.

B. **Concomitant exodeviations.** An outward divergence of the visual axis is an exodeviation. If this divergence is kept latent by single binocular vision, thereby maintaining stereopsis, the condition is termed **exophoria.** A manifest misalignment of the visual axes outward, often with associated suppression area (or scotoma) and loss of stereopsis, is termed **exotropia.** Patients may fluctuate between the two. The **etiology** is considered to be a disturbance in the tonic horizontal vergence that may be neurologic in origin or secondary to anatomic factors such as hypertrophic lateral recti.

1. **Exophoria** of less than 10 pds is often asymptomatic in adults. Even larger degrees of deviation may be asymptomatic in children.

 a. **When symptoms become manifest** they are characterized by vague asthenopia that worsens with prolonged visual tasks, transient diplopia, or momentary blurred vision when the fusional convergence threshold has been exceeded or exhausted. In compensation, a patient may overaccommodate to increase convergence, thereby blurring out visual detail. The symptoms of exophoria will predominate in the field of gaze where the deviation is greatest; i.e., they will be greatest at distance visual tasks if the deviation is greater for distance viewing, and greater for near visual tasks if **convergence insufficiency** is the predominant problem. A common solution to this latter problem is closing one eye during near visual tasks. Exophoric patients have good fusional vergence amplitude and no amblyopia.

   b. **Measurements** of the deviation are discussed in sec. **IV.,** above.

   c. **Exophoria is not treated** if it is asymptomatic. Symptomatic exophoria is often helped by convergence exercise to increase fusional convergence amplitude. For deviation greater at distance, therapy consists of the reading of small detailed distance targets with increasing base-out prism; for near, small print is read to enhance the stimulus of fusional convergence. Overcorrection of any existing myopia will also stimulate accommodative convergence to assist the patient with convergence insufficiency problems. This is useful in younger patients, but adults may suffer asthenopia. Base-in prism spectacles are of greater use in reducing symptoms in older presbyopic patients and in prepresbyopic patients unable to increase their fusional convergence with orthoptic training. The degree of exophoria may be measured at near and distance with Maddox rod and prisms. One-half of this measurement may then be placed as base-in prism in a spectacle correction (one-half of the amount to be put in each lens) along with the normal hypermetropic or myopic correction. When all else fails, surgery may be the answer for exophoria, but may lead to overcorrection.

2. **Intermittent exotropia,** like exophoria, is associated with normal fusional vergence and amplitudes, no amblyopia, and bifixation. Stereopsis is normal during the exophoric phases, but absent when the patient becomes manifestly exotropic.

   a. **Sensory adaptation** in intermittent exotropia is extremely rare but includes suppression scotomas in the temporal fields and possible ARC to avoid the symptoms of diplopia and visual confusion during exotropic phases. As soon as the patient returns to an exophoric phase, however, NRC recurs and bifixation functions at peak level with normal stereopsis. These sensory adaptations must be developed before the age of 10 years or frank diplopia will occur when the exotropia becomes manifest.

   b. **Measurement of exodeviation** must be at near and distance **using a reading chart rather than fixation light** to prevent the patient from using extra accommodative convergence to reduce the exodeviation. A blurred fixation light will not bother the patient, but blurring of print due to overaccommodation will cause the patient to back down on the accommodative effort until vision is clear, thereby revealing the accurate levels of exodeviation. A high AC/A ratio is more frequently found in intermittent exotropia than a low AC/A ratio. Deviations measuring up to 35 pds at distance and 10 pds at near are common in young children but will increase with age at near, causing the near and distance deviation measurements to approximate each other. It is useful to have the patient view the near accommodative target through +3.00 D lenses to reduce accommodative convergence and more accurately measure the near exodeviation. The alternate cover test is used to measure the exodeviation at near and distance. If it is found that the **distance deviation is significantly greater than the near,** a patch should be placed over one eye for at least 45 minutes to thoroughly dissociate the eyes because proximal fusion may be artificially reducing the true amount of exodeviation. Before the patch is removed, the contralateral eye is covered with an occluder. After the patch is removed, it is critical to prevent the patient from using both eyes together even momentarily, because this brief exposure may be sufficient to reestablish binocular vision and reobscure the near deviation by fusional convergence. The prism alternate cover test is performed again at near and measurements are taken. If the angle of deviation at near has then increased to approximate that of the distance measurement, it has been established that convergence is being used to overcome the near deviation. If the measurements at near are still significantly less than distance exodeviation measurements, it has been established that there is a true **divergence excess.** Establishing the difference between divergence excess and simulated divergence excess is instrumental in decisions concerning surgical management.

   c. **Treatment of intermittent exotropia** with surgery is justified if, in the presence of corrected refractive error (anisometropia or myopia), there is still a manifest exodeviation. Surgery of divergence excess is recession of both lateral recti; surgery of a basic exotropia in which near and distance measurements are approximately the same is resection of the MR and recession of the LR on the same eye. If the patient is older than 10 years of age and has not developed suppression or ARC elimination of the divergence angle, surgery will prevent any such sensorial adaptation. **Patients under the age of 10 years are at risk for suppression and possible ARC so long as exotropia exists.**

3. **Exotropia** is constant divergence of one eye and is commonly associated with a normal or low AC/A ratio. Fixation is commonly alternating between the two eyes, thereby preventing amblyopia, although constant exotropia in a patient less than 10 years of age causes a significant increase in the risk of development of amblyopia, suppression, or ARC, because there is no binocular vision present to prevent development of sensorial adaptation.

   a. **The measurement of exotropia** is similar to that described in sec. **IV.,** above.

   b. **Amblyopia.** If, after appropriate refraction and vision testing, amblyopia is found in an exotropic patient, therapy is similar to that described in sec. **VI.D.,** above, and should be undertaken before any surgical correction of the deviation. Patients 10 years of age or younger usually respond to such therapy. The congenitally exotropic child should be thoroughly evaluated and may require a neurologic workup because there is a high prevalence of neurologic problems in this patient population. If normal, early surgery just like with congenital esotropia patients is recommended. Older patients undergo surgery as described in sec. **VII.B.2.c., above.** If one eye has irreversibly reduced visual acuity, a recession of the LR and resection of the MR on the amblyopic eye are recommended.

C. **Concomitant vertical deviations** of up to 4 pds are not uncommon and are often associated with horizontal deviation. In the absence of horizontal deviation, good fusional vergence is present and associated with normal fusion and binocular vision.

   1. **Skew deviations.** Vertical deviations should be differentiated from skew deviations, which are associated with CNS disorders or labyrinthitis. In skew deviation the onset is often abrupt, and the vertical deviation is large and either constant or variable in various positions of gaze.

   2. **Therapy of concomitant vertical deviations** is usually vertical prisms with one-half the correction ground into each lens of a spectacle, base-down over the hypertropic eye, base-up over the hypotropic eye. Optical correction should also be incorporated; if prisms fail, surgical correction may be undertaken. Botulinum injection is rarely used in vertical deviations because of potential lid complications or lack of effect (see sec. **XII.,** below).

VIII. **Dissociated vertical deviation (DVD)** is characterized by an upward turn of the nonfixating eye. The condition is particularly common bilaterally and is often asymmetric. It should not be confused with other imbalances in the vertical muscles.

A. **Clinically** dissociated vertical deviation is recognized by an upward turn of the covered eye on alternate cover testing. Either eye turns up when covered, and the covered eye moves down to fixate as the occluder is moved from the covered to the fellow eye. This occurs in all fields of gaze. Radial limbal vessels may be observed to pick up the **cyclodeviation** that occurs simultaneously with the hyperdeviation in these patients.

B. **The Bielschowsky phenomenon** is found in DVD. This is manifested as a downward movement of the elevated eye, which may infraduct to a level lower than the fixating eye. This is observed by reducing or increasing the light entering the fixating eye only by passing a series of filters of decreasing or increasing density in a filter rack before the fixating eye. When the stimulus threshold is reached in the fixating eye, the downward movement will occur in the contralateral eye.

C. **Therapy of DVD,** when necessary, can be medical or surgical. Patients are often asymptomatic, and the misalignment is brought to their attention by a relative or friend. Medical treatment by switching fixation to the lesser-deviated eye is indicated when the misalignment is quite asymmetric. Surgical treatment consists of bilateral large LR recessions or bilateral IO anteriorization.

IX. **A-V patterns in horizontal strabismus** are manifested by a change of ocular alignment that occurs on upgaze, midline gaze, and downgaze as the eyes move from the primary position. In an **A** pattern, the eyes are closer together in upgaze as compared to downgaze with a 10-pd difference between the two positions. In the **V** pattern, the eyes will be relatively closer together on downgaze and move outward as they progress toward upgaze with a 15-pd difference in the misalignment between the two positions. These patterns may be seen in orthophoric patients or patients with eso- or exodeviation. Compensatory head postures to provide sufficiently good alignment for single binocular vision are often found in these patients.

A. **The V pattern**

1. The **etiology** of V esotropia or exotropia is often associated with overaction of the IO muscles or could be a primary underaction of the SO muscles (or both). As the IO muscles act as abductors in upgaze, the esodeviation decreases and an exodeviation increases on upward movement of the eyes. Alternate mechanisms that have been suggested and that have affected surgical management include overaction of MR muscles. These muscles are most effective in midline downgaze particularly due to their role in convergence. Overaction of the LR muscles has also been proposed as an alternate etiology of **V** exotropia. These muscles are most effective in midline upgaze, because divergence is normally accomplished by looking upward from the down-turned, near-seeing position to view a distant object.

2. **Measurements.** The extent of a **V** pattern may be measured using the alternate cover test and prisms with the patient gazing at a distant fixation object with the chin down and the eyes in upgaze, primary midline gaze, and chin up with gaze downward. Testing of versions may reveal overaction of one or both IOs, underaction of one or both SOs, or overaction of a horizontal rectus muscle.

3. **Head position** in patients who fuse is characteristically chin held down when doing close work in **V** esodeviation. Conversely, a chin-up position may be seen in patients with **V** exodeviation.

4. **Treatment of V esotropia** is recession or disinsertion of the IOs if they are found to be overactive, or recession and downward transposition of the MR muscle(s) if the obliques are normal. Similarly, in **V exotropia,** disinsertion or recession and upward transposition of the lateral recti is indicated if the IOs are overactive. **The principle of upward or downward transposition of horizontal muscles is that the insertions**

are always moved in the direction in which the surgeon wishes to reduce the action of the muscle.

B. The A pattern

1. **The etiology** is most frequently found to be associated with overaction of the SO muscles with or without underaction of the IOs. As the SOs act in abduction in downward gaze, esotropia decreases and exotropia increases in that field of view. In the absence of overaction of the oblique muscles, underaction of LR muscles is suspected.

2. **Measurements.** An A tropia is measured by alternate cover tests and prisms held base-in or base-out, according to the form of horizontal deviation, with the patient looking in upgaze, primary gaze, and downgaze at both distance and near. Versions will often reveal the overacting muscles.

3. **Treatment of A patterns** is not indicated in an asymptomatic patient if the deviation is 10 D or less in primary position and below. In large A patterns, overacting SO muscles may be modified in their action by bilateral weakening procedures such as tenectomy or using the silicone expander in combination with any indicated horizontal surgery. If the oblique muscles appear normal, horizontal muscle surgery may be combined with upward displacement of the MR or downward displacement of the LR. Bilateral SO surgery should be avoided in patients who are foveal bifixators.

X. Strabismic syndromes

A. Microtropia should be suspected when heterophoria is present on the uncover test, but there is an absence of shift on the cover test. The index of suspicion should be raised by the finding of moderate degrees of amblyopia, parafoveal fixation, **harmonious ARC** (ARC adapted to the angle of deviation), and reduced but present stereopsis. In microtropia, there is a sensory and motor adaptation to a primary **small central suppression scotoma** that is rarely found in patients without either anisometropia or a history of esotropia. Clinically, the eyes appear straight and the cover test fails to reveal fixation movement. The visuscope, however, reveals fixation as much as 2 to 3 degrees nasal to the fovea.

B. Monofixation syndrome is characterized by consistent findings of a deviation of 8 D or less, good fusional vergence amplitudes, gross stereopsis, and a macular scotoma within the deviating eye that prevents diplopia. Many patients have no history of manifest strabismus, but frequently have significant anisometropia. The presence of the central scotoma precludes bifixation, but allows active peripheral binocular vision. **Etiologic factors** include small-angle strabismus, anisometropia, unilateral macular lesions, and inherent inability to fuse similar images perceived by the maculae. Strabismic monofixation syndrome is more frequently seen in esotropia than in exotropia, because the constant tropia more frequently seen with the former prevents the establishment of visual bifixation. Anisometropia induces monofixation secondary to a clear image on one macula and a blurred image on the other. The refractive error is often discovered too late to correct the macular image discrepancy and allow for the establishment of bifixation. A unilateral macular lesion produces an organic scotoma precluding binocular vision. Inherent inability to fuse identical macular images is still poorly understood.

1. The **diagnosis** of monofixation syndrome can be made by determining the **area of scotoma** within the binocular field and detecting peripheral fusion and fusional vergence amplitudes. The **cover–uncover test** may reveal a small fixation movement in the nonfixating eye, but the diagnosis of the syndrome can be truly made only by **sensory testing.**

   a. **Fusion** may be evaluated with the Worth four-dot test at near and distance (see sec. **VI.B.,** above). A bifoveal fixating patient will fuse the dots, but the monofixating patient possesses a scotoma in the nonfixating eye that will obscure the dots projected onto that eye. Until the dots are projected onto a retinal area larger than the scotoma, the patient will report either three green dots or two red dots. As the Worth dots are moved closer, the retinal projection area will increase and the patient may suddenly report fusing the four dots.

  b. **The 4-D base-out prism** test may also be used to reveal the central scotoma (see sec. **VI.B.**, above). A shift of both eyes toward the apex of the 4-D prism placed base-out before a fixating eye is a positive test, but a significant number of monofixation patients will not respond to this form of prism testing.

  c. **The Bagolini striated glasses** may also disclose the scotoma (see sec. **VI.C.**, above). The glasses are positioned so that the light streak is seen by the right eye at 135 degrees and by the left eye at 45 degrees. Patients with monofixation syndrome will see a scotoma as a gap surrounding the light in the streak in the nonfixating eye.

 2. **Amblyopia** is found in the majority of patients with monofixation syndrome, but this will vary with the etiology of the syndrome. A minority of the congenital exotropes, most of the primary monofixating patients, most patients with a microstrabismus, and almost all anisometropes with monofixation syndrome will have amblyopia.

 3. **Treatment of monofixation** involves occlusion therapy for improvement of the vision in the amblyopic eye if the decreased vision is nonorganic in origin. Improvement of the motor problems, i.e., the deviation, is usually not necessary because the strabismus is 8 D or less in angle. Treatment is not recommended for adults or children older than 6 years of age because of the risk of intractable diplopia. Younger children respond well to occlusion therapy.

C. **Convergence spasm** may simulate esotropia at near fixation in an otherwise orthophoric patient. A sustained convergence is usually associated with spasm of accommodation. Clinically, the patient will be orthophoric or possibly exotropic at distance. The syndrome classically includes induced myopia, miosis of accommodation, esotropia, and diplopia that increases at near. This spasm may persist for up to 10 minutes after the visual target is removed. The condition may be seen in hysteria, but can also be associated with organic neurologic lesions such Arnold-Chiari malformation, pituitary adenoma, and posterior fossa neurofibroma. **Diagnosis** is made by cycloplegic refraction to rule out true myopia. **Treatment** includes plus lenses in the hyperopic patient or weak minus lenses in the emmetrope, to be used during times of spasm, and psychotherapy to reassure the patient that he or she is not going blind.

D. **Retraction syndrome (Duane syndrome)** is characterized most commonly by the absence of abduction of one eye with some restricted adduction and retraction while attempting to adduct that eye. There may be an associated up or down-shooting of the adducted eye, simulating overaction of an IO or SO muscle. The palpebral fissure is simultaneously narrowed during attempted adduction. Duane syndrome may be unilateral or bilateral and is often hereditary. The **etiology** was initially believed to be fibrosis of the LR muscle(s). Evidence from electromyographic studies has shown anomalies in innervation, namely, paradoxic innervation resulting from anomalous connections at the nuclear level in the CNS. The LR muscle in these patients exhibits no electrical activity on abduction, but is active on adduction. This leads to cocontraction of the MR and LR muscles on attempted adduction that results in retraction of the globe. Other forms include defective abduction only with or without esodeviation, adduction more defective than abduction with or without exodeviation, and vertical retraction syndrome with retraction seen mainly in elevation.

E. **Strabismus fixus** is an extremely large esotropic deviation in both eyes seen in patients with maximum contracture of the MR muscles, secondary to replacement by fibrous tissue. Neither eye may be abducted across the midline even on **forced duction** testing. A similar condition may occur in which the eye is anchored in an abducted position, a fibrous band replacing or present in addition to the LR. **Vertical strabismus fixus** may be unilateral or bilateral. The affected eye is anchored in depression and appears to be associated with a fibrotic IR.

F. **Möbius syndrome** is a multisystem problem. Examination reveals complete or incomplete abduction deficit, facial diplegia, and microglossia. Esotropia is frequently present in various degrees. The presence of an **A** or **V** pattern is not uncommon, and a compensatory head posture up or down may be used by the patient in an effort to avoid diplopia symptoms. This congenital **inability to abduct** either eye may result in a patient maintaining fixation on the lateral target by voluntarily converging. Associated with the **lack of lateral horizontal eye movement,** probably due to sixth nerve palsy, is a **seventh cranial nerve palsy,** manifested by relaxation of the orbicularis muscle, sagging of the lower lids, and pooling of the tears in the lower fornix. There are other associated facial abnormalities, vestibular nystagmus cannot be elicited, and the pupils are normal.

G. **Syndromes inducing limitation of ocular elevation**

1. **Brown syndrome—SO tendon sheath syndrome**—is manifested by an inability to elevate the adducted eye above the midhorizontal plane. The restriction of elevation decreases as the eye moves laterally, but some restriction may persist even in full abduction. There may be slight downshooting of the adducted involved eye mimicking SO overaction. Palpebral fissure widening is associated with elevation restriction on attempted adduction. The **etiology** of this syndrome is probably variable, but the true congenital syndrome is believed to be the result of structural abnormalities of the SO tendon–trochlear complex. Spontaneous resolution of congenital cases has been described. The syndrome may also be acquired postoperatively following the tucking of the SO muscle following trauma or secondary to inflammation. **Forced ductions** are positive in that there is an inability to elevate passively the adducted involved eye. There is often a compensatory head posture. Surgery is usually not indicated unless there is a significant anomalous head posture or hypotropia in primary gaze. **Surgical procedures** directed at the SO tendon have not produced uniformly good results in resolving either the ocular problem or the head position.

2. **Congenital fibrosis syndrome** is usually familial. It is characterized by bilateral ptosis, chin elevation, absence of elevation of both eyes, limited if any depression of both eyes, overconvergence in attempted upward gaze, exotropia or divergence in attempted downward gaze, and limited horizontal eye movements. Most patients have hyperopic astigmatism and amblyopia. The best cosmetic correction comes with freeing up the IR muscles with ipsilateral superior rectus resection plus ptosis surgery.

3. **Orbital floor fracture** causes anatomic nonaccommodative deviation (see sec. **VII.A.2.,** above, and Chap. 4, sec. **VIII.**).

4. **Double elevator palsy** is rare and is due to the combined weakness of contraction of both the IO and SR muscles in the same eye. There is complete inhibition of eye movement in the upper field of gaze. **Treatment** involves transposition of the insertions of both medial and lateral recti to the insertion of the SR muscle, with or without ipsilateral IR recession.

5. **Thyroid ophthalmoplegia** associated with the exophthalmos of thyrotoxicosis is secondary to hypertrophy of the extraocular muscles, reducing the motility of the eyes. Elevation is particularly limited, due to restriction of the IR muscles. During the toxic state, the extraocular muscles become enlarged due to lymphocytic infiltration. An eosinophilic substance and edema will also contribute to the increased size of the extraocular muscle belly. The EOM enlargement can be so severe as to cause a compressive optic neuropathy. Following the acute phase, fibrosis of the muscles may occur. The muscles most commonly affected are the inferior recti, followed by the medial recti, superior recti, and lateral recti. **Forced ductions** are positive for restricted movement of affected muscle. Patients frequently

develop a **chin-up** compensatory head posture. **Treatment** is carried out after the basic disease is stabilized and is usually a generous recession of the involved muscles. Botulinum injection of the IR and MR has been a useful adjunct or alternative to surgery in acute or fairly recent-onset Graves' disease.

6. **Parinaud syndrome.** Paralysis of upward and downward gaze may develop secondary to lesions of the subcortical brain centers for vertical gaze. There may be associated absence of convergence and pupillary reaction to light. Tumors of the pineal gland are the most common **etiology** of this syndrome.

H. **Marcus Gunn ("jaw-winking") syndrome** is a congenital abnormality characterized clinically by unilateral ptosis. On opening the mouth or moving the jaw to the noninvolved side of the head, there is a momentary lid retraction of the ptotic eye. The **etiology** is felt to be an anomalous connection between the nuclei of the external pterygoid muscles of the jaw and the levator muscle of the lid.

I. **Cyclic esotropia (clock mechanism alternate-day squint)** is an unusual form of esotropia that follows a regular rhythm. A 48-hour cycle is most common, although variable cycles have been reported. The patient is orthophoric with normal binocular function on "straight" days and manifestly esotropic with sensory abnormalities on other days. Diplopia is infrequent. Spasm of accommodation is not involved, as demonstrated by normal vision throughout the cycle, and no phoria is present during the orthophoric phase. The cycles continue a few months to years before the esotropia becomes constant. Bimedial surgical recession is successful and does not lead to overcorrection on orthophoric days.

J. **Ophthalmoplegias** are a group of ocular motility disorders associated with temporary or permanent changes at the myoneural junction or within the muscle fiber itself.

1. **Progressive external ophthalmoplegia** is a mitochondrial disorder affecting the extraocular muscles and levator palpebrae. It may progress asymmetrically, but end-stage disease is identical in both eyes. The initial **sign** is acquired ptosis, followed some years later by progressive paresis of the extraocular muscles, usually starting with inability to elevate the eyes. Elevation weakness precedes depression paresis, causing the patient to take on a compensatory **chin-up** posture. As the condition progresses and the eyes become progressively more frozen in primary gaze, the head will return to normal position. There is no involvement of the intraocular muscles of the eye. Chronic progressive external ophthalmoplegia associated with pigmentary retinopathy and cardiomyopathy is called Kearns-Sayre syndrome.

2. **Myasthenia gravis** is a chronic neuromuscular disease characterized primarily by fatigue of muscle groups, usually starting with the small extraocular muscles before involving other larger muscle groups. **Initial findings** usually include ptosis, which becomes progressively more severe as the day wears on. Weakness of convergence and upgaze are seen. Infrequently, isolated paresis of the IR or LR may be noted. The latter may simulate a sixth nerve palsy. **Diagnosis** is by acetylcholine receptor antibody levels, and electromyogram (the myogram becomes silent as action potentials decrease during fatigue). Other important diagnostic tests are the injection of **edrophonium bromide (Tensilon)** or **neostigmine intravenously (i.v.).** The injection causes a transient reversal of clinical findings. Other tests include the muscle fatigue test (which involves the patient looking up for 5 minutes and observing ptosis from fatigue), the sleep test coganis twitch, and the ice test. **Therapy** of systemic and ocular myasthenia is usually pyridostigmine bromide (Mestinon), 60 mg orally (p.o.) tid, but should be managed by a neurologist. Unfortunately, ocular myasthenia is frequently unresponsive to medical therapy. Once stability of the misalignment is documented, strabismus surgery may be helpful.

XI. **Cranial nerve palsy** may involve a single or all three nerves in varying degrees of paresis. It may be congenital, the result of developmental defects in the nuclei of the CNS or peripheral motor nerve fibers, or it may be acquired. **Lyme disease** may cause a variety of extraocular muscle palsies and other inflammatory and neuroophthalmic disorders (see Chap. 5, sec. **IV.L.2.**).

   A. **Third nerve palsies** are characterized as congenital and acquired, although some authorities believe that they are virtually all acquired.

   1. **Congenital third nerve palsy** may variably affect the medial superior and inferior recti and IO, **but never involves** the intraocular muscles (pupil, ciliary body). The levator muscle may also be involved, producing a variable form of ptosis.

      a. **Clinically,** the patients usually have ptosis and exotropia with intact pupillary and accommodative reflexes. There are varied degrees of limitation of elevation, adduction, and depression of the involved eye. By use of a compensatory head turn, many patients develop normal singular binocular vision. In the absence of binocular vision, amblyopia will develop in one eye if the patient does not maintain a compensatory torticollis to avoid the symptoms of diplopia.

      b. The **etiology** is unknown but is presumed to be developmental.

      c. **Forced ductions** are negative, ruling out adhesive problems as etiologic. Because of the hypotropia of the affected eye, an apparent ptosis may in fact be a **pseudoptosis** because the lid position follows eye position. If the hypotropic eye is allowed to fixate, the pseudoptosis will disappear.

      d. **Treatment** requires surgery for the exotropia, hypotropia, and ptosis. Hypotropia is treated by disinsertion of the SO tendon, while maximum recession of the LR and resection of the MR aid in moving the eye to a satisfactory location in the horizontal plane. A frontalis sling is usually indicated for the ptotic lid. The patient should be evaluated for the presence or absence of Bell phenomenon (see Chap. 5, sec. **V.E.**) before any lid evaluation procedure is carried out or the **risk of exposure keratopathy** may be significant postoperatively.

   2. **Acquired third nerve palsy** may be partial or complete, involving intraocular and extraocular muscles together or alone.

      a. **Clinically,** the appearance is similar to congenital third nerve palsy, but if the intraocular muscles are involved, there is a **fixed dilated pupil with paralysis of accommodation.**

      b. **Onset** is usually rapid and maximum with recovery, if any, usually complete by 6 months.

      c. The **etiology** includes unknown, vascular (diabetes, hypertension), aneurysm, head trauma, and neoplasm in decreasing order of frequency. **Diabetic third nerve palsy** rarely involves the pupil and usually recovers 100% of function.

      d. **Other causes of acquired third nerve palsy** may involve both intraocular and extraocular muscles. These include brainstem lesions; inflammatory disease such as meningitis, encephalitis, or toxic polyneuritis; vascular lesions **(painful third nerve palsy with pupillary involvement** is a particularly ominous sign of an **intracranial aneurysm); intracranial tumors** (commonly associated with **aberrant regeneration of the third nerve**); and demyelinating diseases such as multiple sclerosis and trauma.

      e. **Treatment** involves therapy of the underlying disease as an initial step, if warranted. Diplopia is often not a problem if significant ptosis is present; however, elevation of the lid surgically will **produce diplopia** unless the corrective surgical procedures (see sec. **XI.A.1.,** above) are carried out.

   B. **Fourth nerve palsy** can be congenital or acquired.

   1. **Clinically,** a patient with isolated fourth nerve palsy usually presents with a **head tilt to the opposite shoulder** in compensatory movement

against the torsion of the affected eye. Paralysis of the fourth nerve allows the antagonistic IO muscle to extort and elevate the eye. The patient will therefore tilt the head to the opposite shoulder to bring the vertical and torsional alignment of the affected eye parallel with the vertical and torsional alignment of the normal contralateral eye in an effort to avoid diplopia.

2. **The diagnosis of any isolated cyclovertical muscle palsy** such as a fourth nerve paresis is aided by **three evaluative steps (the Parks three-step test):**
   a. **Which eye is hypertropic?** Is it the result of a weak depressor or a weak contralateral elevator, e.g., to a weak IR or SO, or to a weak contralateral SR or IO?
   b. **Determine whether the vertical deviation increases to the right or left gaze.**
   c. **Determine whether vertical deviation increases on tilting the head toward the right or left shoulder,** using the alternate cover test. To best illustrate this, we use the example of a patient with a right hypertropia, worse on left gaze and right head tilt (Fig. 12.5).

   With the head tilted to the right, the left eye will extort and the right eye will intort. The intortors of the right eye are the right SR and the right SO. Because the right SO is weak and cannot depress the eye, the RSR will be unopposed and the right eye will be hypertropic. The paretic muscle, therefore, is the left RSO.

Step 1, an alternate cover test, will reveal a right hypertropia implicating a paretic RSO, RIR, LSR, or LIO.

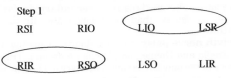

Step 2, evaluating the effects of levoversion and dextroversion, will reveal that vertical deviation increases on left gaze, thereby implicating now only the RSO and the LSR.

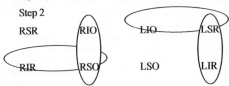

Step 3 indicates that vertical deviation increases with tilting the head to the right because of a upward movement of the right eye secondary to the unopposed action of the RSR.

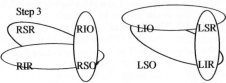

FIG. 12.5. Evaluating vertical deviations.

3. **Head tilt** in patients with fourth nerve palsy will be in the direction of least disparity. **The disparity will increase markedly if the head is forced to be tilted toward the shoulder on the side of the paretic SO (Bielschowsky sign).**

4. **In the presence of a third nerve paralysis,** evaluation of fourth nerve function may be carried out by asking the patient to look down; the iris crypt markings or the radial limbal vessels will reveal a conspicuous intorsion as the SO turns the globe. On attempted superduction, there will be a conspicuous extorsion, noted by examining movements of the iris markings or radial limbal vessels.

5. The **etiology** of congenital fourth nerve palsy is developmental in the nucleus or motor portion, and the etiology of acquired fourth nerve palsy is most commonly closed head trauma. Vascular causes (diabetes, hypertension), intracranial tumors, and aneurysms must be ruled out, however.

6. **Treatment of congenital palsy** with significant head tilt is surgery as soon as possible after diagnosis is firmly established. This is done to prevent a permanent torticollis, facial asymmetry, and scoliosis. **Treatment of acquired fourth nerve palsy,** after underlying disease is ruled out, is watchful waiting to assess the degree of spontaneous recovery until 6 months after onset. The object of surgery is to improve cyclo- and vertical deviations. If there is obvious contraction of the direct antagonist of the paretic muscle, recession of this antagonist should be the first procedure. In the absence of contraction, weakening of the yoke muscle of the palsied muscle or tucking the palsied muscle may be a first procedure.

C. **Sixth nerve palsy** may be congenital or acquired. It produces an esotropia in the primary position that increases on attempted lateral gaze in the direction of the involved muscle. Patients may establish and maintain normal binocular vision by compensatory **head turn** toward the side of the paretic eye. Patients with congenital or recently acquired sixth nerve palsy have a greater primary gaze esotropia (because of **secondary deviation**) when they fixate with the palsied eye than when they fixate with the sound eye **(primary deviation).**

1. **Congenital sixth nerve palsy** is rare and must be distinguished from congenital esotropia and Duane and Möbius syndromes. Trauma to the LR and abducens nerve may be the cause. Primary hypoplasia of the sixth nerve motor nucleus may also be the cause.

2. **Acquired sixth nerve palsy** may be the result of multiple etiologies because of the long intracranial course taken by the postnuclear portion of the nerve. Sixth nerve palsy is not uncommon in vascular disease (diabetes, hypertension), but may also be seen in intracranial neoplasms, head trauma, aneurysm, heavy metal poisoning, a variety of viral diseases inducing intracranial inflammation, and middle ear infection with secondary meningeal irritation and edema affecting the nerve as it passes through the petrospinous area in Dorello canal of the dura.

3. **Treatment** of unilateral sixth nerve palsy after etiologic evaluation is supportive for the first 6 months. Recovery is often noted by 3 months after onset. If there is no improvement after 6 months, surgery is indicated. Botulinum toxin injection to the ipsilateral MR muscle has been advocated to prevent contracture of this muscle. This should be performed within the first 6 months. If recovery of sixth nerve function is not complete or is absent, surgery will consist of a MR recession and LR resection, or a transposition of the vertical recti to the lateral with simultaneous weakening of the medial. The choice of procedure depends on the extent of LR function present at 6 months. If there is 50% function to the paretic LR, resection of the paretic LR will provide some mechanical benefit and may be done as either a primary or a secondary procedure. The **Hummelsheim operation** is used as an alternative procedure to assist the LR by dividing the superior and inferior recti in half and transposing half

of each muscle to the superior and inferior folds of the LR muscle insertion. The MR muscle in the involved eye is recessed at the same time.

XII. **Botulinum A toxin injection for strabismus**

A. **Mechanism of action.** *Clostridium botulinum* exotoxin potently blocks release of acetylcholine and functionally denervates muscle for several weeks. Injection of the toxin into an extraocular muscle, usually under the guidance of an electromyogram, produces temporary paralysis with consequent slight atrophy and stretching of the muscle, and simultaneous functional shortening of the antagonistic muscle, thus moving the globe toward realignment.

B. **Indications.** Botulinum A injection has been most successful in reversing surgical overcorrections, small to medium comitant esodeviations (20 to 30 D), and acute sixth nerve palsies with diplopia. Chronic sixth nerve palsy may also benefit from surgical transposition of the vertical rectus muscles to the LR muscle with injection of toxin into the ipsilateral MR muscle. If esotropia recurs, MR recession or reinjection with toxin may be used effectively. Accommodative esotropia in children with high AC/A ratio is frequently responsive to injection of both medial recti. Similar treatment in infantile esotropia reduces a mean of 35 pds preinjection to a mean of 5 pds postinjection. Conversely, large-angle exotropia is usually only transiently responsive to injection of the lateral recti, and restrictive forms of strabismus such as Duane syndrome are minimally to unresponsive. Adjustable suture surgery is also superior to botulinum for treating horizontal misalignment in adults without fusion. Vertical deviations are more difficult to treat by injection, both because of technical considerations and because of a very high incidence of blepharoptosis in SR injection. Dissociated vertical deviations may be treated with IO or IR toxin, although IR injection may leak to affect the IO adjacent to it. Injection of the IR in **Graves' disease** may be effective in acute disease and a surgical adjunct in the chronic state.

C. **Dosage.** Vertical and horizontal deviations less than 40 pds are treated initially with 2.5 units and horizontal deviations greater than 40 pds are treated with 5.0 units initially in a volume of 0.1 mL. The saline reconstituted lyophilized powder must **not be shaken** or the protein will denature. Reinjections may be titrated down depending on effect achieved from the original injection.

D. **Complications.** No adverse systemic side effects have been reported. Diplopia is very common due to transient overcorrection, but resolves in a few weeks; permanent overcorrection is extremely rare. Blepharoptosis occurs in 25% of children and 16% of adults after horizontal muscle injection (toxin spillage in the orbit), but resolves in several months or less. No amblyopia has been noted in children. Vertical deviations after horizontal muscle injection occur 17% of the time, but only 2% of these persist. Very rare complications are perforation of the globe and vitreous, and retrobulbar or subconjunctival hemorrhage.

XIII. **Nystagmus.** There are more than 38 classifications of nystagmus. The more common forms are discussed in this section.

A. **Latent nystagmus** is a congenital horizontal jerk nystagmus that occurs with monocular occlusion; when both eyes are open the nystagmus may be absent. Occlusion of one eye results in a jerk nystagmus with the fast component away from the covered eye and consequent diminution in visual acuity. There are many **methods to test vision monocularly** without eliciting this nystagmus. One method is to mount a high plus lens before the nonfixing eye without reducing the amount of light entering the eye, but blurring vision in that eye. Binocular vision should always be checked to indicate the best possible vision, although this will not reveal whether one eye sees better than the other. A latent nystagmus may become manifest (manifest latent nystagmus).

B. **Pendular nystagmus** is most frequently associated with sensory deprivation due to reduced central visual acuity, such as that associated with macular scarring (toxoplasmosis), macular hypoplasia (albinism, aniridia), achromatopsia, retinal degeneration (Leber congenital amaurosis), or optic nerve hypoplasia. This horizontal nystagmus is a slow pendular movement in primary gaze, but may change to jerk nystagmus in lateral gaze. It decreases on convergence, persists in the dark with eyes open, but eases on closure of the eyes under any lighting. The primary visual complaint is blurring.

C. **Congenital motor nystagmus** is a horizontal nystagmus that can be pendular, jerk, or circular. It is characteristically decreased by convergence and exhibits a **null point,** at which the nystagmus is decreased or absent. If this point is outside primary gaze, the patient will maintain a head turn to maintain gaze in the position of least eye motion. It is usually not associated with neurologic abnormalities.

D. **Spasmus nutans** is a combination of bilateral symmetric or asymmetric horizontal pendular nystagmus combined with **head nodding** and occasionally torticollis. Rarely, the nystagmus is rotary or vertical. It can be intermittent. Onset is in infancy, and the condition usually self-resolves by childhood; spasmus nutans has been associated with chiasmal tumors and other neurologic disorders.

E. **Acquired pendular nystagmus** may be seen in the only seeing eye of monocular adults who develop decreased visual acuity in that eye, in patients with brainstem dysfunction, or may result from the drug toxicity of sedatives or anticonvulsants.

F. **Acquired jerk nystagmus** may generally be classified as gaze paretic or vestibular.

1. **Gaze paretic nystagmus** is a slow horizontal beat resulting from upper brainstem dysfunction. Compression of the brainstem produces a nystagmus characterized by a slow gaze paretic movement with eyes toward the side of the lesion and a fast jerk nystagmus with eyes away from the side of the lesion.

2. **Vestibular nystagmus (VN)** is the result of malfunction or overstimulation of the eighth nerve vestibular apparatus or its connections, producing a horizontal or rotary jerk nystagmus in the primary position of gaze, or any nystagmus associated with **vertigo. Peripheral VN** is never purely vertical or rotary, but is reduced by visual fixation. **Central VN** is purely vertical or rotary and not affected by fixation.

   a. **Cold water irrigation test.** Such stimulus of the tympanic membrane mimics a **destructive** lesion of the vestibular system, e.g., Ménière syndrome or viral labyrinthitis. A normal response to cold irrigation is a horizontal nystagmus with the fast component away from the side of the stimulus **(cold: opposite; warm: same [COWS]),** vertigo, post-pointing, and a positive Romberg test.

   b. **Warm water irrigation test.** This stimulus mimics an **irritative** lesion. A normal response to warm irrigation is horizontal nystagmus with the fast component toward the side of the stimulus (COWS), vertigo, past-pointing, and a positive Romberg test.

G. **Other nystagmus forms**

1. **Endgaze (physiologic) nystagmus** is a small-amplitude, nonsustained horizontal nystagmus seen in normal patients on far right or left gaze.

2. **Upbeat nystagmus** may be congenital, drug induced, or indicative of posterior fossa disease. In primary position, the fast component is upward.

3. **Downbeat nystagmus** is characterized by the fast component in the downward direction and associated with posterior fossa disease. Compression at the foramen magnum results in marked downbeating on lateral gaze.

4. **Rotary nystagmus** is a torsional jerk movement around the AP axis of the eye and is usually seen with horizontal or vertical nystagmus. It may be congenital or acquired, as in brainstem lesions or in acute vestibular disease.

5. **Dissociated nystagmus** is a horizontal, markedly asymmetric nystagmus most commonly seen in the abducting eye in **internuclear ophthalmoplegia (INO)** (medial longitudinal fasciculus lesions). Sixth nerve paresis should be ruled out as an alternate cause of the eye movement pattern.

6. **Seesaw nystagmus** is a conjugate vertical torsional motion such that the intorting eye rises and the extorting eye falls. It is associated with expanding lesions in the area of the third ventricle or with upper brainstem vascular disease.

7. **Nystagmus blockage syndrome** is seen in patients with discordant nystagmus. This nystagmus is characterized by horizontal increased oscillations on abduction and by decreased oscillations on adduction. To obtain clearest vision, many patients damp or block the nystagmus by fixing with the adducted eye or by converging both eyes, but they will still fix with just one eye and turn the head in the direction of the fixing eye at both near and distance. Many patients with this syndrome have crossed fixation. Some appear orthophoric unless clear vision is required and the focusing mechanism is called into effect. Preferential surgery is on the fixating eye.

8. **Other nystagmoid-like oscillations**
   a. **Ocular myoclonus** is a rhythmic pendular motion, usually vertical, associated with synchronous rhythmic movements of other parts of the body, particularly around the oropharynx and diaphragm. Midbrain lesions are commonly associated with this acquired oscillation.
   b. **Ocular bobbing** is characterized by rapid downward jerks of both eyes followed by slow drift back to midposition. Patients are usually comatose and have massive lesions in and around the pontine area.
   c. **Opsoclonus** or "eye dancing" is involuntary chaotic, arrhythmic horizontal, vertical, and rotating jerks occurring 6 to 12 times per second. In children, the types are neonatal (congenital), encephalitic, and neuroblastoma related. In adults, viral etiology is most common, with occult neoplasm less frequent. Anti-Purkinje cell antibodies suggest an immune etiology. Treatment is removal of the tumor, if present. Systemic steroids are also very effective.
   d. **Ocular flutter** is an involuntary rapid horizontal saccadic oscillation seen in patients with cerebellar disease.

9. **Optokinetic nystagmus** is a physiologic jerk nystagmus elicited by presenting to gaze objects moving serially in one direction, horizontally or vertically, such as the stripes on a spinning optokinetic drum. The eyes will follow a fixed stripe momentarily and then jerk back to reposition centrally and pick up fixation on a new stripe. Clinically, this test may be used as a gross estimate of visual acuity in infants and poorly cooperative patients including malingerers by varying the size of the fixation stripes or pictures. It is also useful in localizing lesions causing homonymous hemianopic field defects. Disease of the parietooccipital region diminishes the optokinetic response when the drum is rotated to the side of the cerebral lesion.

10. **INO** is horizontal nystagmus of an eye on attempted temporal gaze associated with weakness or paralysis of nasal movement of the opposite eye. **Oscillopsia** or **skew deviation** may also be present. In the former, there is an illusory movement of the environment while the head is moving (INO or vestibular disturbance) because of poor compensatory eye movement on head turn. Spontaneous nystagmus may be present with the head still. In skew deviation, either eye may turn upward, but no specific muscle is found at fault. INO is seen in multiple sclerosis and brain stem mass and vascular lesions.

H. **Therapeutic approaches to nystagmus** vary but are sometimes very successful, and include optical, pharmacologic, and surgical (discussed previously) therapies. Treatment is aimed at improving visual acuity by stabilizing the eyes, decreasing any oscillopsia, and shifting the neutral zone in any compensatory head posturing.

1. **Optical** correction of refractive errors is critical to these patients.
   a. **Glasses or contact lenses** may significantly decrease nystagmus in bilateral aphakia.
   b. **Stimulating accommodative convergence** by overcorrecting with minus lenses may improve visual acuity by dampening nystagmus at distance fixation.
   c. **Retinal images** may be **stabilized** in patients with **acquired nystagmus and oscillopsia** by a galilean arrangement of contact lenses and glasses. A converging lens focuses all images at the eye's center of rotation and a high minus (-50 D) refocuses the images on the retina, thus stabilizing them as the contact moves with the eye.
   d. **Base-out prisms** in patients with **congenital motor nystagmus** promote convergence and dampen nystagmus.
   e. **Fresnel stick-on prisms** on glasses may displace the image to the null point in **congenital motor nystagmus,** thus decreasing head posturing and nystagmus when the head is in a normal position. Prisms may also be used vertically to correct head positions in vertical **nystagmus** and acquired downbeat nystagmus. Combination prisms can help in **oblique head turns.**

2. **Pharmacologic treatment**
   a. **Cyclopentolate 1%** one drop bid reduces the amplitude, velocity, and frequency of **latent nystagmus** in about 60% of patients. Visual acuity improves with this cycloplegia and monocular occlusion.
   b. **Baclofen, 5 mg p.o. tid** starting dose, is useful in suppressing acquired **periodic alternating nystagmus** (previously untreatable). If there is no response to the starting dose, dosage is increased every 3 days to a maximum of 80 mg per day. Side effects include dizziness, weakness, headache, and nausea; too rapid withdrawal can produce seizures.
   c. **Botulinum A, 2.5 U** injected into the horizontal muscles under electromyographic control, or 10 to 25 U in 0.1 to 1 mL volume as a retrobulbar injection with a standard 25-gauge, 1.5-in. retrobulbar needle every 3 to 4 months for up to 66 months, dampened **acquired nystagmus and oscillopsia** and improved visual acuity in 66% of patients. Transient ptosis was a common side effect.
   d. **Other useful drugs** include clonazepam for **downbeat nystagmus,** carbamazepine for **SO myokymia,** and propranolol for **opsoclonus.**

13. NEUROOPHTHALMOLOGY: VISUAL FIELDS, OPTIC NERVE, AND PUPIL

Shirley H. Wray and Deborah Pavan-Langston

I. **The visual fields**
   A. **Nerve fiber anatomy.** To examine the visual field efficiently yet quickly, the diagnostic features of a suspected disease must be known. A knowledge of these features is sound only when based on the anatomy of the visual system (Fig. 13.1).
      1. **The retina.** In the retina, the axons of the ganglion cells are arranged in three basic patterns: the papillomacular bundle from the macula, the superior and inferior arcuate nerve fiber bundles from the temporal retina, and radial fibers from the nasal retina (Fig. 13.2).
         a. **The macula,** which lies approximately 3 to 4 mm lateral to the optic disk, contains a disproportionately large number of nerve fiber axons. The axons, the papillomacular bundle, stream medially across the retina and layer out thinly along the lateral margin of the optic disk. They comprise more than 90% of all axons in the optic nerve. The papillomacular bundle subserves the area of central fixation. Its situation corresponds to a spindle-shaped area of the visual field known as the centrocecal area, which lies between the fixation point and the blind spot. Damage to the papillomacular bundle produces two types of visual field defects: central or centrocecal scotoma (Fig. 13.3 D, E).
         b. **The nasal and temporal half of the retina** is divided by an imaginary vertical line drawn through the fovea. It is projected on the visual field on the vertical meridian. The horizontal raphe acts as the boundary between the functional superior and inferior halves of the retina, and it is projected on the visual field on the horizontal meridian.
            (1) **Fibers from the temporal, superior, and inferior zones of the retina** crowd together, sweep over and under the papillomacular bundle, and wedge themselves into the remaining superior and inferior poles of the optic disk. Because of their arcuate course above and below the papillomacular axons, they are referred to as the superior and inferior arcuate bundles, respectively. The arcuate nerve fiber bundles from the temporal retina respect the horizontal raphe (Fig. 13.2A). Consequently, arcuate field defects have a sharp border on the horizontal meridian (Fig. 13.3B).
            (2) **Fibers from the nasal retina** course in a radial pattern directly to the nasal margin of the optic disk (Fig. 13.2A).
      2. **The papilla** and **optic nerve.** The arrangement of the nerve fibers at the disk is maintained in the immediate retrobulbar segment of the optic nerve. The papillomacular bundle occupies the temporal wedge, the arcuate bundles occupy the superior and inferior poles, and the nasal retinal fibers occupy the remaining nasal margin of the papilla (Fig. 13.2A). It is useful to remember this architecture when evaluating optic atrophy. Further posteriorly in the intracanalicular and intracranial segments of the optic nerve, the cross-sectional anatomy of the nerve changes. The papillomacular bundle migrates inward toward the core of the nerve. The axons from the nasal and temporal halves of the retina diverge and segregate. The nasal fibers come to lie in the lateral perimeter of the nerve (Fig. 13.2A).
      3. **The chiasm.** The precise nerve fiber arrangement of the chiasm is not known. It is known, however, that the nasal retinal fibers cross the chiasm and the temporal fibers remain uncrossed. This anatomy is important in relation to chiasmatic field defects (Fig. 13.4). The ratio of crossed to

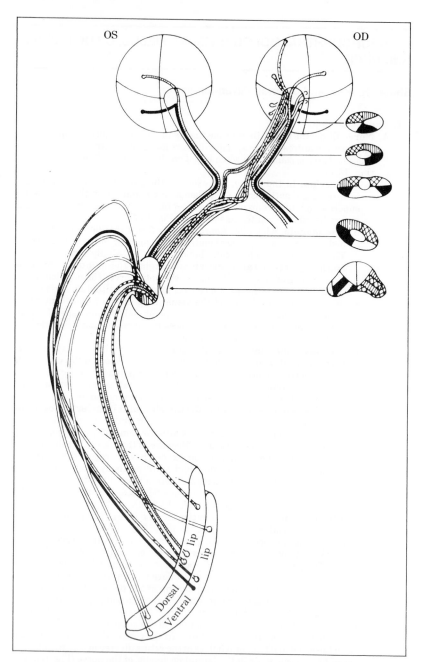

FIG. 13.1. The nerve fiber anatomy of the visual pathways from retina to occipital cortex. Cross sections on right show location of fibers at various levels in the pathway. OS, oculus sinister; OD, oculus dexter. (Modified and reproduced with permission from Donaldson DD.)

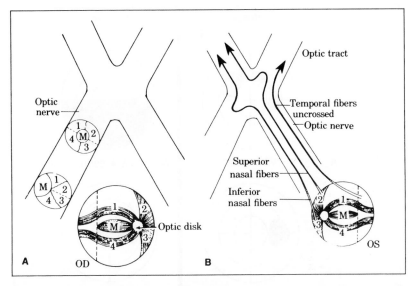

FIG. 13.2. The three basic patterns of retinal nerve fibers: the papillomacular bundle (M), the superior (1) and inferior (4) arcuate nerve fiber bundles from the temporal retina, and radial fibers from the nasal retina (2 and 3). **A:** Right fundus and cross-sectional anatomy of the fibers in the right optic nerve. **B:** Left optic nerve and decussation of the crossing nasal retinal fibers in the chiasm. OD, oculus dexter; OS, oculus sinister.

uncrossed fibers is 3:2. Four points to remember about the **decussation of the nasal retinal fibers are**

   a. **Inferior peripheral nasal fibers** cross in the inferoanterior part of the chiasm and arch first into the medial aspect of the opposite optic nerve for a short distance. This loop is called the anterior knee of von Willebrand. The fibers then course backward into the opposite optic tract (Fig. 13.2B).

   b. **Superior peripheral nasal fibers** cross to the opposite optic tract in the superoposterior part of the chiasm, but arch first for a short distance into the optic tract of the same side. This loop is called the posterior knee of von Willebrand (Fig. 13.2B).

   c. **Fibers arising from the nasal half of the macular area** of the retina fan out into a broad band to cross in the central superior and posterior portions of the chiasm and move upward to lie in a superior wedge of the optic tract.

   d. **Uncrossed temporal retinal fibers** from corresponding upper and lower retina eventually find their mates from the crossing nasal group in the respective medial or lateral portion of the optic tract.

4. **The optic tract.** In the optic tract, nerve fibers from corresponding areas in the two retinas become more closely associated. At the termination of the tract and in the lateral geniculate body, the nerve fibers that started in a superior position in the optic nerve are medial in situation, and the lower fibers in the optic nerve become lateral in the tract and lateral geniculate body (Fig. 13.1). This rotation results in a medial location for fibers from the corresponding upper quadrant of each retina and a lateral location for fibers from the corresponding lower quadrant of each retina. A **central wedge of macular fibers** is insinuated between the lateral lower and the medial upper extramacular fibers in both the tract and the lateral geniculate body.

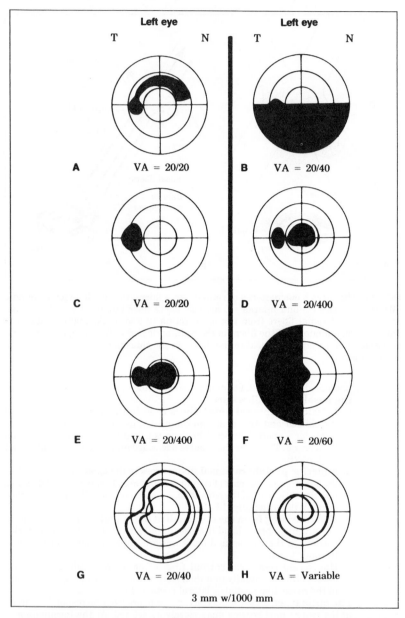

FIG. 13.3. Types of monocular visual field loss in left eye (3-mm white object at 1,000 mm). **A:** Superior arcuate scotoma (inferior nerve fiber bundle defect). **B:** Inferior altitudinal field defect respecting the horizontal meridian (superior nerve fiber bundle defect). **C:** Enlargement of the blind spot in the left eye. **D:** Central scotoma, normal blind spot. **E:** Centrocecal scotoma. **F:** Temporal hemianopia respecting the vertical meridian, but with involvement of central vision. **G:** Generalized constriction of the visual field to 2 isopters. **H:** Nonorganic "corkscrew" field defect (hysteria, malingering) to 1 isopter. VA, visual acuity; T, temporal; N, nasal.

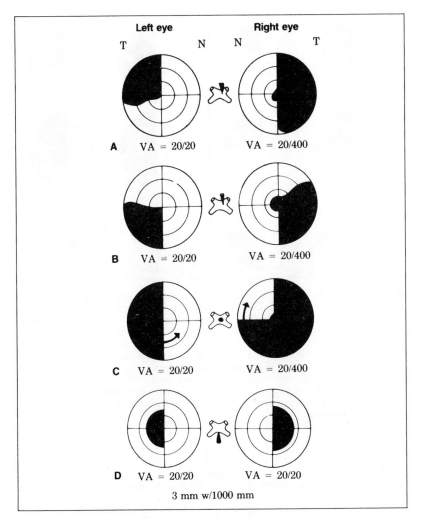

FIG. 13.4. Types of bitemporal field defects (3-mm white object at 1,000 mm). **A:** Central visual fields of a lesion anterior and inferior to chiasm with compression of the optic nerve. **B:** Lesion located anterior and superior to the chiasm affecting predominantly the right side. **C:** Progressive lesion inferior to the chiasm. **D:** Lesion posterior to the chiasm causing bitemporal hemianopic scotomas. VA, visual acuity; T, temporal; N, nasal. (Adapted from Vaughan D, Cook R, Asbury T. *General ophthalmology*. Los Altos, CA: Lange Medical Publications, 1974.)

5. **The lateral geniculate body** consists of six layers, numbered from ventral to dorsal. The lateral geniculate body receives crossed retinal fibers in layers 1, 4, and 6, and uncrossed retinal fibers in layers 2, 3, and 5. There is a vertical alignment of corresponding points of the visual field. The **right side of the brain receives its sensory input from the left side of the visual environment;** thus, the right optic tract and right lateral geniculate body get their input from the left visual field, which must

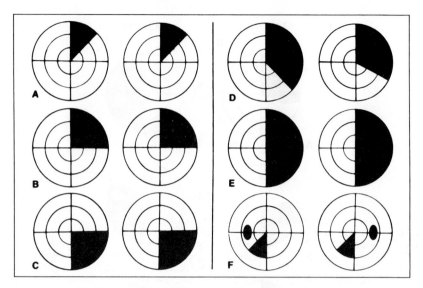

FIG. 13.5. Types of homonymous field defects. **A:** Superior right homonymous quad-rantic defect ("pie in the sky") due to a lesion of the most anteroinferior fibers of the optic radiations in the left temporal lobe (Meyer loop). **B:** Complete right superior homonymous quadrantanopia due to a lesion of the optic radiations in the left tem-poroparietal lobe. **C:** Complete right inferior homonymous quadrantanopia due to a lesion of the superior fibers of the optic radiations in the parietal lobe ("pie on the floor"). **D:** Incongruous right homonymous hemianopia due to a lesion in the anterior optic radiations. **E:** Complete right homonymous hemianopia due to a lesion in the left temporoparietal optic radiations or left visual cortex. **F:** Homonymous hemianopic congruous scotoma abutting fixation in the left inferior quadrant due to a lesion in the right visual cortex.

perforce be from the right half of each retina, i.e., the temporal retina of the right eye, and the nasal retina of the left eye.

6. **The optic radiation.** The nerve fibers of the optic radiation arise from all six layers of the lateral geniculate body.

   a. **All fibers** then sweep laterally and inferiorly around the temporal horn of the lateral ventricle (Fig. 13.1). As the radiation sweeps laterally it as-cends for a short distance in the posterior limb of the internal capsule—an important relationship because a vascular lesion of the internal cap-sule may be expected to produce a **hemiplegia** and a **homonymous hemianopia.**

   b. **The most anteroinferior fibers** of the optic radiation form *Meyer loop*. Meyer loop, which contains projections of the inferior retinal fibers, sweeps forward toward the pole of the temporal lobe. Amputation of the temporal pole in excess of 4 cm produces a homonymous superior quadrantanopia **("pie in the sky").** The defect is always adjacent to the vertical meridian **(Fig. 13.5A).** If 8 cm of the temporal lobe tip is excised, a homonymous hemianopia results.

   c. **Deep in the parietal lobe,** the radiations lie external to the trigone and pass to the medial surface of the occipital lobe (the striate calcarine cortex).

7. **The visual cortex.** The primary visual cortical area lies on the medial surface of each occipital lobe in the interhemispheric fissure. It is situated

both above and below the calcarine and postcalcarine fissures. These two fissures represent the junction between the upper and lower halves of the visual fields (Fig. 13.1).

  a. **The upper dorsal lip** of this fissure receives projections from the corresponding upper quadrant of both retinas that are associated with the lower quadrant of the binocular field on the opposite side.

  b. **The inferior ventral lip** is related to the superior quadrant of the binocular field of the opposite side.

  c. **The periphery of the retina** is represented most anteriorly in the deep rostral aspects of the visual cortex near the splenium of the corpus collosum.

  d. **The macula** is represented posteriorly by an extensive area of visual cortex that extends onto the posterolateral aspect of the occipital lobe. This anatomy is important when considering bullet wounds and similar **traumatic lesions** of the occipital lobe.

  e. **In the evaluation of occipitocortical lesions,** it should always be remembered that there is accurate localization in the occipital cortex; that areas 17, 18, and 19 are interconnected in each hemisphere; and that area 18 may be responsible for pursuit eye movements.

B. **The monocular visual field**

  1. **The visual field** is that area of one's surroundings that is visible at one time. The normal monocular visual field extends approximately 100 degrees laterally, 60 degrees medially, 60 degrees upward, and 75 degrees downward. It is divided into nasal and temporal halves by an imaginary vertical line drawn through the fovea, into superior and inferior altitudinal halves by the horizontal raphe that runs from the fovea to the temporal periphery. Situated in the temporal half field is the normal blind spot, 15 degrees temporal to fixation and 1.5 degrees below the horizontal meridian.

  2. **The blind spot** is represented by an absolute scotoma corresponding to the scleral canal through which the retinal nerve fibers leave the eye at the optic disk.

C. **Visual field tests**

  1. **When is a visual field test indicated?** The ideal is to include a visual field test in every ophthalmic examination, but time is a precious commodity. Perimetry is, however, mandatory when indicated by the clinical history, the eye examination, or brain, computed tomography (CT), or magnetic resonance imaging (MRI) findings.

  2. **Indications for field testing**

    a. **History**

      (1) **A medical history** of headache or amenorrhea–galactorrhea (or both).

      (2) A **neurologic history** of seizures, migraine with visual aura, amaurosis fugax with residual deficit, hemiplegia, head injury, or multiple sclerosis.

      (3) An **ophthalmic history** of blurred vision or loss of vision, bumping into objects, difficulty in reading, exertional amblyopia *(Uhthoff syndrome),* unexplained failure to pass a routine eye test (school, driving), loss of depth perception, loss of color vision, recognition of a blind spot, or double vision.

    b. **Several ocular signs** indicate a need for perimetry testing: optic disk pallor, cupping of the optic disk, papilledema, ischemic optic disk swelling, and retinal diseases such as infarction, degeneration, or detachment.

    c. **Radiologic changes.** Visual field testing is essential when an x-ray of the skull shows enlargement of the sella, J-shaped sella, tumor calcification (particularly suprasellar), enlargement of the optic canals, displacement and calcification of the pineal gland, hyperostosis of the sphenoid bone, or multiple skull fractures, or when a CT scan or MRI documents an orbital or intracranial lesion (see Chapter 1).

3. **Selection of the method of examination.** The choice of the best method of visual field examination and the most suitable equipment for plotting the visual field depends on the clinical condition of the patient, the corrected visual acuity, the type of visual field defect suspected, and the purpose of the examination. The method and equipment must be selected so as to allow the most accurate and reproducible examination in as short a time as possible to avoid patient and examiner fatigue.

A clear distinction should be made between an examination to **determine whether or not a field defect exists** and an examination **to analyze a defect** known to be present. If a defect is suspected, no more than 5 minutes is required to detect and plot its form with one or two targets. From the simple chart thus produced, a diagnosis may often be confirmed. Every defect, however, must be analyzed and as many techniques as necessary used for this analysis, inclusive of kinetic or static perimetric tests. Because this may take 30 or more minutes, it is often advisable to do the locating and the analysis at separate sittings, or to refer the patient to a skilled perimetrist for further testing. In this way, the more complicated field chart, resulting from the analysis of a defect, may be compared on serial examinations of the field, and thus provide vital information about the advance or recovery of disease.

D. **Visual field methods.** All visual field tests are performed with each eye covered in turn (see also Chapter 1, secs. **II.I.,** and Chapter 10, sec. **III.E.**).

1. **The monocular confrontation field test.** Almost all types of visual field defects can be detected with a few colored pins by the monocular confrontation test. This technique is highly recommended for use in the emergency room. Moreover, it is the technique of choice in the bedridden, in those who lack the ability to concentrate, and in children. Sometimes it is the only attainable form of field examination.

   a. **Visual observations by the patient.** In the monocular confrontation field test, the examiner compares the patient's visual field with his or her own. The examiner, sitting face to face with the patient, asks the patient if he or she can see the examiner's face clearly or if some area is missing (face-to-face confrontation). Frequently, an intelligent patient will describe blurring or loss of certain facial landmarks, indicating that he or she has a specific type of field loss. For example, with an inferior altitudinal defect there is loss of clarity of the lower half of the examiner's face. The observation is an invaluable guide to the examiner.

   b. **The peripheral field.** The field is then charted to moving targets. The patient is asked to fixate on the examiner's eye. A white pinhead is moved inward from the periphery. The pin, a 3-, 5-, or 10-mm white hat pin (not a pearl pin), is held about 30 cm from the patient's and examiner's eyes. The patient calls "yes" when he or she catches a glimpse of it without wavering fixation. This is repeated around the circumference of the field, and any defect of the periphery can be detected. Each eye is tested in turn. A homonymous hemianopia is quickly discovered by this method.

   c. **Central fields.** A red pin (5 or 10 mm) is best for exploring the central 20 degrees, particularly on either side of the vertical meridian. If in one spot the red appears pale or hazy, a relative scotoma is present. The central scotoma in optic neuritis is rapidly detected this way. The results are conventionally recorded in the chart as the patient views the world.

   d. **When visual acuity is seriously impaired,** confrontation is limited to a 40-mm white target, to finger counting, to finger or hand movement, or to a flashlight, if necessary. When a defect is found, if possible it should be further analyzed and recorded by using the tangent screen or a perimeter. Both techniques provide a better method of documenting progressive change. Further examination is also necessary when no defect is discovered by confrontation, especially in patients with visual complaints.

2. **The tangent screen (Bjerrum screen)** is a black felt screen on which radial lines and 5-degree concentric circles are inconspicuously marked. It is

used to examine the central field within 30 degrees from the fixation point and to determine the size of the blind spot. By increasing the distance of the patient from the screen, the size of the field defect increases and allows evaluation in greater detail. The hysterical constricted field characteristically remains the same size when charted at different distances. Screens are therefore made for use at 1 or 2 m. A 1-m screen can be accommodated on the wall of most consulting rooms and evenly illuminated.

a. The **method** is simple. The field is charted for each eye alone to one or two sizes of round white targets and occasionally to red or other colors. The traditional method is to fit the colored disk onto a black wand and move the target in from the periphery. The examiner stands in front of the patient to observe fixation and works from each side of the screen in turn. Targets on wands have now largely been replaced by the use of a flashlight especially designed to project a light spot of precise size and luminosity on the screen. Greater versatility is obtained with this technique. A disadvantage is that the examiner, sitting beside the patient, is less able to check the patient's fixation. The blind spot should therefore be charted first to confirm reliability.

b. **Color fields.** When charting the field to a colored target, the point to be recorded is when the patient recognizes the true color of the target, and not when the object is first seen (this is a common error).

c. **The results** on the Bjerrum screen examination can be recorded on a simple chart stamped in one corner of the large perimeter field chart to facilitate quick comparison and filing. This also has merit in reducing the volume of the patient's record.

d. **Field defects detected.** The tangent screen test is particularly valuable for analysis of the following types of visual field defects:

(1) Enlargement of the blind spot (Fig. 13.3C).

(2) Arcuate scotoma (Fig. 13.3A) and altitudinal defects (Fig. 13.3B).

(3) Central scotoma (Fig. 13.3D).

(4) Centrocecal scotoma (Fig. 13.3E).

(5) Paracentral scotoma.

(6) Homonymous scotoma abutting fixation.

(7) Homonymous hemianopia involving the macula (Fig. 13.3F).

(8) Generalized constriction of the visual field (Fig. 13.3G).

(9) Nonorganic (hysterical) constriction of the visual field (Fig. 13.3H).

3. **The Amsler grid** is a name given to a boldly cross-hatched paper. Any rectilinear design can be used for the same purpose. A simple grid with a central fixation point can be drawn on hospital record paper at the bedside. Its principle is the fact that **central retinal lesions often distort geometric patterns, causing metamorphopsia.** In contrast, damage to the optic nerve and chiasm produces hazy defects in central acuity that tend to "fog out" without altering the grid pattern or bending its lines. Often the patient can describe a scotoma very accurately if the examiner keeps a piece of paper of this sort handy and allows the patient to look at it in bright illumination fixing on a central spot. The patient can usually outline or draw the affected area quite adequately. With reading glasses on, if needed, each eye is tested in turn. This technique tests only the central 10 degrees of vision.

4. **The hemispheric projection perimeter (Goldmann perimeter)** is a precision instrument used for testing both peripheral and central fields. It affords a remarkable speed of operation for kinetic perimetry, and luminance of the hemispheric background can be kept precisely controlled to keep retinal light-adaptation constant. The patient is positioned on the hemisphere-shaped machine with the chin on a chin rest and the uncovered eye is aligned with the central fixation point. Fixation is monitored by the perimetrist through a telescope. Projected test spots of constant size and fixed contrast are moved from the periphery in toward the center. The patient presses an electric buzzer when the target is in

view. The same stimulus spot is moved into the visual field along different meridians, and an **isopter**, i.e., a line of equal sensitivity to light contrast, is charted. (An isopter is analogous to a contour line on a map of uneven terrain.) Selection of the speed of the test spot depends on the reaction time of each patient. Five degrees per second gives reproducible results. An orderly rhythmic presentation of the test spot minimizes fatigue. At least two isopters should be charted: one to a large well-visualized spot to aid in training the patient, and the second to the smallest dimmest target he or she can reliably see to permit detection of early defects. Recording several isopters also ensures that all regions of the field are tested in addition to helping to define the **slope** of the borders of a defect. Steep slopes (isopters crowded together) usually indicate that the defect is caused by an acute lesion (frequently vascular); gradual slopes are indicative of a progressive lesion (tumor). The Goldmann perimeter is a large, expensive machine and is not suitable for every examining room. Because of the remarkable reproducibility of the field examination by different examiners, however, the perimeter is essential for use by ophthalmologists who are responsible for the serial evaluation of the visual fields.

5. **Automated static perimetry (Humphrey, Octopus)** is recognized to be a sensitive technique to detect fiber bundle defects in the monocular central visual field. For neuroophthalmic cases, the Octopus 2000 perimeter and program no. 34, which presents 72 points, is used. The method is straightforward and similar to kinetic perimetry. The patient is asked to fix on a central target in a hemisphere with a homogeneous white background, while a nonmoving light of fixed size and brightness is presented at various points in the hemisphere. Brightness is increased until the patient recognizes the presence of the stimulus above background. Thus, static perimetry measures brightness sensitivity at various retinal points. Serial static visual fields can be compared by computer analysis using the DELTA program to determine progression or resolution.

E. **Visual field pathology**

1. **The retina.** Retinal lesions cause visual field defects that may correspond to the pattern of the retinal nerve fibers or to the area of supply of the retinal blood vessels. The defects produced do **not respect the vertical meridian.** Frequently, they correspond to areas of infarction or inflammation or to degenerative lesions seen with the ophthalmoscope. Retinal lesions may thus produce isolated scotomas or extensive altitudinal defects. **Macular lesions** produce central scotomas. **Retinitis pigmentosa** produces constricted fields and equatorial ring scotomas.

2. **Papilla and optic nerve.** Lesions of the optic nerve produce four basic patterns of visual field loss: arcuate scotoma, centrocecal scotoma, generalized constriction, and junctional scotoma.

   a. **Arcuate scotomas** are located in the central portion of the visual field. They appear as annular or cuneate-shaped scotomas. Most paracentral scotomas are actually arcuate. Characteristically, the apex of the scotoma points directly toward or emanates from the blind spot (Fig. 13.3A). Intact field usually surrounds the involved area on all sides, but sometimes the scotoma breaks out into the periphery and produces an **altitudinal defect** (Fig. 13.3B). Arcuate defects have a sharp border on the horizontal meridian. After entering the optic disk, the arcuate nerve fibers remain separate throughout their course in the optic nerve and into the anterior portion of the chiasm. Discrete lesions, frequently ischemic, anywhere along this pathway may produce arcuate field defects. Such lesions include ischemic optic neuropathy, glaucoma, and optic atrophy secondary to papilledema. Rarely, the causal lesion may even be situated as far back as the optic chiasm, i.e., meningioma of the dorsum sellae, pituitary adenoma, or opticochiasmatic arachnoiditis. Careful perimetry of these cases will uncover clear-cut termination of the scotoma at the **vertical** meridian that can be explained anatomically only by a lesion in the anterocentral chiasm, where crossing and non-crossing portions of the nerve fiber bundles separate.

b. **Centrocecal scotoma** results from damage to axons that run within the central core of the optic nerve from the macular and peripapillary retinal receptor zones. Damage to the former produces a scotoma in the area of central fixation; damage to the latter produces an enlargement of the physiologic blind spot. The composite loss of vision with a lesion that affects these two fiber systems is simply a blend of two scotomas. The resultant field defect extends both to fixation and to the blind spot (Fig. 13.3E). The centrocecal scotoma is a specific and common sign of optic nerve disease. It occurs in a variety of conditions both intrinsic (demyelination, infiltrative, metabolic–toxic) and compressive in nature.

c. **Generalized constriction** is a less specific defect and is less reliable in localizing lesions to the optic nerve **unless it is unilateral.** It rarely occurs without concomitant reduction of central vision; therefore, arcuate or centrocecal scotomas are not uncommonly accompanied by a generalized constriction of the field. **Monocular generalized constriction** of peripheral and central isopters without associated local defects suggests diffuse optic nerve involvement (Fig. 13.3G). Constriction of central isopters alone suggests early deterioration of central vision. Progressive generalized constriction of peripheral isopters with relative sparing of central vision may be part of the syndrome of perioptic sheath meningioma. Unlike nonorganic "tubular fields," the outer circumference of the field loss in these patients will appear to enlarge in a physiologic manner as the distance between the patient and the test object is increased.

d. **The junctional scotoma** is one important exception to the rule that unifocal optic nerve lesions produce strictly monocular visual field defects. At the posterior extremity of the optic nerve, the inferonasal retinal fibers from the opposite eye sweep into the optic nerve for a short distance before crossing back into the optic tract (Fig. 13.2B). Thus, a *single lesion situated at the junction of nerve and chiasm can produce visual field defects in both eyes*—an ipsilateral centrocecal scotoma along with a contralateral upper temporal quadrantanopia. The combination of perimetric defects, referred to as the **junctional scotoma of Traquair,** is an important localizing sign *of prechiasmal compression.* It thus behooves the perimetrist to search the upper temporal field of the unaffected eye carefully in cases of unexplained loss of monocular vision, because the most common mistake under these circumstances is for the patient to be told that the condition is the result of chronic retrobulbar neuritis.

3. **The chiasm.** Chiasmal lesions cause field defects with three important characteristics. Frequently, they are bitemporal with sharp borders respecting the vertical meridian. Central vision is usually involved. The defects show considerable variability (Fig. 13.4). The variability is dependent on the position of the chiasm; the varying size, shape, and tilt of the sella; the direction of expansion of the compressing mass; and the distribution of the loops of crossing nasal retinal fibers in the chiasm. The visual field may be monocular or binocular.

a. **Monocular visual field defects** include monocular scotoma, arcuate nerve fiber bundle defects that respect the vertical meridian, and temporal hemianopia. When monocular temporal hemianopia occurs, this rare defect is thought to represent the effects of occlusion or stasis in nutrient chiasmal vessels.

b. **Binocular visual defects** have several different patterns (Fig. 13.4): junctional scotoma, superior bitemporal quadrantanopia, inferior bitemporal quadrantanopia, bitemporal hemianopia, bitemporal hemianopic scotoma, binasal hemianopia, incongruous homonymous hemianopia, and a complete homonymous hemianopia. Each type can provide a clinical clue to the location and type of chiasmal deformation.

c. **In the analysis of topographic localization** of chiasmal field defects, the perimetrist refers to superior, inferior, anterior, and posterior involvement of the chiasm. This classic approach is somewhat oversimplified. A note of caution: Do not neglect the chiasm's tilted orientation and elevated position above the sella. Clearly, "early" vulnerability of the chiasm to compression from "small" pituitary adenomas is a misconception. For practical purposes, the guidelines are as follows:

(1) **Compression of the anterior angle** of the chiasm causes unilateral blindness or a central scotoma plus a contralateral superotemporal defect (junctional scotoma).

(2) **Compression of the median bar** of the chiasm from below (inferiorly) causes a bitemporal superior quadrantanopia or bitemporal hemianopia (Fig. 13.4A).

(3) **Compression of the median bar** from above (superiorly) produces a bitemporal inferior quadrantanopia (Fig. 13.4B), e.g., a craniopharyngioma.

(4) **Compression of the posterior chiasm** from above produces bitemporal hemianopic scotomas (Fig. 13.4D).

(5) **Compression bilaterally of the lateral margin** of the chiasm produces binasal hemianopia; the chiasm actually becomes squeezed and displaced laterally, e.g., an aneurysm.

(6) A mass in the **retrochiasmatic region** impinging on or displacing the optic tract results in homonymous hemianopia of two types: an incongruous homonymous hemianopia or a complete homonymous hemianopia.

d. **Pseudochiasmal defects.** Pseudochiasmal or ocular syndromes mimicking chiasmal lesions include tilted optic disks (see sec. **II.A.4.,** below), drug (chloroquine) toxicity, sector retinitis pigmentosa, and bilateral retinal detachments.

4. **The optic tract.** An anterior optic tract lesion produces an incongruous homonymous hemianopia (Fig. 13.5D), decreased visual acuity, afferent pupil defect **(Wernicke hemianopic pupil),** and atrophy of the optic disks with characteristic bow-tie atrophy in the contralateral eye. A complete homonymous hemianopia results from a lesion of the posterior optic tract (Fig. 13.5E).

5. **Lateral geniculate body.** Lesions of the lateral geniculate body are extremely rare. They produce highly incongruous homonymous hemianopias that may correspond to the laminal organization of the cell layers.

6. **The optic radiation.** Damage to the optic radiations produces a homonymous hemianopia (Fig. 13.5E). Important considerations are congruity, macular sparing, visual attentiveness, and associated oculomotor signs.

a. **Congruity** is said to be present when the edge of the field defect in each eye is identical in shape. Field changes resulting from lesions of the anterior optic radiation tend to be **incongruous.** Those resulting from damage to the radiations close to the visual cortex are **congruous.** Depending on its site, the lesion may involve only the upper or lower fibers of the radiation and thus cause a lower or upper quadrantanopia in the opposite half-field; e.g., temporal lobe radiation lesion causes pie in the sky (Fig. 13.5A), and parietal lobe radiation lesion causes pie on the floor (Fig. 13.5C).

b. **The edges of the field defects** are **steep** or vertical at the onset if the lesion results from ischemic infarction, and **shelving** if the lesion is secondary to compression. The more rapid the growth of a tumor, the more gradual the slope of the margin of the defect.

c. **Macular sparing** in lesions of the optic radiations probably occurs because the macula has such a large area of representation; therefore, destruction of all the macular fibers is uncommon.

d. **A complete hemianopic defect to attention** may occur in lesions of the parietal area. The monocular confrontation test with double simultaneous stimulation of the two half-fields by finger movement is a good method of demonstrating the **extinction phenomenon.**

   (1) **Left temporoparietal lesions** cause defective recognition of visual symbols, alexia, and agraphia.

   (2) **Lesions of the right temporoparietal area** cause impaired judgment of spatial relationships, as in topographic agnosia and constructional apraxia.

  e. **Ocular motility signs** are also associated with parietooccipital lesions. In this situation, a complete homonymous hemianopia is accompanied by **absent optokinetic nystagmus** when the stripes of the drum are rotated horizontally to the side of the cerebral lesion. On **forced eye closure,** the eyes deviate conjugately upward and laterally to the side opposite the cerebral lesion. An examination for these motor signs is essential in the evaluation of the patient with a homonymous hemianopic field defect. The ophthalmologist may then be able to site the lesion along the course of the optic radiations and guide the selection of noninvasive and cerebral angiographic studies.

7. **The visual cortex.** Destruction of the visual cortex of one occipital lobe produces a **contralateral congruous homonymous hemianopia.** This is the most common type of cortical field defect seen and frequently is the result of embolic occlusion of the posterior cerebral artery; however, other patterns of visual loss also occur. These defects permit precise localization. They include congruous homonymous hemianopic scotoma, bilateral altitudinal scotoma, congruous homonymous hemianopia sparing the temporal crescent, or, rarely, a monocular field defect resulting from loss of the temporal crescent, bilateral homonymous hemianopia, cortical blindness, and tunnel or keyhole vision.

  a. **Congruous homonymous hemianopic scotomas** tend to be sector-shaped, filling a triangular area within a quadrant. The apex points toward fixation (Fig. 13.5F). Such a defect indicates damage to the occipital pole. The most common cause is trauma or infarction secondary to embolic occlusion.

  b. **Altitudinal scotomas** result from gunshot wounds or contusion of the occipital lobe following a depressed skull fracture. A bullet produces the defect by passing horizontally through both occipital lobes. Inferior altitudinal defects are more common than superior altitudinal defects, presumably because trauma below the occipital lobe tends to involve the venous sinuses or brain stem or both, and results in death. At initial examination after the trauma, the visual field defect is frequently very extensive; the prognosis for recovery is usually good, however, although not always complete. A guarded prognosis in the early stages is wise.

  c. **Sparing of the temporal crescent** in the presence of a congruous homonymous hemianopia permits exact localization of the site of the lesion to the contralateral visual cortex, with sparing of the most medial group of optic radiation fibers projecting to the most anterior end of the visual cortex. Preservation of a homonymous crescent is not found in the nasal half-field of the opposite eye because the temporal field is larger than the nasal field. In rare instances, the uniocular temporal crescentic area disappears.

  d. **Bilateral homonymous hemianopia** results from bilateral, usually ischemic, lesions of the visual cortex. One occipital lobe is usually infected before the other. The interval between the two strokes may be weeks, months, or years. Prognosis of complete recovery is poor, although there may be a gradual return of vision to light and then to hand movement.

   (1) **Cortical blindness.** In severe cases, when the patient remains blind, the patient may deny that he or she is blind. This condition, cortical blindness or **Anton syndrome,** is characterized by four

important features: bilateral blindness, denial of blindness, normal pupil reflexes, and bilateral occipitocortical lesions.

(2) **Tunnel vision** results after bilateral occlusion of the posterior cerebral arteries and infarction of the occipital lobes, but with sparing of a small central island of vision. The peripheral fields are severely constricted (see also sec. **I.E.8.,** below), but visual acuity is preserved. This situation occurs if the infarction involves only the visual cortex anterior to the posterior pole, preserving a **central keyhole of vision,** or when the middle cerebral artery, which anastomoses with the posterior cerebral artery, provides a vascular supply to the posterior (macular) tip of the cortex.

8. **Nonorganic field defects.** In the absence of optic disk swelling, optic atrophy, and retinal degeneration, bilateral or unilateral constricted fields are often nonorganic. They can result from patient fatigue, lack of attention, misunderstanding, malingering, or hysteria. Spiral or corkscrew fields are also common in hysteria (Fig. 13.3H).

F. **Final analysis of visual field testing.** The task of the ophthalmologist in the evaluation of visual field defects is not over when perimetry and field testing are complete. Two additional steps are mandatory. Step one is to identify the anatomic localization of the site of the lesion by interpretation of the visual field defect. Step two is to determine the nature of the lesion.

1. **Step one** can be facilitated only by a physician with a thorough knowledge of the anatomy of the anterior visual pathways.

2. **Step two** usually requires the prompt referral of the patient to a neuroophthalmologist or neurologist for a neurologic examination and neuroimaging. A contrast **CT scan** of the orbits with coronal views is still one of the best radiologic techniques to study the intraorbital segment of the optic nerves and the orbit contents. A CT scan with bone windows is required to study the base of the brain. MRI of the brain in axial, sagittal, and coronal planes with T1- and T2-weighted images, with and without gadolinium, is beginning to replace the conventional CT scan for the detection of cerebral lesions. The MRI is particularly sensitive in detecting small white matter lesions (plaques) of demyelination seen in cases of idiopathic optic neuritis and multiple sclerosis. MRI studies may also help distinguish between a mass caused by a tumor or aneurysm. Head and neck **magnetic resonance angiography (MRA)** permits visualization of the carotid vessels in the neck and intracerebral circulation by a specialized computer-assisted MRI technique. MRA is a noninvasive procedure recommended for the elderly patient with amaurosis fugax, a carotid or ocular bruit, or both.

II. **The optic nerve head**

A. **Congenital optic disk anomalies** are classified in five groups: optic nerve colobomas, pits, optic nerve dysplasia or hypoplasia, tilted disk (dysversion), and pseudopapilledema. The importance of disk anomalies in neuroophthalmology and pediatric ophthalmology, in particular, cannot be overemphasized. Large disks of the dysplastic type have been associated with congenital forebrain abnormalities, including basal encephaloceles. Small disks of the hypoplastic type have been associated with visual loss, nystagmus, and major concomitant central nervous system (CNS) anomalies. Congenital dysversion is associated with visual field defects, and anomalous disk elevation is associated with the diagnostic dilemma of pseudopapilledema versus papilledema. Such possibilities must be kept in mind by ophthalmologists concerned with the evaluation of the child with poor vision.

1. **Colobomas and pits.** Large anomalous disks are common. They may represent colobomas of the disk contained within peripapillary staphylomas or retinochoroidal colobomas.

a. **Colobomas** are bilateral in more than 60% of cases. Bilateral colobomas may be inherited. The transmission is as an autosomal dominant, the gene varying considerably in its penetrance so that sometimes one or more generations are missed. Congenital colobomatous anomalies, if associated with hypertelorism or other midline facial anomalies, are considered evidence of basal encephalocele until proved otherwise (see Chapter 11, secs. **XI.C.** and **D.**).

  b. **Optic nerve pits,** or craterlike holes in the disks, are a peculiar and relatively rare finding. They occur in association with moderate enlargement and irregularity of the disk and are usually unilateral. There is no evidence of a hereditary pattern. The majority of pits are located in the lower temporal quadrant of the papilla, touching the edge of the disk. The size and depth of the pits vary widely. Often vessels can be observed diving into the pit and emerging to continue their normal course.

 (1) **Visual acuity.** A wide variation in the effect on visual acuity is also noted. Approximately 40% of eyes have good vision, 35% have diminished vision, and 25% have poor vision.

 (2) **Visual field defects.** The characteristic field defect is an arcuate bundle scotoma or central scotoma (present in 60% of cases). Pits are of great significance in the pathogenesis of central serous retinopathy. There appears to be a selective involvement of the papillomacular bundle in the hole-forming process. Both conditions are observed in combination in about 30% of cases.

2. **Optic nerve dysplasia.** Other forms of optic nerve dysplasia illustrate the spectrum of large anomalous disk malformations. For example, the disk may appear enlarged and elevated, enlarged and flat (megalopapilla), or enlarged and excavated with radial vessel array ("morning glory" syndrome).

3. **Optic nerve hypoplasia. Small anomalous disks** resulting from congenital **optic disk hypoplasia** may be unilateral or bilateral and vary in the degree of severity. When hypoplasia is borderline or minimum, good vision is preserved; when hypoplasia is pronounced and the disk is pale, severe impairment of vision is the rule. In one-third of these cases, major concomitant CNS anomalies have been recognized. One of these anomalies, **septooptic dysplasia (de Mosier syndrome),** is characterized by the clinical triad of shortness of stature, nystagmus, and optic nerve hypoplasia. Neurologically, the septum pellucidum is absent. This forebrain dysplasia is also accompanied by a deficiency of growth hormone and even by diabetes insipidus. Early recognition permits correction of the hormonal imbalance and a chance for the child to achieve normal growth and stature.

4. **Tilted disk,** congenital dysversions. The characteristics of the tilted disk syndrome are the tilted appearance (situs inversus) and the small size of the optic disks. In 80% of cases the condition is bilateral, with or without a congenital conus. An inferior conus is the most common variety, with hypopigmentation of the inferonasal fundus contiguous to the crescent.

  a. **Visual acuity.** Refraction shows myopic astigmatism with an oblique axis.

  b. **Visual field** examination shows bitemporal depression with, usually, superotemporal quadrantic defects that fail to respect the vertical meridian and that fail to progress. Occasionally, the field shows an altitudinal defect.

5. **Pseudopapilledema** is a nonspecific term used to describe elevation of the disk similar in appearance to papilledema. When possible, a diagnosis should be made; for example, intrapapillary drusen, hypermetropia, or persistent hyaloid tissue. Medullated nerve fibers, a congenital anomaly, can also be confused with papilledema.

  a. **Optic disk drusen** is an important cause of pseudopapilledema and is the entity that creates the most difficulty, clinically, in the evaluation of the swollen disk.

 (1) **Pathogenesis.** Drusen or hyaline bodies of the optic disk are congenital. Disk drusen are inherited as an autosomal irregular dominant trait.

(2) **Tempo of evolution.** Optic disk drusen are not visible at birth and have rarely been observed in children under the age of 11 years. They erupt on the disk surface in the second or third decade. With increasing age they become more visible and recognizable.

(3) **Ophthalmoscopy.** The ophthalmoscopic appearance of **disk drusen in the child** is atypical. In early life, hyaline bodies remain deep in the nerve (but always anterior to the lamina cribrosa) and are not visible with the ophthalmoscope. When they lie just beneath the surface of the disk, they may be seen partially or not at all. Drusen embedded beneath the surface produce a fullness of the papilla, mild elevation, and blurring of the disk. There may also be an abnormal number of vessels on the disk. Intrapapillary drusen account for 75% of diagnostically troublesome elevated disk anomalies in young children. By the second or third decade, when disk drusen become visible, the condition is less likely to be confused with papilledema. *The ophthalmoscopic appearance in the adult is usually diagnostic.* Both disks are involved in 73% of cases, but an asymmetry in appearance is common. Drusen are recognized on the disk as a small, mulberry-like mass or as a waxy tumor composed of a conglomerate of smaller masses. They may enlarge the nerve head, obliterate the physiologic cup, and give the edge of the disk a crenated appearance. Illumination along the disk margin frequently causes drusen to glow, and red-free light (the green filter on the ophthalmoscope) is often helpful. To retroilluminate drusen, the slit beam of a halogen ophthalmoscope can be used. The color of the disk is gray-yellow and unlike that of hyperemia of papilledema. Drusen, when pronounced, show autofluorescence. Ultrasonography and fundic fluorescein angiography may be helpful in identifying buried drusen.

Overt **disk drusen** may be seen ophthalmoscopically in parents of children with anomalously elevated disks without visible drusen. Examination of family members is mandatory if the distinction between true papilledema and pseudopapilledema in the child is in doubt. Failure to take this simple step is a major cause of misdirected diagnostic studies, including emergency invasive neuroradiologic procedures. When difficulty in fundic diagnosis persists and the patient is otherwise symptom-free and healthy, observe the patient. Reexamine the eyes; reinquire for neurologic symptoms of diplopia, headache, nausea, vomiting, or drowsiness; and arrange for serial fundic photographs. This conservative approach is strongly recommended.

(4) **Visual acuity.** The majority of cases of disk drusen are harmless and remain asymptomatic. There is no associated refractive error. As a rule central vision is intact.

(5) **Visual field defects.** Three patterns of field defects are found: enlargement of the blind spot (60% of cases); arcuate or nerve fiber bundle defects producing sector cuts, ring scotomas, paracentral scotomas, and Bjerrum scotomas; or irregular peripheral contractions. Constriction of the lower nasal field is the most characteristic defect. Typically, the defects progress very slowly.

(6) **Spontaneous hemorrhage** occurring **with disk drusen** may present as peripapillary flame-shaped hemorrhages, intravitreous hemorrhage, or subretinal hemorrhage around the disk that may extend under the macula. Only in this situation should loss of visual acuity and central field be attributed to disk drusen. Blindness is a rare complication. Hemorrhage with optic disk drusen may occur in children.

B. **Acquired elevation of the optic disk** occurs in papilledema, papillitis, optic disk drusen, infiltration of the nerve head by malignant cells, hypotony, and many other ocular conditions. Only papilledema and papillitis will be discussed.

1. **Papilledema** is a term that should be reserved strictly for optic disk swelling resulting from elevation of the intracranial cerebrospinal fluid (CSF) pressure.

   a. **Pathogenesis.** The precise pathogenesis of papilledema is not entirely understood, but it seems clear from experimental autoradiographic and electron microscopic studies that **intraaxonal swelling** with accumulation of mitochondria and **not** extracellular extravasation of fluid is the principal early mechanism resulting from raised intraneural pressure. This results in swelling of prelaminar nerve axons, and early papilledema is simply the result of axoplasmic stasis at the nerve head. The vascular changes, i.e., hyperemia, venous congestion, and hemorrhage, are secondary. In chronic papilledema, in addition to swollen axons there is extracellular accumulation of fluid (edema), vascular engorgement, and ischemia. Papilledema is nearly always *bilateral,* although the degree of severity is often asymmetric. Two ocular conditions protect the eye from papilledema: **high myopia** (5 to 10 diopters [D]) and **optic atrophy.** Therefore, if either of these conditions is present, *no papilledema can develop in the eye.*

   b. **Tempo of evolution and recovery.** Papilledema develops quickly and subsides slowly.

      (1) **Evolution.** Papilledema takes **1 to 5 days to appear** after the intracranial CSF pressure increases. The exception to this is following an acute intracranial hemorrhage, for example, a subarachnoid bleed. In this situation, papilledema with or without subhyaloid hemorrhages may develop rapidly within 2 to 8 hours of the catastrophic event. One might anticipate that there would be a delay in the appearance of papilledema in very young children due to the distensibility of the skull. Although such a delay undoubtedly exists, severe papilledema is found frequently in children, largely as a result of the frequency of posterior fossa tumors in childhood (cerebellar astrocytoma, ependymoma, and medulloblastoma).

      (2) **Recovery** from fully developed papilledema takes 6 to 8 weeks from the time the CSF pressure has returned to normal. Sudden lowering of CSF pressure produces no immediate funduscopic change.

   c. **Ophthalmoscopy**

      (1) **Early signs** of papilledema are the accentuation of the nerve fiber striations of the disk margins (first upper and lower poles, then nasal, lastly temporal), **hyperemia of the disk,** and **capillary dilation.** A reliable and important first sign is **obscuration of the wall of a vessel** crossing the disk margin by swelling of the nerve fiber layer.

      (2) **Fully developed and late papilledema** is characterized by elevation of the disk (3 D is equal to approximately 1 mm of swelling) with partial or complete obliteration of the physiologic cup. Other characteristics are hemorrhage on or near to the disk to form flame-shaped (nerve fiber layer), punctate (outer nuclear layer), or small splinter hemorrhages. Cotton-wool exudate (cystoid bodies) on and around the disk may also occur. **Macular changes** are visible, with edema and star formation and retinal stress lines (concentric striae about the base of the swollen disk). **Spontaneous venous pulsations,** present in 81% of all eyes (being unilateral in 18%), are obliterated. As a general rule, the presence of unequivocal spontaneous venous pulsations on the disk indicates that papilledema is not present (the intracranial pressure is below 180 to 190 mm H_2O). This is not an absolute rule, however, because venous pulsation may occasionally persist even though papilledema is pronounced and the intracranial pressure is high.

It should also be noted that increased venous pressure, as well as increased intracranial CSF pressure, prevents pulsation. When optic disk changes are suspicious for early papilledema, a CT brain scan should always be obtained before the performance of a lumbar puncture to measure the intracranial pressure.

(3) **Long-term changes** of chronic papilledema are the development of **gliosis** surrounding the disk, sheathing of vessels, and progressive optic atrophy. Complete optic atrophy takes 6 to 8 months to develop, but it can occur as early as 4 weeks. Recovery from papilledema takes about 6 to 8 weeks.

d. **The associated ocular symptoms and signs** are transient visual obscurations with preservation of normal visual acuity and diplopia. Chronic papilledema can cause permanent loss of vision and visual field.

(1) **Transient visual obscurations** occur in 25% of patients. The attacks last less than 1 minute, usually 10 to 30 seconds. They are characterized by sudden blurred vision, like a veil, with simultaneous impairment of color vision, or sudden complete darkness or actual blindness. Chronic papilledema accompanied by frequent visual obscurations may portend a poor visual prognosis.

(2) **Diplopia** may be the presenting ocular symptom of increased intracranial pressure, attributable to a unilateral sixth nerve palsy or, occasionally, with a posterior fossa lesion, to a skew deviation.

(3) **Visual acuity loss** develops slowly in some cases of chronic papilledema with optic atrophy. In fact, in the early stages, papilledema is distinguishable from papillitis by the preservation of normal vision. Rarely, acute loss of vision occurs with papilledema resulting from infarction of the severely swollen nerve head.

(4) **Visual field defects** associated with papilledema are enlargement of the blind spot and constriction of the peripheral field. With a 2-mm white target at 2 m, the blind spot width is 7.5 degrees and its height is 9.5 degrees. An increased blind spot size greater than 1 degree is abnormal. Horizontal enlargement is most important. An inferior binasal quadrant field cut is the characteristic early peripheral field defect. In the late stage of papilledema with optic atrophy, the peripheral field is severely restricted to a small temporal island around the blind spot.

(5) **Pupil** size and reactivity are vital signs both to observe and preserve in cases of papilledema. In some instances, however, the diagnosis of papilledema is not easy without inspection of the dilated fundus. If the fundus must be dilated, short-acting mydriatic eye drops must be selected and their use documented in the patient's record.

e. **The associated neurologic symptom** of major importance is **headache.** The headache may be acute or chronic, lateralized or generalized, and mild, moderate, or severe. Characteristically, it is worse on waking in the morning and aggravated by coughing, sneezing, and straining. The condition is particularly serious when accompanied by nausea and vomiting.

f. **The differential diagnosis** involves the important distinction of papilledema from pseudopapilledema, papillitis, optic disk vasculitis, juxtapapillary chorioretinitis, sarcoid of the disk, syphilitic optic perineuritis, uveitis, malignant hypertensive retinopathy, central retinal vein occlusion, and other causes of disk swelling.

g. **Treatment.** Papilledema indicates increased intracranial pressure and a neurologic emergency indicating **immediate admission to a hospital** under the care of a neurologist.

2. **Papillitis** is the term used to describe disk swelling associated with visual loss due to inflammation, infiltration, or vascular disorders of the nerve head. Two types will be discussed: optic neuritis and ischemic optic neuropathy.

a. **Optic neuritis** results from inflammation or demyelination of the optic nerves. Much confusion exists as to nomenclature. The multiplicity of titles is largely due to efforts to indicate the site or extent of the nerve involvement. **Retrobulbar neuritis** refers to lesions of the nerve that acutely show no abnormality in the fundus. **Papillitis** refers to anterior lesions in which the disk is swollen and hyperemic. Fine opacities in the vitreous and venous sheathing may be associated. **Neuroretinitis** has the same connotation as papillitis but indicates that the process extends farther into the adjacent retina and uvea. These clinical terms should not necessarily imply an inflammatory process.

(1) **Pathogenesis. Multiple sclerosis (MS)** is the commonest cause of monosymptomatic acute idiopathic optic neuritis. **Lyme disease** and **neurosyphilis** are specific infectious causes. Characteristically, idiopathic optic neuritis affects young women (mean age, 31 years) more often than men and one eye only. Brain MRI is positive for the presence of multifocal white matter lesions in approximately 80% of cases of idiopathic optic neuritis. Simultaneous bilateral optic neuritis in adults is not common (23% of cases). In contrast, bilateral involvement is the rule in children. In adult cases of idiopathic optic neuritis, the risk of developing multiple sclerosis is approximately 50%. The incidence of clinical signs of MS is greatest within a 2-year period following the attack of optic neuritis.

(2) **Tempo of evolution and recovery**

(a) **Evolution.** Typically, visual acuity is lost progressively over 2 to 5 days concomitant with loss of color vision and depth perception. Chronic progressive visual loss should not be attributed to chronic optic neuritis, a common error. A treatable compressive lesion must be ruled out in every case.

(b) **Visual recovery** usually commences within 1 to 4 weeks. In some patients it may be delayed as long as several months, particularly if severe visual loss is present. Prognosis for full visual recovery should be guarded, even though some improvement in vision is to be expected in 75% of cases. **Serial** ophthalmologic **examinations** should be carried out for a minimum of 8 months. In one patient series, follow-up showed the visual acuity was 20/30 or better after 7 months in 48% of the cases; in another series, visual acuity was 20/60 or better after 7 months in 55% of the cases. Two years is the longest period of visual recovery reported. The **final level of visual acuity** attained is unaffected by the sex of the patient, by unilateral or bilateral involvement, by the presence or absence of pain, or by treatment with intravenous (i.v.) methylprednisolone followed by oral prednisone.

(3) **Ophthalmoscopy**

(a) **Early changes. Papillitis** is present in 38% of cases. The optic disk is normal in 44% of cases. **Temporal pallor,** indicative of a previous optic nerve lesion in the same eye, is observed in as many as 18% of patients at the time of the initial examination. **Early papillitis** is characterized by blurring of the disk margins and by mild hyperemia.

(b) **Fully developed papillitis** is often impossible to tell from papilledema ophthalmoscopically, as there is marked swelling (up to 3 D), obliteration of the physiologic cup, hyperemia, and splinter hemorrhages. Venous sheathing is rarely seen. A slitlamp examination for vitreous cells is valuable.

(c) **Late changes.** In retrobulbar optic neuritis, the disk may remain normal in appearance for as long as 4 to 6 weeks, at which time pallor develops. Following papillitis, there sometimes develops what is described as "secondary optic atrophy." In this condition, the disk margins may be indistinct; there may be glial tissue formation on the disk, and temporal disk pallor. Almost invariably, pallor of the nerve head marks the end stage of optic neuritis. At this stage, nerve fiber atrophy may be observed in the retina with the aid of red-free light.

(4) **Associated ocular symptoms and signs**

(a) **Pain** occurs as the presenting symptom in 63% of cases. It may be mild or quite severe. It is experienced as a dull retroorbital ache or as sharp eye pain provoked by eye movement or by palpation of the globe. In 19% of patients, pain may precede loss of vision by 7 days. More commonly, it occurs only 24 to 48 hours before or simultaneous with visual loss. Pain rarely persists longer than 10 to 14 days. If it does, the diagnosis should be reconsidered. No correlation has been noted between the presence of pain and the severity of the visual loss or the appearance of the fundus (papillitis versus retrobulbar optic neuritis). It is of little prognostic significance. Pain possibly originates from distention of the optic nerve and stretching of the nerve sheath.

(b) **Transient blurring of vision** lasting minutes to a few hours is also experienced in optic neuritis. Factors recognized to produce this symptom include an affective disturbance (16%), exercise, Uhthoff syndrome (29%), temperature change (8%), menstruation (8%), increased illumination (3%), eating (2%), and smoking (0.8%). **Uhthoff syndrome** of intermittent transient blurring of vision on exertion occurs in MS, optic neuritis, and other optic neuropathies. The symptom may also be provoked by emotional stress, temperature change, menstruation, increased illumination, eating, drinking, and smoking. The pathophysiology of Uhthoff syndrome is unknown, although a reversible conduction block in demyelinated nerve fibers secondary to an increase in body temperature or to changes in blood electrolyte levels or pH is believed to play a role. In one study, Uhthoff syndrome was experienced by 40 of 81 (49.5%) patients with idiopathic optic neuritis at some time in the course of the attack, and by 13 of 81 (16%) patients within 2 weeks of the onset of optic neuritis. In this study, Uhthoff syndrome was associated with a significantly greater incidence of recurrent optic neuritis, positive MRI brain scans supportive of MS, and clinical conversion to MS, and, as such, Uhthoff syndrome is considered to be a prognostic indicator for the early development of MS in patients presenting with isolated idiopathic optic neuritis.

(c) **Visual loss** may be mild (20/30 or better), moderate (20/60 or better), or severe (20/70 or less). Vision can even be reduced to light perception. The patient complains of misty or blurred vision, difficulty in reading, a blind spot, a subjective difference in the brightness of light, impaired color perception, loss of depth perception, or transient blurring of vision. In the author's series, 65% of patients had a visual acuity of 20/100 or less at the onset. This high incidence of cases with severe visual loss may reflect the confidence the ophthalmologist feels in following mildly affected patients in the office rather than in the hospital.

(d) **Visual field defects.** A generalized depression of the visual field is the most common type of visual defect. Many other types of field losses are reported, including a centrocecal scotoma, a paracentral nerve fiber bundle defect, a nerve fiber bundle defect extending to the periphery, a nerve fiber bundle defect involving fixation and the periphery, and a peripheral defect only.

With recovery, a centrocecal scotoma gradually shrinks in size and a peripheral field cut or constriction gradually enlarges. After 7 months, 51% of cases may be expected to have normal visual fields.

(e) **Pupil size** is equal in unilateral optic neuritis even when the eye is blind. Invariably, however, an **afferent pupil defect,** characterized by a sluggish or absent constriction to direct light, is present in the ipsilateral eye. The swinging flashlight test is a simple method of detecting the defect. The consensual light reflex and near response is intact. Because the afferent pupil defect can be observed in an optic nerve lesion even in an eye **with 20/15 vision, absence** of this sign in cases of monocular blindness should alert the examiner to the possibility of **nonorganic visual loss.**

(5) **Associated CNS symptoms and signs.** The examiner should inquire for existing or preceding transient CNS symptoms, specifically episodic numbness, paresthesias, burning discomfort, lack of dexterity, weakness, or incoordination of the limbs, as well as any sensory disturbance on the trunk or sphincter difficulties. Attacks of vertigo or trigeminal neuralgia or a psychiatric illness may be significant. In addition, a history of trauma, drug abuse, toxic exposure, or alcoholism is important.

(6) **Family history.** Multiple sclerosis may be familial. The examiner should inquire for CNS disease in the family and also for a history of eye disease.

(7) **Differential diagnosis. Unilateral optic neuritis** must be differentiated from hysterical visual loss (stereopsis intact), optic disk vasculitis, papilledema, juxtapapillary chorioretinitis, uveitis, syphilitic optic perineuritis, lactation neuritis, ischemic optic neuropathy, optic disk drusen, other causes of disk swelling, and other optic nerve lesions, notably, a compressive neuropathy. The examiner should have *a high index of suspicion of a compressive lesion if the patient is older than 40 years,* if **optic atrophy** is present yet the history is short, if the **field defect respects** the **vertical meridian,** if the **tempo of evolution** of visual loss is inappropriate, if there is **no recovery,** and if a careful history reveals other leads, such as headache, amenorrhea, sinus disease, or trauma.

(a) **Neuromyelitis optica** is an important condition to consider in the differential diagnosis of bilateral optic neuritis. Either the optic neuritis or transverse myelitis may appear first. Usually both eyes are affected within hours or a day or each other, and then as long as a week or more may elapse before the transverse myelitis develops, or vice versa. The optic neuritis of the myelitis can recur.

(b) **Bilateral loss of vision without myelitis** may well represent alcohol-nutrition amblyopia, drug toxicity, metabolic disease, syphilitic optic perineuritis, hereditary optic atrophy, cone dysfunction, or one of the rarer forms of optic neuropathy. A treatable compressive lesion must not be overlooked.

(c) **Leber hereditary optic atrophy.** This condition affects males primarily, and is transmitted via female (maternal) carriers through cytoplasmic DNA in the ovum (mitochondrial). Leber optic atrophy is characterized by subacute bilateral central visual loss and ultimately optic atrophy. The age of onset is typically between the ages of 15 and 30 years. There is a male predominance of between 60% and 90%. The visual fields contain scotomas that are initially central and rapidly become cecocentral in location. In acute Leber optic atrophy, the ophthalmoscopic findings are (a) circumpapillary telangiectatic microangiopathy; (b) swelling of the nerve fiber layer around the disk ("pseudoedema"); and (c) absence of leakage from the disk or papillary region on fluorescein angiography with arteriovenous shunting present in the area of the telangiectatic vessels. In chronic Leber optic neuropathy, the optic disk is atrophic. About 15% of patients recover useful vision in one or both eyes many years after the ictus. Cardiac dysrhythmias are also common. Mitochondrial DNA has a single nucleotide replacement mutation at position 11778 in 40% to 60% of Leber families worldwide. Several other mitochondrial DNA point mutations have been identified as causative in Leber hereditary optic neuropathy, but the 11778 mutation has the worst prognosis for visual recovery. Diagnostic centers specializing in genetic analysis for mitochondrial disease screen for the presence of any of these mutations. Leber hereditary optic neuropathy should be considered in the differential diagnosis of any unexplained bilateral optic atrophy regardless of age of onset, patient gender, funduscopic appearance, or family history.

(8) Investigations. MRI of the brain has provided physicians with the means to prognosticate the risk of developing MS after an isolated attack of optic neuritis. For this reason, the investigation of choice in a patient with acute optic neuritis is a brain MRI with T1- and T2-weighted images with and without gadolinium. If the MRI shows multiple focal periventricular white matter lesions, it is read as supportive of a diagnosis of MS. A lumbar puncture is not necessary, although some neurologists still prefer to examine the CSF when the MRI is abnormal.

- **(a) The CSF** in MS optic neuritis may show an elevated protein ($N < 40$ mg per dL), an increased cell count ($N < 5$ cells), an elevated gamma globulin level ($N < 10$ mg per dL), and oligoclonal bands.

- **(b) The visual evoked potential test** can provide solid evidence of a lesion in the optic nerve but not its pathologic nature. The greatest usefulness of the visual evoked response is in detecting damage to the optic nerve when the acuity and disk are normal.

- **(c) Neuroimaging.** The MRI has revealed multifocal periventricular white matter lesions in 90% to 98% of patients with definite clinical MS and 46% to 80% of adult patients with isolated optic neuritis. In optic neuritis, patients whose MRI scan showed two or more periventricular white matter lesions measuring at least 3 mm have a 36% chance of developing MS over the next 2 years. Patients with an MRI showing only one signal abnormality have a 17% chance of converting to MS. Patients whose scan shows no abnormality have only a 3% chance of converting to MS within a 2-year follow-up period. These data are taken from the Optic Neuritis Treatment Trial (ONTT).

(9) Steroid treatment.

- **(a)** The multicenter ONTT results showed that i.v. methylprednisolone followed by oral prednisone accelerated visual recovery but did not improve visual outcome after 1 year. A regimen of oral prednisone alone did not improve visual outcome and was associated with a significant increase in the rate of new attacks of optic neuritis. Within 2 years of follow-up, 30% of the prednisone-treated patients developed new bouts of optic neuritis (in either the affected or fellow eye) compared with 13% of the i.v.-treated and 16% of the placebo-treated patients. Even more important, among oral prednisone-treated patients, the risk of a new optic neuritis attack in the fellow eye was more than double that for the placebo-treated group. *Oral prednisone* *is contraindicated in the treatment of idiopathic optic neuritis.*

(b) **Abnormal MRI** indications for the use of i.v. methylprednisolone followed by oral prednisone are now clarified. A brain MRI is necessary before recommending i.v. steroid therapy. *Immediate i.v. methylprednisolone therapy can then be offered to the patient who has acute monosymptomatic optic neuritis and an abnormal MRI supportive of MS, regardless of the severity of the visual loss.* Each patient should be informed that i.v. methylprednisolone therapy is being used to delay conversion to clinical MS over the next 2-year period. This therapy will not influence the ultimate level of visual recovery, but may shorten the period of visual loss. Because of the risks of steroid side effects, every patient should be fully informed and sign a consent form before undertaking the treatment. Fortunately, i.v. methylprednisolone therapy can be given on an outpatient basis in an i.v. infusion center: methylprednisolone, 250 mg i.v. q6h for 3 days, followed by oral prednisone, 1 mg per kg body weight per day for 11 days.

(c) **Normal MRI.** Indications for i.v. methylprednisolone in acute optic neuritis patients are (a) visual loss in both eyes simultaneously or sequentially within hours or days of each other, (b) when the only good eye is affected, and (c) in rare cases when the tempo of disease is unusual, and slow progressive visual loss continues to occur in the absence of a compressive lesion. The decision to treat or not to treat with i.v. methylprednisolone is best assisted by the hospital-based neuroophthalmologist or neurologist. These specialists are frequently more familiar with the use and risks of i.v. methylprednisolone than the general ophthalmologist. They are also able to provide the very close medical supervision and follow-up required by a steroid-treated patient.

(d) **Long-term prophylaxis therapy** to minimize or prevent recurrent or progression of MS includes *interferon beta-1a* (Avonex), *interferon beta-1b* (Betaseron), and *glatiramer* (Copaxone). Interferon beta-1a is given once weekly intramuscularly (i.m.) to patients with relapsing MS to reduce risk of disability progression, exacerbations, and number and size of active lesions in the brain. Treatment of patients with silent MRI lesions can significantly delay development of disease. Interferon beta-1b is given subcutaneously qod to reduce incidence and severity of exacerbations and to increase time between exacerbations. Glatiramer is given subcutaneously qd to significantly reduce relapse in patients with relapsing–remitting MS.

b. **Ischemic optic neuropathy** results from infarction of the prelaminar anterior optic nerve.

(1) **Pathogenesis.** Infarction results from occlusion of the two main posterior ciliary arteries that supply the optic nerve and choroid. Three causes are giant-cell arteritis (temporal arteritis), nonarteritic arteriosclerosis, and emboli to the ciliary circulation.

(a) Approximately 10% of patients with ischemic optic neuritis have **giant-cell arteritis (temporal arteritis).** This is a disease of the elderly, with onset characteristically over the age of 60 years. Women are more often affected than men.

(b) **Arteriosclerotic ischemic optic neuropathy** tends to occur at a younger age, 46 to 65 years, and the condition is somewhat more prevalent in men. A history of or signs of systemic vascular disease are frequently present (mild hypertension, diabetes mellitus, narrow retinal arteries). Another risk factor is hyperlipidemia.

(c) Attention has also been called to a form of **ischemic optic neuropathy following uncomplicated cataract extraction** with sudden visual loss from 4 weeks to 15 months postoperatively.

(d) **Embolic anterior ischemic optic neuropathy** is a recognized complication of a coronary bypass procedure and may be bilateral.

(2) **Tempo of evolution and recovery**

(a) **Evolution.** Loss of vision is abrupt. It rarely progresses for more than 1 or 2 days. In **giant-cell arteritis** visual loss usually occurs between 3 and 12 weeks after the first manifestation of this systemic disease. Both optic nerves may be involved simultaneously or sequentially. The interval between involvement varies from a few hours to a few days up to several weeks. In **nonarteritic arteriosclerotic ischemic optic neuritis**, both optic nerves are involved simultaneously in 19% and eventually in 49% of cases. The interval between involvement varies between 2 weeks and 17 years, the average being 42 months.

(b) **Recovery.** Visual prognosis is poor in ischemic optic neuritis, but better in nonarteritic ischemic optic neuritis than in giant-cell arteritis. When acuity is impaired it may eventually improve in 33% of cases, especially when the defect in the visual field is a central scotoma or small altitudinal scotoma.

(3) **Ophthalmoscopy**

(a) **Early changes.** Ischemic papillitis (the most frequent form of ocular involvement in giant-cell arteritis [60% of cases]) is characterized by pallor and swelling of the nerve head with small nerve fiber layer hemorrhages in the peripapillary area. Frequently, segmental infarction and swelling of the disk are present. The retinal arteries may appear attenuated. Similar changes are seen in arteriosclerotic ischemic papillitis. In other cases, microinfarction of the retina occurs with cotton-wool patches resulting from focal ischemia of the nerve fiber layer.

(b) **Late changes.** Optic disk cupping similar to that seen in glaucomatous cupping may develop in eyes with ischemic optic neuritis secondary to giant-cell arteritis or arteriosclerosis. Pallor and optic atrophy are usually more severe in these cases than in patients with glaucoma.

(c) **Pseudo-Foster Kennedy syndrome** may be seen in this condition, that is, ischemic **papillitis in one eye** and **optic atrophy in the other.** The clinical setting of acute visual loss in the second eye should help distinguish the case from Foster Kennedy syndrome.

(4) **Associated ocular symptoms and signs**

(a) **Pain** is not a prominent symptom. Pain on eye motion does not usually occur.

(b) **Transient monocular visual loss, amaurosis fugax,** is a prominent symptom in giant-cell arteritis. Characteristically, amaurosis fugax is sudden in onset and short in duration. The typical attack persists for 2 to 3 minutes and rarely longer than 5 to 30 minutes. The patient describes the episode frequently as momentary blurred vision or obscuration of vision by a gray cloud. Less commonly, the patient describes a window shade appearing to be drawn down or across the vision of the affected eye (more typical of amaurosis fugax in extracranial occlusive carotid artery disease). Monocular amaurosis fugax that alternates between the two eyes must be considered to result from giant-cell arteritis until proved otherwise. Amaurosis fugax is due to transient retinal ischemia. It is one of the most important warning symptoms of impending blindness. *If the diagnosis is missed, 40% to 50% of all untreated cases will develop blindness or severe visual loss.*

(c) **Visual loss.** Decreased vision is the presenting complaint. As a rule, loss of vision in giant-cell arteritis is profound. In arteriosclerotic ischemic optic neuritis, 42% of cases have a visual acuity of 20/100 or less. In 35% the vision may remain normal.

(d) **Visual field defects.** Any type of visual field defect characteristic of an optic nerve lesion is seen. In giant-cell arteritis, usually the whole visual field is depressed. In arteriosclerotic ischemic optic neuritis, frequently the defect is an inferior altitudinal defect or arcuate scotoma.

(e) **Pupil.** An afferent pupil defect is present in an eye with severe ischemic papillitis or central retinal artery occlusion. Dilation and paralysis of the pupillary sphincter may indicate severe ischemia of the eye or ciliary ganglion. Tonic pupil may be present.

(f) **Diplopia.** Occasionally, diplopia is the presenting symptom of giant-cell arteritis (12% of cases). In patients with diplopia, 50% are the result of sixth nerve palsy and 50% are from a third nerve palsy with pupil sparing. One pathologic study on a patient who died from giant-cell arteritis with bilateral ophthalmoplegia showed, however, that extraocular muscle ischemia was the mechanism responsible for the ophthalmoplegia.

(5) **Associated systemic symptoms and signs**

(a) The systemic symptoms of **giant-cell arteritis,** in order of decreasing frequency, are temporal pain or headache, jaw claudication, tender temporal arteries, swelling in the temples, fatigue, muscle ache or stiffness, neck pain, anorexia, fever, and weight loss. Some of the symptoms are related to involvement of cranial arteries, and there appears to be a close correlation between the susceptibility to giant-cell arteritis and the amount of elastic tissue in the media and adventitia of the individual arteries of the head and neck. The arteries most commonly affected in 75% to 100% of patients are the superficial temporal, the vertebral (outside the dura), the ophthalmic, and the posterior ciliary arteries. The intracranial arteries are rarely involved. These classic symptoms may be present or absent with the ocular phase.

(b) In contrast, in **nonarteritic arteriosclerotic ischemic optic neuropathy,** symptoms and signs of systemic vascular disease and hypertension are frequently present.

(6) **Management and investigation. Always suspect the diagnosis of giant-cell arteritis in every elderly patient with amaurosis fugax, ischemic optic neuropathy, central retinal artery occlusion, or suggestive systemic symptomatology (jaw claudication, headache, neck ache, exhaustion, sore ears, tender scalp, weight loss, poor temporal artery pulse, thickened temporal arteries). Polymyalgia rheumatica is strongly associated with giant-cell arteritis.**

(a) **Act immediately.** The steps are as follows:

Step 1. **Obtain a stat Westergren sedimentation rate** (normal 35 to 40 mm per hour); 5% to 10% of these may be normal.

Step 2. **Get the results,** whenever possible, **before the patient leaves the office.**

Step 3. **Start high-dose oral steroids if the sedimentation rate is elevated** or if patient must return home before the result is known. Telephone patient to further instruct.

Step 4. **Plan a temporal artery biopsy.**

Step 5. **Refer the patient for an emergency consultation** to a physician in internal medicine for consideration of emergency admission to the hospital.

(b) **Hospital admission** may be advisable because blindness may ensue despite adequate steroid treatment, and the initial dose of prednisone may not be adequate to relieve symptoms immediately and drop the level of the sedimentation rate. Some elderly patients also show visual loss related to postural changes. Most important, however, any patient taking steroids in this age group should be seen and followed by an internist.

(c) **Additional laboratory results** are also of value. An elevation of the fibrinogen level (normal, 200 to 400 mg per dL in plasma) correlates with the increased sedimentation rate. Serum protein electrophoresis may show a marked increase in alpha$_2$-globulin fraction and beta globulins. The white blood count is often increased in association with fever. Fifty percent of patients with giant-cell arteritis show some degree of normocytic hypochromic anemia, which may be responsive to iron, folic acid, and vitamin B12.

(d) **Biopsy of the temporal artery,** occasionally the facial artery, or a superficial posterior occipital artery to the scalp is necessary to confirm the clinical diagnosis. Palpation of the temporal artery, characteristically tender, nonpulsate, and nodular, was normal in more than 50% of positive biopsies in one series of 46 patients. **Skip areas,** though occasionally found, are uncommon if an artery is carefully sectioned serially and if a long (3 to 7 cm) segment is excised. A Doppler ultrasound flow detector can be helpful in selecting the side of the artery biopsy. Biopsy, if done early after steroid therapy, will still show histologic changes of giant-cell arteritis. Though not often reported, patients with classic giant-cell arteritis and elevated sedimentation rates have negative temporal artery biopsies. Nevertheless, a patient with elevated sedimentation rate and symptoms of giant-cell arteritis should have a temporal artery biopsy. A high index of suspicion should be maintained even if the patient's sedimentation rate is normal.

(7) **Treatment**

(a) **Giant-cell arteritis.** Prednisone, 60 to 80 mg orally (p.o.) or methylprednisolone 60 to 80 mg i.m., should be started immediately. After the initial period of treatment with large doses of steroids, the prednisone dose should be tapered over several days to a maintenance dose of 20 mg qd or less. The appropriate **maintenance dose** is *titrated against* the *sedimentation rate,* the *fibrinogen level,* and the patient's *symptoms.* It must be adequate to keep the sedimentation rate in the normal range or at a stable baseline level and to abolish symptoms. **Treatment is continued for at least 6 months.** Once steroids are stopped, the sedimentation rate should be measured at 2-week intervals for 6 weeks to check that it is stable, and the patient should be seen in follow-up by an internist. A few patients may not be in full remission after 6 months of steroid therapy. These patients will develop a high sedimentation rate, clinical symptoms off steroids, or both, and they will need to go back on steroid therapy. Many elderly patients may show a rising sedimentation rate off steroids due to arthritis. In selected cases, a repeat temporal artery biopsy may be required to identify those patients with active temporal arteritis.

Adverse side effects of steroids occur in 40% to 50% of cases of giant-cell arteritis. They include a Cushingoid appearance (40%), symptomatic vertebral compression fractures (26%), proximal muscle weakness (17%), subcapsular cataracts (5%), and increased insulin requirements (2%). In untreated cases, the **mortality** is 12%.

(b) **Nonarteritic arteriosclerotic ischemic optic neuritis.** The ophthalmologist's main concern in the management of nonarteritic ischemic optic neuropathy is to exclude temporal arteritis and bring under control other factors, such as systemic hypertension, hyperlipidemia, diabetes mellitus, or all of these. No therapy for nonarteritic anterior ischemic optic neuropathy has proven effective. The Ischemic Optic Neuropathy Decompression Trial was stopped early to stop the use of surgical treatment. Data showed that **optic nerve sheath decompression in the therapy of nonarteritic ischemic optic neuropathy is not effective and may even be harmful.**

c. **Optic atrophy**

(1) **Pathogenesis.** Three major etiologic types are recognized: heredofamilial optic atrophy, consecutive optic atrophy consequent on death of retinal ganglion cells and axons, and secondary optic atrophy that follows papillitis and chronic papilledema. This classification, while not complete, affords a simple guide.

(a) **Heredofamilial optic atrophy,** which includes a number of important entities, must be considered in the evaluation of insidious visual loss and disk pallor in childhood (see Chapter 11). Table 13.1 documents the major features of **Kjer dominant optic atrophy** and the recessive forms called simple, complicated, and juvenile optic atrophy with diabetes mellitus and deafness. **Leber hereditary optic neuropathy** is discussed in sec. **II.B.2.a.(7)(c),** above.

(b) **Consecutive optic atrophy,** the most frequent form of optic atrophy, includes all diseases that cause *retinal ganglion injury* and *death.* Rare examples are the lipid storage diseases (Tay-Sachs disease), adrenoleukodystrophy, and Menkes kinky-hair syndrome (see Chapter 11, sec. **VII.**). Consecutive optic atrophy also follows more common conditions, such as degenerative, vascular, and toxic lesions, including tobacco–alcohol amblyopia; ethambutol, chloroquine, ethchlorvynol (Placidyl), and other drug-induced neuropathies; and many other conditions associated with loss of optic nerve axons and retrograde degeneration of retinal ganglion cells, including ischemia, trauma, demyelination, and compressive lesions of the anterior visual pathway.

(c) **Nutritional deficiency alcohol amblyopia** is mentioned particularly because it is a *potentially reversible* cause of optic atrophy. It is, however, insidious in onset and frequently undetected in the early stage. Small bilateral **paracentral scotomas** develop between fixation and the blind spot and are initially detectable by response to color targets. Progression leads to loss of color perception, impaired visual acuity, and **bilateral central** or **centrocecal scotoma.** Nerve fiber bundle defects do not occur. As a rule, the fundus is normal. Prognosis for recovery is excellent at this stage, but poor in the chronic case with optic atrophy. **Treatment** consists of a well-balanced diet, B-complex vitamin supplement, and abstinence from alcohol. Thiamine i.m. may be used. Prevention is the key. Every effort should be made to rehabilitate the alcoholic.

(d) **Secondary optic atrophy** follows papillitis and chronic papilledema.

TABLE 13.1. HEREDOFAMILIAL OPTIC ATROPHIES

	Dominant	Recessive			Indeterminate
	Kjer Juvenile (infantile)	Early Infantile (Congenital); Simple	Behr Type; Complicated[a]	Juvenile with Diabetes Mellitus; with or without Deafness	Leber Hereditary Optic Neuropathy
Age at onset	Childhood (4–8 years)	Early childhood[b] (3–4 years)	Childhood (1–9 years)	Childhood (6–14 years)	Early adulthood (18–30 years; up to sixth decade)
Visual impairment	Mild to moderate (20/40–20/200)	Severe (20/200 HM)	Moderate (20/200)	Severe (20/400 FC)	Moderate to severe (20/200 FC)
Nystagmus	Rare[c]	Usual	In 50%	Absent	Absent
Optic disk	Mild temporal pallor (with or without temporal excavation)	Marked diffuse pallor (with or without arteriolar attenuation)[d]	Mild temporal pallor	Marked diffuse pallor	Moderate diffuse pallor; disk swelling in acute phase
Color vision	Blue-yellow dyschromatopsia	Severe dyschromatopsia or achromatopsia	Moderate to severe dyschromatopsia	Severe dyschromatopsia	Dense central scotoma for colors
Course	Variable, slight progression	Stable	Stable	Progressive	Acute visual loss, then usually stable; may improve or worsen

HM, hand motions; FC, finger counting.

[a]See discussion of heredodegenerative neurologic syndromes (sec. VII. and Chapter 11).

[b]Difficult to assess in infancy, but visual impairment usually manifests by age 4 years.

[c]Presence of nystagmus with poor vision and earlier onset suggests separate congenital or infantile form.

[d]Distinguished from tapetoretinal degenerations by normal electroretinogram.

(Modified from Glaser J.S. Heredofamilial disorders of the optic nerve. In: Goldberg M.F. ed. *Genetic and metabolic eye disease.* Boston: Little, Brown, 1974.)

(e) **Lyme disease** and **tertiary syphilis** may cause numerous neuroophthalmic disorders including optic atrophy (see Chapter 5, sec. **IV.L.**).

(2) **Ophthalmoscopy.** Optic atrophy may be difficult to establish by ophthalmoscopic criteria alone. Serial examinations aided by fundus photography are often necessary, as well as screening for signs of optic nerve dysfunction such as reduced visual acuity, field changes, diminished color perception, or sluggish pupil reaction to light.

To evaluate the pale disk, the examiner inspects the retina for attrition of ganglion cells and nerve fibers. (The green filter on the ophthalmoscope provides red-free light.) The disk should be inspected for vascularity (Kestenbaum capillary count) and sector pallor. The pattern of insertion of retinal nerve fibers at the nerve head is important. Sector pallor of the disk should be correlated with an area of retinal nerve fiber atrophy and with the type and extent of the visual field defect. A specific example is illustrated by **bow-tie atrophy,** a horizontal band of pallor of the disk in the eye contralateral to an optic tract lesion.

III. **The pupil.**[1] The pupil is an aperture in the eye formed by the muscles and pigmented stroma of the anterior uveal tract. The muscles are of two types: a circumferential **sphincter** found in the margin of the iris, innervated by the parasympathetic nervous system, and **radial dilator** muscles, which run from the iris margin to the root of the iris, innervated by the sympathetic nervous system.

A. **Afferent limb of the pupillary arc**

1. **Parasympathetic anatomy**

   a. **The afferent limb** of the pupillary light reflex begins in the retina with axons from retinal ganglion cells. No specialization of the retina into "pupil-specific" ganglion cells is known. The **fibers** from each eye **decussate at the chiasm** *with 54% of the fibers* **crossing** *and 47% remaining ipsilateral.* Fibers destined for midbrain connections separate from the optic tract and enter the pretectal nucleus, where they synapse. It is not known whether the axons that subverse pupillary light responses are from their own ganglion cells or are branches of axons. The fibers from the pretectal nuclei hemidecussate via the posterior commissure and synapse in the **Edinger-Westphal nucleus.** The efferent output from the Edinger-Westphal nucleus is cholinergic and receives equal drive from both optic nerves, as a result of the midbrain hemidecussation. The pupilloconstrictor fibers (iris sphincter) are driven by light and near responses. The near reaction has diffuse cortical inputs and projects directly to the Edinger-Westphal nucleus. The **near reaction** consists of accommodation and convergence as well as constriction of the pupil. Both light and near efferents are carried in the parasympathetic Edinger-Westphal outflow.

   b. **Efferent fibers** from the Edinger-Westphal nucleus are carried in the superficial layer of the **oculomotor nerve** and eventually end in its inferior division, where it passes through the superior orbital fissure and synapses in the ciliary ganglion. **Postganglionic fibers,** the short ciliary nerves, enter the globe near the optic nerve and supply the ciliary body and iris sphincter. There is a topographic relationship between cells in the Edinger-Westphal nucleus and sectors of the iris sphincter. For every axon that leaves the ciliary ganglion to supply the light response, 30 axons serve the near response. This 30:1 ratio is important as the **basis for light–near dissociation.** The iris sphincter is smooth muscle and has acetylcholine receptors, as does the ciliary body.

2. **Relative afferent pupil defect (Marcus Gunn pupil).** Because the irides in both eyes respond to light with an equal change in the size of the

---

[1]Reprinted from Corbett JJ, Special Course No. 12, Neuroophthalmology, American Academy of Neurology, 1979, with permission.

pupils, this sensory or afferent limb of the reflex arc can provide evidence for impaired function of the retina or optic nerve.

    a. Testing of the pupillary light response should be done in dim illumination. The patient should be instructed to look into the distance. Using a bright, preferably filament-free light, the examiner shines the light in one eye and then quickly in the other. The normal pupil responds to light with a brief constriction and then slight release to a relatively constant pupil diameter. The light should be alternated from eye to eye, the examiner looking for enlargement of the pupil on the affected ipsilateral side when the light is shone in the affected eye and constriction of the ipsilateral pupil when the light is shone in the nonaffected contralateral eye. In persons with no damage to the retina or optic nerve, the response will be symmetric and there will be no change of pupil size from side to side. **When there is a relative afferent pupil defect, both pupils will be larger as the light is directed into the affected eye and smaller as the light is directed into the unaffected eye.** This *sign is present* when the *sensory retina or optic nerve is damaged,* but is not seen when visual loss is due to corneal, lenticular, vitreous, refractive, or emotional causes.

    The test may occasionally be difficult to interpret in those patients who have large-amplitude physiologic swings in pupil size known as **hippus.** It may require more than one attempt at different times to establish clearly whether or not there truly is a relative afferent pupil defect. Hippus has no pathologic significance.

    b. The pupillary afferent defect can be roughly quantified by the use of **graded neutral density filters.** By placing a neutral filter in front of the normal eye, the examiner can effectively eliminate the relative afferent defect by "balancing" the visual loss in the two eyes. The filter density needed to balance the pupil defect is a measure of the loss of input to the affected eye and can be compared to earlier measurements for evidence of progression of a disease process.

  3. Light–near dissociation. In normal patients, the amplitude of the pupil response to light is essentially equal to the response to near. When the *afferent* pupil fibers are *disrupted* in the *pretectal region,* the response of the pupil to light may be diminished or lost, whereas the reaction to near is preserved. This phenomenon is termed **light–near dissociation.** The pupils tend to be midsized or enlarged, and frequently unequal. This condition has been reported in midbrain lesions in isolation or in association with Parinaud syndrome, with convergence–retraction nystagmus, and limited upgaze.

  4. Argyll Robertson pupil. Another form of **light–near dissociation** is the Argyll Robertson pupil. Here, the pupils are *small* and *respond poorly* or not at all to light, but have a prompt response to near. Both pupils are almost invariably involved, and these pupils *respond poorly to pupil-dilating agents.* This abnormality is probably due to a lesion in the midbrain light reflex path. Although it has been seen in diabetes mellitus and other diseases, the Argyll Robertson pupil should be considered presumptive evidence of neurosyphilis until proved otherwise. In the presence of this sign, a standard serologic test for syphilis as well as a fluorescent treponemal antibody absorption test should be performed (Table 13.2).

B. Efferent cholinergic pupil defects and Horner syndrome

  1. Pupilloconstrictor dysfunction

    a. Compression of the pupilloconstrictor fibers in the subarachnoid space, in the cavernous sinus, or in the orbit may produce a pupil that is unable to constrict to light or near, with or without other elements of a third nerve palsy. The relatively peripheral location of the parasympathetic efferent *pupilloconstrictor fibers on the **third nerve*** makes them particularly vulnerable to compression. This abnormality is produced with some frequency by posterior communicating artery

TABLE 13.2. DIFFERENTIATING COMMON PUPILLARY ANOMALIES

Syndrome	Normal OD	Abnormal OS		Light Reaction	Size	Near Reaction	Comments and Special Tests
Tonic pupil (Adie tonic pupil) (OS)			Dark Light Near Pilocarpine 0.12%	Vermiform, trace, or segmental; best seen under slitlamp	Large, except when old, then small	Strong, slow and tonic; slow redilation	Pilocarpine 0.12% reveals denervation supersensitivity. Adie pupil constricts; normal pupil: no response; areflexia
Horner syndrome (OS)			Dark Light Near *Cocaine 10%*	Normal	Small	Normal	Ptosis, upside-down ptosis, anhidrosis, and early hypotony with conjunctival injection; cocaine 10% positive, i.e., miotic pupil dilates
First- or second-neuron Horner			*Paredrine 1%*				Paredrine 1% fails to dilate third-neuron Horner
Third-neuron Horner							
Argyll Robertson pupil (OU)			Dark Light Near	Trace or absent	Small	Brisk	Rapid plasma Reagin test; fluorescent treponemal antibody absorption test; pupils may be irregular

OS, oculus sinister; OD, oculus dexter; OU, oculi uterque.

aneurysms and internal carotid artery aneurysms, as well as the classic uncal herniation syndrome.

b. The tonic pupil (Adie tonic pupil) results from damage to the **ciliary ganglion** or **postganglion fibers** of the **short posterior ciliary nerves.**

(1) **Dilated pupil.** When these structures are damaged, the pupil becomes enlarged and denervated (usually in a segmental fashion). Because the ratio of cells and fibers that serve the near response is so much greater as compared to those that serve the light response (30:1), the pupil reacts poorly to light but well to near. Furthermore, *the response to near is tonic.* When the patient looks at near and then refixates at distance, the pupil very slowly redilates. In the early phase, observation of a tonic pupil in bright light will accentuate the anisocoria, because the tonic pupil will fail to constrict. Bright light frequently bothers these patients.

(2) **Denervation sensitivity.** The most characteristic part of the tonic pupil is the phenomenon of denervation supersensitivity of the sphincter of the pupil. Use of one or two drops **0.12% pilocarpine** will provide intense constriction of the pupil if there is denervation supersensitivity.

(3) **Accommodation.** In addition to the light–near dissociation, large pupil, and denervation supersensitivity, accommodation is frequently affected with blurred vision at near. Although the pupil rarely recovers much light function following damage to the ciliary ganglion, the high proportion of accommodative fibers ensures reinnervation of the ciliary body.

(4) **Adie syndrome.** The combination of a **tonic pupil** and **areflexia** is known as Adie syndrome. This condition is the most common cause of a tonic pupil, but a multitude of other conditions can damage the ciliary ganglion or short ciliary nerves, resulting in a tonic pupil. After a tonic pupil has been present for years, it becomes smaller and may even be the smaller of the two pupils.

2. Pupillodilator dysfunction (Horner syndrome)

a. Anatomy. The pupillodilator fibers are under the control of the sympathetic nervous system. This neural arc consists of three neurons, beginning in the **posterolateral hypothalamus.** Fibers originating in these areas course caudally through the brain stem in a roughly but diffusely **dorsolateral** location. These first-order axons synapse in the intermediolateral portion of the C8-T2 level of spinal cord known as the **ciliospinal center of Budge.** Second-order axons emerge from the spinal cord at the T-1 level in the *ventral root.* They ascend to cross the apex of the lung, course through (without synapse) the stellate ganglion, the inferior cervical ganglion, around the subclavian artery (anterior loop of the ansa subclavia), and through the middle cervical ganglion. At the level of the angle of the mandible (bifurcation of the carotid, C3-4), these second-order fibers synapse in the **superior cervical ganglion.** From the superior cervical ganglion the third-order neurons form the final common pathway to the pupillodilator muscles. These nerve fibers follow the carotid into the cavernous sinus where they attach to the *ophthalmic division of the trigeminal nerve* and emerge from the cavernous sinus with the *nasociliary branch* and the *long ciliary nerves to the iris.* The neurotransmitter released at the pupillodilator muscle fiber is norepinephrine.

b. Diagnosis of Horner syndrome. Because any dysfunction or damage to the sympathetic chain will decrease the output of norepinephrine in the synaptic cleft of the pupillodilator fiber, the differentiation of Horner syndrome purely by its clinical effects is not always possible. All patients with Horner syndrome have **ptosis** and a **miotic pupil** that **reacts equally to light and near.** Early, they may have ocular hypotony and conjunctival erythema, and they may also have upside-down ptosis or elevation of the lower lid. **Facial anhidrosis** is less easily identified today due to air conditioning, which eliminates the profuse diaphoresis that helped to identify this sign. Three tests are useful in helping to confirm the diagnosis of Horner syndrome and in identifying the level of damage.

  (1) **The cocaine test.** A drop of **cocaine 5% to 10%** ophthalmic is placed in either eye and repeated in 1 minute. Sympathetic damage resulting in a Horner syndrome, no matter at what level, will result in a pupil that dilates poorly to cocaine, which acts to block reuptake of norepinephrine at the synaptic cleft. **The cocaine test confirms or denies the presence of a Horner syndrome. Without it, the diagnosis on clinical criteria alone is presumptive.** Damage to any neuron of the arc will give a positive cocaine test.

  (2) **The Paredrine test. Hydroxyamphetamine 1% (Paredrine)** ophthalmic drops release packets of **norepinephrine** into the synaptic cleft. If the first or second neurons of the oculosympathetic system have been damaged and the final common pathway is intact, the third-order neurons are able to produce, transport, and store norepinephrine. When Paredrine is instilled, the pupils dilate because norepinephrine is released. When the **third-order** neuron (superior cervical ganglion or postganglionic fibers) is damaged, there is no production, transport, or storage of norepinephrine, and when Paredrine is instilled in the affected eye no pupil dilation occurs. Thus, the cocaine test tells whether or not there is a Horner syndrome, and the **Paredrine test can separate a third-neuron Horner syndrome from first- and second-neuron syndromes.** There is no pharmacologic test that can differentiate a first- and second-neuron Horner syndrome. These must be identified clinically by the associated brain stem (first neuron) or spinal cord and lung apex (second neuron) symptoms and signs.

  (3) **Dilation lag.** Recently, a simple, elegant observation has aided in the identification of Horner syndrome. Because the pupillodilator muscle actively dilates the pupil in darkness, damage to the sympathetic nerve supply will result in only passive release of the sphincter rather than active dilation. Thus, the affected pupil will dilate less rapidly in dark as compared to the unaffected side. This is called dilation lag. It is best appreciated in photographs taken at 5 and 15 seconds after turning out the lights, using a flash camera with a close-up attachment. Clinically, it can be appreciated in dim lighting in persons with lightly colored irides.

C. **Simple anisocoria.** About 25% of the normal population will have greater than 0.3 mm of anisocoria from time to time that may even alternate sides. The pupils are otherwise entirely normal and have no light–near dissociation or pharmacologic abnormalities, and they do not demonstrate dilation lag. Because small degrees of ptosis and miosis resulting from simple anisocoria may occur in the same eye, it becomes all the more important to use formal pharmacologic testing to diagnose Horner syndrome.

D. **The fixed dilated pupil.** Pharmacologic blockage may be a real diagnostic dilemma and the fixed dilated pupil can be resolved by history and pharmacologic testing. Accidental or factitious instillation of drugs that cause pupillary dilation is seen most commonly in persons in medical settings. Nurses, doctors, and other paramedic people with access to those drugs may inadvertently rub them into their eyes, producing a dilated pupil. **Pilocarpine 1%** will constrict a pupil that is dilated because of compression but will not overcome pharmacologic blockade. *If the pupil fails to respond to pilocarpine 1% and direct obvious trauma is not the cause of the mydriasis, factitious or accidental mydriasis can be assumed.*

14. REFRACTIVE ERROR, CLINICAL OPTICS, AND CONTACT LENSES*

Sheri Morneault-Sparks and Deborah Pavan-Langston

I. **Physical optics affecting vision and correction of visual refractive errors**

   A. **Wavelength of light.** Electromagnetic radiation exists in many forms. The characteristic of the radiation that determines the form in which it is encountered is the wavelength. Long wavelengths are encountered as radio transmissions or radar; these emit a low energy. Short wavelengths are encountered as cosmic rays and x-rays; these emit a high energy. The visible portion of the electromagnetic radiation spectrum occurs between the ultraviolet and infrared portions, from 380 nm at the violet end of the spectrum to 760 nm at the red end.

   B. **Frequency of light waves.** The frequency of electromagnetic radiation is the number of times a particular position on the wave passes a fixed point in a fixed interval of time. It is inversely related to the wavelength. For example, radio waves, which occur as long wavelength radiation, have a frequency of 10^4 to 10^8 cycles per second (cps), whereas the visible part of the spectrum is in the 10^{14} to 10^{15} cps range, and includes shorter wavelength radiation.

   C. **Velocity of light waves.** The entire spectrum of electromagnetic waves travels at a speed of 3×10^8 m per second (186,000 miles per second) in a vacuum. The wavelength and frequency of light can be spoken of interchangeably because they are related through the following equation: Wavelength × frequency = velocity of light = 3×10^8 m per second.

   D. **Index of refraction.** Although the frequency of light does not vary with the density of the medium through which it is traveling, the speed is reduced in a dense medium. The ratio of the velocity of light in a vacuum to the velocity of light in a particular medium (n/n') is referred to as the index of refraction for that medium. Because the frequency of radiation does not vary with the medium and the speed does, it follows that the wavelength in a dense medium is less than it is in air and is proportional to the change in speed. Each medium, therefore, has a different refractive index for a given wavelength. Short wavelengths, or blue light, are slowed down or refracted more than long wavelengths, or red light. This accounts for the **chromatic aberration** present in the eye or in single-element lens systems. The visible spectrum is defined in relationship to chromatic aberration and is described by the use of the C (red) - F (blue) line.

   E. **Quanta or photons.** The energy in electromagnetic radiation is measured in units called *quanta* or *photons*. The energy of an individual photon is proportional to the frequency or inversely proportional to the wavelength. Therefore, the energy of a photon at 400 nm is twice as great as that of a photon at 800 nm. For example, red light is innocuous, ultraviolet light produces burns, and x-rays produce severe damage to tissues.

   F. **Loss of light by reflection or absorption.** With respect to the eye, the light incident on the retina from a light source is decreased by loss from reflection at the cornea, lens, and retinal surfaces. Although the cornea is quite transparent from 400 to 1,200 nm, the crystalline lens does absorb some of the radiant energy, particularly short wavelengths. The young, healthy lens transmits incident light of 320 nm. Absorption at the blue end of the visible spectrum increases with age as xanthochromic (yellow-brown) proteins accumulate in the lens. Some of the short wavelength radiation is also absorbed by the yellow pigment in the macular region of the retina.

*Updated from Garcia GE, Pavan-Langston D. Refractive errors and clinical optics. In: Pavan-Langston D. *Manual of ocular diagnosis and therapy,* 4th ed. Boston: Little, Brown, 1996: 371–397.

G. **Color of light.** The physical stimulus that is responsible for the sensation of color is the wavelength of the radiation. Wavelength in the region around 430 nm produces a violet sensation, around 460 nm blue, around 520 nm green, around 575 nm yellow, around 600 nm orange, and around 650 nm red. A mixture of wavelengths, such as occurs in sunlight, produces a white sensation.

H. **Reflection.** When light rays strike a smooth surface, they may bounce off the surface, or be reflected, rather than pass through. Reflection from a polished surface is referred to as "regular" or "specular" reflection. This does not occur randomly but follows a simple rule—the angle of reflection is equal to the angle of incidence and lies in the same plane. The angle of reflection and the angle of incidence are measured relative to the surface perpendicular at the point of impact. When light is reflected, a plane or flat mirror reverses the direction of the light rays only and does not effect vergence, so no magnification, minification, or image inversion occurs. Convex or concave reflective surfaces can change the vergence of light rays and focus them, resulting in an altered image. This has a practical significance for spectacle wearers. Reflections from the ocular surfaces of corrective lenses can produce virtual images near the far point plane of the eye, images that can be annoying to the patient. The images can be eliminated by **tilting the lenses** slightly or by using an **antireflective coating** if necessary. The cornea can also be used as a reflective surface. The principal of **keratometry** depends on the anterior surface of the cornea, which acts as a concave mirror. By measuring the size of the reflected image, the radius of curvature can be calculated. The cornea is also employed as a reflecting surface when checking it for irregularity with a **keratoscope.** By examining the reflected images of a series of concentric circles, one can check for distortion. It is also worth noting that objects appear as a particular color because they preferentially reflect wavelengths of that color and absorb the other wavelengths.

I. **Refraction of light.** When rays of light traveling through air enter a denser transparent medium, the speed of the light is reduced and the light rays proceed at a different angle, i.e., they are refracted. The one exception is when the rays are incident perpendicular to the surface (collimated or paraxial light). In this case the speed of the light is reduced but the direction of the light is unchanged.

1. **Snell law of refraction.** The refraction of light at an interface is described whereby the angle of incidence and the angle of refraction are related to the density of the medium for a specific wavelength. When light passes from a medium of low density to a medium of high density, Snell law predicts that the light ray will be bent toward the normal, a line perpendicular to the surface at the point of impact (Fig. 14.1A). In other words, the angle of refraction is less than the angle of incidence when going from a low-density to a high-density medium. Conversely, when light passes from a high-density to a low-density medium (such as out of a tank of water into air), the angle of refraction is greater than the angle of incidence. By bending the surface of a transparent medium that has a high density, such as the cornea or a piece of glass, the angle of incidence can be altered, and by employing Snell law, the deviation of light rays by this altered surface can be predicted. All light rays from real objects diverge from one another; when these rays encounter a medium of high density, they can be made less divergent, parallel to one another, or convergent, depending on the shape and index of the refracting element or lens. By using simple formulas, the point at which the redirected rays come to a focus can be calculated quite easily.

2. **Measurement of lens power.** Lenses are measured in **diopters** (D). The power of a lens in D is the reciprocal of its focal length (f) in meters: $D = 1/f$. For example, a lens that focuses light from an object at infinity (parallel light rays or 0 vergence) at a plane 1 m beyond the lens is a 1-D lens (Fig. 14.1B). If it focuses the light at a plane 0.5 m beyond the lens, it is a 2-D lens: $2 = 1/0.5$.

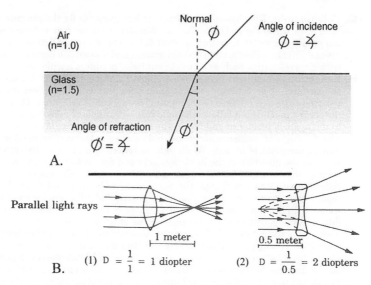

FIG. 14.1. **A:** Refraction of light is the change in direction in passage of light between media of different densities. **B:** Measurement of lens-focusing power in diopters by plus (**A**) and minus (**B**) lenses. D, diopters.

II. Types of corrective lenses
A. Spherical lenses have equal radii of curvature in all meridians.

1. **Convex or plus lenses.** By convention, high-density optical surfaces that are convex are referred to as **plus lenses.** They refract light rays so as to make them more convergent (or less divergent). Plus lenses of the same power can be made with a variety of radii, because it is the relationship of the two surfaces of a spectacle correcting lens that determines the power of the lens (Fig. 14.2A). A **meniscus form,** in which the front surface is more convex than the back surface is concave, results in the most desirable lens form for spectacles, because there is less spherical aberration over a wider area of the lens. A plano–convex-shaped plus lens will also reduce aberration. Plus lenses are used for the correction of **hyperopia, presbyopia,** and **aphakia.** When a nearby object is viewed through a plus lens, the object looks larger. If the lens is moved slightly from side to side, the object appears to move in the direction **opposite** to the movement of the lens. Plus lenses can also be identified by their physical characteristics; they are thicker in the middle and thinner at the edges.

2. **Concave or minus lenses.** High-density optical surfaces that are concave are referred to as **minus lenses.** They refract light rays so as to make them more divergent (or less convergent). As stated previously, it is the relationship of the two surface radii that determines the resultant power. Minus lenses can also be made in many **forms** (Fig. 14.2B). The most common design used in minus spectacle lenses is the **meniscus,** wherein the back or ocular surface is more concave than the front surface is convex. **Myodisc** lenses (biconcave) are used on patients who need very strong minus lenses. They induce less peripheral distortion, but offer a smaller focused central field than the meniscus lens. High-density plastic (polycarbonate) lenses have a higher refractive index than crown glass and may be used to reduce the thickness of high minus lenses. Minus lenses are used to correct **myopia.** When a nearby object is viewed through a minus lens, the object looks smaller. If the lens is moved

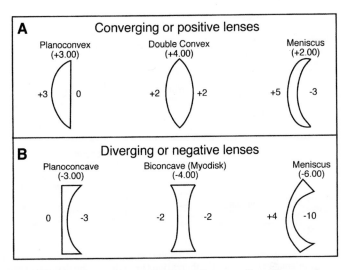

FIG. 14.2. A: Spherical lens designs. Plus lenses for correction of hyperopia or presbyopia. **B:** Minus lenses for correction of myopia.

slightly from side to side, the object appears to move in the **same** direction as the lens. Minus lenses are thin in the middle and thick at the edges.

B. **Toric lenses** are shaped like a section through a football. One meridian is more curved than all of the others, and the meridian at right angles to the steepest meridian is flatter than all of the other meridians. In a toric lens, the meridians of least curvature and the greatest curvature are always at right angles to one another and are referred to as the **principal meridians.** Toric lenses are prescribed to correct **astigmatism.** Toric lenses can be identified by observing a vertical contour such as a window or door frame through the center of the lens and rotating the lens in a vertical plane (parallel to the surface that is being observed). If the lens is a toric lens, the edge of the **vertical contour is broken** or discontinuous in the area viewed through the lens. The image will also appear to rotate clockwise or counterclockwise as the lens is rotated back and forth. If the same vertical contour is viewed through the center of a spherical lens, it remains continuous when viewed within and outside the borders of the lens, and does not appear to rotate when the lens is rotated. Toric lenses can be plus lenses, minus lenses, one principal meridian plus and the other minus, meniscus lenses, or they can be fabricated in a planocylinder form in which one principal meridian has zero optical power. Toric lenses are also referred to as **spherocylinders.**

C. **Prisms.** A prism is an optical device composed of two refracting surfaces that are inclined toward one another so they are not parallel. The line at which the two surfaces intersect is the apex of the prism. The greater the angle formed at the apex, the stronger the prismatic effect [Fig. 14.3A(1)]. Because the two surfaces of a prism are usually flat, they alter the direction of the light rays, but not their vergence. An object viewed through a prism appears to be **displaced in the direction of the prism apex,** but the focus is not altered and no magnification or minification occurs. Prisms are usually prescribed to assist a patient with an **extraocular muscle imbalance,** which results in a deviation of one visual axis relative to the other, so that the patient may achieve single binocular vision or do so more comfortably. They may be oriented in the spectacle correction so as to produce horizontal, vertical, or both horizontal and vertical displacement, as needed. The strength

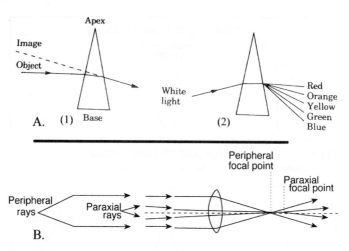

FIG. 14.3. A: Prism effects. **(1):** Prismatic displacement of image for assistance in muscle balance problems. **(2):** Chromatic aberration through varying degrees of refraction of lights of differing wavelength (color). **B:** Spherical aberration induced by varying degrees of light refraction from center of lens to edge.

of a prism is measured in **prism diopters (pds).** The prism power is equal to the displacement in centimeters of a light ray passing through the prism measured 1 m from the prism. (Each diopter displaces a ray of light 1 cm at a distance of 1 m.) Two prism diopters of displacement are approximately equal to 1 degree of arc. See Chapter 12 for prescribing prisms.

   D. Lensometers are precision instruments used to measure the spherical power, cylindrical (toric) power and the corresponding axis, and prism power, if present, of a spectacle or contact lens. Synonyms include: vertometer, vertexometer, dioptometer, and focimeter.

     1. Technique. The lens to be measured is placed on the lensometer stage, and the **power wheel** is turned until the target mires are in focus. The mires cross each other at right angles; there are three lines in one meridian and one in the other. If the mires all focus simultaneously at a given power, no cylinder is present and the lens is completely spherical. The power is read directly off of the power wheel. The second wheel on the lensometer is an **axis wheel,** which can be rotated to turn the mires until they are lined up along the principal meridians of a lens containing a cylinder. Alignment is correct when the crossing lines are perfectly straight (not broken). The power wheel is then turned to focus the strongest plus power of the lens (single line meridian). When this is focused using the greatest plus power (or least minus power), the spherical power component is recorded. The power wheel is turned again to bring the weaker (more minus) meridian into focus (three-line target) and the cylindrical power component is noted as well as the axis of that meridian, which is read directly from the axis wheel. The lens prescription is the strongest plus power minus the **difference** in power between the two settings, and the axis of the cylinder is that of the more minus meridian, as indicated on the axis of the wheel.

     2. Example of *lensometer* calculations
       a. Strongest plus meridian reading: +4.00
         Weaker plus meridian reading: +2.50
         Axis of weaker meridian: 80 degrees
         Final power: +4.00 = −1.50 × 80 degrees.

   b. Strongest plus (weakest minus) meridian reading: -2.00
   Weaker plus (stronger minus) meridian reading: -3.00
   Axis of weaker plus meridian: 40 degrees
   Final power: $-2.00 = -1.00 \times 40$ degrees.

   3. Plus cylinder prescriptions are less convenient and less frequently used, but may be done by reversing the above technique. For example:
   Weakest plus meridian: $+1.00$
   Strongest plus meridian: $+2.50$
   Axis of strongest plus meridian: 50 degrees
   Final power: $+1.00 = +1.50 \times 50$ degrees.

   4. Conversion of minus cylinder prescriptions to plus or the opposite is carried out by reversing the sign of the cylinder, adding the difference between the two lenses, and adding 90 degrees to its axis, e.g., $+3.00 = -2.00 \times 20$ degrees converts to $+1.00 = +2.00 \times 110$ degrees.

   5. Prism power is measured by reading the amount of decentration, from the optical center, of the cross mires. This is measured by counting the number of circles or lines on the eyepiece reticule away from center. Base-in is noted if the power center is located on the nasal side of the lens; base-out is noted if temporal.

III. Refraction techniques. *Refraction* is the term applied to the various testing procedures employed to measure the refractive errors of the eye to provide the proper correction. **Refractive error is by far the most common cause of poor vision.** Fortunately, it is generally the easiest to treat.

   A. Retinoscopy is an objective method of analyzing the optics of the patient's eye to determine the refractive error. A retinoscope is a handheld instrument that the examiner uses to illuminate the inside of the patient's eye and observe the light rays (reflected from the retinal pigmented epithelium and choroid) as they emerge from the patient's eye. This is accomplished by using a mirror to reflect the light along the line connecting the examiner's and the patient's pupils, and by creating a small aperture in the mirror that allows the examiner to view the patient's illuminated pupil. The light reflected from the patient's retina is refracted by the ocular media and focused at the far point of the patient's eye or punctum remotum. The patient must observe an object at 6 m (20 ft) or beyond to control for the accommodative reflex. By placing plus or minus lenses in front of the patient's eye, the patient's focal point can be altered until it is brought to the examiner's pupil, which produces a visible end point. This process involves moving the streak of light back and forth across a series of lenses held in front of the patient's pupil, resulting in a linear light reflex moving in the same (hyperopia) or opposite direction (myopia) as the light. The filling of the entire pupil with light that does not move indicates neutralization of the refractive error in that meridian and is the end point reading for that meridian. The linear streak of light can be rotated 360 degrees through the pupil to examine different meridians of the eye. In the case of astigmatism, the retinoscope linear light must be empirically lined up along a principal meridian (the clearest light streak as the retinoscope light is rotated) and plus or minus lenses put up until movement of light in that meridian is neutralized and the lens power recorded. This is repeated in the meridian 90 degrees away for the second lens and axis. By knowing how far the examiner is from the patient and what lenses are required, it is a simple matter to calculate the amount of ametropia. This technique is highly accurate and useful when used by a skilled retinoscopist, with a pupil of reasonable diameter and clear media. Opacities of the media, tiny pupils, poor fixation by the patient, or distortion of the light reflex can all be troublesome, however. Prescribing lenses on the basis of retinoscopic findings alone can too often result in a prescription that is not well tolerated by the patient.

   B. Subjective refraction is a tool whereby the examiner relies on patient responses to narrow the prescription further. Retinoscopy findings or habitual spectacle power may be the starting guide for subjective refraction. In the absence of astigmatism, the refraction is simply a matter of adding more plus or minus power until the patient reads his or her best visual acuity with the most plus or least minus power. In the presence of **astigmatism,** and to help test for it, the **fogging technique** is very effective (see sec. **VI.B.3.e.,** below). Both retinoscopic and subjective refractions involving astigmatism may be refined by the **Jackson cross-cylinder (JCC) technique** (see sec. **VI.B.3.f.,** below).

C. **Automated refraction.** In recent years, electronic microcircuitry and computer technology have combined to develop sophisticated instruments for refracting patients. Currently, these instruments require a technician to operate them. The standard to which these instruments are compared is retinoscopy or subjective refraction, or both. In general, automated refractometers are reasonably accurate. To provide reliable and valid data, however, the instrument must be properly in line with the patient's visual axis, accommodation must be relaxed, the pupil must be of satisfactory size, and the media must be sufficiently clear. There is no evidence that indicates that automated refraction is better than, and there is considerable controversy as to whether it is as good as, retinoscopy and subjective refraction. The primary role for these instruments at this time would appear to be increasing the efficiency with which eye care can be delivered by indicating the approximate refractive error, which should then be manually refined by the refractionist to give the patient the most satisfactory vision. For example, an automated refractor may indicate cylinder axis of 15 degrees, but the patient has been wearing spectacles at axis 10 degrees without discomfort. It is wiser to give the axis 10 degrees with perhaps some sacrifice of visual clarity than axis 15 degrees, which is clear but feels "uncomfortable."

D. **Cycloplegic refraction.** Cycloplegia is the employment of pharmaceutical agents such as atropine, tropicamide, or cyclopentolate to paralyze the ciliary muscle temporarily to stabilize the accommodative reflex of the eye so that a definitive end point may be measured. It is useful in young patients with highly active accommodation to ensure complete relaxation of the ciliary muscle so that the ametropia can be measured accurately in young hyperopes, thereby avoiding overcorrection. **Methods of inducing cycloplegia** include 1% cyclopentolate or tropicamide, one drop q5min for two or three applications in the office just before refraction, or atropine 1%, one drop tid for 3 days before the refraction.

IV. **Aberrations.** Optical systems generally contain imperfections referred to as *aberrations.* The important aberrations in the visual system and spectacle lenses are chromatic aberration, spherical aberration, radial astigmatism, and distortion.

A. **Chromatic aberration.** The index of refraction for any transparent medium varies with the wavelength of the incident light. This variation is such that blue light is refracted more than red light [Fig. 14.3A (2)]. This accounts for the chromatic dispersion that occurs when white light is passed through a prism and a rainbow effect is produced. In a convex or plus lens, blue light is focused slightly closer to the lens than red light. The same is true of the human eye, in which blue light is focused slightly in front of red light.

B. **Spherical aberration.** In most discussions of optics, certain assumptions are made for the sake of simplicity. Higher-order optics become quite complex and contribute little to the understanding of the visual system or to measuring and prescribing for refractive errors. So far, it has been assumed that all light rays from an object that pass through a lens come to focus at a single image point. A closer analysis reveals that this is true only for light rays that are paraxial, i.e., that pass through the center of the lens. Those light rays that are parallel to the axis but that pass through the periphery of the lens are usually refracted more than the paraxial rays. Peripheral rays will focus closer to the lens (Fig. 14.3B). Every object point on the axis of the lens will then be represented by a blur circle rather than a point focus. The size of this blur circle can be reduced by restricting the passage of light through the lens to the central portion, as is done when an object is viewed through a pinhole aperture. This same effect accounts for the increased depth of focus obtained when the iris diaphragm of a camera is reduced in size or when the pupil of the eye is constricted. Spherical aberration can produce a variable concentric retinoscopic reflex in children, with the peripheral portions of the pupil appearing myopic (against motion) while the central portion is at neutrality.

C. **Radial astigmatism** occurs when light rays pass through a lens obliquely. Instead of focusing a point of light as a point image, two linear images form at right angles to one another with a "circle of least confusion" between them. This form of aberration is of no great significance in the eye; however, it can create considerable blurring of the image formed by spectacle lenses.

D. **Distortion** is the result of differential magnification in an optical system. This occurs because light from some parts of the object is focused by the central portion of the lens, while other parts are focused by peripheral portions of the lens. In other words, the shape of the image formed does not correspond exactly to the shape of the object. For practical purposes, this is not a problem in the eye, but it can be troublesome in higher-powered spectacle lenses. High plus lenses produce "pincushion" distortion, and high minus lenses result in "barrel" distortion.

V. **The eye as an optical instrument.** The analogy of the eye and the camera is a useful one. The focusing elements of the eye are the cornea and the crystalline lens, and the "film" is the retina. To simplify discussions of the eye as an optical instrument, we use some approximations and resort to the schematic or reduced eye, wherein all light rays are assumed to be paraxial and all elements perfectly aligned on the visual axis.

A. **The cornea** contributes approximately two-thirds of the refracting power of the eye. This is true because more deflection of light rays occurs at the air–cornea interface because of the large difference in index of refraction between these two media. The crystalline lens is in fact a more powerful refracting lens than the cornea in air because it is biconvex and each of its surfaces is more convex than the cornea. The lens, however, is in the aqueous–vitreous medium, and the difference in refractive index at the aqueous–lens and lens–vitreous interfaces is much less. The cornea has an index of refraction of 1.376 and contributes **+43 D** to the eye.

B. **The crystalline lens** has an index of refraction that increases from the cortex to the nucleus, but averages 1.41 with a power of **+20 D**. Because these two refracting elements are separated, the **total power of the eye** is not their sum but the equivalent power of **+58.7 D.**

C. **The pupil** is also a significant component of the eye's optical system. It can constrict, reducing the amount of light that enters the eye, decreasing aberrations, and increasing the eye's depth of focus. This accounts for the ability of many people, who require glasses, to get along without them when the illumination is good.

D. **The retina** is a unique kind of film. It contains the "coarse grain" but highly sensitive rods for registering images at very low levels of illumination and the "fine grain" color-sensitive cones for high resolution and discrimination at high levels of illumination. Only one or two quanta of light energy are required to activate the rods. On the other hand, rapid neural adaptation and the more gradual process of adjusting the steady state between bleaching and regeneration of retinal visual pigments enable the retina to function perfectly at extremely high levels of illumination. What other film functions so well both in moonlight and at high noon? The manner in which visual images are formed, transmitted to the visual cortex, and interpreted is a fascinating story but not appropriate to this discussion.

VI. **Refractive errors of the eye (Fig. 14.4).**
A. **Emmetropia.** The eye is considered to be emmetropic if parallel light rays, from an object more than 6 m away, are focused at the plane of the retina when the eye is in a completely relaxed state. An emmetropic eye will have a clear image of a distant object without any internal adjustment of its

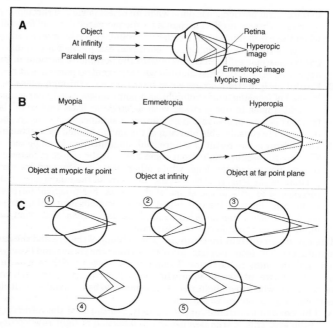

FIG. 14.4. A: Far point (image distance focused on retina in accommodatively relaxed eye) in myopia, emmetropia, and hyperopia. **B:** Focal points of myopic, emmetropic, and hyperopic eye with reference to the retinal plane. **C:** Focal points of astigmatic principal meridians (objects at infinity): **(1)** simple hyperopic astigmatism, emmetropia/hyperopia; **(2)** simple myopic astigmatism, emmetropia–myopia; **(3)** compound hyperopic astigmatism, hyperopia–hyperopia; **(4)** compound myopic astigmatism, myopia–myopia; **(5)** mixed astigmatism, hyperopia–myopia.

optics. Although most emmetropic rays are approximately 24 mm in length, a larger eye can be emmetropic if its optical components are weaker, and a smaller eye can be emmetropic if its optical components are stronger.

B. Ametropias

1. Hyperopia. When the focused image is formed behind the plane of the retina in ametropia, the eye is "too short" and is considered hyperopic. This is also referred to as *farsightedness*. Near images can be blurred unless there is sufficient accommodation, as in a child. Unless the optical system of the eye is actively altered to produce an increase in its power, hyperopic eyes will have blurred images for distant objects also, as any elderly hyperope will confirm. Most children are born about +3 D hyperopic, but this usually resolves by age 12 years.

  a. Structural hyperopia is based on the anatomic configuration of the eye.

   (1) In **axial hyperopia,** the eye is shorter than normal in its anteroposterior (AP) diameter, although the refracting portions (e.g., lens, cornea) are normal. These eyes are more prone to develop **angle-closure glaucoma** because of the shorter anterior segment with crowding of the filtration angle. The optic nerves are also smaller and more densely packed, because they are crowded at the disk. Physiologic cupping is uncommon, and **pseudopapilledema** may be noted. The latter is seen in eyes with greater than +4 D of hyperopia, a normal blind spot on field testing, no venous congestion, and a disk that seems "swollen."

   (2) **Curvature hyperopia** results when either the crystalline lens or the cornea has a weaker than normal curvature and consequently lower refractive power.

   (3) **Index of refraction hyperopia** is the result of decreased index of refraction due to decreased density in some or several parts of the optic system of the eye, thus lowering the refractive power of the eye.

b. **Accommodation in hyperopia** is of greater importance than the structural factors leading to it because accommodation is a key dynamic factor in correcting at least part of the refractive error. It is defined as latent, manifest facultative, and manifest absolute hyperopia.

   (1) **Latent hyperopia** is that part of the refractive error completely corrected by accommodation. It is measurable not by manifest refraction but only with paralysis of accommodation via cycloplegic refraction. Latent hyperopia is the difference in measurement between manifest hyperopia and the results of the cycloplegic refraction, which reveals total hyperopia, latent and manifest.

   (2) **Manifest facultative hyperopia** is that portion of hyperopia that may be corrected by the patient's own powers of accommodation, by corrective lenses, or both. Vision is normal with or without corrective plus lenses, but accommodation is not relaxed without the glasses.

   (3) **Manifest absolute hyperopia** is that part of the refractive error that cannot be compensated for by the patient's accommodation. Distance vision is still blurred no matter how much accommodative power the patient uses. These patients readily accept the aid of plus lenses.

c. **The effect of aging** on hyperopia results from progressive loss of accommodative power, thus moving the eye from latent and facultative hyperopia to greater degrees of absolute hyperopia.

d. **Symptoms of hyperopia**

   (1) **Frontal headaches** worsening as the day progresses and aggravated by prolonged use of near vision.

   (2) **"Uncomfortable" vision** (asthenopia) when the patient must focus at a fixed distance for prolonged periods, e.g., a televised baseball game. Accommodation tires more quickly when held in a fixed level of tension.

   (3) **Blurred distance vision** with refractive errors greater than 3 to 4 D or in older patients with decreasing amplitude of accommodation.

   (4) **Near visual acuity** blurs at a younger age than in the emmetrope, e.g., in the late 30s. This is aggravated when the patient is tired, when print is indistinct, or lighting conditions suboptimal.

   (5) **Light sensitivity** is common in hyperopes, is of unknown etiology, and is relieved by correcting the hyperopia without needing to tint the lenses.

   (6) **Intermittent sudden blurring of vision** is due to a quick change in or **spasm of accommodation.** A shift toward myopia is present (pseudomyopia) and vision temporarily clears with minus lenses. The accommodative spasm may be detected by cycloplegic refraction, which will reveal the underlying hyperopia.

   (7) **"Crossed-eyes" sensation** without diplopia is also due to excessive accommodation in a patient with an esophoria that is being pushed by the accommodation–convergence reflex into a symptom-producing state that "the eyes are crossing."

    e. Treatment of hyperopia is usually most satisfactory when slightly less power (1 D) than the total of facultative and absolute hyperopia is given to a patient with no extraocular muscle imbalance. If an accommodative esotropia (convergence) is present, then the full correction should be given. In exophoria, the hyperopia should be undercorrected by 1 to 2 D (see Chapter 12). If the total manifest refractive error is small, e.g., 1 D or less, correction is given only if the patient is symptomatic.

2. Myopia. When the focused image is formed in front of the plane of the retina in ametropia, the eye is "too long" and is considered myopic. This is referred to as *nearsightedness,* because there is a point less than 6 m in front of the eye that will be coincident with the retina when the optical system of the eye is relaxed.

    a. Types of myopia

        (1) In **axial myopia,** the AP diameter of the eye is longer than normal, although the corneal and lens curvatures are normal and the lens is in the normal anatomic position. In this form of myopia may be found pseudoproptosis resulting from the abnormally large anterior segment, a peripapillary myopic crescent from an exaggerated scleral ring, and a posterior staphyloma.

        (2) In **curvature myopia** the eye has a normal AP diameter, but the curvature of the cornea is steeper than average, e.g., congenitally or in keratoconus, or the lens curvature is increased as in moderate to severe hyperglycemia, which causes lens intumescence.

        (3) Increased index of refraction in the lens due to onset of early to moderate nuclear sclerotic cataracts is a common cause of myopia in the elderly. The sclerotic change increases the index of refraction, thus making the eye myopic. Many people find themselves ultimately able to read without glasses or having gained "second sight." They may usually be given normal distance vision for years simply by increasing the minus power in their corrective lenses, thus avoiding surgery.

        (4) Anterior movement of the lens is often seen after glaucoma surgery and will increase the myopic error in the eye.

    b. Clinical course. Myopia is rarely present at birth, but often begins to develop as the child grows. It is usually detected by age 9 or 10 years in the school vision tests and will increase during the years of growth until stabilizing around the mid-teens, usually at about 5 D or less.

        (1) Pathological (progressive) myopia is a rare form of myopia that increases by as much as 4 D yearly and is associated with vitreous floaters, liquefaction, and chorioretinal changes. The refractive changes usually stabilize at about age 20 years, but occasionally may progress until the mid-30s, and frequently results in degrees of myopia of 10 to 20 D.

        (2) Congenital high myopia is usually a refractive error of 10 D or greater and is detected in infants who seem to be unaware of a visual world beyond their immediate surroundings, but who, fortunately, usually develop normal vision focusing on small objects held an inch or two from their eyes. This myopia is not generally progressive, but should be corrected as soon as discovered to help the child develop normal distance vision and perception of the world.

    c. Symptoms of myopia

        (1) Blurred distance vision.

        (2) Squinting to sharpen distance vision by attempting a pinhole effect through narrowing of the palpebral fissures.

        (3) Headaches are rare, but may be seen in patients with uncorrected low myopic errors.

d. Treatment of myopia

(1) **Children** should be fully corrected and, if under 8 years of age, instructed to wear their glasses constantly both to avoid developing the habit of squinting and to enhance developing a normal accommodation–convergence reflex (see sec. **VI.B.5.,** below). If the refractive error is low, the child may wear the glasses intermittently as needed, e.g., at school.

(2) **Adults** under the age of 30 years are usually comfortable with their full myopic correction. Patients older than 30 years may not be able to tolerate a full correction over 3 D if they have never worn glasses before and may prefer a less than full correction, with resulting undercorrected distance vision but clear reading vision. The patient should be told that full correction might be given in the future if desired. Wearing full correction in a trial frame for about 30 minutes, with the patient both reading and looking at distance in the waiting room, may answer the question of whether to give full correction.

(3) **Undercorrection of myopia** in childhood may result in an adult who has never developed a normal amount of accommodation for near focus. This person will be uncomfortable in full correction and complain that the glasses are too strong and "pull" his or her eyes.

3. **Astigmatism.** The optical systems thus far discussed are spherical, that is, all the meridians of the lenses are of equal curvature, resulting in a surface that resembles a section through a spheroid. Many optical systems, however, are toric surfaces, in which the curvature varies in different meridians, thus refracting light unequally in those meridians and creating the condition known as astigmatism (see sec. **II.B.,** above). Light rays passing through a steep meridian are thus deflected more than those passing through a flatter meridian. This results in the formation of a more complicated image, referred to as the "conoid of Sturm," wherein a point source of light is represented by an image consisting of two lines that are at right angles to one another with a circle of least confusion in a plane midway between them (Fig. 14.5A). The steepest and flattest meridians of the eye are usually at right angles to one another, resulting in regular astigmatism. This is fortunate, because technology makes it possible to generate regular astigmatic surfaces in ophthalmic lenses easily so that astigmatism can be corrected economically.

a. Types of astigmatism

(1) **Corneal toricity** accounts for most of the astigmatism of the eye. If the **vertical meridian is steeper,** it is referred to as astigmatism **"with the rule,"** and if the **horizontal meridian is steeper** it is referred to as astigmatism **"against the rule."** One meridian may be emmetropic and the other hyperopic or myopic, both may be hyperopic or myopic, or one may be hyperopic and the other myopic. In spherical ametropia, only one number is necessary to designate the power of the corrective lens, but in astigmatic corrections, three numbers are required to indicate the power needed in each principal meridian plus the axis to provide the correct orientation of the lens in front of the eye (e.g., $+2.00 = -1.00 \times 180$ is a corrective lens prescription for with-the-rule astigmatism).

(2) **Regular astigmatism** has principal meridians 90 degrees apart and **oblique astigmatism** has them more than 20 degrees from the horizontal or vertical meridians.

(3) **Irregular astigmatism** results from an unevenness of the corneal surface such as in corneal scarring or keratoconus. The principal meridians are not 90 degrees apart and are so irregular that they cannot be completely corrected with ordinary toric lenses (cylinders). The **diagnosis** can be made by shining a light into the eye and observing any irregularity of the pupillary reflex with the

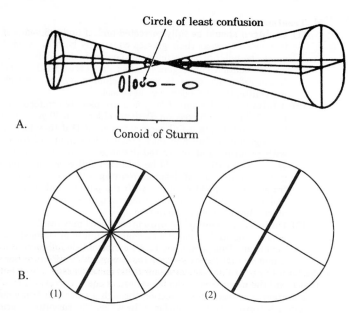

FIG. 14.5. A: Effect of regular astigmatism on focal planes of eye, resulting in least blur (conoid of Sturm). **B(1):** Clock dial as seen by "fogged" patient with astigmatic error; 1 to 7 axis appears darker. **(2):** Two-line rotating dial is set at 1 to 7 position. Axis of correcting **minus** cylinder is 30 degrees (1 × 30). Minus cylinders are placed at 120 degrees (30 + 90 degrees) until all lines appear equal, thus indicating cylinder power and axis needed to correct astigmatic error. Patient is then "defogged."

ophthalmoscope or retinoscope, by the use of a keratometer that measures the corneal curvature, by examination with a slitlamp, or by observing the corneal reflex with either a keratoscope or **Placido disk,** both of which contain concentric circles that are reflected by the surface of the cornea and that appear distorted in cases of irregular corneal astigmatism. Irregular astigmatism cannot be corrected with spectacle lenses, but can frequently be corrected by rigid contact lenses.

    (4) **Symmetric astigmatism** has principal meridians in each eye with similar but opposite axes, e.g., 20 degrees in the right eye and 160 degrees in the left eye, which together add up to 180 degrees.

  b. Symptoms of higher astigmatism (>1.00 D) include:

    (1) **Blurred vision.**

    (2) **Tilting** of the head for oblique astigmatism.

    (3) **Turning** of the head (rare).

    (4) **Squinting** to achieve "pinhole" vision clarity.

    (5) **Reading** material held **close to eyes** to achieve large (as in myopia) but blurred retinal image.

  c. Symptoms of lower astigmatism (<1.00 D) include:

    (1) **Asthenopia** ("tired eyes"), especially when doing precise work at a fixed distance. With-the-rule astigmatism produces more symptoms, but clearer vision than the same amount of against-the-rule astigmatism.

    (2) **Transient blurred vision** relieved by closing or rubbing the eyes (as in hyperopia) when doing precise work at a fixed distance.

(3) **Frontal headaches** with long periods of visual concentration on a task.
d. **Treating astigmatism** depends on the patient's visual needs and symptoms as noted above in terms of whether glasses are worn constantly or intermittently. It is not within the scope of this book to discuss in detail the many methods of measuring astigmatism for corrective lenses such as plus cylinders, Lancaster-Regan charts, or crossed cylinders, but the fogging technique followed by refinement with the JCC is a common method for **measuring regular astigmatic correction** using the clock dial and minus cylinders.
e. **Fogging technique.** Make the patient **artificially myopic (fogged)** to about 20/50 by putting enough plus sphere before the eye to focus all meridians anterior to the retina, i.e., to bring forward compound, simple, or mixed hyperopic astigmatism meridians where both (the former) or one (the latter two) focal plane is posterior to the retina. By making all meridians myopic, the refractionist **inhibits accommodation**, thus stabilizing the refractive error of the eye, and then may use minus cylinders to determine the principal meridians.
(1) Have the patient **identify** the **darkest, most distinct line** on the spokes of the astigmatic clock chart (Fig. 14.5B), e.g., the 1 to 7 o'clock line, and multiply the lower number by 30 degrees to get the proposed axis of the correcting cylinder.
(2) **Switch to a two-line rotating chart** with one line oriented along one principal meridian, e.g., 1 to 7 o'clock. As these lines cross perpendicularly, the other line will be on the opposite principal meridian.
(3) Place **increasing strength minus cylinders** before the eye at an axis 90 degrees from the blackest line, e.g., 4 to 10 o'clock or 120 degrees (30 + 90 degrees). Add one −0.25- to −0.50-D cylinder at a time until both lines are equal in darkness and distinctness. They will still be blurred. For each −0.50 D of cylinder added after the original −0.75 cylinder is in, add a +0.25-D sphere to keep the patient artificially myopic.
(4) Switch to a **distance vision chart** and reduce plus spheres until the patient achieves maximum clarity of vision.
(5) **Example:**
  (a) +2.00 fogs to 20/50.
  (b) 4 to 10 line is darkest.
  (c) 4 × 30 degrees = 120 degrees (axis of correcting cylinder).
  (d) −1.00 × 30 degrees evens out darkness of the two-line chart.
  (e) Reducing plus lenses to +0.25 gives sharpest vision on distant reading chart.
  (f) Final prescription: +0.25 = −1.00 × 120.
(6) **If axis falls between hours** on the clock, multiply by the lowest number plus half, i.e., between 1 and 2 o'clock = 1.5 × 30 degrees = 45 degrees is the correcting cylinder.
(7) **Refine** the final prescription by using the JCC. If the final cylinder correction is greater than 3 D and the patient has never worn glasses before, giving one-half to two-thirds of the cylinder correction may be prudent to avoid intolerance and discomfort from an initial full correction.
f. **The Jackson cross-cylinder (JCC)** is a lens of equal-power plus (white dot) and minus (red dot) plano cylinders with axes 90 degrees apart. Lens powers range from −0.12 to −1.00 cylinder. To test if the patient's **lens axis is correct,** place the JCC before the eye with its handle parallel to the axis of the cylinder in the trial frame. Rotate the handle of the JCC in one direction and then turn it over to the other side, thus changing the combined cylinder axes. Turn the trial frame axis in the direction toward the JCC axis that gives better

vision on the distance chart and repeat the test. The end point is when rotating the JCC handle over makes no change in vision. To ascertain if the **cylinder strength is correct,** place the JCC with its handle at 45 degrees with the axis of the trial frame cylinder such that one axis of the JCC will be parallel to and the other 90 degrees from the trial frame cylinder. If vision is better when similar axes are parallel, e.g., minus over minus, the trial frame cylinder needs to be made stronger and vice versa. If rotating the JCC before the trial frame is equally bad in both directions, the cylinder is correct.

4. **Anisometropia** is a state in which there is a difference in the refractive errors of the two eyes, i.e., one eye is myopic and the other hyperopic, or both are hyperopic or myopic but to different degrees. This condition may be congenital or acquired due to asymmetric age changes or disease.

   a. In anisometropia, the patient may be made visually uncomfortable by
      (1) **Visual acuity differences** between the two eyes.
      (2) **Aniseikonia:** difference in size of the ocular image in each eye (possibly causing retinal rivalry).
      (3) **Anisophoria:** varying heterophoria (muscle imbalance) in different fields of gaze depending on the eye used for fixation.
      (4) **Suppression scotoma, amblyopia,** or **strabismus,** which may develop in young anisometropes. This may be mitigated by the proper refractive correction or even aggravated by the spectacle correction by inducing obstacles to fusion, such as anisophoria and aniseikonia.

   b. **Treatment**
      (1) In **children,** both eyes should receive the best visual correction and any muscle imbalance identified and corrected with prisms or surgically.
      (2) **Adults** should receive the best correction that will not result in ocular discomfort. Usually the more ametropic (poorer) eye is undercorrected.

5. **Accommodation.** The cornea is a static or fixed surface. The crystalline lens, however, is capable of increasing its plus power. This is referred to as *focus,* or *accommodation.* The lens is suspended in the eye by thousands of chemical strands, called *zonules,* that are attached to the ciliary body at one end, and the lens capsule at the opposite end. When the ciliary muscle is relaxed, the zonules maintain a slight tension on the capsule. Since the ciliary muscle is a circular sphincterlike muscle, constriction results in a slight decrease in the diameter of the circle. This reduces the tension of the zonules on the lens capsule, which is elastic. This action squeezes the lens fibers in such a way that the anterior pole, and to a lesser extent the posterior pole, becomes more convex, thereby increasing the power of the lens. This change in power is called *accommodation.* An emmetrope who wants to view a nearby object contracts the ciliary muscle, which results in an increase of power or accommodation to focus the image back to the plane of the retina.

   a. **Amplitude of accommodation** is the range of plus power the lens can produce. This varies with age and is a critical factor in the correction of hyperopia and presbyopia. Table 14.1 indicates a few of the Duane monocular and Donders binocular near point averages of accommodative power at various ages. It is useful to memorize at least the low-, middle-, and high-range figures.

   b. The **near point** or **punctum proximum (PP)** is the nearest point at which a person can see clearly. In the unaided (no glasses) emmetropic eye, the PP and retina are conjugate foci, and the amplitude of accommodation may be measured directly using this distance because it is unaltered by a refractive error. For example, a 20-year-old emmetrope is able to focus clearly at 10 cm, thus indicating a total accommodative power of 10 D by the formula $d = 1/\text{focal distance (m)}$.

TABLE 14.1. AMPLITUDE OF ACCOMMODATION (DIOPTERS)[a]

| Age (years) | Duane Monocular Near Point | | Donders Binocular Near Point |
	Average	Range	Average
10	13	11–16	14
20	11	9–13	10
30	9	7–11	7
40	6	3–8	5
50	2	1–3	3
60	1	1–2	1

[a]Rounded off to nearest whole diopter.

Given the same accommodative power of 10 D, if this patient were a 2-D myope, the total focal length would be 8.3 cm because of the 12-D focal point (10 D accommodation plus 2 D myopic error). A 2-D hyperope with 10 D of accommodation would focus at 12.5 cm (10 D accommodation minus 2 D hyperopic error = 8 D focal length).

c. The **far point** or **punctum remotum** is the farthest point at which a patient can see clearly. In emmetropia, the retina is focused at (conjugate with) infinity. In myopia, the focal point is anterior to the retina; in hyperopia, it is behind the retina, i.e., beyond infinity.

d. **Determining the amplitude of accommodation** may be done by several methods: minus sphere test, Lebensohn target, cycloplegic testing. The simplest method is the **push up method** where, with a distance correction before the eyes (if needed), a fine-print target is gradually moved toward the patient's eyes until the patient notes onset of blurred vision. This test is done monocularly in each eye in the young because of possible extraocular muscle balance effect on the blur distance. The distance at which the blur begins is converted to diopters of accommodative power ($D = 1$/focal distance [m]).

e. **Symptoms of decreased accommodative powers** can occur as a result of presbyopia, exophoria, exotropia, convergence insufficiency, and accommodative insufficiency. Presbyopia (see sec. **VI.B.6.,** below) is most common in patients older than 40 years and includes an inability to read or do close work for prolonged periods of time because of blurring of vision and "tiring" of the eyes. In all causes, intermittent diplopia at near may develop because of the interrelationship between accommodation and convergence. Symptoms are aggravated by fatigue, illness, fever, or other debilitating conditions, and may clear completely as the patient recovers and accommodative powers recompensate.

6. **Presbyopia** is a physiologic decrease in the amplitude of accommodation associated with aging. With time, changes occur in the crystalloids of the lens that result in a decreased elasticity of the lens fibers or a hardening of the lens. When the eye attempts to add plus power to the optical system or accommodate, there is less of a change in the curvature of the lens for each unit of contraction by the ciliary muscle. By the age of the early 40s, accommodative amplitude has usually decreased to less than 5 D, and objects less than 20 cm away cannot be brought into focus.

a. **Symptoms of presbyopia** develop when the amount of accommodation needed to focus at near **exceeds more than half of the total amplitude of the eye.** A 48-year-old emmetropic patient with only 5 D of accommodative amplitude will experience presbyopic symptoms when attempting to read at 33 cm (about 14 in.), because he or she is using 3 D (60%) of the total 5 D available to focus. An uncorrected hyperope and a chronically undercorrected myope who, as a result of the undercorrection, never developed full accommodative powers, will both develop presbyopic symptoms earlier than an emmetropic patient. The hyperope must use excess accommodation to overcome the hyperopia, thus reducing the available reserve for the early presbyopia. Symptoms of presbyopia include:

(1) **Longer reading distance** required.
(2) **Inability to focus on close work**.
(3) **Excessive illumination** required for close work.
(4) **Greater difficulty** with close work **as the day goes on.**

b. **Testing for presbyopia** is done monocularly and binocularly. The latter often requires a weaker correction; this is the more comfortable one for the patient to receive. The patient holds a reading card at the distance desired for work, e.g., typing or closer reading, and the weakest additional plus sphere that will give the patient clear small newsprint or footnote vision is determined. Cards commonly used are the **Snellen, Jaeger,** or **Rosenbaum.** The vision obtained should be recorded for future reference. Visual efficiency may also be calculated based on the best-corrected near vision, e.g., J-2 is 95% efficient (Table 14.2).

c. **Correcting presbyopia** is done through supplementing accommodation with plus lenses that do part of the focusing for the eye. The difference between the distance correction and the strength needed for clear near vision is called the **add.** An effective physiologic rule for prescribing the near correction is to give the add that will leave half of the amplitude of accommodation in reserve.

(1) **The average eyeglass adds for various age levels:**
   (a) 45 years: +1.00 to +1.25 D
   (b) 50 years: +1.50 to +1.75 D.
   (c) 55 years: +2.00 to +2.25 D.
   (d) 60 years: +2.50 to +2.75 D.

(2) **Adjustments for work distance.** The strength of the adds must be adjusted up or down depending on whether the patient wants a longer or shorter working distance. For a patient in his or her late 40s with only 3 D total amplitude left, the following adds give varying work distance and leave a comfortable (50%) amount of accommodation in reserve. (See Table 14.2 for range of adds, working distances, and amplitude reserve.)
   (a) +2.50: 10 in.
   (b) +1.50: 13 in.
   (c) +1.00: 16 in.
   (d) +0.50: 20 in.

7. **Aphakia.** If the crystalline lens becomes sufficiently opaque to interfere with vision, it must be removed by **cataract surgery** so that light may reach the retina. Removal of the lens produces a condition referred to as *aphakia* and results in an eye with one of its major optical elements missing. The eye in this state is extremely farsighted and lacks the ability to accommodate.

a. **Correction of aphakia** is accomplished by prescribing strong plus (convex) lenses. Unfortunately, removing the crystalline lens from within the eye and replacing it with a spectacle lens positioned in front of the eye results in considerable **magnification of the retinal image,** usually 25% to 30%. The aphake is required to make a considerable adaptation to the visual environment, because the larger image of a familiar object is interpreted as indicating that the object is much closer than it really is. In the case of **monocular aphakia,** the difference in the size of the aphakic and phakic images precludes

TABLE 14.2. EQUIVALENT VISUAL ACUITY NOTATIONS FOR NEAR

Visual Angle (Minutes)	Snellen Equivalent	AMA Notation	Decimal Notation	Jaeger Notation	Meter Notation (m)	Central Visual Efficacy for Near (%)
5.00	20/20	14/14	1.00	J1	0.37	100
6.25	20/25	14/17	0.80	J1-	0.43	100
7.50	20/30	14/21	0.66	J2	0.50	95
10.00	20/40	14/28	0.50	J4	0.75	90
12.50	20/50	14/35	0.40	J6	0.87	50
15.00	20/60	14/42	0.33	J8	1.00	40
20.00	20/80	14/56	0.25	J10	1.50	20
25.00	20/100	14/70	0.20	J11	1.75	15
50.00	20/200	14/140	0.10	J17	3.50	2

NECESSARY ADD FOR NEAR-POINT DISTANCES

Total Amplitude of Accomodation	Amplitude of Accomodation in Reserve	Add for 10 in. (4.00 D)	Add for 13 in. (3.00 D)	Add for 16 in. (2.50 D)	Add for 20 in. (2.00 D)	Add for 26 in. (1.50 D)
6.00	3.00	1.00	—	—	—	—
5.00	2.50	1.50	0.50	—	—	—
4.00	2.00	2.00	1.00	0.50	—	—
3.00	1.50	2.50	1.50	1.00	0.50	—
2.00	1.00	3.00	2.00	1.50	1.00	0.50
1.00	0.50	3.50	2.50	2.00	1.50	1.00
0.50	0.25	3.75	2.75	2.25	1.75	1.25

AMA, American Medical Association; M, distance in meters; D, diopters; In., inches.
Type sizes for Jaeger test cards have not been constant thus making a direct comparison between Jaeger and Snellen acuity cards difficult but still adequate for clinical purposes.
(Bureau of Visual Sciences, American Optical Corporation; *The AO Nearpoint Rotochart manual*, 1956; and Garcia G. *Handbook of refraction*, 4th ed, Boston: Little, Brown, 1989.)

combining them in the visual cortex to achieve single binocular vision, and results in double vision resulting from the different image sizes. In addition, strong plus lenses result in a significant increase in lens-induced aberrations that can be very annoying and can limit visual efficiency. It is for these reasons that strong convex contact lenses, and even more frequently, secondary intraocular lenses (IOLs), are being placed in eyes that did not receive them as part of the primary procedure (see Chapter 7).

b. Refraction technique in aphakia may be by retinoscopy (see sec. **III.A.,** above) or by a simple **subjective test** as follows:

(1) Check potential visual acuity on the distance chart with the pinhole test before starting. If no maculopathy or keratopathy is present, the refractionist should be able to achieve approximately the same vision with lenses as by pinhole.

(2) Place a +12-D lens before the eye (trial frame or Phoroptor), making sure the patient's visual axis passes perpendicularly through the plane of the correcting lenses. If the patient preoperatively was a high hyperope, a +14- to +16-D lens may be a better starting lens; if the patient is a high myope, use a +8- to +10-D lens to start.

(3) Increase or decrease the amount of plus sphere until the maximum spherical visual acuity is obtained.

(4) Place a −1.5- or −2.0-D cylinder in front of the plus lens and rotate the cylinder slowly until the axis that gives the patient the clearest vision on the distance chart is reached. If no letters are visible, increase or decrease the plus lens power until some letters are seen, and rotate the cylinder again until they are at their clearest.

(5) Using the JCC technique (see sec. **VI.B.3.f.,** above) increase or decrease the amount of cylinder at the clearest axis found until the patient again feels the vision is clearest.

(6) Increase or decrease the amount of plus sphere, keeping 90% of the plus power closest to the eye, i.e., rear cell of the trial frame, until vision is best. To keep the patient's vision comfortable, maintain a spherical equivalent power by adding +0.25D of power to the sphere for every −0.50 D of cylinder power that the patient accepts.

(7) Note the prescription and the vertex distance (distance between most posterior plus lens and cornea in millimeters) and record both. The vertex distance notation is important and will be used to calculate the final spherical lens strength by the optician.

c. Aphakic contact lenses and monocular aphakia correction. One alternative to the spectacle correction of aphakia is the use of **contact lenses.** By placing the lens element on the surface of the cornea, which is closer to the original site of the crystalline lens, magnification is reduced to between 5% and 10%, and this is usually compatible with fusion of the images in the visual cortex in the monocular aphakic. A contact lens correction results in less alteration of the visual environment by magnification and also eliminates most of the aberrations of aphakic spectacles. The use of a contact lens also restores peripheral vision.

d. IOLs are now by far the most common means of correcting surgical aphakia, with approximately 95% of all cataract surgery today including their implantation. A well-placed IOL has the visual advantages of the original crystalline lens but, as with any surgical device, may also cause complications. These are seen far less frequently now with improved lens design and materials. IOLs are discussed further in Chapter 7.

VII. Glasses in correction of ametropia. Most forms of ametropia can be corrected by spectacles. Plus (convex) lenses are used to correct hyperopia, presbyopia, and aphakia. Minus (concave) lenses are used to correct myopia. Toric lenses are employed for the correction of regular astigmatism. Most corrective lenses are made in the meniscus form to reduce aberrations and to provide a better cosmetic effect.

A. **Safety factors.** Lenses are generally made impact resistant; that is, they must comply with American National Standards Institute (ANSI) standard Z-87.1-1989 and withstand the impact of a 1.5-cm steel ball dropped from a height of 127 cm. Industrial safety glasses must withstand a greater impact and are tested with a 2.9-cm steel ball dropped from a height of 127 cm. Glass lenses are generally made of crown glass with an index of refraction of 1.523, with a minimum thickness of 2 mm, and they are heat-treated or chemically altered to make them shatterproof. Plastic lenses are naturally shatterproof and lighter in weight, but tend to scratch more easily. Because most plastic resins have a density less than that of crown glass, they may be a little thicker than the same diameter glass lens of equal power. Glass and plastic are equally satisfactory for the correction of ametropia but, depending on the power required and the frame style, one may have advantages over the other in certain circumstances.

B. **Lens shapes in extreme corrections.** In high minus lenses a myodisc form may be used to reduce the weight by grinding the peripheral portion of the lens surfaces parallel to one another so that only the central portion is corrective. This also reduces the edge thickness. High plus lenses can be made in a **lenticular form,** wherein only the central portion is corrective and the peripheral surfaces are parallel to one another. High plus and high minus lenses can also be made in an **aspheric form** by modifying the lens curvature peripherally to **reduce aberrations and provide better peripheral vision.**

C. **Tinted lenses.** Lenses may be tinted for comfort, safety, or cosmetic effect. Sunglasses are generally tinted green or gray, according to individual preference. To be effective, they should be dark enough to absorb 60% to 80% of the incident light in the visible part of the spectrum and almost all of the ultraviolet and infrared. Both glass and plastic absorb **ultraviolet** very effectively, but glass lenses are more effective in the infrared range. **Photochromic lenses** that alter their absorptive characteristics according to the amount of ultraviolet exposure are available. It is important to bear in mind that it is the ultraviolet exposure of the lens pigment that alters the absorption of the lens. Because all plastic photochromic lenses will loose a small amount of dye pigment when heated, antireflective coatings or tints should never be added to these, because the additions will reduce the ability of the lens to absorb UV light. **Photochromic lenses will not function as efficiently indoors or in an automobile.** Also, the darkening process occurs quite rapidly, but the lightening process is much slower, requiring 1 minute and 20 minutes, respectively, for a 75% alteration in transmission. Photochromic lenses may be slightly less efficient for night driving and maximum absorption of the lens pigment cannot be varied. Tinted lenses for **industrial applications** are usually highly absorptive and are especially constructed to eliminate ultraviolet and infrared to provide maximum protection for welders, glassblowers, steel processing attendants, and so forth. Light tints for cosmetic effect are not adequate for protection in bright sunlight. If the tints are too dark, they can reduce visual efficiency under conditions of low illumination. **Yellow lenses** absorb all of the ultraviolet and most of the blue light, but none of the infrared. These lenses are designed to improve visual efficiency on hazy, bright, or overcast days, but are not effective as sunglasses and should not be used to improve night vision. **Polarized** lenses are helpful where there is a great deal of reflected glare, such as on the water. In **aphakia,** lightly tinted lenses and ultraviolet absorption are helpful because removal of the crystalline lens results in increased sensitivity to light and decreased ultraviolet absorption.

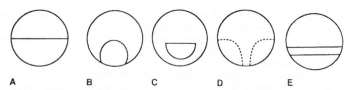

FIG. 14.6. Bifocal styles with segment (reading add) insets in distance correction. **A:** Executive (wide close work field). **B, C:** Insets allowing more inferior peripheral vision than A. **D:** Progressive multifocal lens (dotted lines not visible; denote power channel add of increasing strength inferiorly. **E:** Executive trifocal (may be done in B and C styles also) gives intermediate and close focal lengths in mid and lowest add, respectively.

D. **Single- and multiple-power lenses**
   1. **Single-vision** corrective lenses that have the same correction over the entire surface are referred to as *single-vision lenses* and are used to correct hyperopia, myopia, astigmatism, presbyopia, or aphakia.
   2. **Multifocals.** Lenses can be made with more than one corrective power. If one portion of the lens corrects the distance vision and the other corrects the near vision, as in presbyopia, it is referred to as a **bifocal** lens (Fig. 14.6). If an additional power is added for intermediate-range vision, it is referred to as a **trifocal** lens. The strength of the middle segment of the trifocal is usually 50% that of the net near add (see sec. **VI.B.6.,** above). Bifocals and trifocals can be manufactured by altering the anterior and posterior lens curvature, allowing for multiple powers in one continuous lens, or by fusing a smaller piece of higher-density glass into the crown portion to make a fused multifocal lens. Special occupational multifocal lenses are available.
   3. **Progressive lenses** are multifocal lenses with no visible line separating the distance from the add and no image jump. Although increasingly popular among middle-aged patients because of the cosmetic appearance and ability to focus at about any distance with ease, they are sometimes visually less satisfactory than fused or segmented bifocals for prolonged reading. This occurs because progressive lenses offer a narrower field of view as the eye moves down to look through a stronger part of the lens. Because of this restrictive channel, progressive lenses must be aligned with the eyes with great precision. Improved wider-channel lenses are now available; these minimize the distortion of vision if the patient's eyes move to the right or left of the channel. They also minimize the lateral head movement necessary while reading at close distances. Normal tracking and saccadic eye movements are used for close reading, affording the patient greater comfort (Fig. 14.6).
E. **Prescribing spectacles.** It is important to understand that although prescribing spectacles involves writing a series of numbers on a piece of paper, arriving at the most appropriate set of numbers for a particular patient is not a mathematical certainty. **The amount of ametropia measured and what the patient will tolerate with comfort are frequently not the same.** For example, the young hyperope frequently cannot fully relax accommodation and will not tolerate full correction. The patient with astigmatism that has previously been uncorrected may be uncomfortable if all of his or her astigmatism is corrected at once. Presbyopes of the same age have different body configurations, visual habits, and work requirements, all of which will affect with the appropriate amount of reading correction. The effect of the spectacle correction on extraocular muscle balance via central nervous system mechanisms may also help determine the amount of correction the physician wishes to prescribe. In higher degrees of ametropia, if the distance

at which the spectacle lens is going to rest in front of the cornea varies from the distance at which the ametropia was measured, an adjustment has to be made. In some patients, particularly high myopes and astigmats, altering the form or shape of the corrective spectacle lens, even though the power remains the same, can result in spatial aberrations that can be very annoying. Safety considerations, the use of appropriate tints, **100% ultra-violet screen,** antiglare coat if needed, occupational considerations, and appropriate frame design for the patient's physiognomy must also be taken into consideration. Cosmesis is important, but should not override functional considerations. The dispensing optician should be skilled in advising patients with regard to these aspects of the prescription in addition to ensuring that the prescription is filled accurately.

VIII. **Contact lenses** rest on the surface of the cornea. Different principles of refraction and optics apply to contact lenses than apply to spectacle lenses. The spherical anterior surface of a contact lens and the retro tear film layer actually replace the cornea as a refractive surface. The tear layer that forms behind the lens, in front of the cornea, is called the **lacrimal lens.** Because the indexes of refraction of the lacrimal lens and cornea, as a whole, are basically the same, the anterior aspect of the tear film becomes an artificial optical extension of the corneal surface. The anterior surface of the contact lens is spherical and as a result, the cornea for refractive purposes behaves as a sphere. The remaining refractive error within the eye need only be neutralized with power in the contact lens. Most astigmatism is a result of the toricity on the front corneal surface.

Rigid (hard) contact lenses can completely eliminate corneal astigmatism. Soft lenses however, mold to the surface of the cornea. Given this fact, **astigmatism will persist** and toric correction may need to be added to the contact lens itself. This persistent optical toricity is referred to as **residual astigmatism.** Residual astigmatism is occasionally found with rigid lenses also, especially when the astigmatism is due to toricity in surfaces other than the front surface of the cornea. It is possible to manufacture contact lenses with toric surfaces to correct residual astigmatism. Because contact lenses tend to rotate on the surface of the tear film, methods for stabilizing the toric lens and limiting rotation need to be employed.

In the correction of myopia, the contact lens sits closer to the eye (farther from the far point) than spectacles and is slightly weaker than a spectacle prescription for the same patient. In hyperopia and aphakia, the contact lens is closer to the far point (see secs. **VI.B.1.,5.** and **7.,** above) and consequently has to be stronger than the corresponding spectacle lens correction. In the past several years there has been a gradual evolution in contact lens manufacturing technology. This advanced technology has offered the introduction of new materials and designs that have contributed to high contact lens success rates and many happy patients.

A. **Advantages.** Contact lenses may have optical advantages for most patients in addition to the cosmetic benefit and the convenience of not having to wear glasses. There are many examples of the advantages presented by the use of contact lenses. In high degrees of ametropia, peripheral distortions are reduced with contact lenses. This is due to the small diameter of the lens and the fact that when well centered, the lens will refract paraxial rays without peripheral rays, thereby reducing image distortion. In monocular aphakia, a reduction of the image size with contact lenses generally allows the patient to enjoy the benefits of binocular vision again. Similarly, even binocular aphakics enjoy better peripheral vision, minimal distortion, and reduced magnification while wearing contact lenses. In patients with keratoconus or an irregular cornea for some other reason, satisfactory vision can frequently be achieved with contact lenses when little or no improvement can be obtained with spectacles. The advantages for those engaged in athletics or with special occupational needs are obvious.

B. **Disadvantages.** There are some clear disadvantages to the use of contact lenses. Contact lenses can be expensive and easily lost or destroyed.

Rigid lenses are initially uncomfortable and require a period of adaptation. Soft lenses are more comfortable initially, but they may not be well tolerated by some patients after long-term use. Frequently, soft lenses do not provide satisfactory correction of vision due to residual astigmatism. With the exception of extended-wear lenses, which are asepticized or replaced at prescribed intervals, the daily care and cleaning of contact lenses are important and must be done on a routine basis. Some contact lens wearers are unwilling or unable to follow the required maintenance regimen. Lens wearing time may be limited by physiologic factors, and the patient may still have to wear glasses part of the time. Superficial ocular infections become more significant in the soft contact lens patient. Corneal ulcers may occur with contact lenses; they never occur as a result of wearing spectacles. Foreign bodies may become entrapped under a contact lens instead of being immediately washed away by tears. This can result in significant discomfort and it may require removal of the lens at a highly inconvenient time. In general, it is safe to wear contact lenses for correction of ametropia, provided there are no medical contraindications. Patients should be made aware of their limitations as well as their advantages. **Table 14.3** summarizes contact lens-induced ocular disorders.

C. **Hard lenses** are made of polymethylmethacrylate (PMMA) and are cut with a lathe. They are extremely rigid, very durable, are easy to clean, may be stored wet or dry, and provide excellent correction of vision for the vast majority of patients. PMMA materials boast superior optical properties, but are not flexible and are essentially gas impermeable. Virtually all of the oxygen that reaches the cornea under PMMA lenses does so by means of the tear pump. Given that corneal epithelium has a high metabolic rate and the oxygen solubility in tears is limited, a satisfactory flow of tears must be maintained to prevent corneal epithelial decompensation ultimately resulting in **"overwear syndrome."** This syndrome, a short time after removal of the lenses, causes a patient to experience spectacle blur, injection, and severe pain. All of these symptoms are directly correlated with the degree of corneal swelling present at the time. Hence, PMMA polymers are rarely if ever used today. Finally, the incidence of **infectious ulcerative keratitis** is 2 in 10,000 in PMMA lens wearers and 4 in 10,000 for rigid gas-permeable (RGP) lens wearers.

D. **Gas-permeable lenses.** Technological advancements in contact lens material chemistry have continued to drive **RGP** lens usage for the past two decades.

1. Current **RGP polymers** include fluorosilicone acrylate; cellulose acetate butyrate (CAB); silicone cross-linked with PMMA, as well as others. These materials exhibit varying degrees of oxygen permeability and interfere less with corneal epithelial metabolism than PMMA. They result in little or no corneal edema and few instances of overwear syndrome. In selected cases, lenses designed specifically to enhance gas transmissibility and limit protein and other deposits can be worn for several days or weeks without being removed (although this is not usually advised). Each of the RGP polymers has different properties suitable for different types of applications. Understanding the material properties is important when fitting a lens. This helps to ensure the best possible visual acuity, patient comfort, and eye health.

2. Basic **RGP material properties** include wetting angle, gas permeability, index of refraction, and color.

a. **Wetting angle** is the property that describes how well the tear film will spread across the lens surface. The lower the wetting angle, the better the lens surface will wet. The wetting of the polymer is important to ensure patient comfort.

b. **Gas permeability (D_k)** is the measure of the plastic's ability to allow gasses, particularly oxygen, to pass through it. PMMA plastic does not transmit any oxygen so it has a $D_k = 0$. Commonly used RGP materials have a Dk between 15 and 90. The thickness of the

TABLE 14.3. CONTACT LENS-INDUCED DISORDERS

Disorder	Clinical Signs
Metabolic	
1. Overwear syndrome (acute epithelial necrosis)	Central punctate epithelial erosions or ulcer; with or without stromal edema, hyperemia
2. Tight lens syndrome	As above; ciliary injection; nonmoving lens
3. Epithelial edema (Sattler veil)	Dull corneal reflex, central epithelial edema of overwear
4. Microcystic epitheliopathy	Painful minierosions, clear or opaque epithelial cysts, common in extended-wear soft contact lens wearers
5. Stromal edema	Deep folds associated with severe overwear syndrome
6. Neovascularization (superficial and deep)	Hypoxia-induced vessels; lipid keratopathy with deep vessels
7. Endothelial polymegatheism/ pleomorphism	Hypoxic/acidic-induced polymegatheism/ pleomorphism
Traumatic	
8. Corneal abrasion	Linear or sharp-edged epithelial defect; hyperemia (foreign body under or deposits on lens, poor fit, insertion/ removal trauma)
9. Anterior stromal opacity	Long-term hard lens-related central superficial white stromal opacity; vision change
Toxic/allergic	
10. Enzyme/toxic keratopathy	Painful, widespread epithelial punctate stain; ciliary injection, after inserting proteolytic enzyme/chemically preserved-soaked lens
11. Thimerosal keratopathy	Thimerosal (or other) preservative superior limbal injection, punctate keratitis, superior microcysts, hyperemia
12. Giant lens-related papillary conjunctivitis	Itching; mucoid discharge; upper tarsal hyperemia; fine or cobblestone papillae
13. Lens-related red eye	Hyperemia; punctate keratitis; papillae and follicles
14. Sterile keratitis	Small, often nonstaining, self-limited, peripheral white infiltrates; discomfort; hyperemia
15. Microbial keratitis	Epithelial ulcer over stromal white infiltrate, edema, adherent mucous. *Pseudomonas* suspect in contact lens wearers
Tear resurfacing disorders	
16. 3 and 9 o'clock stain (severe-dellen)	Drying adjacent to lens; punctate stain 3 and 9 o'clock, with or without superficial vascularized scars; interpalpebral hyperemia
17. Incomplete blink stain	Inferior/palpebral punctate stain plus hyperemia
18. Dimple veil	Static air bubbles under lens cause fluorescein pool in epithelial depression

(Adapted from Stapleton F, Dart D, Minassian D. Nonulcerative complications of contact lens wear. *Arch Ophthalmol* 1992; 110:1601.)

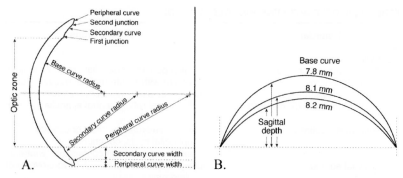

FIG. 14.7. A: The base curve and diameter of a lens are altered to achieve an optimum sagittal depth (sag). As the radius of curvature becomes smaller, the lens becomes steeper and the sag increases. A larger-diameter lens has greater sag than a smaller-diameter lens. The size of the sag helps to determine what the lens will look like on the eye. **B:** The cross section of a contact lens. Note that the peripheral curve radius is longer than the base curve radius. This allows for the gradual flattening of the lens into the periphery.

lens also impacts the amount of oxygen that is transmitted through to the eye. Given the same material, a lens with a thick center (i.e., high plus or biconvex), will transmit less oxygen than a lens of thin center (i.e., high minus or biconcave).

c. **Index of refraction** refers to ability of the material to bend (refract) light (see sec. **I.D.,** above). **Lens color** is best described as a visibility tint. RGP color is not opaque and cannot change the color of the eye. The main reason to tint an RGP is to allow the patient to see the lens more readily (in the case or the sink). RGP materials may also be manufactured with UV protection, which is not detectable to the wearer but offers maximum protection to the eye against UV light. Importantly, aphakic patients should have UV protection in their RGP lenses. Given the absence of the crystalline lens, the retina and posterior structures are offered protection by the RGP.

d. **Specifications.** Once a polymer is chosen, the RGP lens is manufactured with certain prescribed specifications. The basic lens parameters are customized for each patient and will vary from patient to patient. One of the advantages that a RGP lens has over a soft lens is the ability to custom fit the patient. Required contact lens parameters include base curve, lens power, peripheral curve radii, peripheral curve width, optic zone diameter, center thickness, and lenticulation (Fig. 14.7A,B).

(1) The **base curve** defines the radius of curvature to be cut on the posterior surface of the lens. The base curve is selected to ensure a comfortable and healthy fit for the patient. It is also selected to make sure the lens centers on the eye and provides an adequate tear flow to the central corneal surface. The base curve is measured in millimeters or diopters. It can be measured with an instrument called a radiuscope. A typical base curve range is from 8.40 mm (40.25 D) to 7.00 mm (48.25 D).

(2) The **lens power** is generated by controlling the relationship between the front surface curvature of the lens to the base curve. Power is prescribed in diopters. Most powers range from −25.00 to +25.00 D. If a zero power lens is desired, the power is referred to as plano. As a general rule, the higher the power of a plus lens, the steeper the front curve. The reverse is true for a minus

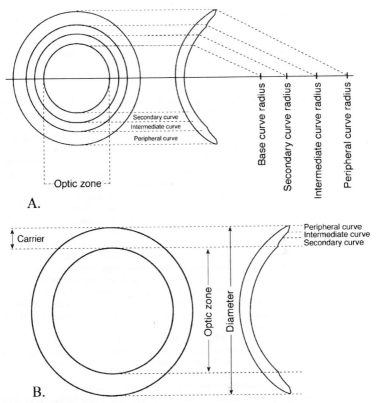

FIG. 14.8. A: The posterior surface of a rigid gas-permeable lens. A lens with a base curve and three peripheral curves is called a tetracurve lens. **B:** The central cornea is similar in shape to a parabola. By adding flatter secondary and peripheral curves, the lens fits the exact shape of the cornea from center to the limbus.

lens; the higher the minus power, the flatter the front curve. Lens power can be measured using a lensometer. When a lens is thick (power greater than +4.50 D), the power reading will be different when measuring the front surface verses the back surface. For this reason, the measurement direction must be specified. Power can be read as front vertex power or back vertex power. Lenses are most often referred to in terms of back vertex power.

(3) **Peripheral curves** are necessary to ensure a good fitting lens and adequate tear exchange. Because the human cornea is not perfectly spherical, the edge of the back surface of the contact lens must be flattened somewhat to sit comfortably on the eye. This is done by cutting a series of curves into the periphery of the lens. The peripheral curve radii are always flatter (larger radius) than the base curve. Peripheral curve radii range between 8.40 and 13.00 mm. The **peripheral curve width** is measured in millimeters along the plane of the lens diameter. Each curve has a width measurement associated with it. These range from 0.10 to 0.45 mm (Fig.14.8A, B).

(4) **The optic zone diameter** is the width of the curve produced by the base curve cut. The optic zone is the area through which the

image will be focused and contains the critical optical properties of the lens. The size of the optic zone ranges between 6.0 and 8.5 mm. The **center thickness** is the measure in millimeters of the lens thickness in the center of the optic zone. The thickness is a function of the lens power and diameter; clinically, it is most desirable to have a lens with a center thickness of less than 0.10 mm, because this enhances patient comfort.

(5) **Lenticulation** of the edge or center of a lens is used to reduce the mass of a lens or limit edge thickness. Lenses with high plus powers will be thick in the center, which will increase the lens mass. A minus lenticular can be ordered and material removed from the anterior center of the lens to reduce the weight of the lens and overall thickness. A plus lenticular is used on high minus lenses to remove material from the anterior edges, producing a thinner edge design.

(6) **The lens designs** that various parameter combinations create can be applied appropriately once the parameters necessary to manufacture an RGP lens are defined. Basically, RGP lenses are designed based on the corneal curvatures, amount of corneal astigmatism, manifest refraction, lid position, and palpebral aperture size of the eye. Lenses can be designed in spherical, back surface toric, front surface toric, and bitoric forms.

(a) A **spherical lens** is the most common and is used to correct simple myopia and hyperopia. A spherical lens has the same radius of curvature from one cross-sectional plane to another. This applies to both the front and back surface of the lens. One base curve radius and one power are used to define a spherical lens.

(b) A **back surface toric** lens has two different base curves and one front curve. Thus, it is defined with two base curves and one power. The angle between the two base curves is always 90 degrees.

(c) A **front surface toric** lens has one toric curve found on the front surface of the lens and one base curve. This lens is commonly used for patients with a small amount of corneal astigmatism (less than 1.00 D) and large amounts of astigmatism in the crystalline lens of the eye.

(d) A **bitoric** lens has toric curves on the front and back surface of the lens. A bitoric lens is defined by listing the two base curves for the back surface and the two power readings for the front surface. This lens type is commonly used for patients with large amounts of corneal and residual astigmatism.

(7) **Tear film patterns.** The primary force that holds the RGP lens against the cornea is the fluid attraction forces produced by the tear layer. The ability of the tear layer to maintain the lens on the eye is directly determined by two factors: (a) the physical characteristics of the tear layer, and (b) the geometric relationship between the posterior lens shape and the corneal surface. It is for this reason that all RGP lens wearers should have a careful examination of the tear film with lenses on the eye. This testing is best accomplished by placing a drop of fluorescein in the eye and examining the contact lens **fluorescein tear exchange pattern.** The tear exchange patterns vary based on the lens and its fitting relationship with the cornea (**see color plates**).

Although RGP lenses represent a significant and exciting part of contact lens practice, there is still some concern among lens fitters. Not all labs manufacture lenses the same way. A lens produced at one lab may fit differently than the same-parameter lens ordered from a different lab. Even when reproducibility at a given lab is good, all lenses must be manually verified by the practitioner to ensure accuracy. Admittedly, this task can be very time consuming. Although many companies are working to achieve the ultimate polymer, a good material for prolonged, continuous wear of RGP contact lenses is still to be identified (see sec. **VIII.C.**, above, regarding ulcerative keratitis).

E. **Daily-wear soft lenses** are made of polymers containing 2-hydroxyethyl methacrylate (HEMA) or related monomers. HEMA is hydrophilic because the free hydroxyl group attached to it bonds with water. All soft lens polymers have a dry phase and a hydrated phase. When hydrated, water swells the polymer network, separating the molecular segments from each other. Hydrogel lenses have the unique characteristic of retaining a large volume of water in the hydrated phase. The water content, which may vary from 30% to 85% with different polymers, makes them relatively comfortable, easy to adapt to, and useful for intermittent wear. These qualities also limit their usefulness in patients with astigmatism. Even patients without astigmatism are sometimes annoyed by slight changes in vision associated with alteration of the lens surface produced by lid movements or changes in hydration. Soft lenses are difficult to clean and sterilize, and have much more of a tendency to accumulate mucus or precipitates than do RGP lenses. Because they are larger and tend to move less than rigid lenses, foreign bodies are generally not much of a problem. They are also less likely to be displaced on the eye or to fall out. Lack of oxygenation to the cornea is of great concern for soft lens wearers because it limits the amount of time the lenses may be worn continuously. The disposable variety, or the so-called "thin lenses," help to minimize problems with oxygenation, but they are more difficult to handle and are more fragile. In some patients, mechanical compression of the blood vessels, as the result of an improperly fitting soft lens, at the corneoscleral junction results in congestion of the limbal vessels and a tendency to **corneal vascularization.**

1. **Conventional soft lenses** are replaced every 8 to 12 months. They must be removed and cleaned with the strongest cleaning systems available, each night. A weekly enzyme treatment is required to remove proteinaceous deposits. They are available for the correction of high myopia, high hyperopia, and low combined astigmatism and presbyopia.

2. **Disposable soft lenses** are worn by the majority of soft lens wearers. Because they are now manufactured in a wide range of powers, a large segment of the population uses them. They are worn for a given time period (1 day, 1 week, or 1 month), discarded, and replaced with a new lens. Disposable lenses should be removed and cleaned nightly or discarded. Their advantages include: convenience, a wide range of powers available, initial comfort, and minimal lens deposit buildup (proteinaceous and other) due to the timely discard of the lens. Replacing the lens on a frequent schedule reduces the incidence of giant papillary conjunctivitis and red eye. Disadvantages of soft contact lens use include a thin lens design. This allows water to evaporate from the lens matrix and increase the chances of dry eye symptomology. In addition, soft lenses are available in a limited number of base curves and have no proven advantage in reducing the microbial keratitis risk.

F. **Extended-wear contact lenses.** The concept of wearing contact lenses continuously, that is, 24 hours a day, has received a great deal of publicity and has achieved some popularity in the patient population. This approach to wearing contact lenses originally developed in response to the needs of **aphakic patients.** Visual rehabilitation of aphakic patients is greatly enhanced by using contact lenses instead of spectacles (see sec. **VI.B.7.c.,** above).

1. Materials used to manufacture lenses with these characteristics fall into three categories: (a) 55% to 80% "high water content" soft lenses; (b) fluorosilicone acrylate or CAB silicone copolymer rigid lenses; and (c) semisoft pure silicone lenses. Although in vitro studies indicate

considerable variation in oxygen permeability for these materials, clinical studies indicate that correctly fit lenses of each type are **successfully worn in approximately 75% to 85% of properly selected patients** fitted for extended wear. Patients with **certain types of corneal diseases,** such as, dry eyes, chronic lid infections, ocular infections, or those who do not have immediate access to medical care, **should not be fit** with continuous-wear lenses. Every patient considering this mode of wear should be evaluated by an optometrist or ophthalmologist for the presence of any medical contraindications.

2. **Ulcerative keratitis** has proved to be the most vision-threatening disadvantage to cosmetic extended-wear contact lenses. The annual incidence of bacterial keratitis is approximately 20 in 10,000 persons using extended-wear lenses as opposed to only 4 in 10,000 persons using daily-wear lenses. In addition, the risk of developing ulcerative keratitis is 10 to 15 times greater in extended-wear lens users who wear them overnight. This is compared with daily-wear users who do not wear the lenses overnight. As a result of this alarming data, the U.S. Food and Drug Administration has recommended a 6-night, 7-day wear schedule for extended-wear lenses followed by removal and discarding of the lens. It is no longer safe, as it was originally thought, to clean extended-wear lenses and reuse them for a given time interval (see Chapter 5, sec. **XI.**).

3. **Problems** encountered with **continuous-wear contact lenses** *include corneal edema, warpage, vascularization, infections, and iritis* (Chapter 5, **XI.C.**). All have been reported with continuous lens wear, along with a "tight lens" syndrome combining many of these findings. Although most of these changes are reversible, they do occur with sufficient frequency and are severe enough to cause concern among physicians and patients alike. Many patients now wear extended-wear soft contact lenses on a daily-wear basis in an attempt to minimize complications. The buildup of proteinaceous or mineral deposits on the surface of continuously worn lenses (especially the soft and silicone-containing lenses) occurs with a great frequency and necessitates frequent lens replacements. Similarly, lost lenses can necessitate change. Although the initial impetus for the use of continuous-wear lenses centered around the needs of aphakic patients, the increasing safety and success of IOLs have diminished this need considerably, because 95% of cataract patients currently have an IOL implanted at the time of surgery (see Chapter 7). New polymers are constantly being studied to improve and provide a more consistent oxygen delivery to the anterior segment, produce less in vivo lens dehydration, and cause less deposition of the organic and inorganic substances, all of which inhibit the healthy wear of extended-use lenses. The high oxygen-permeable silicone-based lenses must be used with caution because lens dehydration can cause large shifts in the fit, leading to lens adherence and loss of the optical characteristics of the lens.

4. **Extended-wear lenses in the phakic patient.** As contact lens companies continue to develop new and improved extended-wear materials, a tremendous advertising and marketing effort is under way to encourage the use of continuous-wear lenses for cosmetic correction. In most instances, this mode of wear is primarily for purposes of convenience; although some phakic patients experience great difficulty handling their lenses, those with high degrees of ametropia experience additional benefits. On balance, the medical risk–benefit ratio is not as favorable for these patients as for the aphakic patients.

G. **Toric soft lenses** are used when spherical soft lenses are inadequate for masking corneal toricity, or when the cornea is spherical and lenticular astigmatism is present. Truncation, thin zones, or prism ballast is used to prevent the soft lens designs from rotating on the cornea. Truncation and thin zones at the top and bottom of the lens result in an asymmetric shape. Prism ballast results in an asymmetric weight distribution. These efforts have met with limited success. Soft toric lenses work best for low to moderate degrees of astigmatism oriented against the rule (flat axis near the 90 degree meridian) or with the rule (flat axis near the 180 degree meridian). These lenses have a very limited application in oblique astigmatism. Fitting fees and replacement costs for these lenses are significantly higher than for spherical conventional lenses.

H. **Bifocal contact lenses.** Several types of bifocal contact lenses currently are on the market in both soft and RGP designs. Bifocal contact lenses are based on two designs: **simultaneous vision** and **alternating vision.**

1. **Simultaneous-vision lenses** are either annular or aspheric in design. The most commonly used **annular design** has a central area to correct for near vision and a peripheral concentric area to correct distance vision. This design is based on the near miotic pupillary response and corresponding distance mydriasis. The **aspheric design** provides simultaneous vision by allowing the wearer to select preferential rays from either distant objects or near ones. The aspheric bifocal lens is similar to the progressive (no line) bifocal spectacle lens, and is formed by altering the anterior and posterior curves to achieve a given power gradient. The simultaneous-vision bifocal lenses are available in soft and RGP varieties.

2. The **alternating design** is only available as an RGP lens. The design is similar to that of a lined bifocal spectacle lens. The wearer uses one portion of the lens for viewing a distant object and another portion for seeing near targets. It is important that the lens fit well and move on the eye, allowing the transition from distance to near viewing and back. The major limitations with all bifocal lenses are stability of vision and maintaining the proper lens position for the visual task at hand. Although blinking and rapid eye movements can alter the position of the lens in relation to the visual axis and the optic zone, a well-fit lens does offer the presbyopic patient excellent visual acuity and the freedom of not having to wear spectacles. Fitting fees and replacement costs for these lenses are significantly higher than those for conventional single-vision lenses. Some presbyopic patients will benefit from a different approach, referred to as monovision, in which the dominant eye is corrected for distance vision and the nondominant eye is corrected for near vision. *Modified monovision* is also a useful technique, where one bifocal lens and one single-vision lens are used to enhance the intermediate range, a range of vision not corrected for by monovision.

I. **Postsurgical uses of contact lenses.** Corneal surgery can occasionally leave a unique corneal shape and poor visual acuity, thus requiring a contact lens correction. Both RGP and hydrogel lenses have been used for this purpose, but each has advantages and limitations. Corneal surgical procedures can leave the cornea with a flattened central area and a steeper periphery. This is the opposite of the usual relationship between the central and peripheral cornea. In addition, for some patients there is a diurnal variation in refraction or changes in vision in low light conditions when the pupil dilates.

1. **Penetrating keratoplasty (PKP, corneal transplantation).** The usual indication for contact lenses following keratoplasty is to achieve better visual acuity than with spectacles. Unfortunately, some transplants leave the patient with a high or irregular astigmatism in the graft. This can also be surrounded by a host cornea with abnormal shape characteristics. The primary consideration in fitting a post-PKP eye is to fit a lens that does not allow pooling of the tears or touch of the posterior lens surface around sutures, suture scars, or any central irregularity. A uniform fluorescein tear exchange is necessary to prevent corneal desiccation and maintain the optical quality of vision afforded by the retro-lens tear layer *(lacrimal lens)*. In most cases, a good optical result is possible using a small RGP lens with a spherical design. In cases of an oblate graft pattern, where the graft is flatter than the host cornea, a highly technical reverse

geometry design (plateau) RGP lens can be fit with difficulty, but this usually results in an adequate retro-lens tear exchange and visual acuity. Because of their relatively low oxygen transmissibility, soft lenses should never be used in patients after PKP. Very occasionally, a soft bandage lens will be used to improve patient comfort, but this application is limited.

2. **Radial keratotomy (RK)** has essentially been abandoned as a refractive technique. For the patients who have had it, however, the fitting of post-RK patients with contact lenses has proven to be a very challenging task. The indications for a contact lens fitting are many and include: undercorrection, overcorrection, anisometropia, induced astigmatism, flare and glare, haloes, and poor visual acuity in low light conditions. Under and overcorrection can be neutralized with a soft lens, but this can lead to numerous complications in the post-RK patient. Most practitioners agree that the RGP lens provides the best modality for fitting the post-RK cornea. RGP lenses provide better visual results than soft lenses because with a properly fit lens, the retro-lens tear film masks or covers up the corneal irregularities, thus correcting astigmatism as well as providing some relief from glare and fluctuating vision. The gas-permeable lens is usually fit with a flat base curve and large diameter so it bridges the central cornea while providing a good fit in the periphery. Care must be taken to avoid a large area of central retro-lens tear pooling, leading to tear stagnation and eventual breakdown of the cornea beneath. In some cases, the reverse geometry design (plateau) lens is indicated (see Chapter 6).

3. **Photorefractive keratectomy (PRK) and laser in situ keratomileusis (LASIK).** Following PRK or LASIK, a contact lens may be necessary. The indications for fitting are similar if not the same as the RK patient. A soft lens is usually the lens of choice after PRK or LASIK surgery, assuming that there are no surface irregularities present which would require the use of a RGP lens for optical reasons, as discussed previously. After fitting a soft lens it is important to watch the cornea for corneal edema and debris entrapment behind the lens. The soft lens should fit with an even drape over the altered corneal contour (see Chapter 6).

J. **Orthokeratology** is a technique of fitting a rigid gas-permeable lens for the purpose of modifying the refractive error, principally in myopes. A series of RGP lenses are fit over an extended period of time, each lens having a progressively flatter base curve. This is employed in an attempt to induce a flattening effect of the cornea and thereby decrease the amount of myopia. When successful, it is frequently necessary for the patient to wear a retainer lens for part of the time to maintain the induced change. The amount of change that can be produced is limited. Studies report about a 1.00- to 2.50-D decrease in myopia with successful orthokeratology. It has been proposed by some that there are significant risks involved in the application of this technique; however, the literature has not reported any such risks to date. In orthokeratology the myopia reduction *effect is transient* and merely reduces the spectacle correction without curing the myopia. Because of the frequency of follow-up examinations and the multiple lens changes required, orthokeratology is quite expensive. Although performed in many practices, it is not widely accepted as a routine procedure at this time.

IX. **Subnormal (low) vision aids.** Many patients have eye diseases that result in subnormal vision that cannot be corrected medically or surgically. In some cases, these patients can be helped by the use of low vision aids. These aids function by enlarging the retinal image and are of benefit primarily in patients with **macular diseases.** In these patients, the resolving power of the retina is decreased centrally. Enlarging the image causes it to fall on adjacent, normally functioning areas. Because the resolving power of paramacular areas is relatively low, this is not a substitute for macular vision, but it does allow patients to perform some visual functions, such as reading, that they would not otherwise be able to perform. Because magnification of the visual image reduces the size of the visual field, some loss of visual efficiency occurs, particularly for distance vision. These devices usually have no value for patients who have normal visual acuity, but have suffered a loss of peripheral vision, such as in advanced glaucoma.

A. **Physical magnification.** If an object is brought closer to the eye, the angle that it subtends at the nodal point of the eye is increased, and the image that falls on the retina is similarly increased. For example, an object 2 mm long when viewed at a distance of 50 cm produces a retinal image of 0.06 mm. The same 2-mm object viewed at a distance of 5 cm produces a retinal image of 0.6 mm, a magnification of $10\times$. This method of magnification is particularly useful in young patients with a large amplitude of accommodation. It also demonstrates the value of **high plus lenses.** These may range from +4 to +20 D, with a progressively shorter reading distance and smaller visual field as the power increases. To a person motivated to read, these disadvantages are tolerable.

B. **Optical magnification.** A wide variety of **telescopic devices** have been developed to aid patients with subnormal vision. Telescopic systems generally have two lenses and are of the terrestrial type to avoid the image inversion that occurs with celestial telescopes. Binocular lens systems of this type are limited by practical considerations to about $2.2\times$ magnification. Beyond this point, the separation of the two lens elements becomes impractical, and reduction of the visual field becomes excessive. Telescopic systems are primarily used to improve distance vision, because high plus single-lens magnifiers are more efficient and provide greater magnification for near vision. For example, a +20-D magnifying lens produces a magnification of $5\times$. In addition, a single-element **magnifier** held close to the eye results in a better field of view. The field size varies directly with the diameter of the magnifying lens and inversely with the distance the lens is held from the eye. For this reason, high-magnification lenses are usually designed as loupes or as special lenses to be held close to the eye rather than at a normal reading distance. Magnification with loupes or high plus lenses is also greatest when the object to be viewed is held just inside the anterior focal point of the lens. Although this is not always the most comfortable reading distance, it does permit the patient to read print that he or she would not otherwise be able to see. A **projection system** or television extends the range of magnification available, but these systems are not very portable and are usually quite expensive. Although other highly expensive and sophisticated optical systems are available as low vision aids, they seldom result in improved visual efficiency, and it is only rarely that the expense is justified.

X. **Surgical correction of refractive errors** is covered in Chapter 6 on refractive surgery.

15. OCULAR MANIFESTATIONS OF SYSTEMIC DISEASE

Deborah Pavan-Langston

I. **Use of tabulated information.** The eyes are frequently involved in diseases affecting the rest of the body. Ocular manifestations in certain multisystem disorders may offer diagnostic clues to aid in identifying the systemic disease. In other instances, the eye involvement may be subtle enough to avoid detection unless the clinician knows to look for it. Once the diagnosis is made, the major element in therapy of the ophthalmic aspect of the systemic disease is often the treatment and cure of the primary disease itself. This is not always the case, however, and an ophthalmic diagnosis may be necessary to determine the cause of local eye involvement, which may require different management. This chapter provides the clinician with a quick reference for symptoms and signs of ocular disorders associated with the more common systemic diseases. Most are discussed in detail in the appropriate chapters. When dealing with cases in which patients have eye symptoms without a known systemic disease, the clinician should refer those individuals to ophthalmologists for a specific ocular diagnosis. If the patient's systemic disease is known, that individual should be referred to an ophthalmologist mainly for confirmation of the diagnosis and treatment of the ocular component.

This chapter is divided into two parts: The first part outlines major ocular regions affected by systemic diseases and lists, in part, the specific diseases affecting each region.

The second part is a series of tables, each devoted to a major systemic disease. The specific disease entities are listed within the larger classification with their ocular manifestations. Associated findings are indicated for each condition. Chapters covering these and additional diseases are listed below each table.

II. **Ocular regions related to systemic diseases**

  A. **Cornea.** The cornea provides a unique opportunity for observation and diagnosis of systemic diseases and abnormal metabolic processes. It is useful to consider the physical and morphologic properties of the cornea to understand how systemic diseases can affect the cornea and conjunctiva.

    1. **Diseases of the skin and mucous membranes.** The corneal epithelium is of ectodermal embryologic origin. Systemic skin and mucous membrane disorders also affect the cornea. Corneal and conjunctival bullae, severe inflammation, and sloughing of the epithelium may occur in the following diseases:

      a. Atopic dermatitis.

      b. Cicatricial pemphigoid.

      c. Epidermolysis bullosa.

      d. Erythema multiforme (Stevens-Johnson syndrome).

      e. Ichthyosis.

      f. Pemphigus.

      g. Phacomatoses.

      h. Psoriasis.

      i. Xeroderma pigmentosa.

    2. **Disorders of collagen metabolism.** The rest of the cornea is of mesodermal embryologic origin. Disorders of collagen metabolism may affect the cornea, possibly inducing keratoconus changes. Two of the most prominent are

      a. Ehlers-Danlos syndrome.

      b. Marfan syndrome.

    3. **Collagen diseases.** Much of the cornea is made of collagen and mucopolysaccharide ground substance. Systemic diseases affecting collagen

may indirectly affect the cornea by way of autoantibodies in the circulation. Marked limbal and marginal corneal ulceration may result. Six systemic diseases affecting collagen that commonly involve the cornea are
   a. Dermatomyositis.
   b. Periarteritis nodosa.
   c. Relapsing polychondritis
   d. Rheumatoid arthritis.
   e. Wegener granulomatosis.
   f. Systemic lupus erythematosus.
4. **Metabolic diseases.** The cornea stores materials made in excess by the body. Damage to the cornea may occur indirectly by accumulation of metabolic products. Systemic metabolic diseases that produce elevated levels of certain precursors and that may opacify the cornea, producing band keratopathy or lipid keratopathy, are
   a. Amyloidosis.
   b. Cystinosis.
   c. Glycogen storage disease.
   d. Gout.
   e. Hyperlipidemia.
   f. Mucopolysaccharidoses (Hurler, Scheie, Hurler-Scheie, Hunter, Sanfilippo, Morquio Maroteaux-Lamy syndromes).
   g. Hypervitaminosis D.
   h. Wilson's disease.
5. **Environmentally caused disorders.** The cornea is the most anterior part of the eye, exposed to environmental harm. Exposure keratitis and infections may occur where there is poor protective function of the cornea. Environmental hazards include:
   a. Exposure (drying, radiant and ionizing energy).
   b. Infectious agents (bacteria, viruses, fungi, and parasites).
B. Cataracts. Cataracts are associated with many systemic diseases. Lens fibers opacify as a response to alterations of the physical and chemical milieu within the semipermeable lens capsule. The exact type of cataract that forms may be distinct from the usual senile lens opacities and may be characteristic for the specific disease entity. Cataracts may be associated with the following systemic diseases:
1. **Chromosomal disorders**
   a. Alport syndrome.
   b. Cri du chat syndrome.
   c. Conradi syndrome.
   d. Crouzon syndrome.
   e. Myotonia dystrophica.
   f. Patau syndrome.
   g. Schmidt-Fraccaro syndrome.
   h. Trisomy 18 (Edwards syndrome).
   i. Turner syndrome.
2. **Diseases of the skin and mucous membranes**
   a. Atopic dermatitis.
   b. Basal-cell nevus syndrome.
   c. Ichthyosis.
   d. Pemphigus.
3. **Metabolic and nutrition diseases**
   a. Aminoaciduria (Lowe syndrome).
   b. Diabetes mellitus.
   c. Fabry's disease.
   d. Galactosemia.
   e. Homocystinuria.
   f. Hypervitaminosis D.
   g. Hypoparathyroidism.
   h. Hypothyroidism.

        i. Mucopolysaccharidoses.

        j. Wilson's disease.

  4. Infectious diseases

      a. Congenital

        (1) Congenital herpes simplex.

        (2) Congenital syphilis.

        (3) Cytomegalic inclusion disease.

        (4) Rubella.

      b. Others

        (1) Cysticercosis.

        (2) Leprosy.

        (3) Onchocerciasis.

        (4) Toxoplasmosis.

  5. Toxic substances introduced systemically (see Chapter 16):

      a. Corticosteroids.

      b. Haloperidol.

      c. Miotics.

      d. Triparanol (MER/29).

C. Glaucoma is not exclusively the result of a hereditary predisposition (as in primary glaucoma). Secondary glaucomas may arise as complications of the systemic disease itself or from its therapy. Systemic diseases that may cause glaucoma are

  1. Hematologic and cardiovascular diseases

      a. Carotid—cavernous fistulas.

      b. Leukemia.

      c. Sickle cell disease.

      d. Waldenström macroglobulinemia.

  2. Collagen diseases

      a. Dermatomyositis.

      b. Periarteritis nodosa.

      c. Relapsing polychondritis.

      d. Rheumatoid arthritis.

      e. Wegener granulomatosis.

      f. Systemic lupus erythematosus.

  3. Diseases of skin and mucous membranes

      a. Atopic diseases (corticosteroid use).

      b. Nevus of Ota.

  4. Infectious diseases

      a. Congenital rubella.

      b. Herpes simplex or zoster.

      c. Onchocerciasis.

  5. Metabolic diseases

      a. Amyloidosis.

      b. Marchesani syndrome.

  6. Musculoskeletal diseases

      a. Conradi syndrome.

      b. Osteogenesis imperfecta.

  7. Neoplastic diseases: metastasis to the trabecular meshwork

  8. Phacomatoses

      a. Neurofibromatosis.

      b. Sturge-Weber syndrome.

  9. Pulmonary diseases: asthma and emphysema (corticosteroid use).

  10. Renal diseases

      a. Lowe syndrome (aminoaciduria).

      b. Wilms tumor.

      c. Renal transplantation (corticosteroid use).

  11. Toxic substances (see Chapter 16)

      a. Amphetamines.

      b. Anticholinergics.

      c. Corticosteroids.
      d. Hexamethonium.
      e. Reserpine.
      f. Tricyclic antidepressants.
    12. Unknown etiology
      a. Sarcoidosis.
D. Uveitis resulting from systemic diseases presents a difficult diagnostic problem. Inflammation of the iris, ciliary body, and choroid may be caused by a wide variety of diseases.
    1. Systemic allergic diseases: hay fever.
    2. Cardiovascular diseases: endocarditis (subacute bacterial).
    3. Collagen diseases
      a. Ankylosing spondylitis.
      b. Periarteritis nodosa.
      c. Reiter syndrome.
      d. Relapsing polychondritis.
      e. Rheumatoid arthritis.
      f. Systemic lupus erythematosus.
      g. Wegener granulomatosis.
    4. Diseases of skin and mucous membranes
      a. Acne rosacea.
      b. Behçet's disease.
      c. Erythema multiforme (Stevens-Johnson syndrome).
      d. Psoriasis.
      e. Vogt-Koyanagi-Harada (VKH) syndrome.
    5. Metabolic diseases
      a. Amyloidosis.
      b. Gout.
    6. Gastrointestinal and nutritional diseases
      a. Regional enteritis.
      b. Peptic ulcer disease.
      c. Ulcerative colitis.
    7. Neoplastic disease
      a. Lymphoma.
      b. Reticulum cell sarcoma.
    8. Toxic substances (see Chapter 16)
      a. Sulfonamides.
      b. Reserpine.
    9. Infectious diseases
      a. Brucellosis.
      b. Gonorrhea.
      c. Leprosy.
      d. Onchocerciasis.
      e. Tuberculosis.
      f. Toxoplasmosis.
      g. Viral infections. (Herpes simplex or zoster, cytomegalovirus, human immunodeficiency virus [HIV]).
    10. Unknown etiology
      a. Sarcoidosis.
E. Retina. The retina is vulnerable to systemic diseases that affect specific retinal tissue elements such as retinal vessels, choroid (microaneurysms, hemorrhages, exudates, hemangiomas, choroiditis), neural tissue (retinitis, exudative retinal detachment, selective rod and cone destruction), and retinal pigment epithelium (loss of pigment, accumulation of toxic substances). The systemic diseases affecting the retina are
    1. Cardiovascular diseases
      a. Aortic arch syndrome (Takayasu syndrome).
      b. Endocarditis.
      c. Hereditary telangiectasia (Rendu-Osler-Weber syndrome).

     d. Hypertension and toxemia of pregnancy.
     e. Occlusive vascular disease.
  2. Collagen diseases
     a. Dermatomyositis.
     b. Periarteritis nodosa.
     c. Reiter syndrome.
     d. Systemic lupus erythematosus.
     e. Temporal arteritis.
     f. Wegener granulomatosis.
  3. Chromosomal disorders
     a. Cri du chat syndrome.
     b. Schmidt-Fraccaro syndrome.
     c. Turner syndrome.
     d. Trisomy 18 (Edwards syndrome).
     e. Deletion of chromosome 18.
     f. Trisomy 13 (Patau syndrome).
     g. Ring-D chromosome.
  4. Endocrine diseases
     a. Diabetes mellitus.
     b. Cushing syndrome.
     c. Hyperthyroidism.
     d. Hypothyroidism.
     e. Hypoparathyroidism.
  5. Diseases of skin and mucous membranes
     a. Behçet's disease.
     b. Ichthyosis.
     c. Incontinentia pigmenti.
     d. Pseudoxanthoma elasticum.
     e. VKH syndrome.
  6. Gastrointestinal and nutritional diseases
     a. Regional enteritis.
     b. Vitamin A deficiency.
  7. Hematologic diseases
     a. Anemias.
     b. Leukemias.
     c. Polycythemia vera.
     d. Sickle cell disease.
     e. Thrombocytopenia.
     f. Waldenström macroglobulinemia.
  8. Infectious diseases
     a. *Candida* retinitis.
     b. Histoplasmosis.
     c. Parasites.
     d. Septicemia.
     e. Viral infections.
     f. Tuberculosis.
     g. HIV.
     h. Herpes simplex or zoster.
     i. Cytomegalovirus.
  9. Phacomatoses: most affect the retina.
 10. Pulmonary diseases
     a. Bronchiectasis.
     b. Cystic fibrosis.
     c. Pneumonia.
 11. Renal diseases
     a. Alport syndrome.
     b. Medullary cystic disease.
     c. Nephrotic syndrome.

   12. **Metabolic diseases**
       a. Albinism.
       b. Amyloidosis.
       c. Cystinosis.
       d. Fabry's disease.
       e. Gaucher's disease.
       f. Niemann-Pick disease.
       g. Lipidoses.
   13. **Neoplastic diseases:** Most can affect the retina.
   14. Unknown etiology
       a. Sarcoidosis.
III. **Specific systemic diseases and their ocular manifestations.** Tables 15.1 through 15.17 list several of the more important systemic disorders that may affect the eye, their clinical ocular manifestations, the clinical and laboratory tests indicated to detect suspected underlying systemic disease, differential diagnosis, and indications for referral to a specialist. **Many systemic conditions, along with others not included in the tables, are also listed in the index or listed in the footnotes of each pertinent table for text page location.** The systemic diseases that may affect the eye are
   A. Systemic allergic diseases. See Chapter 5, sec. **VII.** for atopic eczema, atopic keratoconjunctivitis (hay fever), vernal conjunctivitis, urticaria, and asthma.
   B. Diseases of the skin and mucous membranes (Table 15.1).
   C. Phacomatoses. See Chapter 8, sec. **III.** for angiomatosis retinae (von Hippel's disease) and Chapter 11, sec. **VIII.** for angiomatosis retinae (von Hippel's disease), ataxia—telangiectasia (Louis-Bar syndrome), encephalotrigeminal angiomatosis (Sturge-Weber syndrome), neurofibromatosis (von Recklinghausen's disease), tuberous sclerosis (Bourneville's disease), and Wyburn-Mason syndrome.
   D. Collagen diseases (Table 15.2).
   E. Systemic viral infections (Table 15.3).
   F. Systemic bacterial infections (Table 15.4).
   G. Systemic chlamydial and protozoal infections (Table 15.5).
   H. Systemic fungal infections (Table 15.6).
   I. Systemic cestode and nematode infections (Table 15.7).
   J. Chromosomal disorders (Table 15.8).
   K. Hematologic diseases (Table 15.9).
   L. Cardiovascular diseases (Table 15.10).
   M. Endocrine diseases (Table 15.11).
   N. Gastrointestinal and nutritional disorders (Table 15.12).
   O. Metabolic diseases (Table 15.13).
   P. Musculoskeletal diseases (Table 15.14).
   Q. Pulmonary diseases (Table 15.15).
   R. Renal diseases (Table 15.16).
   S. Neoplastic diseases with ocular metastases (Table 15.17).

TABLE 15.1. DISEASES OF THE SKIN AND MUCOUS MEMBRANES[a]

1. Atopic dermatitis
Conjunctivitis
Posterior subcapsular cataracts
Keratoconus
Associated findings: family history, allergy tests
2. Epidermolysis bullosa
Lid bullae
Lacrimal duct stenosis
Blepharitis
Conjunctival hyperemia
Hypertrichosis
Corneal: bullae, erosions, perforation
Associated findings: family history, skin biopsy
3. Psoriasis
Scaly plaques on lids
Conjunctivitis
Keratitis: punctate, focal stromal opacities, ulcers
Iritis
4. Xeroderma pigmentosum
Lid malignancies
Symblepharon
Keratitis
Associated findings: skin biopsy

---

[a]See also **Chapter 5:** atopic eczema, atopic keratoconjunctivitis, vernal conjunctivitis, urticaria, hay fever, rosacea, erythema multiforme (Stevens-Johnson syndrome), cicatricial pemphigoid.
Chapter 9: psoriasis, Kawasaki's disease, ischemic ocular syndrome, Behçet's disease, Vogt-Koyanagi-Harada syndrome. **Chapter 11:** erythema multiforme, albinism, Ehlers-Danlos syndrome, pseudoxanthoma elasticum.

TABLE 15.2. COLLAGEN DISEASES[a]

1. Dermatomyositis
Diplopia
Extraocular muscle palsy
Lid edema and redness
Retinal hemorrhages and exudates
Associated findings: increased erythrocyte sedimentation rate and creatine
   phosphokinase
Skin biopsy
Electromyography
2. Periarteritis nodosa
Nystagmus
Extraocular muscle palsy
Ptosis
Nodular scleritis
Episcleritis
Peripheral ulcerative keratitis
Uveitis
Retinal hemorrhage
Papilledema
Fever of unknown origin
Arteritis
Associated findings: vasculitis (skin biopsy)
3. Scleroderma
Tense skin, lid margin scars and loss
Keratitis
Peripheral ulcerative keratitis
Retinopathy
Associated findings: skin biopsy
4. Systemic lupus erythematosus
Diskoid skin lesions
Conjunctivitis
Episcleritis
Iritis
Retinal edema, hemorrhages, exudates
Papilledema
Associated findings: antinuclear cytoplasmic antibody, lupus erythematosus
   preparation
5. Wegener granulomatosis
Necrotizing granulomas orbit and nose
Peripheral ulcerative keratitis
Uveitis, retinal arteriolar narrowing, cotton-wool spots, hemorrhages
Papilledema
Associated findings: antinuclear cytoplasmic antibody, biopsy lesion

[a]See also **Chapter 5:** rheumatoid arthritis, lupus erythematosus, pemphigoid, erythema multiforme, scleroderma, periarteritis nodosa, Wegener granulomatosis. **Chapter 9:** ankylosing spondylitis, Reiter syndrome, juvenile rheumatoid arthritis. **Chapter 13:** temporal arteritis (giant cell or cranial arteritis).

TABLE 15.3. SYSTEMIC VIRAL INFECTIONS[a]

1. **Human immunodeficiency virus (HIV)**
   Conjunctival microvasculopathy (microaneurysms)
   Keratitis (punctate, dendritiform)
   Malignancies (Kaposi sarcoma, lymphoma, squamous cell carcinoma)
   Secondary anterior and posterior segment infections (bacterial, viral, fungal, parasitic)
   Retinal cotton-wool spots, intraretinal hemorrhages, Roth's spots, microaneurysms
   Progressive outer retinal necrosis, acute retinal necrosis
2. **Infectious mononucleosis**
   Lid edema
   Conjunctivitis
   Nummular keratitis
   Iritis
   Dacryocystitis
   Vitritis
   Retinal periphlebitis
   Papillitis
   Associated findings: lymphadenopathy; pharyngitis; lymphocytosis; + heterophile;
      + smears, culture
3. **Influenza**
   Extraocular muscle myalgia and palsy
   Mild keratitis
   Iritis
   Retinal hemorrhage and edema
   Optic neuritis
4. **Mumps**
   Conjunctivitis punctate or interstitial keratitis
   Episcleritis
   Scleritis
   Dacryoadenitis
   Extraocular muscle palsy
   Optic neuritis
   Associated findings: parotid gland inflammation
5. **Rubeola (measles)**
   Koplik's spots on conjunctiva
   Conjunctivitis
   Photophobia
   Punctate keratitis and erosions
   Uveitis
   Optic neuritis
   Retinitis
   Associated findings: multinucleated giant cells in scrapings
6. **Rubella (German measles)**
   Congenital: microphthalmos, cataract, glaucoma, strabismus, nasolacrimal duct
      occlusion, corneal clouding, iris atrophy, iritis, chorioretinitis, optic atrophy
   Associated findings: clinical history; rash; cardiac, hearing, genitourinary disorders
7. **Variola or vaccinia (small pox)**
   Pustular lid eruptions
   Symblepharon or ankyloblepharon
   Trichiasis
   Conjunctivitis
   Necrotic keratitis
   Iritis
   Choroiditis
   Optic neuritis
   Preauricular nodes
   Associated findings: cytoplasmic inclusions; epithelial scrapings; + culture

---

+, positive.
[a]See also **Chapter 5:** adenovirus, acquired immunodeficiency syndrome (AIDS), herpes simplex, herpes zoster, vaccinia, varicella. **Chapter 9:** AIDS, cytomegalovirus, herpes simplex, herpes zoster, Epstein-Barr virus. **Chapter 11:** cytomegalovirus, *Chlamydia,* rubella, herpes simplex, subacute sclerosing panencephalitis.

TABLE 15.4. SYSTEMIC BACTERIAL INFECTIONS[a]

1. Brucellosis
Nodular iritis
Choroiditis
Dacryocystitis
Optic neuritis
Associated findings: + blood culture; hemagglutinins
2. Diphtheria
Pseudomembranous or membranous conjunctivitis
Lid edema
Corneal ulcer (*Corynebacterium diphtheriae* can penetrate intact epithelium)
Associated findings: regional adenopathy; + smears, culture
3. Septicemia bacterial metastatic endophthalmitis
Conjunctival hemorrhage
Iritis
Roth's spots
Endophthalmitis
Retinal hemorrhage; chorioretinitis
Associated findings: + blood culture

[a]See also **Chapter 5:** gonorrhea, ophthalmia neonatorum. **Chapter 9:** tuberculosis. **Chapter 11:** gonorrhea, *Chlamydia,* syphilis.

TABLE 15.5. SYSTEMIC CHLAMYDIAL AND PROTOZOAL INFECTIONS[a]

1. Lymphogranuloma venereum (*Chlamydia*)
Rare massive lid edema from lymphatic obstruction
Conjunctivitis
Keratitis with superficial vascularization
Retinal vessel dilation
Regional adenopathy
Associated findings: + cultures; + complement fixation; + Microtrak
2. Malaria
Conjunctivitis
Keratitis
Iritis
Optic neuritis secondary to antimalarials
Associated findings: + blood smears

[a]See also **Chapter 5:** *Chlamydia.* **Chapter 9:** *Toxoplasma, Toxocara,* other parasites. **Chapter11:** *Chlamydia, Toxoplasma.*

TABLE 15.6. SYSTEMIC FUNGAL INFECTIONS[a]

1. **Coccidioidomycosis**
   Lid skin dermatitis
   Phlyctenular conjunctivitis
   Optic neuritis
   Associated findings: + chest x-ray; + complement fixation
2. ***Cryptococcus* (yeast form)**
   Meningitis
   Eye involved secondarily
   Brow lesions
   Rare endophthalmitis
   Retinitis
   Retinal hemorrhages, detachment (rare)
   Papilledema
   Associated findings: + culture and India ink smears for fungus capsules;
   +/− lymphoma

+, positive or −, negative.
[a]See also **Chapter 3:** *Actinomyces, Streptothrix.* **Chapter 5:** *Candida, Actinomyces, Streptothrix.*
Chapter 9: *Candida,* histoplasmosis.

TABLE 15.7. SYSTEMIC CESTODE AND NEMATODE INFECTIONS[a]

1. **Cysticerosis (tapeworm)**
   Iritis
   Cataract
   Vitreous hemorrhage, cyst
   Retinal detachment
   Associated findings: eosinophilia; geographic locale
3. **Echinococcosis (hydatid cyst)**
   Proptosis (orbital cyst)
   Iritis
   Vitreous cyst
   Retinal cyst
   Associated findings: eosinophilia; geographic locale
4. **Trichinosis**
   Periorbital edema
   Pain on eye movement
   Conjunctival chemosis
   Associated findings: eosinophilia; skin and serologic tests; muscle biopsy
4. **Onchocerciasis**
   Microfilaria in ocular tissues
   Conjunctivitis
   Superficial and deep keratitis
   Cataract
   Iritis
   Chorioretinitis
   Optic atrophy
   Associated findings: tissue biopsy; eosinophilia
5. **Loiasis (*Loa loa*)**
   Microfilaria migrate in superficial eye tissue
   Conjunctivitis
   Keratitis
   Iritis
   Associated findings: eosinophilia; filaria occasionally seen in conjunctiva
   or thick blood smear

[a]See also **Chapter 9:** *Toxocara.* **Chapter 11:** *Toxocara.*

TABLE 15.8. CHROMOSOMAL DISORDERS[a]

1. Schmidt-Fraccaro syndrome
Microphthalmos
Strabismus
Iris and retina coloboma
Hypertelorism
Lateral upward lid slant
Cataract
Choroidal coloboma
Associated findings: karyotyping

2. Ring-D chromosome
Microphthalmos
Hypertelorism
Strabismus
Epicanthus
Ptosis
Retrocorneal membrane
Iris coloboma
Optic disk hypoplasia
Associated findings: karyotyping

3. Monosomy-G syndrome
Ptosis
Epicanthus
Hypertelorism
Strabismus
Cataract
Blepharochalasis
Associated findings: karyotyping

4. Deletion long arm chromosome 13
Hypertelorism
Ptosis
Iris coloboma
Associated findings: karyotyping

5. Deletion chromosome 18
Microphthalmos
Ptosis
Hypertelorism
Long arm: congenital glaucoma, cataract, retinal degeneration, optic atrophy
Short arm: posterior keratoconus
Corneal opacity
Associated findings: karyotyping

[a]See also **Chapter 11:** Cri du chat syndrome, DeGrouchy syndrome, Turner syndrome, trisomies 13 (Patau), 18 (Edwards), and 21 (Down).

TABLE 15.9. HEMATOLOGIC DISEASES

1. Anemias
Subconjunctival hemorrhages
Dilated retinal veins, edema, exudates
Associated findings: hemoglobin concentration less than 5 gm/dl
Folate, B_{12} down; red blood cell count indices; marrow biopsy
2. Leukemias
Orbital infiltration
Proptosis
Exophthalmos
Retinal edema, hemorrhages, tortuous vessels
Papillitis
Associated findings: white blood cell count and differential; marrow biopsy
3. Lymphomas
Exophthalmos
Proptosis
Ocular palsy
Lid edema
Iritis
Vitritis
Associated findings: node biopsy; blood smear; complete blood count; x-rays
4. Multiple myeloma
Conjunctival and corneal crystals
Iris and ciliary body cysts
Retinal hemorrhages, dilated veins
Papilledema
Associated findings: urine Bence-Jones proteins; immunoglobulin electrophoresis;
    marrow biopsy
5. Polycythemia vera
Amaurosis fugax
Retinal hemorrhages, dilated vessels
Disk hyperemia
Papilledema
Associated findings: red blood cell count over $6 \times 10^6/\mu l$, red blood cell count indices
6. Sickle cell disease
Comma-shaped conjunctival vessels
Vitreous hemorrhages
Retinal microcirculatory occlusion, peripheral capillary dropout
Black sunburst ischemic chorioretinal scars
Associated findings: hemoglobin electrophoresis, red blood cell count morphology
7. Thalassemia
Rare sickle-type retinopathy
Associated findings: red blood cell count indices; DNA probe; + family history·
8. Thrombocytopenia (idiopathic, thrombotic)
Orbital hemorrhage
Ocular palsy
Retinal edema, hemorrhages, exudates
Associated findings: complete blood count and platelet count, Marrow biopsy
8. Waldenström macroglobulinemia
Sludging conjunctival blood flow
Retinal hemorrhages, dilated veins, cotton-wool spots, vascular occlusion
Associated findings: elevated immunoglobulin M; immunoglobulin electrophoresis

TABLE 15.10. CARDIOVASCULAR DISEASES[a]

1. Arteriosclerosis, chronic hypertension
Arcus senilis
Lipid keratopathy
Retinal copper and silver wire vascular appearance, arteriovenous nicking, vessel tortuosity, arteriolar dilation
Retinal edema, hemorrhages, hard exudates
Star maculopathy
Papilledema
Associated findings: renal and fluorescein angiography; arteriosclerotic vascular disease; increased blood pressure

2. Malignant toxemia of pregnancy
Altered vision
Retinal edema, arteriolar narrowing, hemorrhages, exudates, exudative detachment
Macular edema
Papilledema
Associated findings: pregnancy; increased blood pressure

3. Occlusive vascular disease (*Sudden:* emboli, thrombi, central retinal artery occlusion, cardiac myxoma, cranial arteritis, sickle cell attack)
Amaurosis fugax
Homonymous hemianopia
Anisocoria
Cherry-red spot in macula
Cholesterol plaques in retinal arteriole (Hollenhorst)
Associated findings: + fluorescein angiography; erythrocyte sedimentation rate up (arteritis)

4. Occlusive vascular disease (*Slow:* carotid artery disease, diabetes mellitus, collagen vascular disease)
Transient ischemic attacks
Conjunctival vessel dilation
Ischemic iritis
Rubeosis iridis
Horner syndrome affected side
Retinal arteriolar distention, cotton-wool exudates, venous stasis (punctate hemorrhages, edema)
Unilateral retinopathy
Associated findings: + fluorescein angiography, increased fasting blood sugar/glucose tolerance test; increased blood pressure

5. Venous occlusive disease (thrombosis, oral contraceptive use)
Retinal branch vein occlusion
Focal intraretinal hemorrhages
Central retinal vein occlusion
Rubeosis iridis
Open- or closed-angle glaucoma
Massive intraretinal hemorrhages
Associated findings: visual fields; + fluorescein angiography

(continued)

TABLE 15.10. (*Continued*)

6. Endocarditis
Diplopia
Ocular palsies
Nystagmus
Anisocoria
Conjunctiva petechiae
Roth's spots
Iritis
Metastatic endophthalmitis
Retinal hemorrhages, cotton-wool exudates
Papillitis
Associated findings: + blood culture; anemia; heart murmur; cerebrovascular
accident, Splenomegaly
7. Myxoma
Retinal vascular emboli
Macular cherry-red spot
Associated findings: electrocardiography; chest x-ray; echocardiography
8. Aortic arch syndrome (Takayasu's disease)
Corneal folds
Ischemic iritis
Rubeosis iridis
Cataracts
Vitreous hemorrhage
Retinal neovascularization, hemorrhages, exudates, detachment
Papilledema
Glaucoma
Associated findings: cardiac angiography; fluorescein angiography
9. Thromboangiitis obliterans
Retinal perivasculitis (rare)
Associated findings: smokers; Jewish ancestry; Raynaud's phenomena
**10. Hereditary telangiectasia (Rendu-Osler-Weber syndrome, autosomal
dominant)**
Dilated conjunctival vascular lesions
Vitreous and retinal hemorrhages
Dilated retinal veins
Disk neovascularization
Associated findings: + family history; telangiectasia: face, hands, oral and nasal
mucosa

[a]See also **Chapter 8**: hypertensive retinopathy.

TABLE 15.11. ENDOCRINE DISEASES[a]

1. Cushing's disease (hyperadrenalism)
   Exophthalmos
   Hypertensive retinopathy
   Retinal vessel tortuosity, hemorrhages, exudates
   Papilledema
   Associated findings: high serum glucocorticoids
2. Addison's disease
   Hyperpigmentation skin of lids and conjunctiva
   Papilledema
   Optic atrophy
   Associated findings: high serum potassium, low aldosterone
3. Diabetes mellitus
   Fluctuating refractive error
   Diplopia
   Extraocular muscle palsies (third nerve spares pupil, sixth nerve most frequent)
   Xanthelasma
   Corneal recurrent erosions
   Rubeosis iridis
   Ectropion uveae
   Snowflake cataract
   Retinal dot-blot hemorrhages, hard exudates, neovascularization (+ disk)
   Vitreous hemorrhages
   Lipemia retinalis
   Associated findings: high fasting blood sugar/glucose tolerance test; + fluorescein
      angiography
4. Hyperparathyroidism
   Conjunctival calcification
   Band keratopathy
   Associated findings: high serum calcium
5. Hypoparathyroidism
   Photophobia
   Lid twitch
   Keratitis
   Polychromatic and cortical cataract
   Papilledema
   Associated findings: low serum calcium; tetany
6. Hyperthyroidism
   Extraocular muscle palsy and hypertrophy
   Exophthalmos
   Orbital puffiness
   Lid retraction, lag
   Exposure keratitis
   Superior limbic keratitis
   Papilledema
   Optic atrophy
   Associated findings: high thyroid function tests; orbital ultrasound
7. Hypothyroidism
   Photophobia
   Periorbital and lid edema
   Loss lateral third of brows
   Cortical cataract
   Optic neuritis, atrophy
   Associated findings: cretinism; myxedema; dry hair and skin; low thyroid function tests

[a]See also **Chapter 8:** diabetic retinopathy.

TABLE 15.12. GASTROINTESTINAL AND NUTRITIONAL DISORDERS

1. **Alcoholism (see vitamin B deficiency)**
   Nystagmus, (third and sixth nerve palsies)
   Poor conjugate gaze
   Ptosis
   Iridoplegia
   Optic neuritis
   Associated findings: Wernicke's encephalopathy; low serum vitamin B
2. **Liver disease (nutritional)**
   Scleral icterus
   Night blindness
   Poor color vision
   Keratitis sicca (dry eyes)
   ?Cataract
   Optic atrophy
   Associated findings: abnormal liver enzymes, serum vitamin levels, electroretinogram
3. **Malnutrition**
   Xerophthalmia
   Night blindness
   Lid edema
   Chemosis
   Keratopathy (necrotic)
   Associated findings: abnormal electroretinogram; low Schirmer tests; low serum
   vitamins
4. **Peptic ulcer disease (see vitamin B deficiency)**
   Iritis
   Glaucomatocyclitic crisis
   Associated findings: males; gastroscopy
5. **Pancreatic disease**
   Glaucoma secondary to anticholinergic Rx
   Retinal fat emboli, cotton-wool exudates, hemorrhages
   Associated findings: high serum pancreatic enzymes
6. **Regional enteritis or ulcerative colitis**
   Episcleritis
   Conjunctivitis
   Iritis
   Retinitis
   Macular edema
   Exudative detachment
   Optic neuritis
   Associated findings: gastrointestinal x-rays; arthritis
7. **Vitamin A deficiency**
   Xerophthalmia
   Bitot (dry) spots on conjunctiva
   Keratomalacia (necrotic)
   Retinal perivasculitis
   Degeneration rod outer segments
   Associated findings: low serum vitamin A; abnormal electroretinogram; + conjunctival
   scrapings for xerosis bacillus
8. **Vitamin B deficiency**
   Xerosis of cornea and conjunctiva
   Central scotoma
   Optic neuritis
   Retrobulbar neuritis
   Abnormal color vision
   Associated findings: low serum vitamin B; visual fields
9. **Vitamin C deficiency**
   Subconjunctival and retinal hemorrhages
   Associated findings: Low serum vitamin C; scurvy

(continued)

TABLE 15.12. (*Continued*)

10. Hypervitaminosis A, B, and D
Increased intracranial pressure (A)
Decreased vision (B)
Calcium deposits in conjunctiva and cornea (D)
Cystoid macular edema (B)
Papilledema (A)
Associated findings: elevated serum vitamins

10. Whipple's disease
Extraocular muscle palsies
Iritis
Vitritis
Papilledema
Associated findings: bacillary bodies on electron microscopy; arthritis; malabsorption

?, not definitively documented.

TABLE 15.13. METABOLIC DISEASES[a]

1. **Alkaptonuria (ochronosis, autosomal recessive)**
   Dark pigmentation sclera, conjunctiva, and cornea
   Associated findings: metabolic screening; dark urine; enzyme assays
2. **Amyloidosis (autosomal dominant and recessive)**
   Proptosis
   Extraocular muscle palsies
   Ptosis
   Amyloid nodules in lids, conjunctiva, and corneal stroma
   Iritis
   Glaucoma
   Irregular pupils
   Vitreous opacities
   Retinal hemorrhages
   Optic nerve amyloid
   Associated findings: tissue biopsy; immunoglobulin electrophoresis
3. **Chédiak-Higashi syndrome (autosomal recessive)**
   Photophobia
   Partial ocular albinism
   Nystagmus
   Light-colored lashes and irides
   Albinotic fundi
   Associated findings: blood smear: + polymorphonuclear white blood cells with large
   abnormal granules;   hepatosplenomegaly; lymphadenopathy
4. **Cystinosis (autosomal recessive)**
   Photophobia
   Conjunctival and corneal crystals (anterior stroma)
   Retinal peripheral pigment clumping
   Associated findings: short stature; renal disease; conjunctival biopsy (polarizing light
   to examine crystals)
5. **Fabry's disease (sex-linked)**
   Tortuous conjunctival and retinal vessels
   Vortex pattern corneal epithelial opacities
   Posterior subcapsular cataract
   Retinal hemorrhages
   Macular edema
   Associated findings: enzyme assays
6. **Galactosemia (autosomal recessive)**
   Nuclear or cortical cataract (reversible)
   Associated findings: galactose intolerance; enzyme tests
7. **Gout (hyperuricemia)**
   Episcleritis
   Scleritis
   Corneal uric acid crystals
   Iridocyclitis
   Associated findings: hyperuricemia
8. **Hemochromatosis**
   Brown pigment in conjunctiva
   Diabetic retinopathy
   Associated findings: complete blood count; high serum iron; diabetes; liver cirrhosis
9. **Histiocytosis**
   Exophthalmos
   Infiltrative lesions of bone (eosinophilic granuloma)
10. **Homocystinuria (autosomal recessive)**
    Lens discoloration and downward dislocation
    Associated findings: mental retardation; high serum homocystine and methionine
    levels

(*continued*)

TABLE 15.13. (*Continued*)

11. Lipidoses (arcus senilis or juvenilis)
   Xanthelasma
   Lipid keratopathy
   Lipemia retinalis
   Associated findings: lipid electrophoresis; serum lipid assay
12. Marchesani syndrome
   Secondary glaucoma
   Cataract
   Small lens
   Lens dislocation or subluxation
   Associated findings: short, stocky stature

[a]See also **Chapter 11:** albinism, Gaucher's disease, Marfan syndrome, mucopolysaccharidoses, Niemann-Pick disease, osteogenesis imperfecta, Wilson's disease, other inherited metabolic disorders, developmental disorders, tumors of childhood, retinopathy of prematurity.

TABLE 15.14. MUSCULOSKELETAL DISEASES[a]

1. Albright's disease (fibrous dysplasia of bone)
Proptosis
Strabismus
Chemosis
Exposure keratitis
Optic atrophy
Associated findings: Cafe au lait spots; early epiphyseal closure; + bone x-rays

2. Apert's disease
Proptosis
Lateral upward slant of lids
Exposure keratitis
Keratoconus
Optic atrophy
Chronic papilledema
Associated findings: syndactyly; cranial malformation

3. Conradi syndrome (autosomal recessive)
Hypertelorism
Glaucoma
Heterochromic irides
Iris hypoplasia
Dense cataracts
Optic atrophy
Associated findings: mental retardation; short stature; Micromelia

4. Craniofacial syndromes (Crouzon's, platybasia)
Lid coloboma
Exophthalmos
Nystagmus
Exotropia
Exposure keratitis
Papilledema
Optic atrophy
Myelinated nerve fibers
Associated findings: + skull x-rays

5. Facial deformity syndromes (Goldenhar, Treacher Collins, Pierre-Robin, Hallermann-Streiff-François)
Coloboma lower lids
Lateral upward lid slant
Microphthalmos
Preauricular appendages and epibulbar dermoids (Goldenhar)
Nystagmus
Strabismus
Cataract
Associated findings: + skull x-rays

6. Muscular dystrophy disorders
Ptosis
External ophthalmoplegia
Dry eyes
Polychromatic cataract
Pigmentary retinopathy
Associated findings: electromyography and muscle enzymes

7. Myasthenia gravis
Lid twitch sign
Ptosis
Diplopia
Paradoxical lid retraction
Pseudogaze palsy
Associated findings: exertional weakness; + Tensilon test

(continued)

TABLE 15.14. (*Continued*)

8. Paget's disease
Extraocular muscle palsy
Choroidal sclerosis
Retinal angioid streaks
Optic atrophy
Associated findings: skull x-rays; high serum alkaline phosphatase

[a]See also **Chapter 11:** osteogenesis imperfecta.

TABLE 15.15. PULMONARY DISEASES[a]

1. Asthma
Stellate cortical cataract
Steroid cataract and glaucoma
2. Bronchogenic carcinoma (see Table 15.17)
Metastasis to iris, choroid, and retina
Associated findings: Chest x-ray; bronchoscopy
2. Bronchiectasis
Retina: vessels dilated, tortuous; edema, hemorrhages
3. Cystic fibrosis and pancreatic disease
Retinal vascular dilation, edema, hemorrhages
Macular holes
Papilledema
Optic neuritis
Associated findings: + Sweat test (high sodium); pancreatic enzyme and stool
  fat tests
5. Emphysema
Steroid cataract and glaucoma
Papilledema
Associated findings: smoker: + chest x-ray, pulmonary functions
6. Pneumonias
Roth's spots
Septic retinitis

[a]See also **Chapter 9:** tuberculosis.

TABLE 15.16. RENAL DISEASES

1. **Alport syndrome (autosomal dominant)**
   Anterior lenticonus and polar cataract
   White retinal dots
   Optic nerve drusen
   Associated findings: nerve deafness; proteinuria; hypertension; abnormal
   electroretinogram
2. **Azotemia (acute and chronic pyelonephritis)**
   Retinal edema, hemorrhages, cotton-wool exudates
   Nonrhegmatogenous detachment
   Papilledema
   Associated findings: high blood urea nitrogen, renin; hypertension
3. **Lowe syndrome (recessive sex-linked)**
   Congenital cataract
   Small lenses
   Posterior lenticonus
   Congenital glaucoma
   Associated findings: aminoaciduria
4. **Medullary cystic disease (dominant or recessive)**
   Decreased vision
   Nystagmus
   Retinitis pigmentosa
4. **Nephrotic syndrome (acute glomerulonephritis,
   diabetic kidney, systemic lupus erythematosus)**
   Mild retinopathy, edema
   Papilledema
   Associated findings: normal blood urea nitrogen
   and blood pressure; + proteinuria
6. **Renal transplantation**
   Steroid cataract and glaucoma
7. **Wilms tumor**
   Aniridia
   Orbital mass
   Associated findings: x-rays of abdomen

TABLE 15.17. NEOPLASTIC DISEASES WITH OCULAR METASTASES[a]

1. Blood (leukemia, lymphoma)
Orbital infiltration (lymphoma, granulocytic leukemia)
Uveitis (reticulum cell sarcoma)
Retinal nerve fiber layer damage, Roth's spots, macular hemorrhage, vascular lesions
Associated findings: Ultrasound; fluorescein angiography; phosphorous (radioactive)
uptake; aqueous cytology; complete blood count
2. Breast (high incidence ocular metastasis)
Orbital metastasis
Iris or angle metastasis
Choroidal metastasis
3. Colon
Orbit and anterior segment metastasis rare
Choroidal and retinal metastasis
4. Kidney
Orbit and anterior segment metastasis rare
Choroidal and retinal metastasis
5. Lung (high incidence ocular metastasis)
Orbital metastasis frequent
Iris or angle metastasis common
Choroidal and retinal metastasis
6. Genital organs (ovary or cervix; testis or prostate)
Rare exophthalmos
Ocular palsies
Hyphema
Posterior segment metastasis
7. Gut (stomach or pancreas)
Unusual orbital or anterior segment metastasis
Choroidal and retinal metastasis
8. Thyroid
Rare anterior segment or chorioretinal metastasis

[a]See also potential findings in metastatic lesion of the eye: visible mass, pain, redness, hyphema, exophthalmos, ocular palsies, blurred vision, loss of field. Clinical characteristics of ocular metastases: pale gray or yellow color, flatness (not usually elevated), faster growth rate than primary malignant melanoma, poor ocular prognosis.

16. OCULAR TOXICITY OF SYSTEMIC DRUGS

Deborah Pavan-Langston

I. **General considerations.** Many undesired side effects on the ocular tissues have been reported involving various drugs used for both the treatment of systemic medical disorders and for local ophthalmic problems. The types of adverse effects of drugs on the eye may be mild and transient, such as temporary decreased visual acuity, impairment of accommodation, abnormal pupillary responses, and color vision disturbances. Other effects, such as eye movement abnormalities, glaucoma, cataracts, and retinal damage, may seriously reduce ocular function. To recognize and prevent vision-threatening complications from adverse effects of drug reactions, it is necessary for the clinician to obtain a careful history, with particular attention to specific medications used. The clinician must then be aware of certain oculotoxic drugs and their side effects to recognize the drug-related eye disorder.

II. **Pretreatment examination.** For certain drugs with potential ocular toxicity, a careful pretreatment examination should be performed before the drug is administered, particularly if (a) the drug will be used for a long period of time (isoniazid, streptomycin, quinine, and indomethacin), or (b) it is known to have severe toxic effects (ethambutol, hydroxychloroquine, and thioridazine). Patients taking drugs that are not as toxic may not require the complete baseline examination before therapy, but they should undergo frequent monitoring examinations so that if symptoms do arise, the drug can be withdrawn immediately. Reversible effects can likewise be observed while the patient is not taking the drug, and later, after resolution of the effects, the drug regimen may be judiciously reinstituted at a lower dose. The pretreatment examination should include the following steps, which are described in greater detail in Chapter 1.

A. **Visual acuity with glasses.** Test acuity screening at near and distance with and without pinhole testing.

B. **Pupillary responses.** Test pupil size, briskness of reactions (direct and consensual) to light, and convergence reflex.

C. **Ocular motility examination.** Test complete motility in all fields of gaze with ductions, versions, and convergence.

D. **Intraocular pressures.** Periodic tonometry should be performed.

E. **Slitlamp examination (biomicroscopy).** Drugs may affect the **conjunctiva, cornea,** and **lens** during the course of therapy. Loupe or slitlamp examination is indicated. **Tear film** adequacy should be tested.

F. **Dilated ophthalmoscopy.** Drugs may cause changes in the **retina, macula, blood vessels,** and the **optic nerve.**

G. **Special examinations for retinal function.** Other tests may be performed to provide supplemental data on retinal function. These examinations include:

1. Photography of the fundus.
2. Electroretinography.
3. Visual fields.
4. Color vision tests.
5. Visual evoked potential.
6. Fluorescein angiography.

III. **Repeat eye examinations** should be performed and followed judiciously if there is any clinical change noted during the course of the patient's therapy.

IV. Ocular manifestations of systemic drug toxicity

   A. Reduced visual acuity may result from transient changes in refractive errors, or anterior or posterior segment toxicity.

   B. Blurred vision may be caused by dilated pupils (mydriasis) and impairment of accommodation (cycloplegia) as well as anterior or posterior segment toxic changes.

   C. Color vision disturbances include hallucination, altered perception, and diminished sensitivity.

   D. Ocular motility abnormalities include neuromuscular myesthenic block, paralytic strabismus, diplopia, and oculogyric crisis.

   E. Conjunctival inflammation and **corneal opacification** may occur.

   F. Glaucoma may occur in those individuals with shallow anterior chamber angles who use drugs causing mydriasis, or in deep open angles depending on the offending agent.

   G. More serious are those adverse drug effects that occur in the crystalline **lens** (cataract) and the **optic nerve.**

   H. There are still other oculotoxic conditions, such as **exophthalmos, retinal** hemorrhages, vasculopathy, retinal pigment epitheliopathy, and **macular** edema.

V. Drugs and their ocular toxicity. Tables 16.1 through 16.18 represent major drug classifications under which are listed specific drugs and their potential adverse ocular side effects. Also tabulated are associated symptoms and signs according to specific ocular structures:

   A. Analgesics (Table 16.1).

   B. Antiarthritics (Table 16.2).

   C. Anesthetics–general (Table 16.3).

   D. Antihistamines (Table 16.4).

   E. Antiinfectives: antibiotics (Table 16.5).

   F. Antivirals–systemic (Table 16.6).

   G. Antineoplastic agents (Table 16.7).

   H. Cardiovascular drugs (Table 16.8).

   I. Central nervous system (CNS) drugs (Table 16.9).

   J. Dermatologic agents (Table 16.10).

   K. Diuretics and osmotics (Table 16.11).

   L. Gastrointestinal agents (Table 16.12).

   M. Hematologic agents (Table 16.13).

   N. Hormonal agents (Table 16.14).

   O. Immunosuppressant agents (Table 16.15).

   P. Neuromuscular agents (Table 16.16).

   Q. Vaccines (Table 16.17).

   R. Vitamins (Table 16.18).

   For a more extensive listing, see Fraunfelder FT, Fraunfelder FW. *Drug-induced ocular side effects,* 5th ed. Boston: Butterworth Heineman, 2001.

VI. Examples of drugs in each category are given usually by generic name but occasionally by commercial name for reader orientation. It should be noted that not all drugs in each category have been reported as causing every side effect within that category. The potential for a given side effect in any category should be borne in mind, however, even if not previously reported for a specific agent.

Abbreviations Used in Tables 16.1–16.18.

<, decreased; >, increased; ?, not definitively documented; IOP, intraocular pressure; DPT, diphtheria-pertussis-tetanus.

TABLE 16.1. ANALGESICS

1. Nonnarcotic (acetaminophen, phenacetin)
    < Color vision
    < Vision
    Yellow vision
    Visual hallucinations
    Lid or conjunctiva: irritation, allergy, redness, edema
    Green or brown conjunctival vessel discoloration
    Subconjunctival heme
    Mydriasis
    < Pupil light reflex

2. Narcotic and narcotic antagonists (methadone, propoxyphene [Darvon], codeine, fentanyl [Duragesic], heroin, hydromorphone, morphine, meperidine [Demerol], pentazocine [Talwin], morphine opioids [levallorphan, nalorphine, naloxone])
    < Vision
    Visual hallucinations
    Diplopia
    Myopia
    Photophobia
    Yellow vision
    Color vision defects
    Lid edema
    Tearing (withdrawal)
    Dry eyes
    Miosis
    Mydriasis or anisocoria (withdrawal)
    Paralysis of accommodation
    Extraocular muscle paralysis
    Nystagmus
    Optic atrophy
    Visual field scotomas or constriction
    < Spontaneous eye movements

TABLE 16.2. ANTIARTHRITICS AND NONSTEROIDAL ANTIINFLAMMATORY DRUGS (NSAIDS)

1. Antigout (allopurinol colchicine)
< Vision
Lid or conjunctiva: allergy, redness, edema, ulceration, subconjunctival heme
Lash or brow loss
Scleritis
Corneal: keratitis, ulcers, scarring, recurrent erosions, dellen
Retinal hemorrhages
Macular edema
Retinal? hemorrhages,? exudates
Papilledema
Diplopia
Extraocular muscle paresis

2. Gold salts (auranofin, aurothioglucose, gold sodium thiomalate)
Photophobia
Corneal ulcers
Lid or conjunctiva: allergy, redness, edema, photosensitivity, symblepharon
? Lash or brow loss
Iritis
Diplopia
Myesthenic block
Extraocular muscle paresis
Ptosis
Gold deposits (red, brown, violet): lids, conjunctiva, pancorneal, lens
Retinal hemorrhages
? Papilledema

3. NSAIDs (fenoprofen, flurbiprofen, ibuprofen, indomethacin, ketoprofen, naproxen, phenylbutazone, piroxicam, salicylates)
< Vision
Red-green color vision defect
Blue or yellow vision
Visual hallucinations
Scintillating scotomas
Myopia
Photophobia
< Dark adaptation
Extraocular muscle paralysis
Diplopia
Lids or conjunctiva: redness, edema, discoloration, subconjunctival heme, photosensitivity
? Brow or lash loss
Dry eyes
Corneal subepithelial whorls, erosions, deposits, ulcers, vessels (indomethacin, naproxen, phenylbutazone)
Mydriasis
Paralysis of accommodation
Retinal hemorrhages
Serous retinopathy
Abnormal electroretinogram
Macular edema, degeneration
Retinal pigment epithelium disturbance
Papilledema
Optic neuritis/atrophy
Extraocular muscle paralysis
Toxic amblyopia
Visual field: constriction, paracentral, cecocentral scotomas, hemianopia
Nystagmus

TABLE 16.3. ANESTHETICS: GENERAL

1. Chloroform, ether, ketamine, methoxyflurane, nitrous oxide, trichloroethylene
  < Vision
  Visual hallucinations
  Diplopia
  Color vision defects
  > or < Tearing
  < Intraocular pressure (deep anesthesia)
  Mydriasis (light anesthesia)
  Miosis (deep anesthesia)
  Abnormal electroretinogram
  Eso- or exotropia
  Extraocular muscle paralysis
  Nystagmus
  Scotomas (central or paracentral)
  ? Cortical blindness

TABLE 16.4. ANTIHISTAMINES

1. Pheniramines, triprolidine, diphenhydramines (Benadryl), antazolines, pyrilamine, phenothiazine analogs (azatadine)
  < Vision
  Visual hallucinations
  Diplopia
  Dry eyes
  Lid or conjunctiva: redness, photosensitivity, blepharospasm
  Subconjunctival heme
  Punctate keratitis
  Mydriasis
  Anisocoria
  < Pupil light reflex
  Paralysis of accommodation
  Nystagmus
  Retinal hemorrhages

TABLE 16.5. ANTIINFECTIVES

Antibiotics
1. Aminoglycosides (amikacin, gentamicin, kanamycin, neomycin, streptomycin, tobramycin)
  < Vision
  Visual hallucinations
  Diplopia
  Afterimaging
  Color vision defects
  Yellow vision
  Lash or brow loss
  Lid or conjunctiva: ptosis, allergy, redness, edema
  Subconjunctival heme
  < Pupil light reflex
  Extraocular muscle paralysis
  Retinal hemorrhages
  Papilledema
  Optic or retrobulbar neuritis
  Nystagmus
  Pseudotumor cerebri
  Toxic amblyopia
  Scotomas
2. Cephalosporins (cefaclor, cefotaxime, ceftazidime, ceftriaxone, cefuroxime, cephalothin, cephamandole, imipenem, moxalactam)
  Visual hallucinations
  Diplopia
  Color vision defects
  Lid or conjunctiva: allergy, redness, edema, subconjunctival heme
  Corneal peripheral edema
  Retinal hemorrhages
  ? Retinal pigment epithelium disturbance
  ? Papilledema
  ? Nystagmus
3. Chloramphenicol
  < Vision
  Color vision defects
  Yellow vision
  Lid or conjunctiva: allergy, redness, edema
  Paralysis of accommodation
  Mydriasis
  < Pupil reflex
  Retinal pigment epithelium disturbance
  Retinal edema, hemorrhages
  Retrobulbar or optic neuritis
  Optic atrophy
  Toxic amblyopia
  Scotomas
  Visual field constriction
4. Clindamycin, erythromycin, lincomycin, vancomycin
  Ptosis
  Extraocular muscle paralysis
  Color vision defects
  Yellow vision
  Lid or conjunctiva: allergy, redness
  Photosensitivity
  Subconjunctival heme
  Retinal hemorrhages
  Extraocular muscle paralysis

(continued)

TABLE 16.5. (*Continued*)

5. Colistin
Diplopia
Mydriasis
Extraocular muscle paralysis
6. Erythromycin: see clindamycin
7. Nalidixic acid (NeGram), nitrofurantoins
Glare
Scintillating scotomas
Colored vision (multi)
Lid or conjunctival photosensitivity
Mydriasis
Paralysis of accommodation
Retinal hemorrhages
Papilledema
Pseudotumor cerebri
Extraocular muscle paralysis
Nystagmus
8. Penicillins (benzathine, potassium); semisynthetic (amoxicillin, ampicillin, carbenicillin, dicloxacillin, methicillin, nafcillin, oxacillin, piperacillin ticarcillin)
Diplopia
Lid or conjunctiva: allergy, blepharoconjunctivitis, edema, photosensitivity, subconjunctival heme
9. Quinolones (ciprofloxacin, ofloxacin, levofloxacin, norfloxacin, sparfloxacin)
> Vision
Eyelids (hyperpigmentation, edema, allergy, vasculitis, urticaria, photosensitivity)
Photophobia
Tearing
Visual hallucinations
Myasthenia (diplopia, extraocular muscle paralysis)
Abnormal VER
Nystagmus
Toxic optic neuropathy
Retinal hemorrhages
Papilledema (pseudotumor cerebri)
Extraocular muscle (EOM) paralysis
10. Sulfonamides (sulfadiazine, sulfamethazine, sulfamethoxazole, sulfisoxazole)
< Vision
< Depth perception
< Adduction at near
Myopia
Photophobia
Color vision defects
Yellow vision
Visual hallucinations
Lid or conjunctiva: ptosis, tearing, allergy, redness, photosensitivity
Keratitis
Anterior chamber shallowing
Iritis
Retinal hemorrhages
Papilledema
Optic atrophy
Optic neuritis
Extraocular muscle paralysis
Diplopia
Periorbital edema
Scotomas
Visual field constriction
Cortical blindness
? Toxic amblyopia

(*continued*)

TABLE 16.5. (*Continued*)

11. Tetracyclines (doxycycline, minocycline, oxytetracycline, tetracycline)
< Vision
Photophobia
Diplopia
Color vision defect
Yellow vision
Myopia
Visual hallucinations
Lids or conjunctiva: edema, redness, yellow discoloration, ptosis, hyperpigmentation,
  photosensitivity, subconjunctival heme
? Lash loss
Retinal hemorrhages
Extraocular muscle paralysis
12. Vancomycin: see clindamycin
Antifungals
  1. Penicillin derivatives (griseofulvin)
  < Vision
  Lid or conjunctiva: allergy, redness, edema, conjunctivitis, photosensitivity, ulceration
  Subconjunctival heme, ? lash loss
  Scleritis
  Corneal: keratitis, ulcers, scarring
  Retinal hemorrhages
  Macular edema,? degeneration,? exudates
  2. Polyenes (amphotericin B, nystatin)
  < Vision
  Diplopia
  Subconjunctival heme
  Retinal exudates and/or hemorrhages
  Optic neuritis
  Extraocular muscle paralysis
  3. Imidazoles: see antiprotozoals (antiparasitics)
Antileprosy drugs
  1. Phenazines (clofazimine)
  < Vision
  Lids or conjunctiva: red tears, hyperpigmentation
  Corneal polychromatic crystals
  Macular retinal pigment epithelium mottle
  2. Sulfones (Dapsone)
  < Vision
  Visual hallucinations
  Lid or conjunctiva: edema, hyperpigmentation, subconjunctival heme
  Optic atrophy
  Retinal hemorrhages
  3. Ethionamide, rifampin: see antituberculosis drugs
Antiparasitics
  1. Amebicides (quinolones, alkaloids [emetine])
  < Vision
  Diplopia
  ? Corneal opacities
  Optic atrophy/neuritis
  Macular edema/degeneration, retinal pigment epithelium mottle
  Toxic amblyopia
  Nystagmus

(*continued*)

TABLE 16.5. (*Continued*)

2. Antihelminthics (antimonials, thiabendazole, quinacrine, piperazine [diethylcarbamazine])
< Vision
Variable color vision
Color vision defects
Photophobia
Visual hallucinations
Flashing lights
Lid or conjunctiva: edema, yellow or black pigmentation, subconjunctival heme
Yellow sclera
Dry eyes
Punctate keratitis
Corneal multicolor deposits
Nonreactive pupils
Mydriasis
Miosis
Paralysis of accommodation
Iritis
Extraocular muscles paralysis
Retinal hemorrhages
Optic neuritis
Chorioretinitis
Nystagmus
Toxic amblyopia
Scotomas

3. Antimalarials (chloroquine, quinines)
< Vision
Photophobia
Night blindness
Visual hallucinations
< Dark adaptation
Flashing lights and waves
Lids or conjunctiva: poliosis, yellow discoloration, photosensitivity, hyper- or depigmentation, madarosis, subconjunctival heme
Corneal: whorl deposits, iron lines
Dry eyes
Cataracts: anterior snowflake and posterior subcapsular
Paralysis of accommodation
Retina: pigment or doughnut retinopathy, diffuse degeneration, vasoconstriction, hemorrhages, exudates
Optic neuritis/atrophy
Extraocular muscle paralysis
Toxic amblyopia
Scotomas: central, annular, paracentral, constriction
Vertical nystagmus

4. Antiprotozoals (imidazoles, tryparsamide, suramin)
< Vision
Photophobia
Visual hallucinations
Shimmering lights
Diplopia
Lid or conjunctiva: tearing, edema, subconjunctival heme
Corneal vortex whorls
Superficial punctate keratitis
Iritis
Optic neuritis or atrophy
Retinal hemorrhages
Oculogyric crisis
Toxic amblyopia
Antituberculosis drugs

(*continued*)

TABLE 16.5. (*Continued*)

1. Ethambutol
   < Vision
   Photophobia
   Color vision defects
   Retinal or macular edema, hemorrhages, vascular dilation, spasm
   Extraocular muscle paralysis
   Toxic amblyopia
   Scotomas: annular, central, cecocentral
   Visual field: constriction hemianopia, > blind spot
2. Paraaminosalicylates
   < Vision
   Red-green color defect
   Lid or conjunctiva: allergy, inflammation, edema, subconjunctival heme
   Paralysis of accommodation
   Retinal hemorrhages
   Optic neuritis/atrophy
   Scotomas
3. Cycloserine
   < Vision
   Visual hallucinations
   Flickering vision
   Lids or conjunctiva: allergy, inflammation, photosensitivity, subconjunctival heme
   ? Paralysis of accommodation
   Retinal hemorrhages
   ? Optic neuritis/atrophy
4. Isoniazid, ethionamide
   < Vision
   Diplopia
   Photophobia
   Color vision defect or > color vision
   Visual hallucinations
   Red-green color defect
   Lids or conjunctiva: allergy, edema, subconjunctival heme
   Keratitis
   Mydriasis
   < Pupil light reflex
   Paralysis of accommodation
   Retinal hemorrhages
   Optic or retrobulbar neuritis/atrophy
   Papilledema
   Extraocular muscle paresis
   Toxic amblyopia
   Visual field scotomas, hemianopia
   Nystagmus
5. Capreomycin, rifampin
   < Vision
   Flashing lights
   Red-green color vision defect
   White vision
   ? Visual hallucinations
   Lid or conjunctiva: angioneurotic edema, tearing, hyperemia, blepharoconjunctivitis,
      yellow or red discoloration, subconjunctival heme
   Iritis
6. Streptomycin: see antibacterials

TABLE 16.6. ANTIVIRALS: SYSTEMIC

1. **Antiherpes: acyclovir, ganciclovir, famciclovir, vidarabine, valacyclovir)**
   < Vision
   Visual hallucinations
   Lid spasm, erythema
   Subconjunctival heme
   Retinal hemorrhages
2. **Antiherpes: cidofovir**
   Iritis
   Ocular hypotony
2. **Anti-HIV agents (didanosine, zidovudine, dideoxyinosine)**
   > Vision
   Hypertrichosis
   Eyelids (urticaria, rashes, vasculitis)
   Color vision abnormalities
   Hyperpigmentation of lids and conjunctiva
   Diplopia
   Visual hallucinations
   Nystagmus (overdose)
   Retinal pigment epithelial disturbance
   Choriocapillaris atrophy
   Diminished electrooculogram
   Visual field defects
   Night blindness
   Optic neuritis/atrophy

HIV, human immunodeficiency virus.

TABLE 16.7. ANTINEOPLASTIC AGENTS

1. Alkaloids (busulfan, chlorambucil, cyclophosphamide, dacarbazine, melphalan, uracil mustard)
< Vision
Photophobia
Visual hallucinations
Lids or conjunctiva: allergy, redness, tearing, hyperpigmentation, photosensitivity, edema, lash or brow loss, dry eyes, subconjunctival heme
Nonspecific pain, burning
Retinal hemorrhages, vascular occlusion
Optic neuritis/atrophy
Papilledema
Pseudotumor cerebri
2. Antibiotics—antineoplastics (bleomycin, daunorubicin, mitomycin): see alkaloids–antiparasitic amebicides
3. Antimetabolites (fluorouracil, mercaptopurine, thioguanine)
< Vision
Photophobia
Diplopia
Color vision defects
Lids or conjunctiva: tearing, hyperemia, edema, burning, pain, cicatricial ectropion, hyperpigmentation, photosensitivity, ulcers, lash or brow loss, subconjunctival heme
Paralysis of accommodation
Retinal hemorrhages
? Optic neuritis
< Convergence or divergence
Nystagmus
4. Thiotepa
Lids or conjunctiva: redness, edema, lash or brow loss, subconjunctival heme
? Iritis
Retinal hemorrhages
5. Folic acid antagonists (methotrexate): see alkaloids
Keratitis
Extraocular muscle paralysis
Periorbital edema
6. Heavy metals (cisplatinum): see alkaloids
Plus: extraocular muscle paralysis
Oculogyric crisis
Orbital pain
Cortical blindness
Hemianopia
7. Interferon
< Vision
Visual hallucinations
Lid or conjunctiva: > lash or brow growth or loss, conjunctivitis
Retinal hemorrhages
Cystoid macular edema
Papilledema
Abnormal electroretinogram, electrooculography, visual evoked potential
< Extraocular muscle movement
8. Nonsteroidal antiestrogens (tamoxifen, capecitabine)
< Vision
Subepithelial corneal whorl opacities
Retinal or macular: hemorrhages, edema, yellow-white refractile opacities, degeneration, retinal pigment epithelium disturbances
Visual field constriction
Paracentral scotomas   *(continued)*

TABLE 16.7. (*Continued*)

9. **Vinca alkaloids (vinblastine, vincristine): see alkaloids (antiparasitics, amebicides)**
    < dark adaptation
    Corneal deposits or ulcers
    Scleritis
    Iritis
    Extraocular muscle paralysis
    ? Nystagmus
    Visual field constriction
    Scotomas: central or paracentral
    Hemianopia
    Cortical blindness

TABLE 16.8. CARDIOVASCULAR DRUGS

Antianginal agents (amiodarone, calcium channel blockers [nifedipine, verapamil], lidocaine analogs, analogs, nitrates, nitrites)
< Vision
Color vision defect
Halos
Photophobia
Visual hallucinations
Diplopia
Myopia
Yellow or blue vision (nitrates, nitrites)
Lid or conjunctiva: inflammation, photosensitivity, edema, discoloration, brow or lash loss
Dry eyes
Corneal: ulcers, < reflex, brownish-yellow epithelial whorl deposits (amiodarone)
Periorbital edema
Mydriasis
< or > Intraocular pressure (transient)
Retinal hemorrhages
Papilledema
? Optic neuritis
Pseudotumor cerebri
Nystagmus
Visual field defects
Antiarrhythmics
1. Anticholinergics (disopyramide)
< Vision
Visual hallucinations
Photophobia
Diplopia
Dry eyes
Lid or conjunctiva: redness, photosensitivity
Mydriasis
Paralysis of accommodation
Extraocular muscle paralysis
2. Beta-adrenergic blockers (oxypranolol, practolol, propranolol): see antihypertensives
< Vision
Visual hallucinations
Photophobia
Lids or conjunctiva: < or > tearing, allergy, redness, ptosis, conjunctivitis, edema, hyperpigmentation
< Corneal sensation
Severe dry eye
> Vascularity (practolol)
Corneal: yellow or white stromal opacities (practolol)
Ocular pain
Paralysis of accommodation
Extraocular muscle paresis
< Intraocular pressure
Ocular pseudotumor
3. Quinidine
< Vision
Color vision defect
Photophobia
Diplopia

(continued)

TABLE 16.8. (*Continued*)

Night blindness
Visual hallucinations
Lids or conjunctiva: allergy, hyperpigmentation, photosensitivity, edema,
  subconjunctival heme
Dry eyes
Corneal deposits
Iritis
Mydriasis
Retinal hemorrhages
Optic neuritis
Extraocular muscle paralysis
Toxic amblyopia
Antihypertensives
1. **Alpha-adrenergic agonists (clonidine)**
   < Vision
   Visual hallucinations
   Lids or conjunctiva: burning, edema
   Dry eyes
   Miosis (toxic)
   < Pupil reflex
   ? Retinal or macular degeneration
2. **Beta-adrenergic blockers (atenolol, nadolol, pindolol, timolol, guanethidine, methyldopa)**
   < Vision
   Visual hallucinations
   Diplopia
   Photophobia
   Lids or conjunctiva: redness, inflammation, ocular pain, subconjunctival heme
   Dry eyes
   Retinal hemorrhages
   Extraocular muscle paralysis
   Hemianopia (methyldopa)
3. **Angiotensin-converting enzyme (ACE) inhibitors (captopril, enalapril)**
   < Vision
   Visual hallucinations
   Lids or conjunctiva: redness, inflammation, edema, brown discoloration,
     photosensitivity, subconjunctival heme
   ? Paralysis of accommodation
   Retinal hemorrhages
4. **Ganglionic blockers (hexamethonium, mecamylamine)**
   < Vision
   Red-green color defect
   Ptosis
   Dry eyes
   Conjunctival edema
   Mydriasis
   < Intraocular pressure
   Paralysis of accommodation
   Retinal vasodilation
   Macular edema
   Optic atrophy
5. **Monoamine oxidase inhibitors (paragyline): see central nervous system (CNS) drugs–antidepressants**
6. ***Rauwolfia* alkaloids (deserpidine, reserpine)**
   < Vision
   Color vision defects

(*continued*)

TABLE 16.8. (*Continued*)

Yellow vision
Lids or conjunctiva: tearing, redness
Mydriasis
? Iritis
< Intraocular pressure
Retinal hemorrhages
Oculogyric crises
< Spontaneous eye movements
Abnormal conjugate gaze
Jerky pursuit
Antimigraine agents
1. Ergot alkaloids (ergotamine, methysergide)
< Vision
Red-green color vision defect
Red vision
Visual hallucinations
< Dark adaptation
Lids or conjunctiva: allergy, redness, edema
Miosis
< Intraocular pressure
Paralysis of accommodation
Retinal vascular spasm, occlusion
Abnormal electroretinogram
Optic neuritis
Scotomas
Hemianopia
? Cortical blindness
Cardiac glycosides
1. Deslanoside, digitoxin, digoxin, gitalin, ouabain
< Vision
Color vision defect
Yellow, green, blue, or red vision
Halos
Flickering yellow or green vision
White, brown, or orange "snow glare" to objects
Photophobia
Visual hallucinations
Diplopia
Lids or conjunctiva: ptosis, allergy, edema
Mydriasis
Accommodative spasm
Abnormal electroretinogram
Retrobulbar or optic neuritis
Extraocular muscle paralysis
Scotomas: central or paracentral
Toxic amblyopia
Peripheral vasodilators
1. Alpha-adrenergic blockers (tolazoline), nicotinic acids
Lid or conjunctiva: ptosis, redness
Miosis
< or > Intraocular pressure
Retinal hemorrhages
Vasopressors/bronchodilators

(*continued*)

TABLE 16.8. (*Continued*)

1. **Sympathomimetic amines (albuterol, ephedrine, epinephrine, methoxamine, phenylephrine)**
   < Vision
   Visual hallucinations
   Red-green color defect
   Green vision
   Photophobia and diplopia (norepinephrine)
   Lids or conjunctiva: > tearing, redness, edema
   Mydriasis
   < Intraocular pressure
   Rebound redness
   Hemianopia
   Nystagmus (horizontal)

TABLE 16.9. CENTRAL NERVOUS SYSTEM (CNS) DRUGS

Alcohols
1. (Chloral hydrate, ethanol)
  Miosis
  Mydriasis
  Tearing
  Ptosis
  Diplopia
  Paralysis of accommodation
  Nystagmus (downbeat and peripheral gaze)
  Conjunctivitis
  < Convergence
  Color vision defects
  Blue vision
  Toxic amblyopia
  Visual field constriction
  Extraocular muscle paralysis
  Strabismus
  Oscillopsia
  Central scotomas
Alcohol antagonists
1. Disulfiram
  < Vision
  Visual hallucinations
  Color vision defects
  Lid or conjunctiva: redness
  Mydriasis
  Anisocoria
  Retrobulbar or optic neuritis
  Extraocular muscle paralysis
  Toxic amblyopia
  Nystagmus
  Scotomas (central or cecocentral)
Anorexiants
1. Amphetamines
  < Vision
  Visual hallucinations
  Blue vision
  Lash loss
  Blepharospasm
  Paralysis of accommodation
  Mydriasis
  < Pupil reflex
  < Convergence
  Retinal vein occlusion
  Optic neuritis
  Nystagmus
Anxiolytics, muscle relaxants
1. Benzodiazepines (Xanax, Valium), carbamates
  < Vision
  < Depth perception
  Diplopia
  Visual hallucinations
  Color vision defects
  Photophobia
  Lash loss
  < Corneal reflex

(continued)

TABLE 16.9. (*Continued*)

Extraocular muscle paralysis
Oculogyric crisis
Nystagmus
Jerky pursuit
Retinal hemorrhages

Anticonvulsants

1. Valproic acid, phenytoin, Dilantin, methadiones
"White snow" vision
Night blindness
Color vision defects
Diplopia
Photosensitivity
Extraocular muscle paralysis
Scotomas
Nystagmus
Retinal hemorrhages

Antidepressants

1. Carbamazepines, monoamine oxidase inhibitors, fluoxetines, trazodones, tricyclics (desipramine, amitriptylene, nortriptyline)
< Vision
Color vision defects
Photophobia
Visual hallucinations
Diplopia
Extraocular muscle paralysis
Oculogyric crisis
Nystagmus
Jerky pursuit
Tearing
Blepharospasm
< Corneal reflex
Dry eyes
Paralysis of accommodation
Mydriasis
Toxic amblyopia

Antipsychotics and tranquilizers

1. Haloperidols, droperidol (Inapsine), fentanyl (Innovar), phenothiazines: chlorpromazine (Thorazine), fluphenazine, prochlorperazine (Compazine), lithiums
< Vision
Photophobia
Visual hallucinations
Night blindness
Color vision defects and halos
Yellow or brown vision
> Tearing
Corneal hyperpigmentation
Mydriasis
Miosis
< Pupil light reflex
Cataracts
Diplopia
Oculogyric crisis
Myesthenic block
Extraocular muscle paralysis
Nystagmus

(*continued*)

TABLE 16.9. (*Continued*)

Jerky pursuit
Retinal hemorrhages
Retinal pigment epithelium disturbance
Optic atrophy
Papilledema
Toxic amblyopia
Scotomas: annular, central, paracentral
Visual field constriction
Exophthalmos
Psychedelic drugs
1. Marijuana, LSD
< Vision
Visual hallucinations
Color vision defect or > perception
Yellow or violet vision
< Dark adaptation
Flashing colored lights
Prolonged after-images
Ptosis
< or > Intraocular pressure
Paralysis of accommodation
Miosis
Anisocoria
< Pupil and corneal reflex
Nystagmus
Jerky pursuit
Oculogyric crisis
Sedatives and hypnotics
1. Barbiturates, paraldehyde, glutethimide, bromides
< Vision
Color vision defects
Yellow or green vision
Visual hallucinations
Photophobia
Ptosis
Blepharoclonus
Diplopia
Oscillopsia
Nystagmus
Vertical gaze palsy
Extraocular muscle paresis
Jerky pursuit
Paralysis of accommodation
< Convergence
Dry eyes
< Corneal and pupil reflex
Mydriasis
Miosis
Anisocoria
Hippus
Retinal hemorrhages
Optic neuritis
Papilledema
Optic atrophy
Toxic amblyopia
Scotomas
Visual field constriction

TABLE 16.10. DERMATOLOGIC AGENTS

Germicides
1. Hexachlorophene (skin absorption, accidental ingestion)
   < Vision
   Diplopia
   Lids or conjunctiva: redness, photosensitivity
   Mydriasis
   Miosis
   Absent pupil light reflex
   Retinal hemorrhages
   Papilledema
   Optic atrophy
   Extraocular muscle paralysis
   Pseudotumor cerebri
   Toxic amblyopia
Psoriasis or cystic acne therapy
1. Chrysarobin (skin absorption)
   Nonspecific ocular irritation
   Lids or conjunctiva: redness, brown-violet discoloration
   Keratoconjunctivitis
   Punctate keratitis
   Gray corneal opacities
2. Retinoids (etretinate, isotretinoin [Accutane])
   < Vision
   Myopia
   < Dark adaptation
   Dry eyes
   Lids or conjunctiva: redness, inflammation, edema, hyperpigmentation, photosensitivity,
      ? brow or lash loss
   < Contact lens intolerance
   Corneal: opacities, keratitis, ulcers
   Papilledema
   Optic neuritis
   Abnormal electroretinogram
   Pseudotumor cerebri
Vitiligo therapy
1. Psoralen (methoxsalen, trioxsalen), skin absorption
   Photophobia
   Dry eyes
   Lids or conjunctiva: redness, hyperpigmentation, photosensitivity
   Keratitis
   Pigmentary glaucoma
   Scotomas: central

TABLE 16.11. DIURETICS AND OSMOTICS

Diuretics
1. Spironolactone
    < Vision
    Myopia
    Lid or conjunctiva: redness
    < Intraocular pressure
2. Ethacrynic acid
    < Vision
    Subconjunctival heme
    Retinal hemorrhages
    Nystagmus
3. Sulfonamides (furosemide)
    < Vision
    Yellow vision
    Visual hallucinations
    ? Photophobia
    Lids or conjunctiva: allergy, photosensitivity, subconjunctival heme
    ? Paralysis of accommodation
    < Intraocular pressure
    < Contact lens tolerance
    Retinal hemorrhages
4. Thiazides (benzthiazide, hydrochlorothiazide, indapamide, metolazone,
quinethazone)
    < Vision
    Myopia
    Yellow vision
    Yellow spots on white background
    Visual hallucinations
    Dry eyes
    Lids or conjunctiva: allergy, conjunctivitis
    Photosensitivity, subconjunctival heme
    < Intraocular pressure
    Paralysis of accommodation
    Retinal hemorrhages
    ? Cortical blindness
Hyperosmotics
1. Glycerin, isosorbide, mannitol, urea
    < Vision
    Visual hallucinations
    Lids or conjunctiva: edema, subconjunctival heme
    < Intraocular pressure
    Retinal hemorrhages
    ? Nystagmus

TABLE 16.12. GASTROINTESTINAL AGENTS

Antacids
1. Bismuth salts
< Vision (toxic)
Visual hallucinations (toxic)
Lids or conjunctiva: blue discoloration, subconjunctival heme
Corneal deposits
2. Histamine (H2) blockers (cimetidine [Tagamet], ranitidine [Zantac], famotidine [Pepsid])
< Vision
Visual hallucinations
Lids or conjunctiva:? brow loss, redness, conjunctivitis, subconjunctival heme
Mydriasis (toxic)
< Pupil light reflex
Retinal hemorrhages
Antiemetics
1. Compazine: see CNS agents–antipsychotic agents
2. Metoclopramide (Reglan), cyclizine, meclizine (Antivert, Bonine)
< Vision
Color vision defect
Photophobia
Diplopia
Visual hallucinations
< Tearing
< Contact lens tolerance
Lids or conjunctiva: edema
Mydriasis
< Pupil light reflex
Oculogyric crisis
Extraocular muscle paralysis
Strabismus
Antispasmodics
1. Anticholinergics (atropine [Donnatal], homatropine, scopolamine), quaternary NH 4 compounds (Bentyl, clidinium [Quarzan], Librax, propantheline [Pro-Banthine])
< Vision
Photophobia
Micropsia
Diplopia
Visual hallucinations
Color vision defect
Red vision
Flashing lights
Dry eyes
Lids or conjunctiva: allergy,? lash loss
Paralysis of accommodation
Mydriasis

TABLE 16.13. HEMATOLOGIC AGENTS

Anticoagulants
1. Coumarins (dicumerol, warfarin), heparin, phenindiones
   < Vision
   Color vision defect
   Lids or conjunctiva: allergy, conjunctivitis,? lash or brow loss
   > Lacrimation, subconjunctival heme
   Hyphema
   Paralysis of accommodation (phenindiones)
   Retinal hemorrhages

TABLE 16.14. HORMONAL AGENTS

Adrenal steroids
1. Androgens (Danazol)
< Vision
Diplopia
Lids or conjunctiva: redness, edema, photosensitivity,? lash or brow loss
? Cataracts
Papilledema
Extraocular muscle paresis
Pseudotumor cerebri
Visual field defects
2. Corticosteroids: glucocorticoids and mineralocorticoids (aldosterone, betamethasone, dexamethasone, fluprednisolone, hydrocortisone, prednisone, triamcinolone)
< Vision
Myopia
Diplopia
Color vision defects
Visual hallucinations
Lids or conjunctiva: ptosis, redness, edema, < tear lysozyme, subconjunctival heme
> Intraocular pressure
Posterior subcapsular cataracts
Delayed wound healing
Mydriasis
Ciliary body epithelial microcysts
Retinal hemorrhages, edema
Abnormal electroretinogram or visual evoked potential
Papilledema
Exophthalmos
Extraocular muscle paralysis
Myesthenic block
Toxic amblyopia
Pseudotumor cerebri
Visual fields: scotomas, constriction, glaucoma field defects
Antihyperglycemics
1. Insulin
< Vision
Diplopia
Lids or conjunctiva: allergy, redness, inflammation, < tear lysozymes
Mydriasis
Absent pupil light reflex
< or > Intraocular pressure
Extraocular muscle paresis
Strabismus
Nystagmus
2. Sulfonylureas (chlorpropamide, tolazamide, tolbutamide)
< Vision
Diplopia
Photophobia
Color vision defect
Lids or conjunctiva:? lash loss, allergy, redness, conjunctivitis, edema
Retinal hemorrhages
Retrobulbar or optic neuritis
Extraocular muscle paresis
Scotomas: central or cecocentral

(continued)

TABLE 16.14. (*Continued*)

Antithyroid drugs
1. Iodines
< Vision
Color vision defect
Green vision
Visual hallucinations
Lids or conjunctiva: allergy, > tearing, pain, burning, redness, edema, nodules
Paralysis of accommodation
Mydriasis
Punctate keratitis
Hypopyon
Hemorrhagic iritis
Vitreous floaters
Retinal or macular degeneration or edema
Retrobulbar neuritis
Optic atrophy
? Exophthalmos
Visual fields: scotomas, constriction, hemianopia
Toxic amblyopia
2. Thiouracils
Lids or conjunctiva: allergy, conjunctivitis, depigmentation,? brow or lash loss,
    subconjunctival heme
Dry eyes
Keratitis
Retinal hemorrhages
Exophthalmos
Nystagmus
Thyroid replacement
1. Thyroxines, liothyronine, thyroglobulin, thyroid
< Vision
Photophobia
Visual hallucinations
Lids or conjunctiva: ptosis, edema, redness, spasm
? Cataracts
Papilledema
? Optic neuritis/atrophy
Myesthenic block
Extraocular muscle paralysis
Exophthalmos
Pseudotumor cerebri
Visual field constriction
Scotomas: central
Hemianopia
Oral contraceptives
1. Estrogen—progesterone combinations
< Vision
Diplopia
Myopia
Color vision defects
Blue vision
Colored halos
Lids or conjunctiva: ptosis, allergy, edema, hyperpigmentation, photosensitivity,? lash
    or brow loss
< Contact lens tolerance
Dry eyes
Iritis

(continued)

TABLE 16.14. (Continued)

Mydriasis
Anisocoria
? Cataracts
Retinal vascular: occlusion, hemorrhage, edema, vasospasm
Macular edema
Optic or retrobulbar neuritis
Papilledema
Extraocular muscle paralysis
Visual field constriction
Scotomas: central or paracentral, quadrantanopia or hemianopia
Pseudotumor cerebri
Nystagmus
Ovulatory drugs
1. Nonsteroidal antiestrogens (clomiphene)
< Vision
Flashing or colored lights
Wave or glare image distortion
Phosgene stimulation
Prolonged afterimages
Photophobia
Diplopia
Lids or conjunctiva, allergy
? Lash loss
< Contact lens tolerance
? Posterior subcapsular cataracts
? Retinal vasospasm
? Optic neuritis
Visual field constriction
Scotomas

TABLE 16.15. IMMUNOSUPPRESSANT AGENTS

1. Cyclosporine, azathioprine, methotrexate, cyclophosphamide
< Vision
Visual hallucinations
Lids or conjunctiva: redness, conjunctivitis, subconjunctival heme, hypertrichosis
? Lash or brow loss
Retinal hemorrhages
Retinal pigment epithelium disturbances
? Cortical blindness (cyclosporine)

TABLE 16.16. NEUROMUSCULAR AGENTS

Antiparkinsonian drugs and muscle relaxants
1. **Polyalcohols (mephenesin, methocarbamol)**
   < Vision
   Diplopia
   Lids or conjunctiva: ptosis, ciliary flush, redness
   < Intraocular pressure
   Extraocular muscle paralysis
   Nystagmus: rotary, horizontal, vertical
2. **Anticholinergics (benztropine, biperiden, cycrimine, caramiphen)**
   < Vision
   Visual hallucinations
   Paralysis of accommodation
   Mydriasis
   < Pupil light reflex
   Retrobulbar neuritis
3. **Beta-adrenergic blockers (levodopa, dantrolene): see cardiovascular drugs**
4. **Baclofen, amantadine**
   < Vision
   Diplopia
   Visual hallucinations
   Lid photosensitivity
   Corneal edema
   Punctate keratitis
   Mydriasis
   Miosis
   Strabismus
   Oculogyric crisis

Myasthenia gravis drugs
1. **Anticholinesterases (ambenonium, edrophonium, pyridostigmine [Mestinon])**
   < Vision
   Diplopia
   Lids or conjunctiva: tearing, blepharoclonus (toxic)
   Miosis
   Ptotic eye up
   Nonptotic eye down

TABLE 16.17. VACCINES

1. **Tuberculosis, diphtheria—pertussis—tetanus (DPT), influenza,
   measles— mumps—rubella, polio, rabies, smallpox, tetanus**
   < Vision
   Diplopia
   Photophobia
   Visual hallucinations
   Color vision defect (influenza)
   Lids or conjunctiva: pain, redness, allergy, edema, inflammation, subconjunctival heme
   Iritis
   Mydriasis
   ? Paralysis of accommodation
   Retinal hemorrhages, retinitis
   Papilledema
   Optic neuritis
   Myasthenic block
   Extraocular muscle paresis
   Nystagmus
   Visual field defect (DPT)
   Pseudotumor cerebri (DPT)
   Scotomas (rubella)

TABLE 16.18. VITAMINS

1. Vitamin A (retinol)
   Diplopia
   Yellow vision
   Red dyschromatopsia
   Lids or conjunctiva: yellow or orange discoloration, conjunctivitis, lash or brow loss,
      subconjunctival heme, drug in tears
   ? Calcium deposits in conjunctiva, cornea, sclera
   Miosis
   < Intraocular pressure
   Retinal hemorrhages
   Optic atrophy
   Papilledema
   Exophthalmos
   Strabismus
   Extraocular muscle paralysis
   Nystagmus
   Scotomas
   Pseudotumor cerebri
**2. Vitamin D (calcitriol, cholecalciferol or ergocalciferol) toxicity primarily in
   infants**
   Diplopia
   Visual hallucinations
   Lids or conjunctiva: subconjunctival heme
   ? Calcium deposits in conjunctiva, cornea, sclera
   < Pupil light reflex
   ? Cataracts
   Retinal hemorrhages
   Papilledema
   Optic atrophy
   ? Optic neuritis
   Small optic disks
   Strabismus
   Narrowed optic foramina
   ? Extraocular muscle paresis
   Nystagmus
   ? Hemianopia

Deborah Pavan-Langston

Note: Names in parentheses are a partial list of proprietary names of drugs. Concentrations of drugs in combination antibiotics may vary slightly among manufacturers. Major differences are so indicated.

I. **Antiallergy**
   A. **Decongestant drops. Usual dose:** qd to qid.
      1. Naphazoline (AK-Con, Albalon, Naphcon-A, Clear Eyes, Vasoclear, Vasocon Regular).
      2. Oxymetazoline (Visine LR, Ocuclear).
      3. Phenylephrine HCl (AK-Nefrin, Eye Cool, Prefrin Liquifilm, Relief).
      4. Tetrahydrozoline HCl (Collyrium Fresh, Murine Plus, Visine).
   B. **Decongestant/astringent drops. Usual dose:** qd to qid.
      1. Naphazoline—zinc sulfate (Clear Eyes ACR).
      2. Phenylephrine—zinc sulfate (Zincfrin).
      3. Tetrahydrozaline—zinc sulfate (Visine Allergy Relief).
   C. **Antihistamine—decongestant drops. Usual dose:** qd to qid.
      1. Naphthazoline—antazoline (Vasoncon A).
      2. Naphthazoline—pheniramine (Naphcon A, Opcon A).
   D. **Nonsteroidal antiinflammatory (NSAID) drops. Usual dose:** bid to qid.
      1. Ketorolac (Acular); also useful in cystoid macular edema.
      2. Diclofenac (Voltaren).
   E. **Antihistamine drops (H1 antagonist). Usual dose:** bid to qid.
      1. Levacobastin (Livostin).
      2. Emedastine (Emedine).

   F. **Mast-cell stabilizer drops. Usual dose:** qid.
      1. Lodoxamide (Alomide).
      2. Cromolyn (Crolom).
   G. **Mast cell stabilizer—antihistamine drops. Usual dose:** bid to tid.
      1. Olopatadine (Patanol).
   H. **Mast cell stabilizer—antihistamine—NSAID drops. Usual dose:** bid.
      1. Nedocromil (Alocril).
      2. Pemirolast (Alamast).
      3. Azelastine (Optivar).
      4. Ketotifen (Zaditor).
   I. **Oral. Antihistamines (nonsedating).**
      1. Fexofenadine (Allegra) 60 mg p.o. bid.
      2. Loratadine (Claritin) 10 mg p.o. qd.
      3. Cetirizine (Zyrtec) 5 to 10 mg p.o. bid.
II. **Topical anesthetic solutions. Usual dose:** One to two drops for temporary (15 to 20 minutes) anesthesia to allow ocular examination and manipulation.
   A. Cocaine 1% to 4%.
   B. Proparacaine HCl 0.5% (AK-Tcaine, Ophthaine, Ophthetic).
   C. Tetracaine HCl 0.5% (Tetracaine, Pontocaine).
III. **Topical antibiotic solutions and ointments Usual dose:** bid or qid for 1 to 2 weeks (see also Chapter 5, secs. III. and IV.).
   A. Bacitracin: ointment, 500 U per g (AK-Tracin).
   B. Chloramphenicol: ointment 1%; solution 0.5% (AK-Chlor, Chloroptic, Chloromycetin, generic).
   C. Ciprofloxacin solution or ointment 0.3% (Ciloxan).
   D. Erythromycin: ointment 0.5% (Ilotycin, generic).
   E. Gentamicin: ointment or solution 0.3% (Garamycin,

Genoptic, Gentacidin, Gentak, generic).

F. Levofloxacin solution 0.3% (Quixin, Sariten).

G. Neomycin 0.35%; polymyxin B 10,000 U; and bacitracin 500 U per g, ointment (Neosporin, AK-Spore, generic). Neomycin—polymyxin B—gramicidin 0.0025% solution (AK-Spore, Neosporin, generic).

H. Norfloxacin solution 0.3% (Chibroxin).

I. Netilmicin solution 0.3% (Nettacin).

J. Ofloxacin solution 0.3% (Ocuflox).

K. Polymyxin B 10,000 U, and bacitracin 500 U per g, ointment (AK-PolyBac, Polysporin).

L. Polymyxin B 10,000 U per mL or g, and neomycin 0.35%, solution and ointment (Statrol).

M. Polymyxin B—oxytetracycline ointment 10,000 u–5 mg/g (Terramycin, Terak).

N. Sulfacetamide: ointment 10%; solution 10%, 15%, or 30% (AK-Sulf, Bleph-10, Isoptocetamide, Sulamyd, Sulf-10, generic).

O. Tobramycin: ointment or solution 0.3% (Tobrex, Tobralcon, generic).

P. Trimethoprim 0.1% and polymyxin B, 10,000 U per mL (Polytrim).

IV. Topical antiinflammatory agents: corticosteroids. Usual dose: See text on specific disease entity.

A. Prednisolone:
1. Acetate suspension 0.12% (Pred Mild, Econopred, generic) or 1.0% (AK-Tate, Econopred Plus, Pred Forte, generic).
2. Sodium phosphate solution 0.12% (AK-Pred, Inflamase), 1% (AK-Pred, Inflamase Forte, generic).

B. Dexamethasone:
1. Phosphate solution 0.1% (AK-Dex, Decadron, generic).
2. Suspension 0.1% (Maxidex).
3. Phosphate ointment 0.05% (AK-Dex, Decadron, generic).

C. Fluorometholone suspension 0.1% (FML, Fluor-Op, generic), 0.25% (FML Forte).

D. Fluorometholone acetate suspension 0.1% (Flarex, Eflone).

E. Loteprednol suspension 0.2% (Alrex), 0.5% (Lotemax).

F. Rimexolone suspension 1% (Vexol).

G. Medrysone 1.0% (Hydroxymedrysone) (HMS).

V. Topical antiinflammatory agents: corticosteroid—antibiotic combinations. Usual dose: based on desired corticosteroid dose; see text on specific disease.

A. Hydrocortisone 1%; polymyxin B 10,000 U per g; bacitracin 400 U per g; and neomycin ointment (Cortisporin); suspension (Cortisporin).

B. Prednisolone 0.2% and sulfacetamide 10% suspension (Blephamide); ointment with 0.2% prednisolone (Blephamide) or 0.5% prednisolone (AK-Cide).

C. Prednisolone 0.5%, neomycin 0.35%, and polymyxin B, 10,000 U per mL, suspension (Polypred).

D. Prednisolone 1% and gentamicin 0.3% suspension or ointment (Pred-G).

E. Dexamethasone 0.1% with neomycin 0.35% (NeoDecadron); with neomycin 0.35% and polymyxin B, 10,000 U per mL (Maxitrol, AK-trol), suspension or ointment.

F. Dexamethasone 0.1% and tobramycin 0.3% suspension (Tobradex).

VI. Topical antiinflammatory agents: NSAIDs

A. Diclofenac (Voltaren) **Usual dose:** qid for 2 weeks for postoperative inflammation; also useful qid for many weeks in cystoid macular edema (see Ketorolac).

B. Ketorolac (Acular) **Usual dose:** bid to qid (see sec. **I.**, above).

VII. **Topical and systemic antifungal agents. Usual eye drop dose:** Every 1 or 2 hours initially; see text on specific disease entity for regimen and systemic doses. Only natamycin is U.S. Food and Drug Administration (FDA) approved for the eye. (See Chapter 5, sec. **IV.N.**).

  A. Amphotericin B 0.075% to 0.3% in distilled water, or dextrose 5% in water solution (made up by pharmacy). i.v.: 1 to 1.5 mg per kg over 4 hours qd. Start with low dose and pretreat with 50 mg hydrocortisone and a narcotic to minimize adverse reactions.

  B. Clotrimazole 1% solution (made up by pharmacy).

  C. Fluconazole (Diflucan) oral 400 mg loading dose then 200 to 400 mg per day.

  D. Flucytosine (Ancobon) solution 1% (made up by pharmacy). Oral 100 to 150 mg/kg/d in four divided doses.

  E. Itraconazole (Sporanox) 1% drop (made up by pharmacy). Oral 200 mg bid.

  F. Miconazole solution 1% (made up by pharmacy).

  G. Natamycin suspension 5% (Pimaricin).

VIII. **Antiglaucoma agents: topical and systemic**

  A. **Beta-adrenergic blockers Usual dose: qd to bid.**
  Selective
  Betaxolol 0.25% solution (Betoptic-S).
  Nonselective
  Timolol 0.25% to 0.5%, solution (Timoptic, Timoptic XE gel, Betimol, Timolide).
  Carteolol 1% solution (Ocupress, Cartrol).
  Levobunolol 0.25% to 0.5% solution (AK Beta, Betagan, generic).
  Metipranolol 0.3% solution (Optipranolol).

  B. **Alpha$_2$-adrenergic agonists. Usual dose:**
  Apraclonidine 0.5% to 1% solution (Iopidine).
  Brimonidine 0.2% solution (Alphagan).

C. **Carbonic anhydrase inhibitors**
  Oral
  1. Acetazolamide 125- or 250-mg tablets (Diamox). **Usual dose:** up to qid.
  Acetazolamide 500-mg capsules (Diamox). **Usual dose:** q12h.
  Acetazolamide 250 to 500 mg per 5 to 10 mL in distilled water (Diamox). **Usual dose:** 500 mg i.v. q12h.
  2. Dichlorphenamide 50-mg tablets (Daranide). **Usual dose:** up to qid.
  3. Methazolamide 25- or 50-mg tablets (Neptazane, Glauctabs, MZM, generic). **Usual dose:** up to tid.
  Topical. Usual dose: tid.
  4. Brinzolamide 1% solution (Azopt).
  5. Dorzolamide 2% solution (Trusopt).

D. **Hyperosmotic agents**
  1. Glycerin 50% (Osmoglyn). **Usual dose:** 1.0 to 1.5 g per kg body weight p.o. (on ice with juice preferably).
  2. Isosorbide 45% (Ismotic). **Usual dose:** 1.5 g per kg body weight p.o.
  3. Mannitol 5% to 20% (Osmitrol). **Usual dose:** 1 to 2 g per kg i.v. over 30 to 60 minutes.
  4. Urea powder or 30% solution. **Usual dose:** 0.5 to 2 g per kg i.v. (Ureaphil).

E. Miotics **(pupillary constrictors)**
  1. Carbachol solution 0.75%, 1.5%, 2.25%, 3% (Isoptocarbachol). **Usual dose:** bid or tid.
  2. Echothiophate iodide (phospholine iodide) solution 0.03%, 0.06%, 0.125%, 0.25%. **Usual dose:** qd to bid.
  3. Pilocarpine 0.25%, 0.5%, 1%, 2%, 3%, 4%, 6%, 10% (Akarpine, Isoptocarpine, Pilocar, Piloptic, Pilogen, Pilostat, generic; Ocusert P 20 or P 40 insert; Pilopine 4% gel).

Usual dose: two to four times daily. Ocusert P 20 qd.

F. **Prostaglandin agonists. Usual dose: qd.**
1. Bimatoprost 0.03% solution (Lumigan).
2. Latanoprost 0.005% solution (Xalatan).
3. Travaprost 0.004% solution (Travatan).

G. **Prostaglandin derivatives. Usual dose: qd.**
1. Unoprostone 0.12% solution (Rescular).

H. **Sympathomimetics. Usual dose: qd to bid (mild dilators).**
1. Dipivalyl epinephrine solution 1%[2] (AKPro, Propine, generic).
2. Epinephrine[2]; borate, bitartrate, or HCl 0.25%, 0.5%, 1.2% (Epifrin, Epitrate, Epinal, Eppy/N, Glaucon).

I. **Combination antiglaucoma drugs**
1. Dorzolamide plus timolol (Cosopt) qd to bid.
2. Latanoprost plus timolol (Xalcom) qd to bid.

IX. **Antiviral agents** (see Chapters 5 and 9).
Systemic.
A. Acyclovir 200-, 400-, or 800-mg tablet (Zovirax). **Usual dose: herpes simplex infection:** 400 mg tid for 7 to 10 days. **Prophylaxis** 400 mg bid for 1+ years times per day (see text). Acute **herpes zoster** 800 mg p.o. five times per day for 7 days.
B. Famciclovir (Famvir). **Usual dose: herpes simplex infection:** 250 mg p.o. tid for 7 days (see text). **Prophylaxis** 125 to 250 mg p.o. bid for 1 year. Acute **herpes zoster:** 500 mg p.o. tid for 7 days.
C. Valacyclovir (Valtrex). **Usual dose: herpes simplex infection:** 1 g p.o. bid. **Prophylaxis** 500 mg p.o. qd for 1 year (immunocompetent only). Acute **herpes zoster:** 1 g p.o. tid for 7 days.

D. Foscarnet (Foscavir). **Usual dose:** 60 mg per kg adjusted for renal function i.v. over 1 hour, q8h for 14 to 21 days acutely. Maintenance: 90 to 120 mg per kg i.v. over 2 hours qd.
E. Ganciclovir (Cytovene). **Usual dose:** 2.5 mg per kg i.v. q8h for 10 days, then 5 mg/kg/day followed by ganciclovir, 500 mg p.o. six times per day or 1,000 mg p.o. tid after i.v. stabilization of cytomegalovirus (CMV) retinitis (see text).
F. Valganciclovir (Valcyte) 900 mg p.o. bid for active CMV retinitis, 900 mg p.o. qd maintenance.
Topical
A. Acyclovir 3% ointment (Zovirax). Not available in United States. **Usual dose:** five times per day for 14 days.
B. Idoxuridine, solution 0.1% (Herplex). **Usual dose:** solution–qh during the day, q2h at night for 10 to 14 days.
C. Trifluorothymidine solution 1% (Viroptic). **Usual dose:** nine times per day for 10 to 14 days.
D. Vidarabine ointment 3% (Vira A) five times per day for 10 to 14 days.

X. **Artificial tears and lubricants for dry eyes**[3] (partial listing)
A. Methylcellulose or ethylcellulose base:
1. Bion Tears.[1]
2. Celluvisc.[1]
3. Genteal.[1]
4. Isopto Tears.
5. Murocel.
6. Ocucoat.
7. Tearisol.
8. Theratears.[1]
9. Tears Renewed.
10. Tear Guard.
11. Tears Natural Free[1], Tears Natural II.
12. Lacrisert[1] (biodegradable insert).
B. Polyvinyl alcohol based solutions:
1. AKWA Tears.
2. Hypotears, HypoTears PF.

3. Liquifilm.
4. Murine.
5. Puralube.
6. Refresh.[1]

C. Longer-lasting mucoadhesive or increased viscosity agents.
1. AquaSite[1] (polycarbophil, dextran).
2. Bion Tears[1] (methylcellulose).
3. Celluvisc[1] (methylcellulose).
4. OcuCoat[1] (methylcellulose).
5. Refresh Plus[1] (methylcellulose).

D. Polyvinylpyrrolidone polymer base: adsorbonac sodium chloride 2% or 5% (hyperosmotic).

E. Tear ointments:
1. AKWA Tears.[1]
2. Dry eyes.
3. Duolube.[1]
4. Duratears Naturale.
5. Hypotears.[1]
6. Lacrilube.[1]
7. Refresh PM.[1]

XI. **Dilating and cycloplegic agents. Usual dose:** qd to qid.
A. Atropine ointment 0.5% or 1%, or solution 0.5%, 1%, 2%, 3% (atropine sulfate, Atropisol, Isopto-Atropine, generic).
B. Cyclopentolate solution 0.5%, 1%, 2% (AK-Pentolate, Cyclogyl, Pentolair, generic).
C. Homatropine solution 2% or 5% (Homatropine HBr, Isopto Homatropine, AK-Homatropine, Homatrine).

[1]Preservative free. Commercial names given for simplicity.

D. Phenylephrine solution 2.5% or 10% (AK-Dilate, Mydfrin, Neo-Synephrine [ophthalmic], generic). **Usual dose:** qd to tid.
E. Scopolamine solution 0.25% (Isopto Hyoscine).
F. Tropicamide solution 0.5% or 1% (Mydriacyl, Tropicacyl, generic).

XII. **Miotics (pupillary constrictors)** (see sec. **VIII.E.,** above).

XIII. **Ocular decongestants for uninfected, red eyes** (partial listing)
A. Naphazoline hydrochloride (AK-Con, Albalon, Clear Eyes, Degest 2, Naphcon, Opcon, Vasoclear, Vasocon Regular).
B. Phenylephrine hydrochloride (AK-Nefrin, Isopto Frin, Prefrin Liquifilm, Efricel, Eye Cool, Relief, Tear Efrin, Velva-Kleen).
C. Tetrahydrozoline hydrochloride (Murine Plus, Soothe, Visine, Tetracon, Collyrium).

XIV. **Decongestant—astringents**
A. Naphazdine—zinc SO_4 (Clear Eyes).
B. Phenylephrine—zinc SO_4 (Prefrin Z, Zincfrin).
C. Tetrahydrozoline—zinc SO^4 (Visine AC).

XV. **Postsurgical alpha-adrenergic blocker (miotic)**
A. Dapirazole HCl (Rev Eyes). **Usual dose:** Two drops followed 5 minutes later by two drops to reverse mydriasis by phenylephrine and tropicamide.

Appendix B. DOSAGES OF ANTIMICROBIAL DRUGS USED IN OCULAR INFECTIONS

APPENDIX B TABLE

Drug	Adults		Children			Usual Divided Dose Interval Dose/Day	Usual Maximum	Organism Susceptibility Guide
	Oral Daily Dosage	Parenteral Daily Dosage	Oral Daily Dosage	Parenteral Daily Dosage				
Acyclovir	200 mg q4h × ⑤ or 400 mg	5–15 mg/kg	20 mg/kg	5–20 mg/kg		q8h	4 g oral 45 mg/kg i.v.	Herpes simplex, Herpes zoster
Amikacin		15 mg/kg		15 mg/kg		q8–12h	1.5 g	Pseudomonas, Escherichia coli, Herellea, (Mima), Enterobacter, Proteus, Klebsiella, Serratia marcescens, Staphylococcus aureus, S. epidermidis
Amoxicillin/ clavulanic acid[a]	0.75–1.5 g[2]	—	20–40 mg/kg	—		q8h	1.5 g	S. aureus, S. epidermidis, Streptococcus sp, Haemophilus, H. ducreyi, Neisseria gonorrhoeae, E. coli, Klebsiella
Amphotericin B/sulfate complex	—	3–4 mg/kg	—	3–4 mg/kg		q24h	4 mg/kg	Aspergillosus, blastomycosis, Candida, coccidiomycosis, cryptococcosis, histoplasmosis, mucomycosis, paracoccidiomycosis, sporotrichosis
Ampicillin	2 g	2–8 g	50–100 mg/kg	100–200 mg/kg		q6–8h	12 g	Streptococcus sp, Streptococcus pneumoniae, Neisseria, Staphylococcus sp, H. influenzae, Salmonella, Shigella, E. coli, Proteus
Azithromycin[1]	250–1,000 mg	500 mg	5–12 mg/kg	—		q24h	500 mg	Chlamydia, Mycoplasma, Legionella, S. pneumoniae, H. influenzae, Mycobacterium avium (in HIV-positive with other antibiotics)

(continued)

APPENDIX B TABLE (Continued)

Drug	Adults Oral Daily Dosage	Adults Parenteral Daily Dosage	Children Oral Daily Dosage	Children Parenteral Daily Dosage	Usual Divided Dose Interval Dose/Day	Usual Maximum	Organism Susceptibility Guide
Carbenicillin[a] (382 mg/tablet)	4–8 tablets	—	15–25 mg/kg		q4–6h	3 g	Pseudomonas, Proteus Klebsiella, E. coli, Serratia, non-penicillinase-producing Staphylococcus, Neisseria sp, B-hemolytic Streptococcus, S. pneumoniae, Streptococcus faecalis, anaerobes (Bacteroides, Clostridium, Peptostreptococcus)
Cefaclor (1)[b,c]	0.75–1.5 g	—	20–40 mg/kg	—	q8h	4 g	Staphylococcus sp including penicillinase producers, S. pneumoniae, and Streptococcus pyogenes, but not S. faecalis, Haemophilus, Escherichia, Proteus, Klebsiella N. gonorrhoeae, Propionibacterium, Peptostreptococcus
Cefamandole[b,c]	—	1.5–12 g	—	50–150 mg/kg	q4–8h	12 g	S. aureus, S. epidermidis, Streptococcus sp (except enterococci; e.g., S. faecalis), Enterobacter, Haemophilus sp, E. coli, Klebsiella, Proteus sp, Clostridium, Bacteroides, Peptostreptococcus
Cefazolin[b,c]	—	1–6 g	—	25–100 mg/kg	q6–8h	6 g	See cefaclor
Cefixime	200 mg q12h or 400 mg q24h	—	4 mg/kg q12h or 8 mg/kg q24h	—	See dose	400 mg	See cefazolin (but poor vs Staphylococcus)
Cefotaxime[b,c]		2–12 g		100–200 mg/kg	q4–8h	12 g	See cefamandole

Drug							Spectrum
Ceftazidime		500 mg–6 g		30–50 mg/kg	q8–12h	4 g	See cefamandole, plus covers *Pseudomonas* sp, *Serratia*
Ceftriaxone[b,c]		1–4 g		50–100 mg/kg	q12–24h	4 g	See cefamandole, *Neisseria meningitidis*, and *N. gonorrhoeae*
Chloramphenicol	50–100 mg/kg			50–100 mg.kg	q6h	4 g	*H. influenzae*, *Salmonella*, *S. pneumoniae*, *Neisseria* sp
Cidofovir		5 mg/kg once/week ×② then 5 mg/kg every other week					Cytomegalovirus, molluscum contagiosum
Ciprofloxacin	0.5–1.5 g	200–400 mg			q12h	2 g	*Staphylococcus* sp (including methicillin-resistant strains), *Streptococcus* sp, *Haemophilus*, *Pseudomonas*, *Proteus*, *Escherichia*, *Klebsiella*, other Enterobacteriaceae, anaerobes, *Legionella*, *N. gonorrhoeae* and meningococcus, *Serratia*, *Chlamydia*, *Acinetobacter*, *Bacillus cereus*, *Salmonella*
Clindamycin[d]	0.6–1.8 g	0.6–3.6 g	10.25 mg/kg	10–40 mg/kg	q6–8h	4.8 g	*S. pneumoniae*, *S. pyogenes*, *Streptococcus viridans*, *S. aureus* except methicillin-resistant strains, *Bacteroides*, *Actinomyces*

(continued)

| Drug | Adults | | Children | | | | Organism Susceptibility Guide |
	Oral Daily Dosage	Parenteral Daily Dosage	Oral Daily Dosage	Parenteral Daily Dosage	Usual Divided Dose Interval Dose/Day	Usual Maximum	
Cloxacillin	2–4 g		50–100 mg/kg		q6h	4 g	Penicillinase-resistant Staphylococcus, S. pneumoniae S. pyogenes
Dicloxacillin[a]	1–2 g		12.5–25.0 mg/kg		q6h	4 g	See cloxacillin
Doxycycline[a]	100–200 mg	100–200 mg	1–2 mg/kg	1–2 mg/kg	q12–24h	200 mg	Some Staphylococcus and Streptococcus, Escherichia, Enterobacter, Acinetobacter, Haemophilus, Klebsiella, Pasteurella, Rickettsia, Borellia, Bacteroides, Brucella
Erythromycin	1–2 g	1–4 g	30–50 mg/kg	15–50 mg/kg	q6h	4 g	Streptococcus pneumococcus, Mycoplasma, Treponema pallidum, see azithromycin
Famciclovir[2]	500 mg q8h					1.5 g	Herpes simplex, Herpes, zoster
Fluconazole	50–400 mg q24h	100–400 mg			q24h	400 mg	Candida, coccidomycosis cryptococcosis, histoplasmosis, sporotrichosis
Flucytosine	12.5–37.5 mg/kg q6h		12.5–37.5 mg/kg q6h		See dose	150 mg/kg	Aspergillus, Candida, cryptococcosis, Cladosporium
Foscarnet[3]		60 mg/kg q8h or 90 mg/kg q12h					Herpes simplex, Herpes zoster, cytomegalovirus
Ganciclovir[4]	1,000 mg q8h or 500 mg × ⑥ doses	5 mg/kg q12h		5 mg/kg q12h	See dose	10 mg/kg	Herpes simplex, Herpes zoster, cytomegalovirus
Gentamicin		3–7 mg/kg		3.0–7.0 mg/kg	q8h	7 mg/kg	See amikacin

Drug			Pediatric dose	Interval	Max dose	Organisms/Uses
Imipenem[a,e]		1–4 g		q6–8h	4 g	Methicillin-sensitive *S. aureus*, *S. pneumoniae*, *Streptococcus* groups A and B, some *S. faecalis*, *N. gonorrhoeae*, *N. menmgitidis*, *H. influenzae*, *E. coli*, *Klebsiella*, *Pseudomonas*, *Bacillus sp*, *Moraxella*, *Eikenella*, *Brucella*
Isoniazid	300 mg		10–20 mg/kg	q24h	300 mg	*M. tuberculosis*
Itraconazole	100–200 mg q12–24h	200 mg q12h ×4 then 200 mg q24h	5 mg/kg q24h	See dose	400 mg	Blastomycosis, *Candida*, histoplasmosis, cryptococcosis, pseudallescheriasis, sporotrichosis
Ketoconazole	200–400 mg q12h–24h		3.3–6.6 mg/kg q24h	See dose	1 g	Blastomycosis, coccidioimycosis, histoplasmosis, paracoccidioidomycosis, pseudallescheriasis
Levofloxacin	500 mg	500 mg		q24h	500 mg	See ciprofloxacin
Miconazole		600–1200 mg q8h	6.6–13.3 mg/kg q8h	See dose	3.6 g	*Actinomyces*, *Alternaria*, *Aspergillus*, *Coccidioides*, *Candida*, *Cladosporium*, *Histoplasma*, *Fusarium*, *Paracoccioides*, *Penicillium*, *Phialophora*, *Rhodotorula*

(continued)

Drug	Adults		Children				Usual Maximum	Organism Susceptibility Guide
	Oral Daily Dosage	Parenteral Daily Dosage	Oral Daily Dosage	Parenteral Daily Dosage	Usual Divided Dose Interval Dose/Day			
Minocycline	100 mg	2 mg/kg					200 mg	See cloxacillin
Nafcillin[a]	2–4 g	2–9 g	50–100 mg/kg	100–200 mg/kg	q6h		12 g	Staphylococcus, S. pneumoniae, other Streptococcus sp, Neisseria sp, Peptostreptococcus
Norfloxacin	400 mg q12h				See dose		800 mg	See ciprofloxacin
Ofloxacin	200–400 mg q12h	200–400 mg q12h			See dose		800 mg	See ciprofloxacin; less active against Pseudomonas; single dose for gonorrhea; 7 d dose for Chlamydia
Oxacillin[a]	2–4 g	2–12 g	50–100 mg/kg	100–200 mg/kg	q6h		12 g	Staphylococcus, Str. pneumoniae, other Streptococcus sp, Neisseria sp, Peptostreptococcus
Oxytetracycline	1–2 g	0.75–1.0 g (over 8 years of age)	20–50 mg/kg (over 8 years of age)	10–20 mg/kg	q12h		2 g	See doxycycline
Penicillin G	250–500 mg q6h	1.2–24.0 million U/d K+ or Na+ penicillin: procaine or benzathine penicillin	25–50 mg/kg q6h	100,000– 250,000 U/kg/d q2–12h	See dose		24 million U 4.8 million U	S. pneumoniae, S. pyogenes, S. viridans, non-penicillinase-producing S. aureus, N. meningitidis, N. gonorrhoeae, Clostridium, many Bacteroides, Enterobacteriaceae Actinomyces, Treponema

Drug				Interval	Maximum	Spectrum
Penicillin V	1–2 g	25–50 mg/kg		q6h	4 g	See penicillin G; less active against N. gonorrhoeae
Piperacillin	12–24 g		200–300 mg/kg	q4–6h	24 g	See carbenicillin, especially Pseudomonas and Klebsiella
Rifampin[f]	0.6 g	0.6 g	10–20 mg/kg	q12–24h	0.6 g	S. aureus, S. epidermidis, Streptococcus sp, N. meningitidis, N. gonorrhoeae, H. influenzae, Legionella, Mycobacterium sp, Chlamydia
Spectinomycin[d]	2 g once		40 mg/kg once	qd	2 g	N. gonorrhoeae
Streptomycin	1–2 g		20–30 mg/kg	q12h	2 g	Mycobacterium tuberculosis, some Gram-negative bacilli
Sulfisoxazole[a]	1–2 g	100 mg/kg		q6h	8 g	Staphylococcus, S. pyogenes, N. meningitidis, Chlamydia, Toxoplasma, Nocardia
Tetracycline (HCl)	1–2 g	25–50 mg/kg (over 8 years of age)	10–20 mg/kg (over 8 years of age)	q6h	2 g	See doxycycline
Ticarcillin	1–2 g	200–300 mg/kg	200–300 mg/kg	q4–6h	16 g	See Carbenicillin, Bacillus fragilis, but most resistant Klebsiella

(continued)

APPENDIX B TABLE (Continued)

Drug	Adults		Children		Usual Divided Dose Interval Dose/Day	Usual Maximum	Organism Susceptibility Guide
	Oral Daily Dosage	Parenteral Daily Dosage	Oral Daily Dosage	Parenteral Daily Dosage			
Tobramycin		3–5 mg/kg q8h		6.0–7.5 mg/kg q8h	See dose	5 mg/kg	See Amikacin
Trimethoprim-sulfamethoxazole (TMP-SMX)[a,d]	4 tablets (80 mg TMP + 400 mg SMX tablet)	8–20 mg/kg (TMP)	8–20 mg (TMP)	8–20 mg/kg (TMP)	q6–12h	1,200 mg TMP with 600 mg, SMX	S. aureus, S. epidermidis, S. pneumoniae, S. viridans, H. influenzae, Bacteroides, E. coli, Enterobacter, Klebsiella, Proteus, Serratia, Pneumocystis
Trovafloxacin	200 mg		200–300 mg		q24h	300 mg	See ciprofloxacin
Valacyclovir[5]	3 g				q8h	3 g	Herpes simplex, Herpes zoster

HIV, human immunodeficiency virus; HSV, herpes simplex virus; CMV, cytomegalovirus.

[a]Active against penicillinase-producing staphylococci.

[b]Number in parentheses indicates cephalosporin generation.

[c]Second- and third-generation cephalosporins are less active than first-generation against staphylococci and streptococci, but more active against Gram-negative bacilli and anaerobes. Pseudomonas, indole-positive Proteus, Acinetobacter (Mima, Herellea), and most Serratia are resistant to all cephalosporins.

[d]Penicillin-allergy alternate.

[e]A beta-lactam. Imipenem is the most active drug against all pathogenic bacteria.

[f]Not U.S. Food and Drug Administration approved for ocular disease.

[1]Azithromycin—Adults: 500 mg day one and 250 mg/days 2–5; 1 g once for Chlamydia trachomatous urethritis.

[2]Famciclovir—For herpes zoster. First genital herpes dose is 250 mg q8h ×10 days. For herpes simplex recurrence, dose is 125 mg q12h for 10 days. For prophylaxis of HSV 250 mg p.o. q12h.

[3]Foscarnet—For CMV give induction dose over 1 h. For maintenance 90–120 mg/kg daily over 2h.

[4]Ganciclovir—For CMV induction i.v. over 1 h for maintenance 5 mg/kg 7d/w or 6 mg/kg 5d/w.

[5]Valacyclovir—For herpes zoster. First herpes simplex 1 g q12h ×7–10 days. Recurrent HSV infection 500 mg q12h ×7d. Prophylaxis HSV 1 g q12h.

For topical subconjunctival, and intravitreal dosages see Tables 5.5, 5.6, 5.7, and Table 9.7.
(Adapted in part from Abramowicz M, ed. Handbook of antimicrobial therapy. New Rochelle, NY: Medical Letter, 2000.)

SUBJECT INDEX

Page numbers followed by *f* indicate figures; those followed by *t* indicate tabular material.

A

A esotropia, 350
A exotropia, 350
Abduction, 334
 tests for, 349–350
Aberrations, 404–405
 chromatic aberration, 402*f*, 404
 distortion, 402*f*, 405
 radial astigmatism, 402*f*, 405
 spherical aberration, 402*f*, 404–405
Abetalipoproteinemia
 (Bassen-Kornzweig
 syndrome), 185, 330
Absorption of light, 398
Acanthamoeba, 101–102
Acanthocytosis, 185
Accommodation, 196, 412–413
 amplitude of, 412, 413*t*
 hyperopia and, 407
 symptoms of decreased, 413
Accommodative esodeviations,
 347–349
Accommodative esophoria, 347
Accommodative esotropia, 347
 clinical evaluation of, 347
 therapy for, 348–349
Acetazolamide, 33, 63, 161, 215, 260,
 274
Achromatopsia, 310
Acid burns, 61
Acinetobacter infection, in corneal
 ulcers, 84*t*
Acne rosacea, 111–112
 chronic conjunctivitis with, 73
 facial eruption in, 111
 ocular findings in, 111
 punctate epithelial lesions in, 81
 treatment of, 78, 79, 111–112
Acquired immunodeficiency syndrome
 (AIDS), 219–220
 conjunctival involvement with, 95
 corneal herpes simplex virus (HSV)
 infection and, 89
 cotton-wool spots in, 168
 cytomegalic inclusion disease (CID)
 and, 218
 diagnosis of, 220
 endophthalmitis, 240
 herpes zoster and, 92
 molluscum contagiosum virus and,
 95

therapy of, 220
 uveitis in, 197, 199*t*, 204, 217, 221
Actinic keratopathy, 105
Actinomyces infection
 of lacrimal system, 55, 101
 treatment of, 101
Acute angle-closure glaucoma, 231,
 272–275. *See also*
 Angle–closure glaucoma
 corneal edema with, 117
 differential diagnosis of, 201
 direct ophthalmoscopy in, 11, 41
Acute posterior multifocal placoid
 pigment epitheliopathy
 (APMPPE), 184
 uveitis with, 199*t*, 203*t*, 232
Acyclovir, 89, 93, 94, 217
Adduction, 334
Adenoid cystic carcinoma, 62
Adenoviral infection
 conjunctivitis and keratitis, 71,
 94–95
Adie syndrome, 396
Adie's tonic pupil, 396
 differential diagnosis of, 395*t*
 examination in, 9
Afterimage testing, 344, 345
Age-related macular degeneration
 (AMD), 179–182
 treatment of, 180–182
 types of, 180
Aging
 absorption of light and, 398
 choroid and, 246–247
 drusen changes and, 179
 eyelid changes with, 49
 hyperopia and, 407
 lens and, 137
 macular holes and, 183–184
 miosis and, 246
Aicardi syndrome, 310–311
Air puff noncontact tonometer, 11
Airway obstruction, with chemical
 burns, 33
Alan-Thorpe lens, in gonioscopy, 20
Albinism, 309–310
Albipunctate dystrophy, 329
Alcohol, toxicity and side effects of,
 471*t*–472*t*
Aldose reductase inhibitors, in
 cataract, 150

Fusion, 336
Fusional reserve measurement, for
    strabismus, 341

G

Galactokinase deficiency, 308
Galactosemia, 308
    cataract and, 145
Ganciclovir, 218–219
Gastrointestinal agents, toxicity and
    side effects of, 476*t*
Gaucher's disease, 306
Gaze, 335
    cardinal positions of, 4, 335, 335*f*
    primary positions of, 335
    secondary positions of, 335
Genetic counseling, 298–300, 302–303
Genetics
    inheritance modes and, 298
    principles of, 297–298
Genetics and genetic counseling,
    297–300
Genotype, 297–298
Giant papillary conjunctivitis, 123–124
Giant-cell arteritis, 177, 387–391
Glaucoma, 251–285
    angle-closure. *See* Angle-clousure
        glaucoma
    angle-recession, 279, 280
    and changes in macula, 254
    childhood, 325–329
        history taking in, 329
        rubella and, 291
        secondary to inflammation,
            328–329
    contusion to eye and, 278–279
    corticosteroids and, 215, 282
    crystalline-lens induced, 282–283
    definition, 251
    erythroclastic, 192
    examination in, 253–257
        angle rating system in, 252*f*, 257
        anterior chamber depth
            estimation in, 252*f*
        flashlight in, 253
        Fuchs's heterochromic, 230,
            280–281
        glaucomotocyclitic crisis
            (Posner-Schlossman's), 230,
            280
        gonioscopy in, 20, 257
        intraocular pressure (IOP)
            measurement in, 9–11, 253–254
        ophthalmoscopy in, 254–256
        slit-lamp biomicroscopy in, 253
        visual fields in, 256–257
    glaucomatocyclitic crisis in, 280
    gonioscopy in, 20

infancy and childhood, 325–329
infantile, 325–327
inflammatory, 279–281
intraocular inflammation causing,
    279–281
intraocular lenses (IOL) and, 283
lens-induced, 230, 282–283
low-tension, 277
malignant, 276
neovascular, 169, 281
normal tension, 277
open-angle. *See* Open-angle
    glaucoma
perforating injuries and, 284
physiological mechanism of,
    251–253, 252*f*
pigmentary, 277–278
pseudoexfoliation, 278
risk factors for, 251
secondary
    inflammation and, 328–329
    luxation and subluxation of lens
        and, 44
    steroids and, 34
    subchoroidal hemorrhage with, 43
    traumatic angle recession and, 44
    uveitis, 215
therapy of, 487–488
    lasers in, 267–269
    medical treatments in, 258–266
    principles of, 257–258
    surgical approaches to, 269–270
trauma and
    blunt, 329
    penetrating, 329
uveitis with, 215
viscoelastic, 283–284
Glaucomatocyclitic crisis, 280
Glioma, optic nerve, 57, 62, 321
Goblet cells, 67
Goldenhar syndrome, 317
Goldmann lens, in gonioscopy, 19, 20
Goldmann perimeter, 15
Goldmann-Favre syndrome, 330
Gonioplasty, in glaucoma, 268
Gonioscopy, 1, 19–20
    in glaucoma, 20, 257, 327–328
    technique of, 20
Goniotomy, 327
Gonorrhea. *See* Neisseria
Granular dystrophy, 114
Granulomatous colitis, 238
Graves' disease, ophthalmic, 58–59
    anatomic tests for, 59
    clinical signs and symptoms of,
        58–59
    thyroid tests for, 59
    treatment of, 59
    Werner's classification of signs of, 59

O